The Massage Connection
ANATOMY AND PHYSIOLOGY

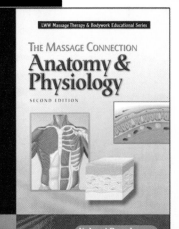
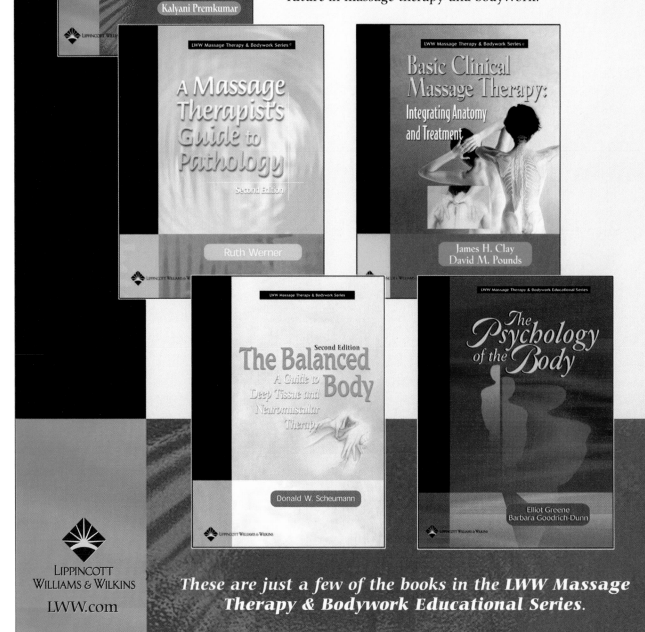

SECOND EDITION

The Massage Connection
ANATOMY AND PHYSIOLOGY

Kalyani Premkumar M.B.B.S., M.D., MSc. (Med Ed.), C.M.T., Ph.D.
University of Calgary & Mount Royal College
Canada

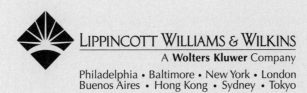

LIPPINCOTT WILLIAMS & WILKINS
A **Wolters Kluwer** Company

Philadelphia • Baltimore • New York • London
Buenos Aires • Hong Kong • Sydney • Tokyo

Editor: Pete Darcy
Managing Editor: Eric Branger
Marketing Manager: Christen DeMarco
Production Editor: Christina Remsberg
Art Director: Jonathan Dimes
Artwork: Dragonfly Media Group, Mark Miller Medical Illustration, Kim Battista, Mary Anna Barratt, and Susan Caldwell
Compositor: Graphic World
Printer: RR Donnelly-Willard

351 West Camden Street
Baltimore, Maryland 21201-2436 USA

530 Walnut Street
Philadelphia, PA 19106

The publisher is not responsible (as a matter of product liability, negligence, or otherwise) for any injury resulting from any material contained herein. This publication contains information relating to general principles of medical care that should not be construed as specific instructions for individual patients. Manufacturers' product information and package inserts should be reviewed for current information, including contraindications, dosages, and precautions.

Printed in the United States of America

Library of Congress Cataloging-in-Publication Data
Premkumar, Kalyani.
    The massage connection anatomy and physiology / Kalyani Premkumar.-- 2nd ed.
        p. cm.
    Includes index.
    ISBN 0-7817-3476-2
    1. Human physiology. 2. Human anatomy. 3. Massage. I. Title.

QP31.2.P74 2003
612--dc21

2003050653

The publishers have made every effort to trace the copyright holders for borrowed material. If they have inadvertently overlooked any, they will be pleased to make the necessary arrangements at the first opportunity.

To purchase additional copies of this book, call our customer service department at **(800) 638-3030** or fax orders to **(301) 824-7390.** International customers should call **(301) 714-2324.**

Visit Lippincott Williams & Wilkins on the Internet: http://www.LWW.com. Lippincott Williams & Wilkins customer service representatives are available from 8:30 am to 6:00 pm, EST.

05 06 07
2 3 4 5 6 7 8 9 10

To my dad, D.I. Paul, and my mother, Stella Paul, who lovingly supported me (financially and otherwise) throughout my undergraduate and postgraduate education and to my parents-in-law, A.G. Vedasundararaj and Helen Vedasundararaj, who believed that I could use my medical education for the good of others.

About The Author

Dr. Premkumar is a Physician and a Medical Educator with a doctorate in Educational Technology and over 20 years experience in teaching.

Currently, she instructs massage therapy students at the Center for Complementary Health Education, Mount Royal College, Calgary, Canada. She is also an Adjunct Assistant Professor at the University of Calgary, Faculty of Medicine and a Tutor at Athabasca University.

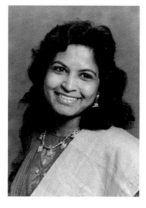

She is the President of Meducational Skills, Tools & Technology Inc., Canada and Meducational Skills, Tools & Technology Pvt. Ltd., India, a company that develops medical education resources and courses.

She is a recording artist and has two Christian music albums to her credit.

Dr. Kalyani Premkumar is also the author of *Pathology A to Z – a Handbook for Massage Therapists* and *Understanding Medical Terminology – a Beginner's Guide.*

corporated into any textbook; the second edition strives to do so. The proven effects of massage on each body system have been added at the end of every chapter, based on current findings along with references for further reading.

In recent years, massage therapy schools and associations have taken steps to reform the curriculum. This required revisiting the curriculum for the second edition. Based on curriculum changes, detail has been added to every chapter. Major revisions have been made to the chapters dealing with the muscle, skeletal, and nervous systems. Tables have been added that include origin, insertion, action, and innervation of muscles, together with illustrations of individual muscles. Tables listing muscles that produce specific movements across joints give the student a different perspective of muscles. Illustrations of muscles grouped together, bones indicating origins and insertions of various muscles, and photographs with bony landmarks are features that massage therapy students will find useful.

The comprehensive index and the glossary at the end of the book have been specifically designed for ease in locating important terms, topics, and concepts.

By converting to hard cover, the book is now sturdier to withstand frequent handling. This change was based on feedback from students and practitioners who used the previous edition as a text. In addition to the new features for students and practitioners, new resources have been created for instructors. Instructors will find the images from the book and PowerPoint slides for each chapter on the connection companion **website** http://connection.lww.com. Also available is the Test Generator for The Massage Connection: Anatomy and Physiology, 2nd Edition. This CD-ROM contains test questions and answers for all twelve chapters and allows users to design their own tests and answer keys. With the software, instructors are able to select, delete, edit, or add questions to the tests they create.

It is encouraging that the public is increasingly turning to alternative and complementary practitioners for their health care needs. As such changes occur, it is important that the education of these practitioners be reformed to meet this societal need. It is envisaged that this new edition, written for massage therapists and including all the relevant content that they need to practice, will move therapists in this direction.

Preface

The first edition of this book was written to meet the specific needs of massage therapy students and professionals and to simplify the learning and teaching of anatomy and physiology. It was a result of having shared the intense frustration of massage therapy students as they tried to weed out irrelevant details from texts written for medical and nursing students and focus on what they needed to know for their profession.

The specific requirements for the book were painstakingly determined by scrutinizing the curriculums of many massage therapy schools in the United States and Canada. In addition to personal experience, the input from massage therapy students and therapists was used to organize the objectives and contents of the book. The first edition was well received.

As with any product, there is always scope for improvement; however, improvements are best made based on feedback from all stakeholders. Changes and additions made to the second edition are based on feedback from those who actually use the book—the massage therapy students, instructors, practitioners, and policy makers.

The first edition was organized into three major divisions—anatomy and physiology—system-wise; topics in pathology; and case studies in relation to each body system. Based on feedback, the second edition is compiled as one major section, with each chapter discussing one body system. Important pathology topics and relevant case studies have been incorporated into each chapter.

A chapter outline in the table of contents and a detailed list of objectives are given at the beginning of each chapter, to help the student construct a conceptual framework and identify the key points. Each chapter is interspersed with information boxes that describe pathologies relevant to the anatomy and physiology topic under study. Also included are boxes that give specific information relevant to massage therapists. All new terms and key terms are shown in boldface throughout the text. New to this edition is the inclusion of additional illustrations—and colorful ones at that. Color was significantly absent in the previous edition.

Extensive review questions, with answers and pictures for labeling and coloring, are given at the end of each chapter to assess the understanding of basic concepts introduced. Case studies, giving typical scenarios that the therapist may encounter in the clinic, have been included. This will place the study of each system in the right context and encourage problem solving. The case studies may be used for discussion after the study of the chapter or used as a starting point for the study of individual systems.

Exciting advances have been made in the field of massage therapy since the publication of the first edition. Additional books have been published. A number of authentic studies have been published on the use and effects of massage therapy on the body. Systematic studies on the effects of specific massage techniques for various diseases and conditions are also underway. It is important for these findings and advances to be in-

✓ Superficial and Deep Fascia

The **superficial fascia,** also known as **subcutaneous tissue,** is made up of fat and connective tissue. Its main function is to reduce heat loss from the body. Superficial veins, lymph glands, and cutaneous nerves are found in this region. In some areas of the body—especially over bony prominences—the superficial fascia is modified into **subcutaneous synovial bursae.** For example, bursae may be found over the bony prominence in the posterior aspect of the elbow or over the knee joint. In certain areas where the skin is moved, cutaneous muscles are present in the fascia. The facial muscles, the superficial muscle in the scrotum (dartos), the neck and facial muscle (platysma) are examples of these muscles.

The **deep fascia** is a tough layer of connective tissue that lies over the muscles and attaches to bony prominences that are subcutaneous by fusing with the outer layer of the bone. In some regions, skeletal muscle is partly or fully inserted into the deep fascia. For example, the gluteal muscle (gluteus maximus) inserts into a thick fascia in the lateral part of the leg (the iliotibial tract).

Sheets of deep fascia often pass between groups of muscles before they blend with the periosteum (outer covering) of the underlying bone. These **intermuscular septa** divide the limb into different compartments, apart from providing a larger surface area for the attachment of muscles.

In regions over joints, the deep fascia forms tough sheets that hold tendons in place. For example, such sheets (e.g., flexor retinacula) are found anterior to the wrist joint.

Deep fascia plays an important role in blood circulation. Because of the effect of gravity, blood in the veins tends to pool in dependent parts. The deep fascia is particularly tough in these regions, preventing muscle mass distention.

---

collagen fibers, reticular fibers, or **elastic fibers.** The proportion of different fibers in the ground substance is responsible for the different texture and property.

Collagen Fibers

Collagen fibers are the most common type. They are long, straight, and unbranched. They are made up of protein strands tightly wound together like rope and held together by hydrogen bonds, giving connective tissue flexibility. Collagen, however, is strong and can withstand a lot of force if applied from both ends. Tendons and ligaments, which withstand a lot of force as muscle contracts, are made up almost entirely of collagen. The flexibility of collagen also allows joints to move as the tendons and ligaments go across them.

Collagen fibers can be arranged in ways to alter the property of the tissue, dictated by the ground substance and the local tissue. They may be arranged

randomly, forming sheets (e.g., **fascia**); systematically stacked (e.g., **aponeurosis**); spun loosely (e.g., **subcutaneous tissue**); or arranged in parallel (e.g., **tendon**).

Reticular Fibers

Reticular fibers are also proteins, but they are much thinner, forming branching networks. This gives the connective tissue flexibility. At the same time, these fibers are tough and can resist force applied in different directions. Because of these properties, reticular fibers are more abundant in areas where cells and organs must be kept together. Reticular fibers hold blood vessels and nerves in place.

Elastic Fibers

Elastic fibers are branched, wavy fibers containing the protein elastin. The special characteristic of elastin is that it can be stretched and it will return to its original size when released.

Ground Substance

The ground substance is the medium in which the cells and protein fibers are suspended. Usually clear and colorless, it has the consistency of thick syrup. Proteoglycan, which gives ground substance its viscous property, is formed by the interaction of polysaccharides and proteins secreted by fibroblasts into the extracellular fluid.

Substances moving in and out of cells have to pass through the ground substance before they enter blood vessels. The consistency of ground substance varies from region to region. In tissue where mobility is required, the major component of ground substance is hyaluronic acid. In tissues where support is the major function, chondroitin sulfate is the major component.

Depending on how loose or dense they appear, connective tissue proper can be classified as **loose connective tissue** or **dense connective tissue.**

Loose connective tissue has more ground substance and less protein fibers and cells. It is the "packing material" that fills the space between organs, providing support and absorbing shock. For example, it is the presence of loose connective tissue that keeps the skin in place. At the same time, it allows the skin to be pinched up and separated to some extent from the underlying tissue. Along with the adipose tissue, this

✓ Rolfing

The techniques used by this method of manipulation have an effect on the body by exerting pressure and varied forces on the connective tissue.

Special Consideration Boxes

Key topics relevant to massage therapy or areas that need further elaboration are highlighted in **Special Consideration Boxes,** indicated by checkmark icons.

SUGGESTED READINGS

Andrade CK, Clifford P. Outcome-Based Massage. Baltimore: Lippincott Williams & Wilkins, 2001.
Goats GCK. Connective tissue massage. Br J Sports Med 1991; 25(3):131–133.
Goats GC. Massage—the scientific basis of an ancient art: Part 1, Part 2. Br J Sports Med 1994;28(3):149–155.
Juhan D. A Handbook for Bodywork: Job's Body. New York: Station Hill Press, 1987.
Kenney RA. Physiology of Aging: A Synopsis. 2nd Ed. Chicago: Year Book Medical, 1989.
Kotzsch RE. Restructure the body with rolfing: deep massage that realigns the human form. East West Nat Health 1992;22(6):35–38.
Premkumar K. Pathology A to Z. 2nd Ed. Calgary: VanPub Books, 1999.
Sandler S. The physiology of soft tissue massage. J Bodywork Movement Ther 1999;3(2):118–122.

🔵 Review Questions

Multiple Choice

1. Which structure separates the thoracic cavity from the abdominopelvic cavity?
   A. Diaphragm
   B. Visceral peritoneum
   C. Liver
   D. Parietal pleura
   E. Rib cage

2. Which of the following is NOT a characteristic of a person in anatomical position?
   A. Feet together
   B. Arms at sides
   C. Body erect
   D. Eyes directed forward
   E. Palms facing posteriorly

Fill-in-the-Blank

1. The levels of organization from larger to smaller are:

   Organism _____ → _____ → _____ → _____ → _____ → Chemicals

2. In each situation, determine if water would move into the cell (I); out of the cell (O); or neither (N). Mark each situation with I, O, or N.

   Solute (chemical substance dissolved in water) more concentrated around the cell _____

   Solute less concentrated around the cell _____

   Solute concentration is the same as in the cell _____

3. Completion
   a. Within the nucleus of the atom, there are positively charged particles called _____ and uncharged particles called _____.
   b. If you subtract the atomic number from the mass number, you will identify the number of _____.
   c. In the _____ bond, a pair of electrons is shared.
   d. In the _____ type bond, a weak link between a hydrogen atom and another atom, such as oxygen or nitrogen, is formed.
   e. The ratio of hydrogen to oxygen in all carbohydrates is _____ : _____.

Review Questions

Each chapter contains a variety of **Review Questions** to help you reinforce understanding of key concepts introduced. Put your knowledge to the test with matching, short answer, multiple choice, fill-in-the-blank, true/false questions. Answers to the questions are included so you can check your work.

---

6. Fill in the blanks, using the appropriate membrane type: a. mucous, b. serous, c. cutaneous, and d. synovial.
   a. Membrane found in joints, such as the knees and shoulders
   b. Membrane that lines the mouth
   c. Membrane lining of the thoracic cavity
   d. The skin is considered to be this type membrane

7. Below is a classification of connective tissue. Fill in the blanks with the appropriate type.

True or False

(Answer the following questions T, for true; or F, for false):

1. Diffusion, osmosis, and facilitated diffusion are all passive transport processes.
2. Plasma membranes consist of a double layer of carbohydrate molecules with proteins embedded in the bilayer.
3. Oxygen, water, NaCl and glucose are inorganic compounds.

Matching

A.
a. _____ parasagittal plane
b. _____ midsagittal plane
c. _____ transverse plane
d. _____ frontal plane

1. This plane divides the body into superior and inferior parts.
2. This plane divides the body into equal right and left portions.
3. This plane divides the body into anterior and posterior portions.
4. This plane divides the body into unequal right and left portions.

B.
a. _____ lateral
b. _____ medial
c. _____ superficial
d. _____ inferior
e. _____ anterior

1. Toward or near the surface of a structure or body.
2. Away from the midline of a structure or body.
3. Toward the front of a structure or body.
4. Toward the lower part of a structure or body.
5. Toward the midline of a structure or body.

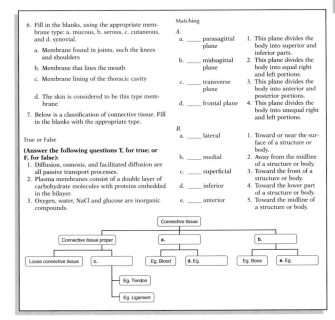

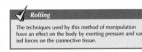

Connective tissue
Connective tissue proper — a. — b.
Loose connective tissue — c. — Eg. Blood — d. Eg. — Eg. Bone — e. Eg.
Eg. Tendon
Eg. Ligament

---

10. The cardinal signs of inflammation include all of the following **except**
    A. sweating
    B. swelling
    C. redness
    D. increased temperature
    E. pain

11. The cells in the epidermis that are involved in immunity are
    A. Merkel cells
    B. melanocytes
    C. Langerhans cells
    D. keratinocytes

Fill-In-the-Blanks

1. In the condition known as _____, the skin takes on a blue color. The blue coloration is due to the pigment _____.
2. The dermis is organized into two layers. They are the _____ and the _____.
3. The muscle that causes the hair to stand on end is the _____.

True–False
(Answer the following questions T, for true; or F, for false):

1. The subcutaneous layer is primarily made up of blood vessels and nerves that respond to stimulation of skin.
2. The accessory structures are located in the dermis.
3. Lipid-soluble substances are more easily absorbed through the skin than water-soluble substances.

Matching

A. _____ a yellow discoloration of mucous membrane as a result of liver dysfunction
B. _____ a type of skin cancer that spreads rapidly
C. _____ a condition where the cells of the epidermis migrate to the surface more rapidly than normal
D. _____ a condition where there is dysfunction of melanocytes
E. _____ a condition where the skin takes on a bluish tinge
F. _____ a solid elevation of epidermis and dermis
G. _____ loss of epidermis

1. psoriasis
2. cyanosis
3. jaundice
4. melanoma
5. ulcer
6. vitiligo
7. papule

Short Answer Questions

1. Describe the role of white blood cells in inflammatory reactions.
2. List the different ways by which inflammation may resolve.
3. Compare and contrast acute and chronic inflammation.
4. Describe the mechanical effects of massage.
5. Give examples of some reflex effects of massage.
6. Identify the manipulative techniques that primarily affect the superficial and deep fascia.

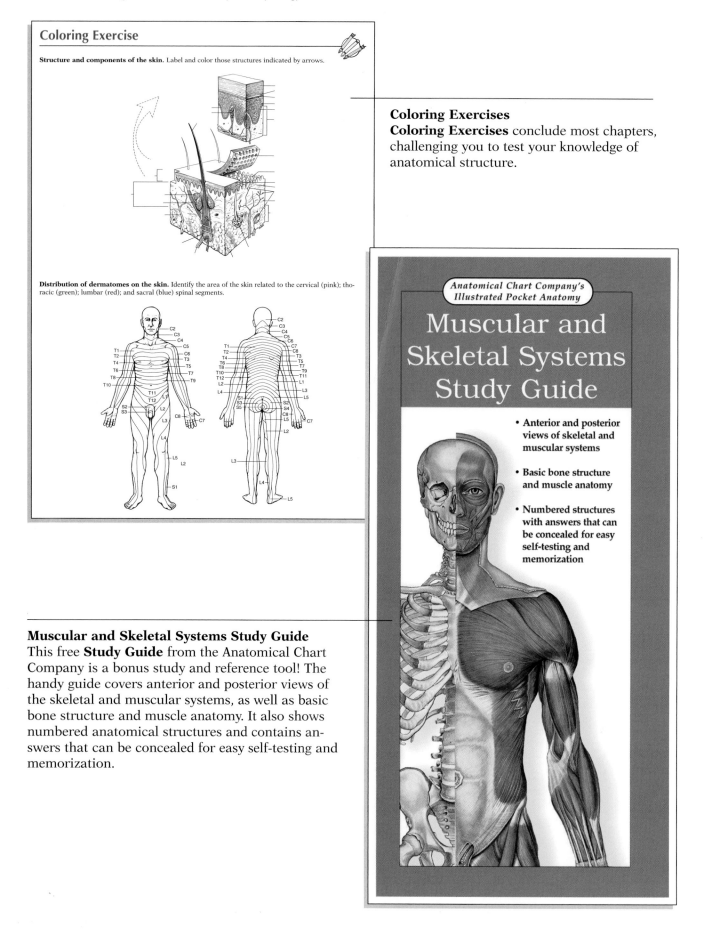

Coloring Exercise

Structure and components of the skin. Label and color those structures indicated by arrows.

Distribution of dermatomes on the skin. Identify the area of the skin related to the cervical (pink); thoracic (green); lumbar (red); and sacral (blue) spinal segments.

Coloring Exercises
Coloring Exercises conclude most chapters, challenging you to test your knowledge of anatomical structure.

Anatomical Chart Company's Illustrated Pocket Anatomy

Muscular and Skeletal Systems Study Guide

- Anterior and posterior views of skeletal and muscular systems

- Basic bone structure and muscle anatomy

- Numbered structures with answers that can be concealed for easy self-testing and memorization

Muscular and Skeletal Systems Study Guide
This free **Study Guide** from the Anatomical Chart Company is a bonus study and reference tool! The handy guide covers anterior and posterior views of the skeletal and muscular systems, as well as basic bone structure and muscle anatomy. It also shows numbered anatomical structures and contains answers that can be concealed for easy self-testing and memorization.

How To Use This Book

User's Guide

The Massage Connection: Anatomy & Physiology, Second Edition gives you a well-rounded understanding of anatomy and physiology as it pertains to massage therapy. This user's guide shows you how to put the book's features to work for you.

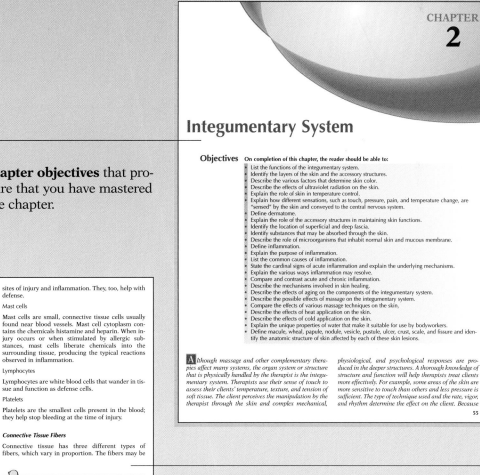

Integumentary System

Objectives On completion of this chapter, the reader should be able to:

- List the functions of the integumentary system.
- Identify the layers of the skin and the accessory structures.
- Describe the various factors that determine skin color.
- Describe the effects of ultraviolet radiation on the skin.
- Explain the role of skin in temperature control.
- Explain how different sensations, such as touch, pressure, pain, and temperature change, are "sensed" by the skin and conveyed to the central nervous system.
- Define dermatome.
- Explain the role of the accessory structures in maintaining skin functions.
- Identify the location of superficial and deep fascia.
- Identify substances that may be absorbed through the skin.
- Describe the role of microorganisms that inhabit normal skin and mucous membrane.
- Define inflammation.
- Explain the purpose of inflammation.
- List the common causes of inflammation.
- State the cardinal signs of acute inflammation and explain the underlying mechanisms.
- Explain the various ways inflammation may resolve.
- Compare and contrast acute and chronic inflammation.
- Describe the mechanisms involved in skin healing.
- Describe the effects of aging on the components of the integumentary system.
- Describe the possible effects of massage on the integumentary system.
- Compare the effects of various massage techniques on the skin.
- Describe the effects of heat application on the skin.
- Describe the effects of cold application on the skin.
- Explain the unique properties of water that make it suitable for use by bodyworkers.
- Define macule, wheal, papule, nodule, vesicle, pustule, ulcer, crust, scale, and fissure and identify the anatomic structure of skin affected by each of these skin lesions.

Although massage and other complementary therapies affect many systems, the organ system or structure that is physically handled by the therapist is the integumentary system. Therapists use their sense of touch to assess their clients' temperature, texture, and tension of soft tissue. The client perceives the manipulation by the therapist through the skin and complex mechanical, physiological, and psychological responses are produced in the deeper structures. A thorough knowledge of structure and function will help therapists treat clients more effectively. For example, some areas of the skin are more sensitive to touch than others and less pressure is sufficient. The type of technique used and the rate, vigor, and rhythm determine the effect on the client. Because

55

Chapter Objectives

Each chapter opens with **chapter objectives** that provide clear goals to help ensure that you have mastered the material presented in the chapter.

Macrophages

Macrophages are defense cells that have wandered into the connective tissue from the blood. Scavenger cells, they remove dead cells and foreign agents. Certain macrophages may be fixed to a site (**fixed macrophages**), as found in the liver and spleen. Others are wanderers, attracted to injured areas by chemicals liberated by injured tissue. These are the **free macrophages.**

Microphages

Microphages are other types of white blood cells (neutrophils and eosinophils) that are attracted to

sites of injury and inflammation. They, too, help with defense.

Mast cells

Mast cells are small, connective tissue cells usually found near blood vessels. Mast cell cytoplasm contains the chemicals histamine and heparin. When injury occurs or when stimulated by allergic substances, mast cells liberate chemicals into the surrounding tissue, producing the typical reactions observed in inflammation.

Lymphocytes

Lymphocytes are white blood cells that wander in tissue and function as defense cells.

Platelets

Platelets are the smallest cells present in the blood; they help stop bleeding at the time of injury.

Connective Tissue Fibers

Connective tissue has three different types of fibers, which vary in proportion. The fibers may be

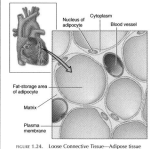

FIGURE 1.24.   Loose Connective Tissue—Adipose tissue

CAPSULES

The body defends itself from disease and microorganisms by forming a connective tissue capsule around infected areas. A pustule or abscess is a typical example. The microorganisms, defense cells (both dead and alive), together with secretions, are cordoned off by a connective tissue capsule, which contains the infection to the local area and prevents it from spreading.

Information Boxes

Indicated by a light bulb icon, the **Information Boxes** highlight additional facts, precautions, and guidelines relevant to bodyworkers.

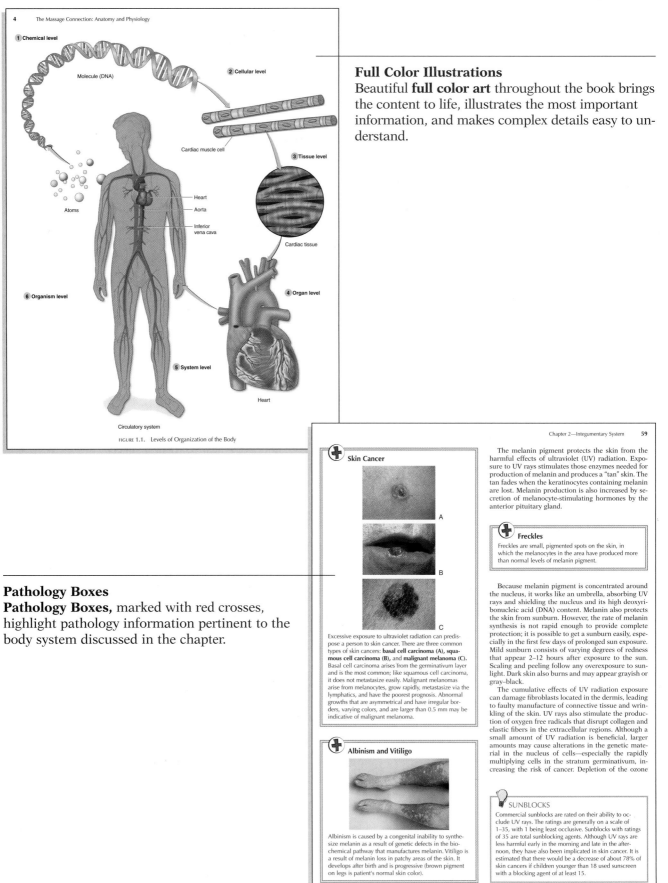

① Chemical level

Molecule (DNA)

② Cellular level

Atoms

Cardiac muscle cell

③ Tissue level

Heart
Aorta
Inferior
vena cava

Cardiac tissue

⑥ Organism level

④ Organ level

⑤ System level

Heart

Circulatory system

FIGURE 1.1.   Levels of Organization of the Body

Full Color Illustrations
Beautiful **full color art** throughout the book brings the content to life, illustrates the most important information, and makes complex details easy to understand.

Pathology Boxes
Pathology Boxes, marked with red crosses, highlight pathology information pertinent to the body system discussed in the chapter.

✚ Skin Cancer

A

B

C

Excessive exposure to ultraviolet radiation can predispose a person to skin cancer. There are three common types of skin cancers: **basal cell carcinoma (A), squamous cell carcinoma (B),** and **malignant melanoma (C).** Basal cell carcinoma arises from the germinativum layer and is the most common; like squamous cell carcinoma, it does not metastasize easily. Malignant melanomas arise from melanocytes, grow rapidly, metastasize via the lymphatics, and have the poorest prognosis. Abnormal growths that are asymmetrical and have irregular borders, varying colors, and are larger than 0.5 mm may be indicative of malignant melanoma.

✚ Albinism and Vitiligo

Albinism is caused by a congenital inability to synthesize melanin as a result of genetic defects in the biochemical pathway that manufactures melanin. Vitiligo is a result of melanin loss in patchy areas of the skin. It develops after birth and is progressive (brown pigment on legs is patient's normal skin color).

The melanin pigment protects the skin from the harmful effects of ultraviolet (UV) radiation. Exposure to UV rays stimulates those enzymes needed for production of melanin and produces a "tan" skin. The tan fades when the keratinocytes containing melanin are lost. Melanin production is also increased by secretion of melanocyte-stimulating hormones by the anterior pituitary gland.

✚ Freckles
Freckles are small, pigmented spots on the skin, in which the melanocytes in the area have produced more than normal levels of melanin pigment.

Because melanin pigment is concentrated around the nucleus, it works like an umbrella, absorbing UV rays and shielding the nucleus and its high deoxyribonucleic acid (DNA) content. Melanin also protects the skin from sunburn. However, the rate of melanin synthesis is not rapid enough to provide complete protection; it is possible to get a sunburn easily, especially in the first few days of prolonged sun exposure. Mild sunburn consists of varying degrees of redness that appear 2–12 hours after exposure to the sun. Scaling and peeling follow any overexposure to sunlight. Dark skin also burns and may appear grayish or gray–black.

The cumulative effects of UV radiation exposure can damage fibroblasts located in the dermis, leading to faulty manufacture of connective tissue and wrinkling of the skin. UV rays also stimulate the production of oxygen free radicals that disrupt collagen and elastic fibers in the extracellular regions. Although a small amount of UV radiation is beneficial, larger amounts may cause alterations in the genetic material in the nucleus of cells—especially the rapidly multiplying cells in the stratum germinativum, increasing the risk of cancer. Depletion of the ozone

💡 SUNBLOCKS
Commercial sunblocks are rated on their ability to occlude UV rays. The ratings are generally on a scale of 1–35, with 1 being least occlusive. Sunblocks with ratings of 35 are total sunblocking agents. Although UV rays are less harmful early in the morning and late in the afternoon, they have also been implicated in skin cancer. It is estimated that there would be a decrease of about 78% of skin cancers if children younger than 18 used sunscreen with a blocking agent of at least 15.

REVIEWERS

John Balletto
Center for Muscular Therapy
Providence, RI

William J. Ryan
Department of Exercise and
Rehabilitative Sciences
Slippery Rock University of
Pennsylvania

Mary Sinclair
Professional Institute of Massage Therapy
Saskatoon, Saskatchewan

Nadine Forbes
Steiner Education Group
Pompano Beach, FL

William Rahner
Desert Institute of Healing Arts
Tuscon, AZ

Stuart Watts
Academy of Oriental Medicine
Austin, TX

Acknowledgments

I am greatly indebted to many individuals who helped with the preparation of the book. I wish to acknowledge Pete Darcy, Eric Branger, and the rest of the team of professionals at Lippincott Williams & Wilkins for their assistance and support with the transformation of the first edition into its present format.

I wish to thank the administrators of various schools and associations who shared their curriculum and objectives. A special thanks to the reviewers for their useful comments, without which it would have been difficult to modify the contents of the first edition and better meet the needs of this audience. I would also like to acknowledge the massage therapy students of Mount Royal College, Calgary, for their useful feedback and suggestions for improvement as they used the first edition as their textbook.

I would especially like to thank Ms. Nobuko Pratt, my efficient and able research assistant, for the excellent job of identifying and compiling relevant journal articles and for administrative assistance as I revised the book. Last, but certainly not least, I wish to thank my husband and children for their encouragement and great support.

Figure Credits

In addition to the artwork created by Dragonfly Media Group, Mark Miller Medical Illustrations, Kim Battista, Mary Anna Barratt, and Susan Caldwell, liberal use has been made of illustrations from the following Lippincott Williams & Wilkins sources:

Agur MRA, Lee MJ. Grant's Atlas of Anatomy, 10th Ed. Lippincott Williams & Wilkins, 1999.

Anderson M, Hall SJ. Sports Injury Management, 2nd Ed. Lippincott Williams & Wilkins, 2000.

Bear M, Conner B, Paradiso M. Neuroscience, 2nd Ed. Lippincott Williams & Wilkins, 2000.

Cipriano J. Photographic Manual of Regional Orthopaedic and Neurological Tests, 2nd Ed. Lippincott Williams & Wilkins, 1991.

Cohen BJ, Wood DL. Memmler's The Human Body in Health and Disease, 9th Ed. Lippincott Williams & Wilkins, 1999.

Cormack DH. Essential Histology, 2nd Ed. Lippincott Williams & Wilkins, 2001.

Daffner RH. Clinical Radiology, 2nd Ed. Lippincott Williams & Wilkins, 1998.

Dean D, Herbener TE. Cross-Sectional Human Anatomy. Lippincott Williams & Wilkins, 2000.

Gartner H. Color Atlas of Histology, 3rd Ed. Lippincott Williams & Wilkins, 2001.

Goodheart HP. Photoguide of Common Skin Disorders, 2nd Ed. Lippincott Williams & Wilkins, 2003.

Hamill J, Knutzen K. Biomechanical Basis of Movement, 2nd Ed. Lippincott Williams & Wilkins, 2003.

Hendrickson T. Massage for Orthopedic Conditions. Lippincott Williams & Wilkins, 2002.

Kendall FP, McCreary EK, Provance PG. Muscles: Testing and Function with posture and pain, 4th Ed. Lippincott Williams & Wilkins, 1993.

McArdle WD, Katch FI, Katch VL. Essentials of Exercise Physiology, 2nd Ed. Lippincott Williams & Wilkins, 2000.

Moore KL, Agur AMR. Essential Clinical Anatomy, 2nd Ed. Lippincott Williams & Wilkins, 2002.

Moore K, Dalley AF. Clinically Oriented Anatomy, 4th Ed. Lippincott Williams & Wilkins, 1999.

Oatis CA. Kinesiology. The Mechanics and Pathomechanics of Human Movement. Lippincott Williams & Wilkins, 2003.

Pillitteri A. Maternal and Child Health Nursing, 4th Ed. Lippincott Williams & Wilkins, 2002.

Porth CM. Pathophysiology Concepts in Altered Health States, 6th Ed. Lippincott Williams & Wilkins, 2002.

Rubin E. Essential Pathology, 3rd Ed. Lippincott Williams & Wilkins, 2000.

Sadler T. Langman's Medical Embryology, 9th Ed. Lippincott Williams & Wilkins, 2003.

Smeltzer SCO, Bare BG. Brunner and Suddarth's Textbook of Medical-Surgical Nursing, 9th Ed. Lippincott Williams & Wilkins, 2002.

Snell R. Clinical Neuroanatomy. Lippincott Williams & Wilkins, 2001.

Stedman's Concise Medical Dictionary for the Health Professions, 3rd Ed. Lippincott Williams & Wilkins, 2001.

Stedman's Medical Dictionary, 27th Ed. Lippincott Williams & Wilkins, 2000.

Tweitmeyer A, McCracken T. Coloring Guide to Human Anatomy, 3rd Ed. Lippincott Williams & Wilkins, 2001.

Westheimer R, Lopater S. Human Sexuality. Lippincott Williams & Wilkins, 2003.

Contents

An Introduction to the Human Body

Objectives **On completion of this chapter, the reader should be able to:**

- Define anatomy and physiology and identify some of the subdivisions.
- Identify word roots, prefixes, and suffixes and combining forms.
- List the organizational levels of the body.
- List the major organ systems of the body and explain the function of each system.
- Describe the anatomic position.
- Identify the abdominal regions and quadrants.
- Identify the organs located in each abdominal region.
- Define the principal directional terms and body planes.
- Name the cavities of the body and identify the major organs contained in each cavity.
- Differentiate intracellular, extracellular, interstitial, and intravascular body fluids.
- Define homeostasis.
- Identify the components of a feedback system.
- Describe how a physiologic feedback mechanism maintains homeostasis.
- Differentiate between positive and negative feedback mechanisms; give examples of each.
- Define atoms and molecules.
- Describe the different chemical reactions.
- Define enzymes and explain their functions.
- List the factors that affect enzyme activity.
- Define pH.
- Define buffers. Provide examples of buffer systems in the body.
- Distinguish between organic and inorganic compounds and provide examples for both compound types.
- Give a brief description of the structure and biologic functions of carbohydrates, lipids, proteins, and nucleic acids and provide examples.
- Give a brief description of DNA structure and the genetic codes.
- Give a brief description of protein synthesis regulation and the steps involved in the process.
- Describe the structure of a cell and the functions of each organelle.
- Describe the structure of the cell membrane.
- Describe the different ways transport occurs across a cell membrane.
- Define chromosomes.
- Give a brief description of mitosis and meiosis.
- Classify tissue.
- Describe the structure and function of each tissue type; identify some locations where each type is found.
- Describe and compare the different types of connective tissue.
- Describe the structure of collagen.

- Describe the different types of cartilage and identify locations for each type.
- Differentiate between skeletal, cardiac, and smooth muscle.
- Describe the structure and function of nervous tissue.
- Describe the inflammation process and tissue repair.
- Describe the different outcomes of tissue repair.
- Identify the different types of membranes and give the locations where each type may be found.
- Describe the effects of aging on different types of tissue.
- Describe the possible effects of massage on healthy tissue.

*W*ith the recognition of massage as an alternative or complementary form of therapy, the demands made of the therapist are increasing. Although massage is more involved with the knowledge and use of physical skills and techniques, the knowledge of anatomy, physiology, and pathology is also necessary for the therapist to effectively use those learned massage skills. The therapist is certainly not required to know the field as thoroughly as medical professionals because diagnosis is not involved; however, the therapist should have the knowledge to understand how the body functions and how different parts of the body integrate.

With this foundation, a therapist should understand how various diseases affect specific functions and how to recognize those conditions in which treatment may be detrimental to the client. Therapists should also be able to recognize conditions that may be harmful to his or her well-being.

In addition, the therapist must have a thorough knowledge of various standard medical terms that are accepted and used in the medical field. This will help the therapist effectively discuss a client's condition with other health professionals, a situation that often occurs. The correct terminology will also help the therapist keep up with the rapidly increasing knowledge in health-related fields relevant to massage.

Chapter 1 gives an overview of the organization of the body and introduces basic anatomy and physiology terms.

The definition of the term **anatomy,** meaning "cutting open," originates from the ancient Greek. Although the study of anatomy need not involve "cutting," it is the study of the external and internal structures of the body and the physical relationship between the parts of the body. Anatomy answers the questions: What? Where? **Physiology,** also of Greek origin, is the study of the functions of the various parts of the body. It answers the questions: Why? How? For example, anatomy describes the location of a muscle; physiology describes how the muscle

contracts. Remember that the structure of any body is adapted to its functions; therefore, anatomy and physiology are closely related.

Anatomy can be divided into many subtypes. **Microscopic anatomy** involves structures that cannot be visualized with the naked eye. **Macroscopic,** or **gross anatomy,** considers structures that can be visualized without aid. **Surface anatomy** involves the study of general forms and superficial markings on the surface of the body. **Regional anatomy** focuses on the superficial and internal features of a specific area. **Systemic anatomy** is the study of structures that have the same function. **Developmental anatomy** involves changes that occur during the course of physical development. **Embryology** is a study of changes that occur during development in the womb. **Histology** involves the examination of tissues, groups of specialized cells, and cell products that work together to perform specific functions. **Cytology** involves the analysis of the internal structure of individual cells.

Physiology can also be divided into subtypes. **Cell physiology** relates to the study of the cell function, and **systemic physiology** considers the functioning of structures that serve specific needs, such as respiration and reproduction. **Pathophysiology** is the study of how disease affects specific functions.

Levels of Organization—an Overview

The body is made up of millions of individual units called **cells.** Cells are the smallest living part of the body. The cells, in turn, are made up of **chemicals**—atoms (e.g., carbon, hydrogen, oxygen, nitrogen, and

Think It Through. . .

Would you consider massage therapy to be alternative therapy, complementary therapy, or both?

AUTOPSY

Autopsy is the examination of all of the organs and tissues of the body after death. Autopsies are of value because they often determine the cause of death or reveal disease or structural defects. They can be used to check the effectiveness of a particular drug therapy or surgery.

phosphorus), molecules, and compounds (proteins, carbohydrates) organized in different ways to form the structures inside the cell. A collection of cells having the same function is called **tissue.** For example, a collection of cells that produce contraction is called muscle tissue. Different tissues that are grouped together and perform the same function are called **organs.** For example, the stomach, which helps with food digestion, is made up of muscle tissue that helps move the food, connective tissue that binds the muscle tissue, blood vessels and glands, epithelial tissue that lines the inside of the stomach, and nervous tissue that regulates the movement and secretion of glands. Organs that perform certain functions together are grouped together as **systems.** For example, the respiratory system includes organs that help deliver oxygen to the body; the reproductive system includes organs that help the organism reproduce. Sometimes, an organ may be part of more than one system. The body may be considered to have six different levels of organization—**chemical, cellular, tissue, organ,** and **systemic** (see Figure 1.1) The highest level of organization—the **organismal level**—is the living body.

The Holistic Approach

Although it is easier to teach and learn anatomy and physiology by dividing the body into organs and systems, it has to be understood that the body is complex and highly integrated. Each system is interdependent and works together as one—the body. In the Bible, the analogy of the human body is used in a different context; however, it aptly describes the working of the body: ". . . the body is a unit, though it is made up of many parts; and though all its parts are many, they form one body . . . if one part suffers, every part suffers with it; if one part is honored, every part rejoices with it." (*Life Application Study Bible.* Tyndale House Publishers, 1997:I Corinthians 12:12-27.)

What happens to one tissue affects the whole body and what happens to the body affects all of its parts. It is this holistic concept that alternative/complementary therapy, of which massage is one, adopts. To extend this further, the manipulation of soft tissue in one area potentially affects the whole body.

The best learning approach for anatomy and physiology is to view the body "holistically." Although ideal, the body is too complex for the beginning student to fully appreciate how the different parts integrate. This book, therefore, addresses individual systems or parts of the body with the hope that, in the end, the entire picture will fall into place.

Homeostasis

Traditionally, the body has been divided into many systems, according to specific functions. The ultimate purpose of every system, however, is to maintain a constant cell environment, enabling each cell to live. Fluid surrounds every cell of the body, and all systems are structured to maintain the physical conditions and concentrations of dissolved substances in this fluid. The fluid outside the cell is known as the **extracellular fluid** (ECF), and the fluid inside the cell is known as **intracellular fluid** (ICF) (see Figure 1.2). The extracellular fluid inside the blood vessel is known as the **intravascular fluid,** or **plasma.** The fluid outside of the cells and the blood vessels is known as the **interstitial fluid.** Because the interstitial fluid surrounds the cells, it is known as the **internal environment;** the condition of constancy in the internal environment is called **homeostasis.** In short, all systems maintain homeostasis by regulating the volume and composition of the internal environment.

Each system continuously alters its active state to maintain homeostasis. The maintenance of homeostasis can be compared to the working of a baking oven. When the temperature is set, the heating element (the **effector**) is switched on—indicated by a red light—to heat the oven. When the desired temperature is reached, the heating element is switched off and the light goes out. When you open the oven door (without switching off the oven, of course) to check the food that is baking, the light comes on again—have you noticed that? When you open the oven door, the heat escapes and the temperature drops slightly. This drop in temperature is detected (**receptor**) and conveyed to the thermostat (the **control center**) in the oven and the heating element is switched on.

Similarly, the body has various detectors to detect changes in specific elements. Let's take, for example, the oxygen content in the blood. If the detectors (receptors) find the level of oxygen becoming lower, they stimulate the system(s) that bring oxygen into the body—the respiratory system works harder until the oxygen level reaches the normal range.

Imagine many similar detectors located all over the body—monitoring calcium, hydrogen, and sodium levels; volume of blood; blood pressure; hormone levels; and body temperature. Can you picture each of these regulators monitoring specific elements and bringing about an appropriate action or change in various systems—all at the same time! You expect chaos. Instead, the body is orchestrated so beautifully that all systems work in harmony with one aim—to maintain homeostasis. When a person is ill, therefore, the body must be treated as a whole and

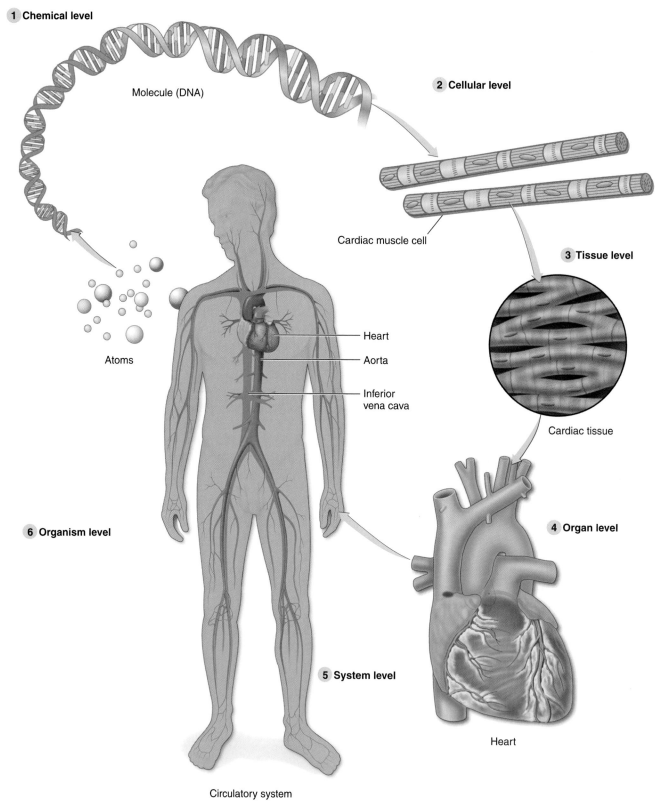

1 Chemical level

Molecule (DNA)

2 Cellular level

Cardiac muscle cell

Atoms

3 Tissue level

Cardiac tissue

6 Organism level

Heart
Aorta
Inferior
vena cava

4 Organ level

5 System level

Heart

Circulatory system

FIGURE 1.1.   Levels of Organization of the Body

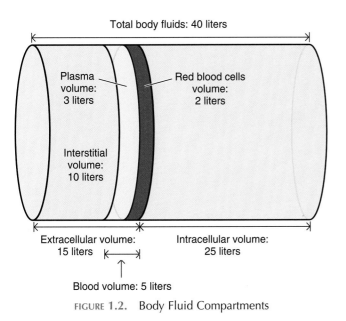

Total body fluids: 40 liters

Plasma volume: 3 liters

Red blood cells volume: 2 liters

Interstitial volume: 10 liters

Extracellular volume: 15 liters

Intracellular volume: 25 liters

Blood volume: 5 liters

FIGURE **1.2.**   Body Fluid Compartments

not as individual systems. Massage therapy, to bring about complete healing, should treat the entire person and not only the diseased part or state.

FEEDBACK SYSTEMS

The sequence of events that result in maintaining homeostasis is known as a **feedback system.** In a feedback system, a particular variable is constantly monitored. Changes are instituted to decrease or increase the level of the variable to maintain the level within the normal range. Numerous feedback systems are involved in the regulation of the internal environment. The variable in question is known as the **controlled condition.** Any factor that changes the level of the variable is known as the **stimulus.** The **receptor** in the body monitors the variable and sends input to the

control center in the brain. The control center determines the normal range of values. Depending on the change in the level of the variable, the control center sends out messages to structures that help nullify this effect. These structures are known as the **effectors.**

When you stand up from a lying down position, for example, blood pools in your lower limbs and your blood pressure drops as a result of the effects of gravity. This drop in pressure is detected by receptors located in the blood vessels' walls in your neck. The receptors convey the change in blood pressure to the brain (control center) via the nerves, and the brain sends messages to the blood vessels (effectors) to constrict. With constriction, the volume decreases and the pressure inside the blood vessels increases, bringing the blood pressure back to the normal range. Here, the **feedback loop** has nullified the change that occurs. This feedback mechanism is known as **negative feedback** (see Figure 1.3A).

Rarely, changes in the variable are enhanced. In such a feedback loop, change produced in the variable is conveyed to the control center, and the control center intensifies the change. This feedback mechanism is known as **positive feedback** (see Figure 1.3B). For example, at the time of labor, the head of the baby descends and stretches the cervix (the lower end of the uterus). The stretch is detected by receptors and conveyed to the pituitary gland located in the brain. The pituitary gland secretes a hormone (oxytocin) that produces uterine contractions. The uterine contractions push the baby down, further stretching the cervix. This process continues until the baby is born and the cervix is no longer stretched. Because positive feedback *reinforces* the change, it is not a feedback mechanism commonly used by the body.

When all the components of every feedback system work well and homeostasis is maintained, the body remains healthy.

Systems of the Body

This book, for convenience, divides the body into the **integumentary, skeletal, muscular, nervous, cardiovascular, lymphatic, respiratory, endocrine, reproductive, digestive,** and **urinary systems** (see Figure 1.4). At times, the skeletal and muscular are considered together as musculoskeletal system.

The integumentary (skin) system includes the skin and all of its structures, such as sweat glands, nails, and hair. The major function of this system (see Figure 1.4A) is to protect the body from environmental hazards and to maintain core temperature. For an example of how skin maintains homeostasis, consider the effects of an increase in atmospheric temperature.

✓ *Regulatory Mechanisms*

Try this simple experiment. Hold your breath for one minute and then start breathing. You will notice that you breathe more rapidly for a short while after you stop holding your breath. This increase in breathing is caused by regulatory mechanisms. The detectors, which noticed that the carbon dioxide and hydrogen ion levels were increasing in your body, conveyed that information to the control center in the brain, which, in turn, made your respiratory muscles (effectors) work more actively. When the carbon dioxide and hydrogen ion levels reach the normal range, it is detected by the receptors and conveyed to the control center, which, in turn, reduces the activity of the respiratory muscles.

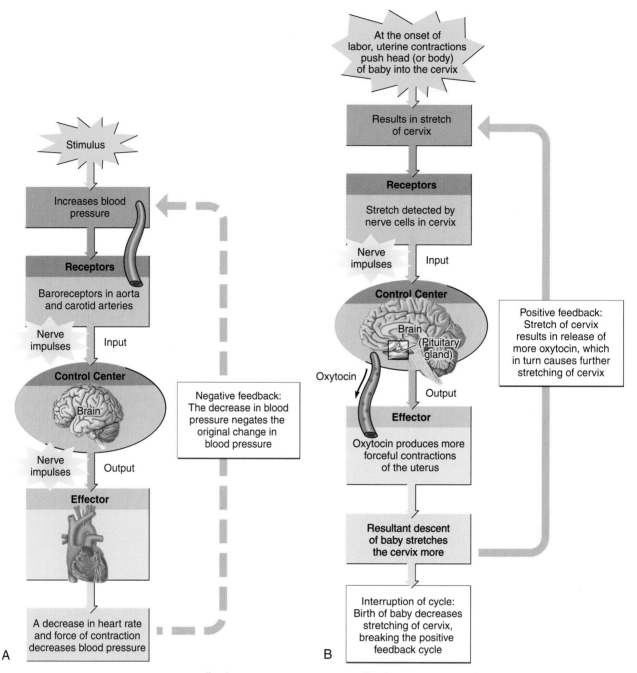

FIGURE 1.3. Feedback Systems. **A,** Negative Feedback; **B,** Positive Feedback.

The skin possesses sensors (nerve receptors) that detect temperature change. When a rise in temperature is detected, the network of blood vessels in the skin, aided by the nervous system, dilate and more blood reaches closer to the surface of the body where heat can be removed by conduction, convection, and radiation. The sweat glands increase production, and the body is cooled by sweat evaporation until body temperature reaches normal values. Other skin functions include manufacturing vitamin **D** and eliminating waste products.

The **skeletal system** (see Figure 1.4B) comprises the bones, bone marrow, and joints of the body. The skeletal system's major functions are to support the body, provide an area for muscle attachment (bones), and allow movement in various planes (joints). In addition, this system protects tissue and organs—for example, the ribs protect the lungs and heart, which are located in the chest. Minerals, including calcium, are deposited in the bones and are mobilized when the blood levels of these minerals are lower than the normal range. Different parts of the bones also manufacture blood cells.

The **muscular system** (see Figure 1.4C) is responsible for any form of movement. It includes all the muscle tissue of the body. The skeletal, cardiac, and smooth muscle are three types of muscle tissue. This system allows the organism to move in the external environment. In addition, internal muscles help move blood inside the body (e.g., the heart). The blood volume in any region can be altered by muscle contractions, which narrow or dilate the vessel, in the blood vessels walls. Muscles in the tube walls of the respiratory tract alter the size of the tubes. Food is moved down the gut by the contraction and relaxation of muscles. Urine is expelled from the body by

contraction of the muscles of the urinary bladder. The process of muscle contraction also produces heat and helps maintain body temperature.

The **nervous system** (see Figure 1.4D) consists of structures that respond to stimuli from inside and outside of the body, integrating the sensed stimuli and producing an appropriate response. Nervous system structures include the brain, the spinal cord, the nerves, and the supporting tissue. The nervous system coordinates the activities of all other organ systems. For example, the nervous system senses the change in temperature when you enter a cold room and, by making the hair on your arms stand on end and your muscles shiver (rapid contraction and relaxation), produces heat.

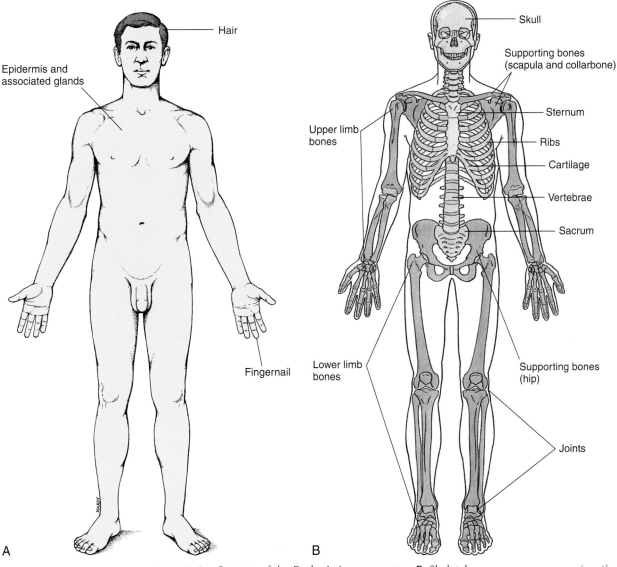

FIGURE 1.4. Systems of the Body. **A,** Integumentary; **B,** Skeletal   *(continued)*

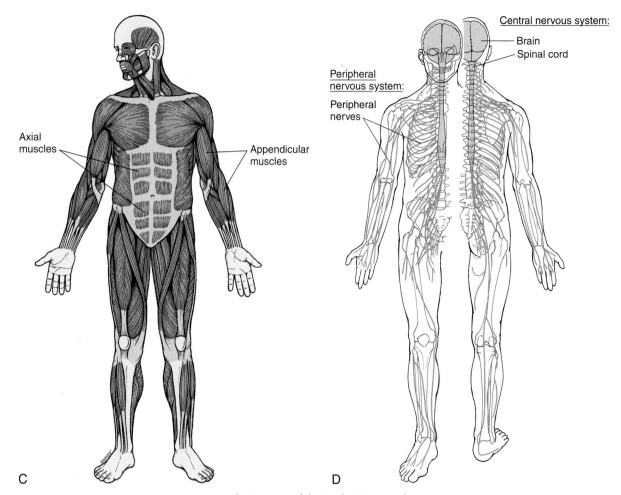

Axial muscles

Appendicular muscles

Central nervous system:
- Brain
- Spinal cord

Peripheral nervous system:

Peripheral nerves

C

D

FIGURE **1.4.**, cont'd   Systems of the Body. **C,** Muscular; **D,** Nervous   (continued)

The organs of the **cardiovascular system** (see Figure 1.4E) are responsible for the circulation of blood. This system includes the heart, blood vessels, and the blood. It helps transport oxygen, nutrients, and hormones, among others, throughout the body to various tissue, according to the needs of the tissue. Conversely, it carries waste products from the tissue to other areas for excretion.

The **lymphatic system** (see Figure 1.4F) consists of lymph vessels, lymph nodes, and lymphoid tissue in such areas as the tonsils, spleen, and thymus. It is responsible for defense against infection and disease and to help remove excess water from the tissue spaces.

The **respiratory system** (see Figure 1.4G) works closely with the cardiovascular system and includes the nose and nasal cavities and the pharynx, larynx, trachea, bronchial tubes, and lungs. Although the respiratory system brings oxygen to the site where exchange can take place (i.e., between air and the blood), it is the cardiovascular system that circulates the blood and enables the tissue to access the

oxygen. The respiratory system also allows carbon dioxide, a byproduct of metabolism, to be released in the air.

The **endocrine system** (see Figure 1.4H) works closely with the nervous system. Through the use of hormones, it produces long-term changes in various organ and system activities. Hormones are the chemicals secreted by the organs of the endocrine system, which include the pituitary, thyroid, parathyroid, and adrenal glands and endocrine part of the pancreas, ovary, and testis. The blood carries these chemicals to other receptive organs and, in turn, produces change. For example, during a pregnant woman's labor, the hormone oxytocin is secreted by an endocrine organ in the brain (pituitary) and is carried by the blood to the uterus. The uterus, in turn, responds by contracting.

The **reproductive system** (see Figure 1.4I) is responsible for the propagation of the species and includes organs, such as the ovary and testis, that manufacture sperms or eggs and secrete sex hormones. Other organs include the fallopian tubes and uterus

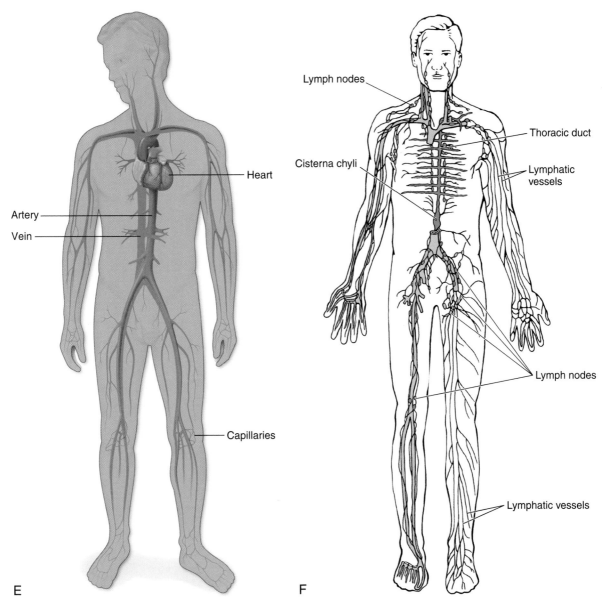

Lymph nodes

Thoracic duct

Cisterna chyli

Lymphatic vessels

Heart

Artery

Vein

Capillaries

Lymph nodes

Lymphatic vessels

E   F

FIGURE **1.4., cont'd**   Systems of the Body. **E,** Cardiovascular; **F,** Lymphatic   *(continued)*

in women and the vas deferens and accessory glands in men. The hormones, together with the genetic make up, are responsible for the male or female characteristics of the body.

The **digestive system** (see Figure 1.4J) also works in coordination with the cardiovascular system. While it is responsible for breaking down the food eaten into a form that can be utilized by the body, it is the cardiovascular system that carries the nutrients to the tissues that need it. The digestive system includes the mouth, pharynx, esophagus, stomach, and small and large intestines.

The **urinary system** (see Figure 1.4K) eliminates excess water, salts, and waste products. When the

body is dehydrated, this system helps conserve water and salt. In addition, together with the respiratory system, the urinary system maintains the body fluid pH. Its structures include the kidney, ureter, urinary bladder, and urethra.

Planes of Reference

To study the relationship of one structure to the other or to accurately explain its position, certain standard planes of references are used. Three planes are described here. The **sagittal plane** runs from front to

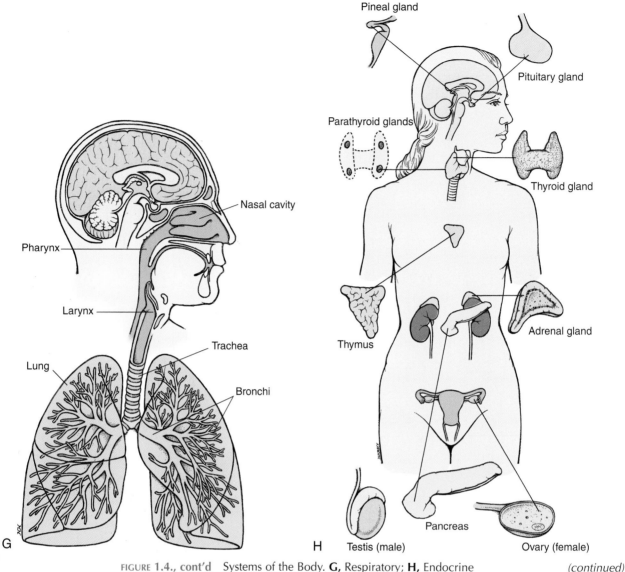

FIGURE **1.4., cont'd**   Systems of the Body. **G,** Respiratory; **H,** Endocrine   *(continued)*

back, dividing the body into right and left parts. The **coronal** or **frontal plane** runs from left to right, dividing the body into front and back portions. The **transverse** or **horizontal plane** runs across the body, dividing it into top and bottom portions. These planes help to orient the position of studied structure (see Figure 1.5).

Anatomical Position

Because the body can move in different ways, it is difficult to describe the position of a structure without agreeing on a standard body position. This standard position is called the **anatomical position.** All structures are described in relationship to this position. In

the anatomical position, the body is erect, with the feet parallel to each other and flat on the floor; the arms are at the sides of the body, with the palms of the hands turned forward and the fingers pointing straight down. The head and eyes are directed forward (see Figure 1.6).

Directional References

In the anatomical position, a structure is described as **superior/cranial** or **cephalic** when it lies toward the head, or top, and **inferior** or **caudal** when it lies toward the bottom, or away from the head (Figure 1.6). For example, the tip of the nose is superior to the lips; the chin is inferior to both. A structure lying in front

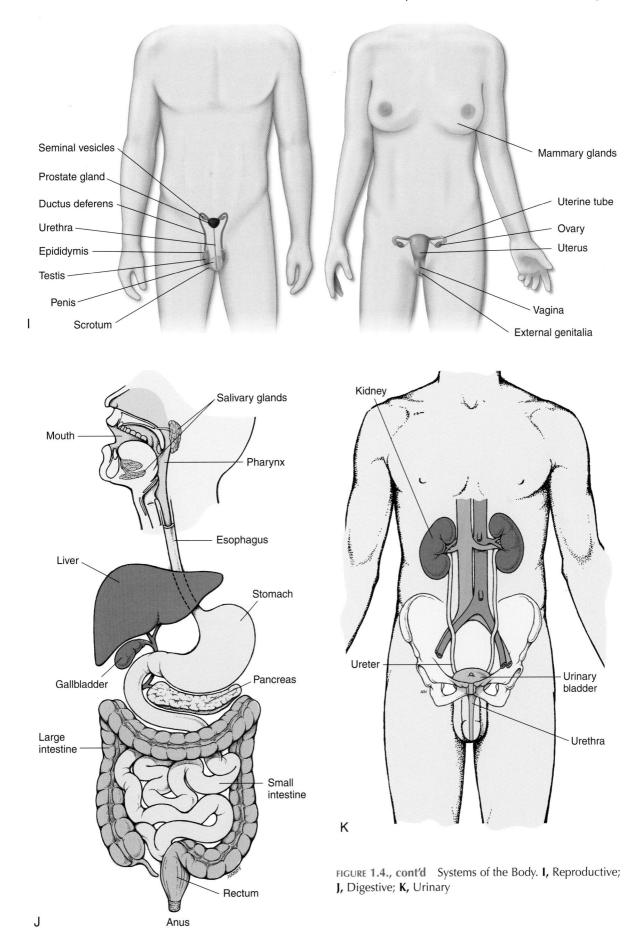

Seminal vesicles

Prostate gland

Ductus deferens

Urethra

Epididymis

Testis

Penis

Scrotum

I

Mammary glands

Uterine tube

Ovary

Uterus

Vagina

External genitalia

Salivary glands

Mouth

Pharynx

Esophagus

Liver

Stomach

Gallbladder

Pancreas

Large
intestine

Small
intestine

Rectum

Anus

J

Kidney

Ureter

Urinary
bladder

Urethra

K

FIGURE **1.4., cont'd**   Systems of the Body. **I,** Reproductive;
J, Digestive; **K,** Urinary

of another is **anterior** or **ventral**. A structure lying behind another is **posterior** or **dorsal**. For example, the ear is posterior to the cheek, and the cheek is anterior to the ear.

Those structures lying closer to an imaginary line passing through the middle of the body in the sagittal plane are said to be **medial**, while those away from the middle are **lateral**. For example, my belly button will always be medial to my widening waistline.

A structure lying away from the surface of the body is considered to be **deep** or **internal**, while a structure closer to the surface is considered **superficial** or **external**. For example, the skin is superficial to the muscles; however, the bone is deep to the muscles. **Proximal** describes structures closer to the trunk (chest and abdomen) and **distal** describes structures away from the trunk. For example, the elbow is proximal and the finger is distal to the wrist.

Body Regions

The body is divided into many regions (see Figure 1.7). Knowledge of these regions helps health care professionals identify different areas of the body. Because each region is related to specific internal organs, problems in internal organs often present as pain or swelling in these regions. For easy identification, the major body regions are also shown in the photographs. The major body regions are the **head, neck, trunk, upper extremity,** and **lower extremity.**

HEAD AND NECK

The **head** is divided into the **facial** region, which includes the eyes, nose, and mouth and the **cranial** region—the top and back of the head. The **neck,** also known as the **cervical** region, is the area that supports the head. Specific areas of the face are referred to by different terms. The forehead region, **frontal;** eye, **orbital;** ear, **otic;** cheek, **buccal,** nose, **nasal;** mouth, **oral;** and chin, **mental.**

TRUNK

The **trunk** refers to the combination of the **chest** and the **abdomen**. The chest is also known as the **thorax** or **thoracic** region and includes the **mammary** area (the region around the nipples), the **sternal** region (the area between the mammary regions), the **axillary** or armpit region and, posteriorly, the **vertebral** region. The shoulder blade region is referred to as **scapular** because it is the location of the bone scapula.

The abdomen is the region below the chest. The belly button (navel, or **umbilicus**) is located in the center of the abdomen. The **pelvic** region is the lowermost part of the abdomen and includes the **pubic** area and the **perineum** (the region containing the external genitalia and the anus). The lower back area is

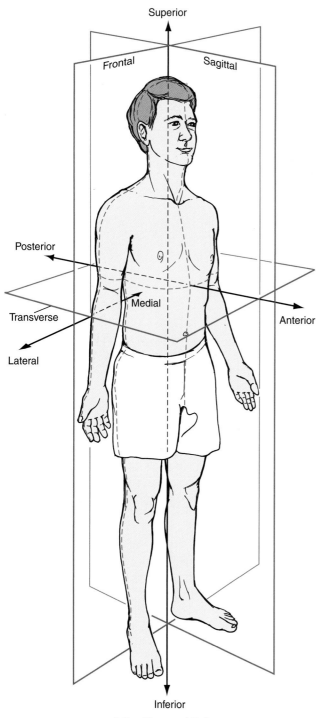

FIGURE 1.5.   Planes of Reference

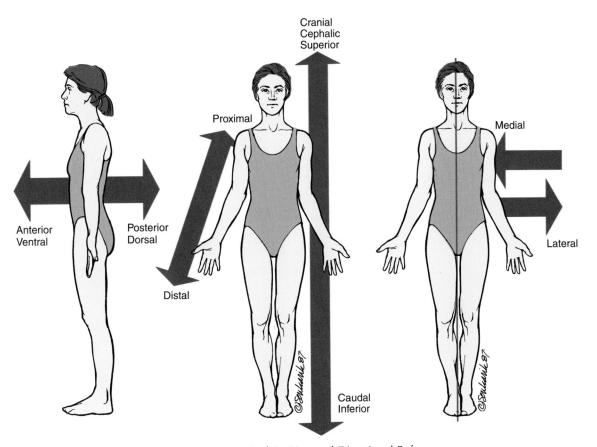

FIGURE **1.6.**   Anatomical Position and Directional References

known as the **lumbar** region, and the large hip area is known as the **buttock** or **gluteal** region. The lowermost, central region of the back is called the **sacral** region. To locate and relate pain and other problems of the organs lying inside, the abdomen has been divided into many subregions.

The abdomen is often divided into four regions—described as the **right upper, left upper, right lower,** and **left lower quadrants** (see Figure 1.8). At times, the abdomen is divided into nine regions, drawing two vertical imaginary lines just medial to the nipples and two horizontal lines, one at the lower part of the rib cage and one joining the anterior prominent part of the hip bones. The nine regions (on the right) are the **right hypochondriac, right lateral** or **lumbar,** and **right inguinal** or **iliac** (lowermost region on the right); (in the middle) **epigastric, umbilical,** and **hypogastric** regions; (on the left) **left hypochondriac, left lateral,** and **left inguinal** or **iliac regions** (lowermost region on the left).

UPPER EXTREMITY

The upper extremity is divided into the **deltoid, acromial** or **shoulder** region, **brachium** or **upper arm,**

antebrachium or **forearm,** and **manus** or **hand** regions. Between the upper arm and forearm is the **elbow** or **cubital** region. The front of the elbow is known as the **cubital fossa.** If you have had blood taken, it is likely that the needle was introduced into the blood vessel in the cubital fossa. This region is also known as the **antecubital** region. The back of the elbow is the **olecranal** region; the wrist is the **carpal** region; the front of the hand is the **palm,** and the back of the hand is the **dorsum.** The fingers are known as the **digital** or **phalangeal** region.

LOWER EXTREMITY

The lower extremity is divided into the **thigh, knee, leg,** and **foot** regions. The upper part of the extremity—the thigh—is known as the **femoral** region. The front of the knee is the **patellar** region and the back of the knee (similar to the front of the elbow) is called the **popliteal fossa.** The anterior part of lower leg is known as the **crural** region. The **shin** is the bony ridge that can be felt in the anterior part of the lower leg. The prominent, posterior, muscular part of the lower leg is the **calf** or **sural** region. The joint between the leg and foot is the **ankle.** Because the ankle is the

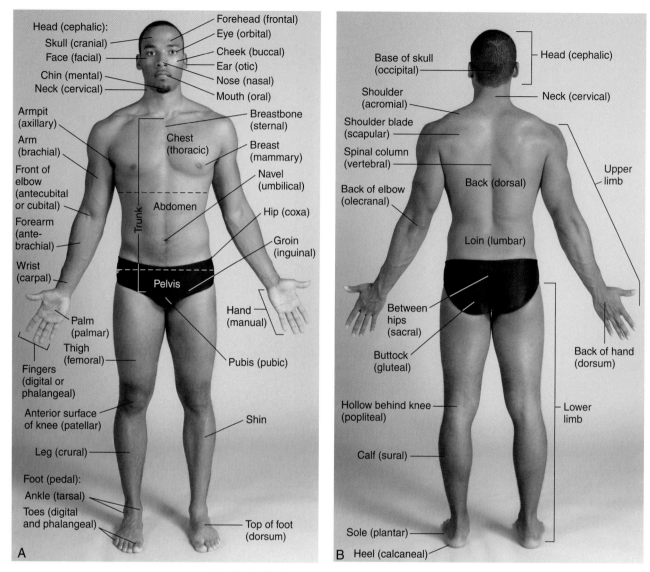

FIGURE **1.7.**   Body Regions. **A,** Anterior view; **B,** Posterior view

location of the tarsal bones, this region is also referred to as the **tarsal** region. The posterior part of the foot is the **heel** or **calcaneal** region. The part of the foot that faces the ground is the **sole,** or **plantar surface,** of the foot. The superior surface is referred to as the **dorsum** of the foot. The fingers of the hands and toes of the foot are called **digits**.

Body Cavities

Although massage is given on the surface of the body, it affects the structures located deep inside the body. If an imaginary cut is made in the sagittal plane to look inside the body, many confined spaces or body cavities containing the organs will be seen (see Figure

1.9). Posteriorly, the brain and the spinal cord lie in the **cranial** and **vertebral,** or **spinal cavities,** respectively. The cranial and vertebral cavities are continuous with each other.

Anteriorly, in the chest, is the **thoracic cavity.** Inside the thoracic cavity, the two lungs lie in the **pleural cavity** and the heart lies in the **pericardial cavity.** The thoracic cavity is separated from the **abdominopelvic cavity** below by the diaphragm. This cavity extends from the diaphragm into the pelvis. The abdominopelvic cavity can be divided into the **abdominal** and the **pelvic cavity.** The major organs in the abdominal cavity are the liver, gallbladder, stomach, small and large intestines, pancreas, kidneys, and spleen. The uterus (in women), the urinary bladder, and the lower part of the large intestines are some organs that lie in the pelvic cavity.

Levels of Organization

There are many ways to view the human body. Each view gives a different perspective on how the makeup of the body and how the body works. It is similar to viewing a flower. We can look at a flower's colors, with its green calyces and colorful petals, or we can view its shape (the shape of its petals or how they are arranged) or we can consider the flower's smell. We can pull the flower apart and view the individual parts. To go further, we can put the flower under a magnifying glass and scrutinize the pollen. If we are really curious, we can take it to a laboratory and analyze the flower's chemical makeup. So many different ways—each giving a different view and perspective.

Similarly, for a full understanding of the human body, we can study it in many ways. Here, we choose to view the organization of the body at the chemical level, cellular level, tissue level and, finally, the systemic level. More time will be spent at the systemic level, with each system being addressed as one chapter.

CHEMICAL LEVEL OF ORGANIZATION

Although a therapist seems to work at the systemic level, the benefits of therapy are a result of changes produced at the chemical and cellular levels. Diseases, although they produce symptoms such as pain, fever, and edema, are actually caused by dysfunction at the cellular and chemical levels. Small changes in chemical makeup can have serious effects. For example, in a disease known as sickle cell anemia, the protein in the hemoglobin molecule is slightly different from normal. This small change has drastic effects on the properties of hemoglobin. The hemoglobin in sickle cell anemia, unlike normal hemoglobin, changes into a more solid form in an environment with less oxygen, resulting in red cells that become sickle-shaped and break up easily. The final outcome—less red cells, less oxygen available to the cells—the patient has difficulty performing normal, day-to-day activities. All because of a slight change in the protein structure in hemoglobin.

Water, which makes up 50–60% of body weight, has properties that are used to cool the body by

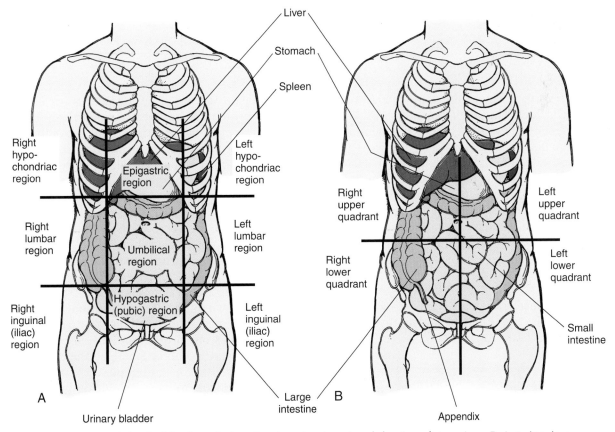

FIGURE 1.8. Abdominal Regions. **A,** Anterior view showing nine abdominopelvic regions; **B,** Anterior view showing abdominopelvic quadrants

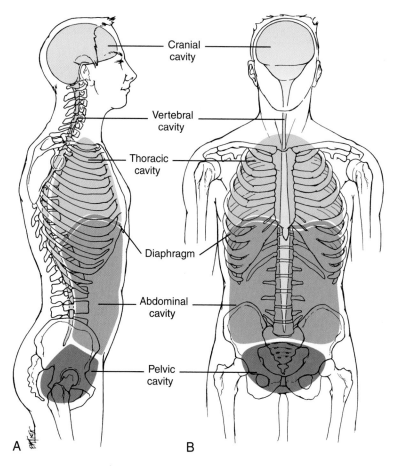

Cranial cavity

Vertebral cavity

Thoracic cavity

Diaphragm

Abdominal cavity

Pelvic cavity

A   B

FIGURE 1.9.   Body Cavities. **A,** Right lateral view; **B,** Anterior view

evaporation. Water is the medium in which ions dissolve and cells float. The acidity and alkalinity of this medium determine how well the various chemical reactions of the body occur. Therapists use water properties to their advantage. Water is used for heat and cold application. During rehabilitation, water exercise has been found to be beneficial. Knowledge of the body at the chemical level and the chemical properties of water and other common substances are, therefore, beneficial to therapists.

The Atom

At the chemical level, the smallest unit of matter is the **atom** (see Figure 1.10). All living and nonliving things

ELECTRICITY AND IONS IN THE BODY
The detrimental effects of lightening and electric shock are a result of the presence of ions in the internal environment. The ions conduct electricity easily.

are made up of atoms. The characteristics of each substance result from the types of atoms involved and how they are combined. An atom is made up of three different types of particles—**protons, neutrons,** and **electrons.** Protons carry a positive (+) electrical charge; neutrons have no charge; and electrons carry a negative (-) charge. The protons and neutrons are almost the same size and mass, while the electrons are much lighter. Hence, the weight of the body is equal to all the neutrons and protons combined.

Normally, because positive charges attract negative charges, an atom carries an equal number of protons and electrons. The number of protons in an atom is known as the **atomic number.** For example, a hydrogen atom has an atomic number of 1, meaning that it has one proton and one electron. The positively charged proton is usually in the center, an area which is called the **nucleus** and the negatively charged electron moving around it in an orbit referred to as the **electron shell.**

At times, the electrons may not equal the number of protons in an atom. In this case, the chemical may have more positive charges or more negative charges.

The chemical then tends to attract or repel other chemicals, depending on their charges. This is the basis for the movement of an electrical impulse down the nerves.

All atoms are assigned to groups called **elements,** based on the number of protons they carry or, in other words, on their atomic number. Elements are substances that cannot be split into simpler substances by ordinary chemical means. (An atom is the smallest unit of matter that has the properties and characteristics of elements.) There are 92 elements in nature. As a standard, each element is given a **symbol.** Many symbols are connected to their English names, while other symbols to their Latin names. The symbols and percentage of body weight for thirteen of the most abundant elements in the human body are given in Table 1.1. These elements are mostly combined with other elements (discussed later). Note that the elements oxygen, carbon, hydrogen, and nitrogen contribute to more than 90% of body weight. In addition to these elements, the body has minute quantities of other elements (**trace elements**), such as silicon, fluorine, copper, manganese, zinc, selenium, and cobalt.

Table 1.1		
The Name and Body Weight Percentage of the Elements in the Body		
Element (Atomic Number)	**Symbol**	**Body Weight (%)**
Oxygen (8)	O	65
Carbon (6)	C	18.6
Hydrogen (1)	H	9.7
Nitrogen (7)	N	3.2
Calcium (20)	Ca	1.8
Phosphorus (15)	P	1.0
Potassium (19)	K	0.4
Sodium (11)	Na	0.2
Chlorine (17)	Cl	0.2
Magnesium (12)	Mg	0.06
Sulfur (16)	S	0.04
Iron (26)	Fe	0.007
Iodine (53)	I	0.0002

Isotopes

The atoms of the same element may have different numbers of neutrons in the nucleus. Although this difference in number does not affect the property of the atom, the weight of the atoms may differ (remember, neutrons are of the same mass and size as protons). Hydrogen, for example, may have a proton and no neutrons or one neutron or two neutrons in the nucleus. The atoms of an element that has a different number of neutrons in the nucleus are known as **isotopes.** Isotopes are referred to by the combined number of protons and neutrons (i.e., **mass number**). The mass number is the number of protons and neutrons in an atom. In the above example, hydrogen with one proton is hydrogen-1 (^{1}H); with one proton and one neutron, hydrogen-2 (^{2}H); and with one proton and two neutrons, hydrogen-3 (^{3}H).

Some of the isotopes of certain elements contain nuclei that spontaneously emit subatomic particles known as **radioisotopes.** Radioisotopes are said to be radioactive. These emissions can be dangerous as they can damage or destroy cells and exposure to these emissions increases the risk of cancer. In medicine, radioisotopes are used for medical imaging and destroying cancerous cells.

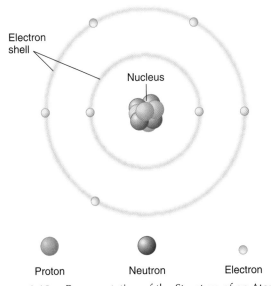

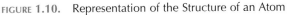

FIGURE **1.10.**   Representation of the Structure of an Atom

RADIOACTIVE EMISSIONS

By carefully directing emissions on cancerous areas, radioactive isotopes are used to kill cancerous cells. This is referred to as radiation therapy.

Exposure to radioactive emissions is dangerous, as it can also destroy rapidly multiplying living cells. For this reason, pregnant women should ensure that they are not exposed to radiation as it may affect the developing fetus.

Electrons, Energy Levels, and Chemical Bonds

Generally, atoms have the same number of protons and electrons (an equal number of positive and negative charges) and are considered electrically neutral.

Even when the protons and electrons in an atom are equal, not all electrons can orbit in the same electron shell. Each electron shell can hold only a specific number of electrons. For example, the first shell (closest to the nucleus) can hold two electrons; the second shell, eight electrons; the third shell, eight electrons; the fourth shell, 18 electrons, and so on. Imagine a circular theatre, with a stage in the center and chairs arranged in successive circular rows. Not all of the audience can sit in the first row. If there are only a few people, even the first row may not get filled. If there are more people in the audience, the first row gets filled and may spill over to the second row. Depending on the number of people, the second row may or may not get filled. Similarly, there are many electron shells (referred to here as **energy levels**) in an atom. The first energy level can have only two electrons in its orbit, and the second level can have only eight. The number of electrons in the energy level affects the property of the atom. Atoms with energy levels that are not full react with other atoms and try to fill the level. For example, the hydrogen atom has an atomic number of 1 (one proton and one electron). Because the first energy level is lacking one electron, it tries to attract another electron to fill the level. In this way, atoms with outer energy levels that are not full gain, lose, or share electrons to fill the outer energy level. This interaction involves the formation of **chemical bonds** that hold the interacting atoms together, maintaining stability. Atoms with full outer shells are stable—they do not take part in these reactions—and are said to be **inert.**

When atoms are held together by chemical bonds, the property of this "particle" is different from that of the individual atoms. Water, for example, forms by bonding two hydrogen atoms and one oxygen atom. The product (water) has completely different properties than hydrogen or oxygen. A chemical structure formed with two or more elements is referred to as a **compound**—a substance that can be broken down into its elements by ordinary chemical means. When atoms held together by bonds share electrons, the resulting substance is called a **molecule.** A molecule may have atoms of the same element or of different elements.

When atoms are bonded together, the resulting substance is denoted by a **molecular formula.** The formula indicates the involved elements by their chemical symbol. The number of each element involved in forming the molecule or compound is de-

noted, in subscript, beside the element. For example, water is made up of two hydrogen atoms and one oxygen atom. The molecular formula for water is H_2O.

Chemical Bonds

Atoms can interact in three ways; therefore, there are three types of chemical bonds—**ionic bonds, covalent bonds,** and **hydrogen bonds.**

Ionic Bonds

Some atoms may lose or gain an electron when bonding with another atom. In the first case, this atom has one electron less than the number of protons, meaning that there are more positive than negative charges. This atom is referred to as a **cation** (positively charged). In the second case, this atom gains an electron and has more electrons than protons, meaning that there are more negative charges than positive charges. This atom is referred to as an **anion.** Both cations and anions, with their unequal number of protons and electrons, are known as **ions.** Ions are denoted by their chemical symbol, with positive or negative signs given in superscript. For example, sodium ion is represented as Na^+; chlorine as Cl^-. Being positively charged, cations attract anions and vice versa. This type of bonding is known as **ionic bonds.** Ionic bonds and ions are especially important in nerve conduction and brain activity.

SALT

A **salt** is an ionic compound consisting of any cation other than a hydrogen ion and any anion other than a hydroxyl ion. This means that, in chemistry, the term salt does not imply table salt as it does in the kitchen.

The formation of salt—table salt is a good example (see Figure 1.11). The chemical name of table salt is sodium chloride (NaCl); it is made up of sodium and chlorine. Sodium has an atomic number of 11. This means that it has 11 protons (and 11 electrons) to be neutral. Of the eleven electrons, two occupy the first energy level and eight occupy the second energy level and fill it. The remaining one electron (2 + 8 = 10) orbits alone in the third energy level. Because the outer energy level is not full, the sodium atom is reactive and tends to donate its electron to another atom.

Chlorine has an atomic number of 17. This means it has 17 protons and 17 electrons, making it neutral. Of the electrons, two occupy the first energy level, eight occupy the second level, and seven occupy the outer level. One more electron will fill its outer energy level; chlorine has a tendency to attract an electron.

By ionic bond, sodium and chlorine come together to satisfy each other's needs. By donating and accepting electrons, the positively charged sodium is attracted to the negatively charged chlorine and they stay together to form the compound sodium chloride—table salt. When sodium chloride is dissolved in water, the ions separate—**ionize**—and positively charged sodium ions (Na+) and negatively charged chloride ions (Cl-) are found.

Covalent Bonds

In some cases, atoms share their electrons rather than gain or lose them. Such bonds are known as covalent bonds (see Figure 1.12). The resultant chemical is termed a **molecule.** A good example is the element hydrogen. Hydrogen has an atomic number of 1 (i.e., 1 proton and 1 electron). However, the outer shell needs another electron to be complete. Therefore, one hydrogen atom shares its electron with another hydrogen atom, completing their energy levels and forming a molecule. This is how hydrogen normally exists—in pairs, and is referred to as hydrogen molecules. A hydrogen molecule is symbolized as H_2.

Similarly, many different elements may bond together. Carbon dioxide gas has one carbon atom and two oxygen atoms bonded covalently (CO_2). Water has two hydrogen atoms and one oxygen atom bonded covalently (H_2O). Elements may share one, two, or three electrons. In the human body, covalent bonds are the most common.

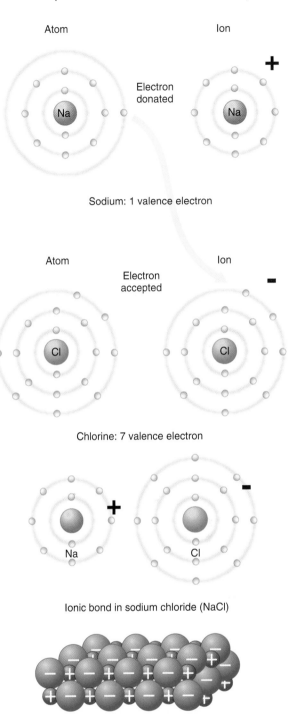

FIGURE 1.11. Representation of Ionic Bond Formation (e.g., sodium chloride [table salt])

ELECTROLYTES

Soluble inorganic molecules with ions that conduct an electrical current in solution are known as **electrolytes.**

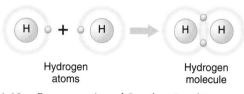

FIGURE 1.12.   Representation of Covalent Bond Formation (e.g., hydrogen molecule)

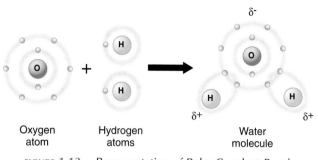

FIGURE 1.13.   Representation of Polar Covalent Bond

When covalent bonds are formed, the electrons may be shared equally or unequally between the specific atoms. When shared equally, these bonds are known as **nonpolar covalent bonds.** Sometimes, one atom attracts the shared electron more than the other atom. In this case, the atom that attracts the electron to a greater degree would be slightly more negatively charged than the other atom. The other atom will be slightly more positively charged. These charges are represented with the symbol δ^+ or δ^- (see Figure 1.13). These covalent bonds are known as **polar covalent bonds.**

Hydrogen Bonds

Other than ionic and covalent bonds, weak attractions may be present between atoms of the same molecule or compound or between atoms in other molecules. The most important of these weak attractions are hydrogen bonds, in which a hydrogen atom involved in a polar covalent bond is attracted to oxygen or nitrogen involved in a polar covalent bond by itself. This attraction is important. Although molecules are not formed through the hydrogen bonds, this bonding can alter the shape of the molecules. For example, it is this weak attraction that holds water together and makes it form a drop. We refer to this force as **surface tension** (see Figure 1.14). At the molecular level in the body, these hydrogen bonds can alter the properties of proteins, making them change their shape and structure.

Matter exists as solids, liquids, or gases as a result of the degree of interaction between the atoms and molecules. For example, hydrogen molecules do not attract each other and, therefore, exist as gas. Water, however, has more interactions and exists as liquid throughout a wide temperature range.

Chemical Reactions

There is a constant reaction in the human body between atoms and molecules. Cells control these reactions to stay alive. In the chemical reaction, new bonds form between atoms or present bonds break down to form a different compound. The term **metabolism** refers to all the chemical reactions that oc-

cur in the body. When a chemical reaction occurs, energy may be expended or released.

What is energy? **Energy** is the capacity to work, and **work** is movement or a change in the physical structure of matter. Energy can be in two forms—**potential energy** or **kinetic energy.** For example, imagine an elastic band stretched across two poles. The stretched elastic band has potential energy. If the band comes undone from one pole, it springs back to its original length. This is kinetic energy. Of course, kinetic energy was initially used to stretch the elastic band and tie it to the two poles. Remember that energy cannot be lost, it is only converted from one form to another.

During chemical reactions, much of the energy in the body is converted to heat, which maintains the core body temperature. When the body is cold, metabolism (chemical reactions) increases and more heat is produced. That's why we shiver. The muscles quickly contract and relax (shivering), and the chemical reactions that occur during this process generate the needed heat.

The body "captures" energy in the form of high-energy compounds. These compounds require energy to build up; however, when broken down, they release a lot of energy. This high-energy compound is **adenosine triphosphate** (ATP). ATP is formed from the

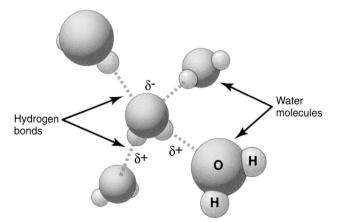

FIGURE 1.14.   Hydrogen Bonds Holding Water Molecules Together

chemicals **adenosine monophosphate** (AMP) and **adenosine diphosphate** (ADP) by combining with phosphate. For example, chemical reactions in the body break glucose down into smaller compounds. The energy that is released is "captured" by combining ADP with organic phosphate to form ATP. When mechanical energy is needed to walk, ATP is broken down to release energy and ADP and phosphate.

Types of Chemical Reactions in the Body

Many types of reactions take place in the body. Some reactions occur to break down compounds into smaller bits. This is a **decomposition reaction.**

$$AB \rightarrow A + B$$

This is what happens when food is broken down and digested. Similarly, when a person loses weight, fat is broken down into smaller fragments. Within the cell, chemical reactions break down substances and the energy released is used to do work. This process is known as **catabolism.**

Building up, or **synthesis,** is the opposite of decomposition. In this process, kinetic energy is invariably used to form compounds from fragments. The kinetic energy is converted to potential energy to be used later in a decomposition reaction when work is needed. The process of building up is known as **anabolism.**

$$A + B \rightarrow AB$$

Another reaction that occurs in the body is **exchange.** In this process, the fragments get shuffled.

$$AB + CD \rightarrow AD + CB$$

Some reactions can proceed in both ways. The direction in which the reaction proceeds is altered by many factors, referred to as **reversible reactions.**

$$AB \rightarrow A + B \rightarrow AB$$

Reversible reactions may be represented as:

$$AB \rightleftharpoons A + B$$

The Role of Enzymes

The various chemical reactions in the body would proceed too slowly to be of any use if they did not have mechanisms in place to speed up the reaction. The enzyme is one of the mechanisms that help that process. Enzymes are proteins and, although they do not actually participate in the chemical reaction itself, facilitate the reaction. Enzymes do not get consumed or altered in the process. The body has numerous enzymes that speed up specific chemical reactions. The importance of specific enzymes is realized when one of them is deficient in the body.

✓ Different Types of Mixtures

When different elements or compounds are blended together without forming chemical bonds, a **mixture** is formed. For example, if you mix salt and sugar together, you form a dry mixture. Now, if you add some water, you form a liquid mixture. In both, no chemical bonds are formed.

Three different mixtures can be formed in liquids—**solution, colloid,** and **suspension.** In a solution, the elements/compounds mixed with water are small and evenly dispersed. Hence, a solution appears clear. The fluid in the solution is known as the **solvent,** and the dissolved elements/compounds are known as **solutes.**

In a colloid, the elements/compounds are larger particles; they tend to scatter light and make the mixture less clear or transparent. Although the particles are large, they do not settle down if the mixture is left undisturbed. Milk is an example of a colloid.

In a suspension, the particles are very large and tend to settle down to the bottom of the container if left undisturbed for some time. An example of a suspension is a mixture of sand particles of different sizes in water. If the mixture is left undisturbed, the sand particles settle to the bottom, according to the mass. In the body, blood is an example of a suspension. If undisturbed, the larger particles—the cells—settle to the bottom of the container.

Enzyme activity can be modified by various factors, such as temperature, acidity, or alkalinity. For example, the activity of many enzymes is significantly reduced when the temperature drops, slowing down chemical reactions. Similarly, an acidic environment is detrimental to enzymes. When muscle activity is increased, many chemical reactions are triggered to produce energy for contraction. One of the metabolites formed, especially if oxygen supply is inadequate, is lactic acid. If this metabolite is not rapidly removed, the muscle environment becomes acidic and the activity of various enzymes slows down or stops and muscle fatigue results.

Acidity and Alkalinity

For the purpose of enzyme activity and to maintain the shape and structure of the proteins, the body

---

💡 ACIDS AND BASES

The body has both inorganic and organic acids and bases. An acid is any solute that dissociates in solution and releases hydrogen ions, lowering the pH. A base is a solute that removes hydrogen ions from a solution and, thereby, increases the pH.

must maintain the right state of acidity and alkalinity. If there are more H^+ (hydrogen ions), a solution is acidic. If there are more OH^- (hydroxyl ions), the solution is alkaline. The acidity and alkalinity of a solution is measured in terms of **pH** (hydrogen ion concentration). As the quantity of hydrogen ion is so small, it is cumbersome to express in actual numbers. If needed, the number would be something like 0.0000001. To make it easier, this is expressed by pH. The pH is actually a measure of hydrogen ion concentration in the body fluid; the pH scale extends from 0 to 14. Water is considered to be a pH of 7.0; a neutral pH. This means that water contains 0.0000001, or 1×10^{-7} of a mole of hydrogen ions per liter. If the pH is lower than 7.0, it denotes that the fluid has more hydrogen ions or that it is acidic. For example, if a solution has a pH of 5.0, it contains 0.00001 or 1×10^{-5} of a mole of hydrogen ions per liter (i.e., more hydrogen ions than a solution of pH 7.0). If a solution has a pH above 7.0, it has fewer hydrogen ions than water and is alkaline.

The pH of the body is 7.4 (range, 7.35–7.45) (i.e., slightly alkaline). For body enzymes to be active and for chemical reactions to proceed optimally, it is vital that pH be maintained at this level. This implies that the body needs regulatory mechanisms that monitor the hydrogen ion levels carefully and get rid of them as and when they form above normal levels.

One of the body's compensatory mechanisms is the presence of many **buffers**. Buffers are compounds that prevent the hydrogen ion concentration from fluctuating too much and too rapidly to alter the pH. The body uses buffers to convert strong acids (that dissociate easily into hydrogen ions) to weak acids (that dissociate less easily). Proteins, hemoglobin, and a combination of bicarbonate and carbonic acid compounds are a few of the buffers present in body fluids. The latter is an important buffer. The following chemical reaction indicates how a combination of bicarbonate and carbonic acid compounds work as buffers.

$$HCO_3^- + H^+ \rightleftarrows H_2CO_3 \rightleftarrows H_2O + CO_2$$

In this chemical reaction, HCO_3 (bicarbonate), a weak base, combines with the hydrogen ions to form H_2CO_3 (carbonic acid), a weak acid. This weak acid can be further broken down to CO_2 (carbon dioxide), which can be breathed out, and H_2O (water), which can be used for other reactions or excreted by the kidneys. Alternately, if the pH becomes alkaline, the weak carbonic acid H_2CO_3 can break down to form HCO_3^- (a weak base) and H^+ (hydrogen ions).

Important Organic Compounds in the Body

Organic compounds are compounds that have the elements carbon, hydrogen and, usually, oxygen. Many

True Meaning of Organic

The term "organic" is often used to denote something natural from nature, without it being contaminated by synthetic, man-made substances. According to the scientific definition, organic compounds are chemical structures that always have carbon and hydrogen as part of their basic structure.

Inorganic compounds are chemical structures that, in general, do not have carbon and hydrogen atoms as the primary structure.

of the compounds have the carbon atoms in chains, linked by covalent bonds. There are four important organic compounds in the body—**carbohydrates; proteins; fats** or **lipids;** and **nucleic acids.** The first three are vital sources of energy in the body. The structure of the body is mostly made up of proteins. Lipids are needed for building certain structures, such as cell membranes. Lipids are also stored and used as an energy reserve. Nucleic acids are used to form genetic material.

Carbohydrates

Carbohydrates are organic compounds that have carbon, hydrogen, and oxygen in a ratio of 1:2:1. Sugars and starches are typical examples. Carbohydrates are typical sources of energy for the cell and can be easily broken down by the cells of the body. Carbohydrates may be simple or complex.

Simple sugars or monosaccharides contain 2–7 carbon atoms. Glucose, for example, has six carbon atoms. Fructose, found in fruits, is another example. Simple sugars dissolve easily in water and are easily transported in the blood. Complex sugars are formed by the combination of two or more simple sugars. They are broken down by the digestive tract into its simplest form before being absorbed into the body.

Simple sugars that are absorbed are reconverted by chemical reactions in the presence of enzymes into various complex forms by the liver, muscle, and other tissues. Glycogen is one form of complex carbohydrate. This form of carbohydrate is insoluble in body fluids. When the demand for energy goes up, glycogen is broken down into its simple form and transported by blood to the needed areas.

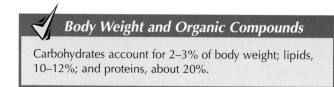

Body Weight and Organic Compounds

Carbohydrates account for 2–3% of body weight; lipids, 10–12%; and proteins, about 20%.

Lipids

Lipids are organic compounds that have carbon, hydrogen, and oxygen atoms, however, in a different ratio than carbohydrates. These compounds are insoluble in water and must be transported in the blood by special mechanisms. For example, in blood, lipids combine with proteins and are carried as **lipoproteins.** Lipids are used to form important structures, such as cell membranes and certain hormones, and are an important source of energy. When there is more lipid supply than needed, it is stored in various regions for future use. The properties of lipids make them important body insulators. Fatty acids, glycerides, steroids, and phospholipids are some of the important lipids found in the body.

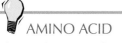

SATURATED AND UNSATURATED FAT

A small change in the chemical bond in fatty acids alters their properties. There are two forms of fatty acids of importance—saturated and unsaturated fatty acids. Although the body can break down both types, the presence of increased amount of saturated fatty acids in the diet increases the risk of heart disease. Ice cream, fatty meat, and butter have a high content of saturated fatty acids.

Proteins

Proteins are the organic compounds that are most abundant in the body. All proteins contain carbon, hydrogen, oxygen, and nitrogen. In addition, some proteins may contain sulfur.

Proteins form the structural framework for the body. The bulk of our muscles are made of proteins. The enzymes that facilitate chemical reactions are proteins, as are some of the buffers. The blood contains protein in the plasma. Hemoglobin is a protein used to transport gases. The antibodies are plasma proteins used in defense. Many of the hormones are made of proteins.

AMINO ACID

The word amino is derived from the presence of amino group (nitrogen and two hydrogen atoms—NH_2) and an acid group (carbon, two oxygen, and hydrogen—COOH).

Proteins consist of organic molecules chains known as **amino acids**. There are about 20 significant amino acids in the human body. Different proteins in the body are formed by combining amino acids, using covalent bonds in different sequences. A protein chain may have any number of amino acids and is known as a **polypeptide**. Some proteins may have 100,000 or more amino acids. Each amino acid has a different chemical structure and this, in turn, alters its properties.

The shape of a protein is one property that may be altered. Certain proteins may be flat and appear as a long chain; certain proteins are more complex and form spirals. Others may be folded or coiled to form complex three-dimensional structures (e.g., hemoglobin). The structural properties are determined by the sequence in which the amino acids are arranged. The alteration of just one amino acid sequence can alter the function of the protein drastically, as in the example of sickle cell anemia given earlier.

Nucleic Acids

Nucleic acids are large organic molecules containing carbon, hydrogen, oxygen, nitrogen, and phosphorus. Found in the nucleus of the cell, they are important for storing and processing information in every cell. Nucleic acid is the major component of ova and sperm and conveys such information as shape, eye color, and sex. There are two types of nucleic acid— **DNA (deoxyribonucleic acid)** and **RNA (ribonucleic acid)**.

DNA is in the form of a double helix (i.e., two spirals, parallel to each other). The two strands are held together by hydrogen bonds. A small segment of DNA molecule forms a **gene.** Each gene determines the traits we inherit from our parents. They also control protein synthesis in each cell. The RNA conveys the message from the gene to the cell and determines the amino acids sequence when proteins are synthesized.

High-Energy Compounds

All cells require energy to carry out their functions. This energy is derived by catabolism of organic substances in the presence of enzymes. The energy liberated is stored as potential energy in the form of **high-energy bonds.** High-energy bonds are covalent bonds created in specific organic substrates in the presence of enzymes. When the cell needs energy, these bonds are broken and the energy harnessed.

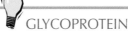

GLYCOPROTEIN

Some organic compounds exist as a combination of proteins and carbohydrates. An example is glycoprotein, a large protein with small carbohydrate groups attached. Antigens are examples of glycoproteins.

AMP is the most important organic substrate used by the cells to form covalent bonds. The cells use the energy liberated by nutrient breakdown to convert AMP to ADP, which is then converted to ATP. Both ADP and ATP are formed by attaching phosphate groups by covalent bonds.

$$ADP + \text{phosphate group} + \text{energy} \rightarrow ATP + H_2O$$
$$ATP \rightarrow ADP + \text{phosphate group} + \text{energy}$$

As the body needs energy, ATP is broken down. Other compounds with high-energy bonds exist, but ATP is the most abundant.

CELLULAR LEVEL OF ORGANIZATION

So far, we have viewed the body at the chemical level and reduced it to a collection of chemicals. Such fragmentation is useful in understanding the physical properties of the body and how the chemical structures contribute to the property. However, the body is much more than a mixture of chemical compounds. It is a dynamic, living being with its functional unit, the cell, behaving like a miniature human, responding to internal and external stimuli.

The human body has two classes of cells—**somatic cells** and **sex cells.** The somatic cells include all cells other than ova and sperm.

Typically, cells are surrounded by a medium known as **extracellular fluid.** Of the extracellular fluid, the fluid that actually surrounds the cells (i.e., fluid not inside blood vessels) is known as the **interstitial fluid.** The inside of the cell is separated from the interstitial fluid by the **cell membrane,** which plays many important roles—it serves as a physical barrier between the inside of the cell and the extracellular fluid; it controls the entry of nutrients and other substances; and it contains special receptors that respond to specific stimuli and alter the functioning of the inside of the cell. Connections between cell membranes of adjacent cells help stabilize the tissue.

Cytoplasm

The material enclosed by the cell membrane is known as **cytoplasm** (see Figure 1.15). The cytoplasm contains the **nucleus** and special structures, or **organelles,** floating in the fluid. The fluid inside the cell is known as the **intracellular fluid,** or **cytosol.** Ions, soluble and insoluble proteins, and waste products can be found in the cytosol. The major difference between the intracellular fluid and extracellular fluid is that the intracellular fluid has more potassium ions and proteins. In addition, the intracellular fluid has stored nutrients in the form of glycogen and amino acids.

Organelles

The cell has many organelles. Some of the organelles are enclosed in a lipid membrane, separating them from the cytosol; others are in direct contact with the cytosol (Figure 1.15). The membranous organelles include the **mitochondria, endoplasmic reticulum, the Golgi apparatus, lysosomes,** and **peroxisomes.** The nonmembranous structures include the **cytoskeleton,** the **microvilli, centrioles, cilia, flagella,** and **ribosomes.**

Mitochondria

The mitochondria are double-membrane structures, which may be long and slender or short and fat. The number of mitochondria vary from cell to cell, from red blood cells, having no mitochondria, to liver cells, which are packed with them. The presence of mitochondria indicates the demand for energy by specific cells.

The inner membrane of the mitochondria is thrown into folds to increase the surface area. The inside of the mitochondria contains the enzymes required for breaking down nutrients to liberate energy for cellular function; 95% of the ATP requirements are provided by mitochondrial activity.

Endoplasmic Reticulum

The endoplasmic reticulum, as the term suggests, is a network of intracellular membranes (which are in the form of tubes and sacs) that is connected to the nuclear membrane. It contains enzymes and participates in protein and lipid synthesis. Some endoplasmic reticula appear smooth—smooth endoplasmic reticulum—while others appear rough as a result of the presence of ribosomes (discussed later).

The function of the endoplasmic reticulum varies from cell to cell. The rough endoplasmic reticulum helps manufacture, process, and sort proteins. Smooth endoplasmic reticulum helps manufacture fats and steroids. In muscle cells, it stores the calcium required for muscle contraction. In liver cells, it contains enzymes that help detoxify harmful agents such as drugs and alcohol.

Golgi Apparatus (Golgi Complex)

The Golgi apparatus appears as flattened membrane disks known as **saccules.** If considered similar to a factory, Golgi complex serves as the packaging center of the cell. Chemicals manufactured by the endoplasmic reticulum enter the Golgi complex where they are processed, sorted, and packaged in secretory

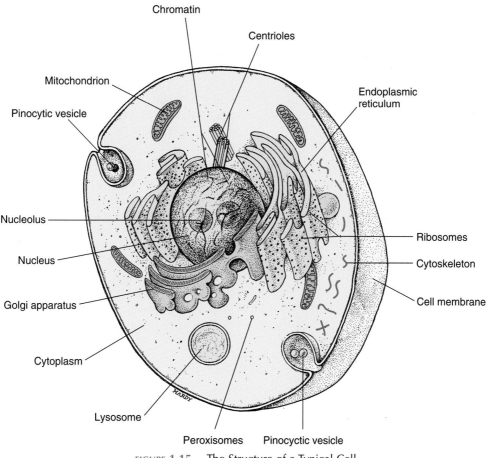

FIGURE **1.15.**   The Structure of a Typical Cell

vesicles ready for dispatch to the outside of the cell, or for storage inside the cell as storage vesicles. Secretions, such as hormones and enzymes, are packaged by this structure.

Lysosomes

Lysosomes are vesicles filled with digestive enzymes. The lysosomes are manufactured in the Golgi apparatus. The lysosomes' enzymes are activated when they fuse with damaged organelles or other vesicles containing contents to be destroyed. On fusion, the enzymes become activated and digest the contents. Substances that can be recycled diffuse back into the cytosol. Unwanted contents are expelled into the extracellular fluid by exocytosis. In sperm cells, lysosomal enzymes are secreted outside and help the sperm penetrate the ovum.

Peroxisomes

Peroxisomes are similar to lysosomes, except they help detoxify substances, such as alcohol and hydro-

gen peroxide, that are produced by the cell. In this way, peroxisomes protect the cell from the harmful effects of toxic substances.

Cytoskeleton

The cytoskeleton is actually a framework of proteins located inside the cell that gives the cell its flexibility and strength. The cytoskeleton is in the form of **filaments** (threadlike structures) and **tubules** (microtubules). The filaments help anchor organelles inside the cell, as well as anchor the cells to surrounding areas. Tubules help maintain the shape of the cell and help transport substances within the cell.

Microvilli

Microvilli are small fingerlike projections of the cell membrane that increase the surface area. They are found in those cells involved in absorbing substances from the extracellular fluid. Unlike the processes created by the cell membrane in endocytosis, the microvilli are more stable and are anchored to the cytoskeleton of the cell. The microvilli present on the surface of intestinal cells increase the surface area for absorption by 20%.

The Centrosome

The centrosome is a structure located close to the nucleus. It consists of the pericentriolar area, which is composed of protein fibers and centrioles. The centrioles are two, short, cylindrical structures composed of microtubules. They are only found in those cells capable of dividing. Muscle cells, neurons, mature red blood cells, and cardiac muscle cells—all cells not capable of multiplying—lack centrioles. The centriole is important at the time of cell division to separate DNA material.

Cilia

Cilia are projections from the cell membrane found in certain cells, such as those in the respiratory tract. Cilia have nine pairs of microtubules, surrounding a central pair. They move rhythmically in one direction and move mucus and other secretions over the cell surface.

Flagella

Flagella (singular, flagellum) can be considered longer cilia. Rather than moving the fluid over the cell surface like the cilia, flagella help move the cell in the surrounding fluid. A good example of a cell with flagella is the sperm cell of the testis.

Ribosomes

Ribosomes are tiny organelles that manufacture proteins. They may be fixed to the endoplasmic reticulum (rough endoplasmic reticulum) or float freely in the cytosol.

The Nucleus

The nucleus of the cell is a denser area found in most cells (mature red blood cells do not contain a nucleus). Some cells, such as skeletal muscle cells, may have more than one nucleus. A membrane known as the **nuclear membrane,** or **nuclear envelope,** resembling the plasma membrane, surrounds the nucleus. Channels in the nuclear membrane control the movement of substances in and out of the nucleus. The nucleus contains a denser structure called the **nucleolus,** in which ribosomes (containing RNA) are assembled.

The nucleus contains all the information required for the cell to function and controls all cellular oper-

ations. The nucleus has the information needed for the manufacture of body proteins. It also controls which proteins will be synthesized and in what amounts in a given time.

The information required by the cell is stored in **DNA** strands. The DNA strands are found in threadlike structures known as **chromosomes.** Each human cell has 23 pairs of chromosomes.

DNA is actually a double-helix strand, with the two strands held together by hydrogen bonds (see Figure 1.16). The **genetic code** in the DNA is in the sequence of nitrogenous bases. The nitrogenous bases adenine, thymine, cytosine, and guanine are arranged in different ways to form the genetic code. Three of the bases, arranged in a specific way, code for a specific amino acid. In this way, the DNA has codes that give the sequence of arrangement of amino acids needed to form a specific protein. The lineup of bases that code for a specific protein is known as a **gene,** and a gene exists for every type of protein manufactured in the body.

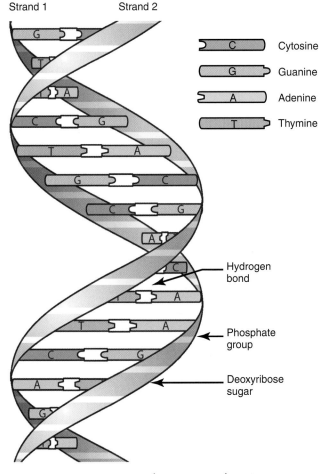

FIGURE **1.16.** The Structure of DNA

When the gene is activated, it begins to manufacture proteins with the help of the ribosomes and RNA. The RNA carries the template of the genetic code to the cytoplasm and assembles the amino acids in the right sequence to form the protein.

Protein Synthesis

It should be noted that the proteins determine the characteristics of the cells, tissues, and the organism itself. Therefore, a large part of cellular activity is synthesizing different proteins; the instructions for the sequence of amino acids in the proteins are carried by the DNA.

The genetic code for a specific protein, present in the DNA, is used as a template to copy the sequence of amino acids for that protein. The copy is in the form of RNA. This process is called **transcription.** The RNA moves out of the nucleus into the cytoplasm. In the cytoplasm, with the help of ribosomes and using the template on the RNA, amino acids are lined and bonded in the right sequence to form the specific protein needed. This process is known as **translation.**

Cell Membrane (Plasma Membrane)

The cell membrane (Figure 1.17) is a thin, delicate layer that is made up of lipids, carbohydrates, and proteins. It is referred to as a **phospholipid bilayer** because it is made up of two layers of phospholipids. The phospholipids are lined in such a way that the end of the molecules containing the phosphate group that have an affinity for water—hydrophilic end—faces the outside of the cell membrane. The hydrophobic ends that contain the fatty acids face each other in the middle of the cell membrane. This arrangement of the cell membrane prevents most water-soluble substances from crossing the lipid portion of the cell membrane. This arrangement is used because the composition of the cytoplasm of the cell is different from that of the fluid around it. These differences have to be maintained if the cell is to survive.

The phospholipid bilayer is interrupted in certain areas by proteins that go completely through the wall or are integrated into the wall with part of the protein molecule projecting into or out of the cell. These are known as **membrane proteins.** Because of the presence of a large number of different proteins (mosaic) in the "sea" of phospholipids, the structure of the cell membrane is referred to as the **fluid mosaic model.**

The membrane proteins that go completely through the wall are referred to as **integral proteins.** The others are referred to as **peripheral proteins.** The membrane proteins have many functions. Some proteins serve as **anchors** or **linkers** and connect the cell membrane to surrounding structures to stabilize the cell. Others serve as **recognition proteins,** or

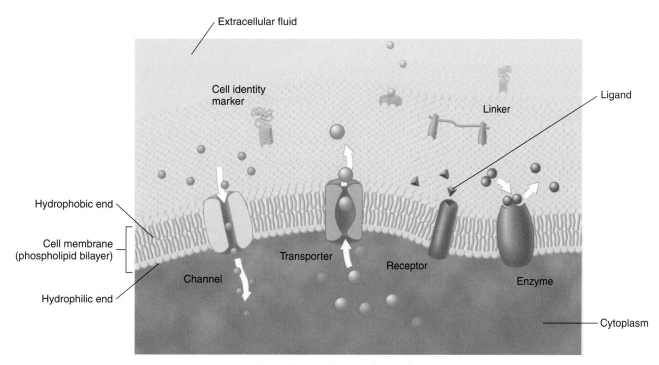

FIGURE **1.17.**   The Cell Membrane with membrane proteins.

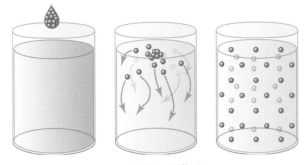

FIGURE 1.18.   Diffusion

identifiers, or **cell identity markers.** These are usually glycoproteins that project out of the membrane and help the immune cells identify the cell as self or nonself. Some of the proteins are **enzymes** and facilitate chemical reactions inside or outside the cell, depending on their position; others are **receptors.**

Receptor proteins are specific and have an affinity for specific hormones and other substances. The specific extracellular molecules that stimulate the receptors are referred to as **ligands.** Each cell may have receptors for more than one ligand, and the receptors vary from cell to cell. In this way, hormones, which are carried throughout the body by the blood, affect only cells that have receptors for the specific hormone.

Certain proteins located in the cell membrane may serve as **carriers** or **transporters.** If a specific solute becomes attached to the carrier, the protein carrier changes shape and transports the solute across the cell membrane. This may occur with or without the use of active energy. Certain integral proteins work as **channels** or **gates;** forming small paths across the cell membrane and allowing water and specific ions to pass through. The channels may be opened by changes in potential or by binding of ligands.

The carbohydrates in the membrane, although only contributing about 3% of the weight of the cell membrane, project outward and help form a layer that protects the cell membrane.

Membrane Transport

The cell membrane determines which substances enter or leave the cell and is said to be **impermeable** if it does not allow any substance to pass through. A cell membrane can also be **selectively permeable.** It may be impermeable to one substance and freely allow another to pass through. A typical cell membrane is selectively permeable. Because of its selective permeability, the cell can maintain a different concentration of substances inside the cell than outside the cell. For example, there are more sodium ions outside the cell compared with inside. This difference in

chemical concentration is known as the **chemical gradient.** If the inside and outside electrical charges are compared, the inside of the cell is more negative than the outside. This is known as the **electrical gradient.** Many factors determine whether a substance can pass through and the direction of movement.

Factors Affecting Transport

To some extent, the *size* of the substance plays a part, with the membrane being less permeable to those substances that are larger. The *electrical charge* of the substance has an effect on whether it is transported. At rest, the inside of the cell is more negative than the outside. Substances that carry negative charges, therefore, find it more difficult to pass. The *molecular shape* of the substance also has an effect. Substances that are *lipid-soluble* pass through the membrane easily because the membrane is made up of phospholipids. The direction of movement is determined by the electrical and chemical gradients (**electrochemical gradient**). Transport may be affected by a combination of one or more factors.

The transport across the membrane may occur with or without the use of energy. Transport without use of energy is referred to as **passive transport.** For the transport of some substances, energy in the form of ATP must be used. This is known as **active transport.** In both of these transport types, transporters may or may not be involved—known as **mediated** or **unmediated transport,** respectively. There are many mechanisms by which passive transport occurs.

Passive Transport

Some mechanisms used for passive transport are **diffusion, osmosis, filtration,** and **carrier-mediated transport.**

Diffusion

Diffusion (see Figure 1.18) is the movement of ions and molecules from an area of higher concentration to one of lower concentration. This difference in concentration is known as the concentration gradient. Substances that are lipid-soluble diffuse directly through the phospholipid bilayer. Other substances, such as ions, diffuse through specific channels, if the channels are open. This passive process—diffusion—is important in the body. When the blood reaches the tissue, nutrients move from inside the blood vessels into the interstitial fluid by diffusion. The opposite also occurs by diffusion. Waste products from the cell move along the concentration gradient into the blood. Similarly, carbon dioxide and oxygen between the air and blood move by diffusion.

The rate of diffusion depends on the *distance* that separates the two solutions. To increase efficiency in the body, the distance of the cells from the blood is only about 125 micrometers (μm). The difference between the *concentrations* of the two solutions also plays an important part. Oxygen in the body moves more rapidly into the tissue when the tissue has been active and the concentration of oxygen is much lower than in the blood.

Molecule size affects diffusion. Smaller particles tend to move at a faster pace than larger particles. Other than distance and concentration gradient and size, the *electrical charges* on the two substances affect diffusion, as the interior of the cell is negative. Even if a concentration gradient exists, a negatively charged substance finds it more difficult to enter the negatively charged cell. *Temperature* is another factor that affects diffusion. Higher temperatures increase the diffusion rate.

Substances that are *lipid-soluble,* such as alcohol, fatty acids, and steroids, enter the cell easily through the lipid cell membrane if there is a concentration gradient. Substances that are water-soluble, however, must rely on the presence of channels to pass through, even if a concentration gradient exists. The *surface area* available for diffusion also determines the rate of movement. Because channels occupy only a small percentage of the cell membrane, diffusion through channels is comparatively slower than direct diffusion across the phospholipid bilayer.

Osmosis

Osmosis (see Figure 1.19) is the net diffusion of water from a region of lower concentration of solute (particles) to a region of higher concentration of solute across a semipermeable membrane. Conversely, the

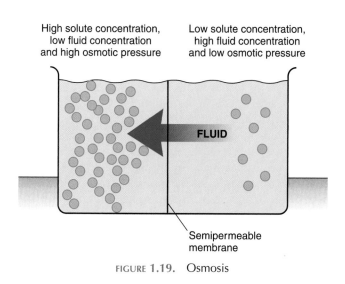

High solute concentration, low fluid concentration and high osmotic pressure

Low solute concentration, high fluid concentration and low osmotic pressure

FLUID

Semipermeable membrane

FIGURE **1.19.**   Osmosis

movement of water from a region of higher concentration (of water) to a region of lower concentration.

Three important characteristics of osmosis are:

- Osmosis is the diffusion of water molecules across a membrane.
- Osmosis occurs across a selectively permeable membrane that allows water to freely move through it; not the solutes.
- The movement of water is toward the solution with the higher concentration of solutes.

In the body, the fluid inside the cell (intracellular fluid) and the fluid outside the cell (extracellular fluid) have dissolved substances. Each of these substances tend to diffuse as if they were the only substance in the solution. For example, if sodium and chloride are present, they each move along their own concentration gradient. The changes in the concentration gradient of chloride do not affect the movement of sodium.

In general, the total concentration remains the same on both sides. If the concentration of ions and molecules vary between the inside and outside of the cell, water is drawn by osmosis to the side that has more ions and molecules and less water.

Red blood cells can be used to illustrate osmosis. When placed in a glass of water, water rushes (by osmosis) into the red blood cells because they have more particles inside. The cells swell and immediately rupture. If the cells are placed in a glass of water into which two spoonsful of table salt was mixed, water from the cell moves out and the cells shrink. **Osmotic pressure** of a solution is an indication of the force of water movement into that solution as a result of its solute concentration.

Filtration

In filtration, water is forced across a semipermeable membrane as a result of **hydrostatic pressure.** For example, it is equivalent to the pressure that pushes water out of a nick in a garden hose through which water is flowing. By filtration, fluid moves out of capillaries. Similarly, fluid filtered from the blood into the renal tubules of the kidney finally forms urine. The movement of larger particles, along with water, by filtration depends on the size of the pores present in the membrane.

Carrier-Mediated Transport

In this method of transport, integral proteins bind to specific ions, or other substances, and carry them across the cell membrane into the cell. Each carrier on the cell membrane is specific (i.e., it binds to only one specific substance). The amount of substance carried into the cell depends on the number of carriers present for that substance and the concentration gradient. Some carriers can carry two different substances. Both substances may be carried in the same direction or one substance may be carried out of the cell while the other is simultaneously brought into the cell.

Substances, such as glucose and amino acids, are transported by carriers because they are insoluble in lipids and are too large to be transported through channels. Carriers specific for these substances bind to them and move them into the cell along the concentration gradient. Here, no energy is used. It should be noted that it is a diffusion process, except that it is facilitated by carriers. This type of transport is referred to as **facilitated diffusion.** The rate at which they move into the cell depends on the number of carriers present on the cell membrane.

A unique property of carriers is that hormones can regulate them. Certain carrier activity is facilitated by the binding of hormones. In this way, hormones regulate the movement of specific substances into the cell. For example, the hormone insulin facilitates the movement of glucose into the cell.

Active Transport

Active transport is the transport of substances into or out of the cell using energy. Energy is needed for this kind of transport because it occurs against the concentration gradient, unlike diffusion. The carriers involved in this transport are referred to as **ion pumps.** All cells have specific ion pumps that transport sodium, potassium, calcium, and magnesium. Ion pumps are specific (i.e., a pump is specific for one ion). There are certain pumps that transport one ion inside as another is sent outside. These special carrier proteins are known as **exchange pumps.** The most common exchange pump is the **sodium–potassium exchange pump,** or **sodium–potassium ATPase.**

Normally, the extracellular fluid has more sodium than the inside of the cell; potassium is the opposite. Sodium tends to diffuse in slowly along its concentration gradient, while potassium moves out. To maintain homeostasis, the sodium–potassium pump uses energy to pump out sodium and pump in potassium. This pump uses energy by consuming about 40% of the ATP produced in a resting cell.

Vesicular Transport

With vesicular transport, vesicles or small membrane-lined sacs are used to bring substances into or out of the cell. The process of bringing substances in by forming vesicles is known as **endocytosis.** Transport of substances out of the cell in this manner is referred to as **exocytosis.**

Endocytosis

Substances outside the cell that are too large to enter via channels are "engulfed" by a depression in the cell membrane. The cell membrane folds to form two processes, similar to two arms in an embrace, and the processes fuse with each other to form a vesicle inside the cytoplasm (see Figure 1.20A). In some types of endocytosis, the substance initially binds to receptor proteins before a vesicle is formed.

After endocytosis, at times, the contents are digested by enzymes (stored in vesicles) present in the cytoplasm. This process is known as **phagocytosis** (cell eating). Most defense cells kill microorganisms by phagocytosis.

Exocytosis

Exocytosis is the opposite of endocytosis (see Figure 1.20B). Here, vesicles floating in the cytoplasm fuse with the cell membrane and extrude their contents into the extracellular fluid. Mucus secretion, secretory products of certain glands, and nerve endings extrude the contents of vesicles in this way.

Transmembrane Potential

All cells have more negative charges inside as compared with the outside. This difference in charges is maintained by the presence of a cell membrane that is selectively permeable and ionic pumps that move substances by active transport. This difference in electrical charge is known as the **transmembrane potential.** Transmembrane potential is measured in millivolts (mV). The membrane potential of a neuron, for example, is -70 mV. The maintenance of transmembrane potential is important, as it is required for many functions, such as transmission of nerve impulses, muscle contraction, and gland secretion.

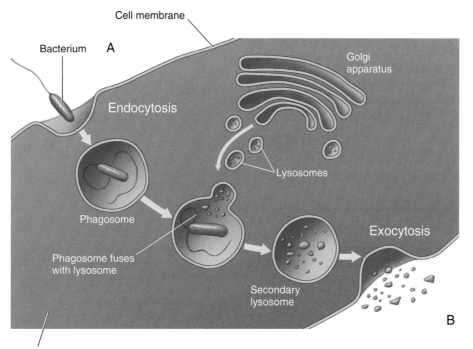

FIGURE **1.20.**   Vesicular Transport. **A,** Endocytosis; **B,** Exocytosis

Pinocytosis = cell "drinking."

The Cell Life Cycle

From fertilization to physical maturity, the cells undergo many divisions. When a single cell divides, it forms two daughter cells that are identical to the original cell. A cell may live from a few days to many years, depending on the cell type. Most cells have a gene, which triggers the cell to self-destruct at a specific time.

Cells divide in two ways: **mitosis** and **meiosis.** Mitosis is common and is the process of division seen in somatic cells, involving the separation of the duplicated chromosome into two identical nuclei. The cytoplasm and the nucleus then separate into two new cells.

Meiosis can be seen in the testis and ovary during the formation of sperm and ova, in which the daughter cells end up with half the number of chromosomes found in somatic cells. When the ovum and sperm fuse during fertilization, the fused cell then has the right number of chromosomes.

When cells are not dividing, they continue to function fully. This phase is known as the **interphase.** Cells that do not multiply after birth, such as neurons, are said to be in the interphase.

Cell division is regulated by peptides known as **growth factors,** which are present in the extracellular fluid. Growth factors bind to receptors in the cell membrane and trigger cell division. Growth hormone, nerve growth factor, epidermal growth factor, and erythropoietin are a few of the growth factors identified.

Phagocytosis = cell "eating."

Specific genes, known as **repressor genes,** oppose cell division. When the rate of growth exceeds that of inhibition, the tissue enlarges. If uncontrolled cell growth occurs, a **tumor** or **neoplasm** results.

TISSUE LEVEL OF ORGANIZATION

Because of the complexity of the human body, it is not possible for every cell to do all the functions required. Instead, some cells become specialized to do specific functions. Together, all these differentiated cells are able to fulfill the needs of the body. As a result of specialization, the cells, although they have the basic organelles, appear different, taking on different sizes and shapes with modifications according to function. A collection of cells that does the same function is known as **tissue.**

The body basically consists of four main tissue types—**epithelial tissue, connective tissue, muscle tissue,** and **neural tissue.** Muscle tissue is described in **Chapter 4;** neural tissue in **Chapter 5.** The epithelial and connective tissues are described below.

Epithelial Tissue

Epithelial tissues cover surfaces that are exposed to the environment, line internal passages and chambers, and form glands. They are found in the skin, lining the respiratory, reproductive, digestive, and urinary tracts. They also line the inner walls of the blood vessels and heart. Epithelia are found lining the various body cavities, such as the cerebral, spinal, pericardial, pleural, and peritoneal cavities.

Structure

As the major function of epithelia is to form a barrier, they are found in layers, with individual cells bound to adjacent cells, unlike other tissues that may be found scattered individually in the extracellular material. Cells may be bound to each other by fusion of cell membranes to form **tight junctions.** Tight junctions prevent movement of water and other substances between the cells. In some epithelia, the binding between the cells may be in the form of **gap junctions.** Gap junctions have small passages that allow movement of substances between adjacent cells. Other cells, such as those in the skin, are bound together by **desmosomes.** These connections are strong and help to maintain the cell layers in sheets.

One surface of epithelial cells is exposed to the external surface, such as the atmosphere or passage they line (**lumen**). This surface is the **apical surface.** The other surface faces the inside of the body and is known as the **basal surface.** The basal surface of the epithelia is attached to a thin, fibrous membrane known as the **basement membrane.**

As the cells of the epithelia are closely packed, they do not have blood vessels supplying them. Instead, they rely on nutrients brought by diffusion from blood vessels in adjacent tissues. The cells closer to the lumen may obtain nutrients by diffusion from the lumen. Being exposed to the environment, epithelial cells are constantly being damaged and lost; however, the stem cells located in the epithelia multiply rapidly and replace these cells constantly.

The epithelia located in areas of absorption or secretion, are modified to increase the surface area for this function. The modification is in the form of microvilli. Such epithelia are found in the digestive and urinary tract. Certain epithelia have cilia, which enables them to move secretions and other fluid over the surface. Ciliated epithelia are found in the respiratory tract.

Functions

As previously mentioned, a major function of the epithelia is to form a barrier and protect the body from

dehydration, injury, and destruction by chemicals and foreign agents. Because the epithelia are selectively permeable to substances, they control the entry of substances into the body.

Almost all epithelia have a good nerve supply, which enables them to sense changes in the environment and convey that information to the brain for suitable action. Some epithelia have a secretory function and form the glandular epithelium.

Epithelia Classification

As epithelia have common features as mentioned above, they are subtly modified to suit specific functions. Epithelia have been classified in accordance with the modifications in numbers of layers and with the shape of cell.

According to the number of layers, they are classified as **simple epithelium** (one layer) or **stratified epithelium** (multilayered). According to cell shape, epithelia are classified as **squamous, cuboidal, transitional,** and **columnar.**

Simple Epithelium

Simple epithelium has only one layer of cells over the basement membrane. Being thin, epithelia are fragile and found only in areas inside the body that are relatively protected, such as the lining of the heart and blood vessels and the lining of body cavities. They are also found lining the digestive tract and in the exchange surfaces of the lungs, where their thinness is an advantage for speedy absorption.

Stratified Epithelium

A stratified epithelium has many layers and forms an effective protection from mechanical and chemical stress. They are found in the skin and lining the openings of lumens such as the mouth, anus, vagina, and urethra. The squamous, cuboidal, and columnar epithelium may be simple or stratified.

Squamous Epithelium

The squamous epithelium consists of cells that are flat and thin and somewhat irregular in shape. **Simple squamous epithelium** (see Figure 1.21A) is found in protected regions (being thin and delicate) where absorption takes place or where friction must be minimal. A specific name is given to the epithelium that lines body cavities—**mesothelium.** The simple epithelium lining blood vessels and heart are called **endothelium.**

A **stratified squamous epithelium** has many layers (see Figure 1.21B). The skin is a good example. In areas such as the skin, where the barrier formed by

---

💡 EXAMINATION OF EPITHELIA

Bits of epithelia are often used for investigations. For example, scrapings from unusual looking epithelia are examined for cancerous changes. Epithelia shed into the amniotic fluid are studied for genetic abnormalities in the fetus.

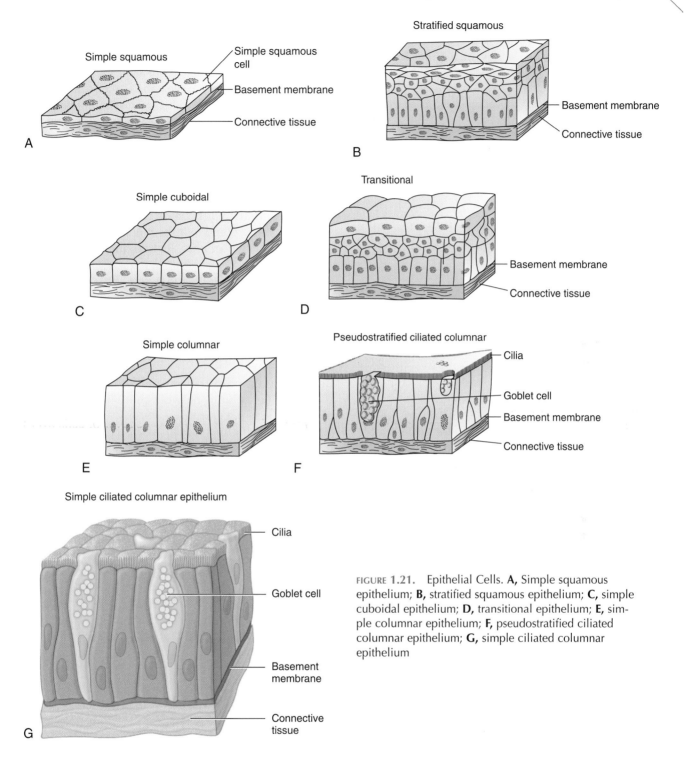

FIGURE **1.21.** Epithelial Cells. **A,** Simple squamous epithelium; **B,** stratified squamous epithelium; **C,** simple cuboidal epithelium; **D,** transitional epithelium; **E,** simple columnar epithelium; **F,** pseudostratified ciliated columnar epithelium; **G,** simple ciliated columnar epithelium

the epithelium also protects the body from dehydration, the most superficial layers are packed with a protein known as **keratin.** Such epithelia are referred to as **keratinized;** those without keratin are said to be **nonkeratinized.**

Cuboidal Epithelium

Cuboidal epithelium (see Figure 1.21C), as the name suggests, appear like a cube in section. They are

found in areas where absorption or secretion takes place, such as the pancreas, salivary glands, and thyroid glands. **Stratified cuboidal epithelia** are rare and found in the large ducts of the mammary glands and sweat glands.

Transitional Epithelium

Transitional epithelium (see Figure 1.21D) is the type of epithelium in which the cells seem to change shape. They are found in the lining of the urinary bladder. When the bladder is full, the cells are stretched and appear flat. When the bladder is empty, the cells appear multilayered.

Columnar Epithelium

The cells of columnar epithelium (see Figure 1.21E) appear as if they are columns—long and slender. These cells are found in regions where absorption or secretion occurs. Some columnar epithelia, such as those in the respiratory tract, appear to be in layers, but they actually are not. These are referred to as **pseudostratified columnar epithelium** (see Figure 1.21F). In the respiratory tract, these epithelia also have cilia and are an example of **ciliated epithelium** (see Figure 1.21G).

Glandular Epithelium

Many epithelia that have cells that produce secretions are known as **glandular epithelium** (see Figure 1.22). The structures lined with glandular epithelium are known as **glands.** Two types of glands—the **exocrine** and **endocrine**—exist in the body.

The exocrine glands release secretions on the epithelial surface. Tubes, known as **ducts,** usually convey the secretions to the surface. Tear glands, sweat glands, and salivary glands are a few examples. The secretions may be released from the cell by exocytosis (**merocrine secretion**); by the apical region of the cell, packed with vesicles being detached (**apocrine secretion**); or by the entire cell rupturing and releas-

ing the contents (**holocrine secretion**). Merocrine secretion is the most common. Apocrine secretion is found in sweat glands in the armpit. Holocrine secretion is used by sebaceous glands near the hair follicles.

Exocrine glands are classified according to the type of secretion they produce. They are classified as **serous glands** if they secrete a watery secretion containing enzymes and **mucous glands** if they secrete the slippery, lubricating, glycoprotein—**mucus.** Some glands are **mixed** and secrete both serous and mucus secretions.

The glands may be either **unicellular**—just one secretory cell in the epithelia or **multicellular,** forming simple or more complex tubes that secrete.

The endocrine glands secrete their products directly into the blood. The thyroid gland, pituitary gland, adrenal glands are a few examples of endocrine glands.

Connective Tissue

Structure

Connective tissue is the most abundant of all tissue, forming a continuous network thoughout the body. If all other tissue was removed, connective tissue would form the three-dimensional framework of the body, much like cellulose in plants. Connective tissue, such as bone, blood and fat, appear to be different from each other, but they have some common features that place them under this classification. All connective tissue have three characteristics—they have specialized **cells;** protein **fibers** that are present outside the

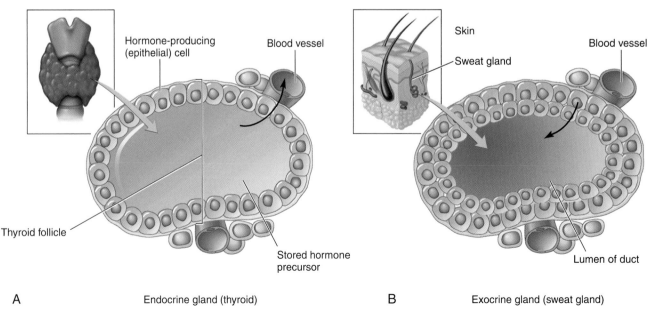

A   Endocrine gland (thyroid)   B   Exocrine gland (sweat gland)

FIGURE **1.22.**   Glandular Epithelium. **A,** Endocrine gland; **B,** exocrine gland

Remember that collagen fibers are not actually living tissue. They are protein fibers secreted by fibroblasts into the ground substance. This implies that where there is a large proportion of collagen in tissue, there is not much demand for blood supply (as the fibers are just secretions).

Unfortunately, areas with less blood supply take longer to heal. That is why injured tendons and ligaments heal slowly. Because cartilage does not have a direct blood supply, it also heals slowly.

Connective Tissue—Like Marmalade?

An apt analogy of connective tissue is marmalade. The thick translucent base of marmalade is similar to ground substance. The orange peel and other ingredients floating in the base are similar to the protein fibers and cells found in connective tissue. Like marmalade, connective tissue becomes thicker in consistency when cooled and becomes more fluid when warmed or when more water is present.

cells; and a fluid known as **ground substance,** in which the fibers and cells are suspended. The fibers and the ground substance combined are referred to as the **matrix** that surrounds the cells.

Unlike epithelia, the cells in connective tissue are scattered. Connective tissue is not exposed to the exterior and most connective tissue is vascularized (i.e., they have a good supply of blood vessels). Many types of connective tissue have nerve endings that respond to various sensations, such as touch, pressure, pain, and temperature changes.

Function

Connective tissue has many functions. It forms the structural framework for the body and helps support, surround, and interconnect various organs and tissues. It also helps transport fluid and substances from one region to the other (e.g., blood). Certain connective tissue protects the organs and certain tissue has special cells scattered in them that help kill invading organisms. Connective tissue may serve as a storage site for nutrients (e.g., fat).

Classification

Connective tissue may be classified as **connective tissue proper, fluid connective tissue,** and **supporting connective tissue.** The three types differ in the type of cells, fibers, and ground substance. The proportions also vary, altering the consistency.

Connective Tissue Proper

This type of connective tissue (see Figure 1.23) has many different types of cells suspended in the matrix. The properties and proportions of fibers also vary.

Cells

Connective tissue proper has cells that help with repair, healing, and storage, as well as other cells that help with defense. **Fibroblasts** and **mesenchymal cells** repair injured tissue; **adipocytes** store fat. Other cells in connective tissue proper that have the capability of migrating to injured areas are **macrophages, microphages, mast cells, lymphocytes,** and **plasma cells.**

Fibroblasts

Fibroblasts are the most abundant cells. They secrete a polysaccharide known as **hyaluronic acid** and proteins into the ground substance, which gives connective tissue its thick consistency. Fibroblasts also secrete proteins that interact and form the protein fibers in the ground substance that is responsible for the strength, flexibility, and elasticity of connective tissue.

Mesenchymal Cells

Mesenchymal cells are the mother cells that differentiate into fibroblasts and other cells when there is injury.

Adipocytes

Adipocytes (see Figure 1.24) are fat cells in which the cytoplasm is filled with a huge, fat droplet. The number of adipocytes varies from region to region and from one person to another.

Connective Tissue and Hormones

Growth hormone secreted by the pituitary gland stimulates fibroblasts and other cells. As a result, it increases the formation of ground substance and protein fibers. **Cortisone** secreted by the adrenal cortex has an inhibitory effect in the formation of connective tissue. For this reason, cortisone (steroids) is used to reduce inflammation and adhesion formation in injured tissue.

Contractures

When muscles are not used, they are replaced by connective tissue, making the muscles stiff. Contractures are observed in people who are paralyzed because their muscles and joints have been in a fixed position for a long time.

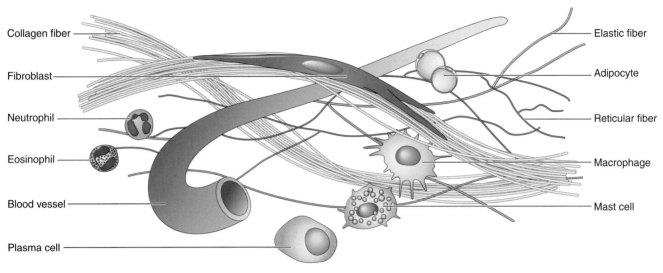

FIGURE 1.23.   Connective Tissue Proper

Macrophages

Macrophages are defense cells that have wandered into the connective tissue from the blood. Scavenger cells, they remove dead cells and foreign agents. Certain macrophages may be fixed to a site (**fixed macrophages**), as found in the liver and spleen. Others are wanderers, attracted to injured areas by chemicals liberated by injured tissue. These are the **free macrophages.**

Microphages

Microphages are other types of white blood cells (neutrophils and eosinophils) that are attracted to

sites of injury and inflammation. They, too, help with defense.

Mast cells

Mast cells are small, connective tissue cells usually found near blood vessels. Mast cell cytoplasm contains the chemicals histamine and heparin. When injury occurs or when stimulated by allergic substances, mast cells liberate chemicals into the surrounding tissue, producing the typical reactions observed in inflammation.

Lymphocytes

Lymphocytes are white blood cells that wander in tissue and function as defense cells.

Plasma cells

Plasma cells are small cells that develop from a type of white blood cell. They are involved in immunity.

Connective Tissue Fibers

Connective tissue has three different types of fibers, which vary in proportion. The fibers may be

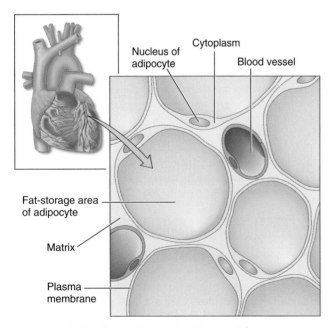

FIGURE 1.24.   Loose Connective Tissue—Adipose tissue

CAPSULES

The body defends itself from disease and microorganisms by forming a connective tissue capsule around infected areas. A pustule or abscess is a typical example. The microorganisms, defense cells (both dead and alive), together with secretions, are cordoned off by a connective tissue capsule, which contains the infection to the local area and prevents it from spreading.

✓ *Superficial and Deep Fascia*

The **superficial fascia,** also known as **subcutaneous tissue,** is made up of fat and connective tissue. Its main function is to reduce heat loss from the body. Superficial veins, lymph glands, and cutaneous nerves are found in this region. In some areas of the body—especially over bony prominences—the superficial fascia is modified into **subcutaneous synovial bursae** (see page 127). For example, bursae may be found over the bony prominence in the posterior aspect of the elbow or over the knee joint. In certain areas where the skin is moved, cutaneous muscles are present in the fascia. The facial muscles, the superficial muscle in the scrotum (dartos), the neck and facial muscle (platysma) are examples of these muscles.

   The **deep fascia** is a tough layer of connective tissue that lies over the muscles and attaches to bony prominences that are subcutaneous by fusing with the outer layer of the bone. In some regions, skeletal muscle is partly or fully inserted into the deep fascia. For example, the gluteal muscle (gluteus maximus) inserts into a thick fascia in the lateral part of the leg (the iliotibial tract).

   Sheets of deep fascia often pass between groups of muscles before they blend with the periosteum (outer covering) of the underlying bone. These **intermuscular septa** divide the limb into different compartments, apart from providing a larger surface area for the attachment of muscles.

   In regions over joints, the deep fascia forms tough sheets that hold tendons in place. For example, such sheets (e.g., flexor retinacula) are found anterior to the wrist joint.

   Deep fascia plays an important role in blood circulation. Because of the effect of gravity, blood in the veins tends to pool in dependent parts. The deep fascia is particularly tough in these regions, preventing muscle mass

collagen fibers, reticular fibers, or **elastic fibers.** The proportion of different fibers in the ground substance is responsible for the different texture and property.

Collagen Fibers

Collagen fibers are the most common type. They are long, straight, and unbranched. They are made up of protein strands tightly wound together like rope and held together by hydrogen bonds, giving connective tissue flexibility. Collagen, however, is strong and can withstand a lot of force if applied from both ends. Tendons and ligaments, which withstand a lot of force as muscle contracts, are made up almost entirely of collagen. The flexibility of collagen also allows joints to move as the tendons and ligaments go across them.

   Collagen fibers can be arranged in different ways to alter the property of the tissue, dictated by the ground substance and the local tissue. They may be arranged randomly, forming sheets (e.g., **fascia**); systematically stacked (e.g., **aponeurosis**); spun loosely (e.g., **subcutaneous tissue**); or arranged in parallel (e.g., **tendon**).

Reticular Fibers

Reticular fibers are also proteins, but they are much thinner, forming branching networks. This gives the connective tissue flexibility. At the same time, these fibers are tough and can resist force applied in different directions. Because of these properties, reticular fibers are more abundant in areas where cells and organs must be kept together. Reticular fibers hold blood vessels and nerves in place.

Elastic Fibers

Elastic fibers are branched, wavy fibers containing the protein elastin. The special characteristic of elastin is that it can be stretched and it will return to its original size when released.

Ground Substance

The ground substance is the medium in which the cells and protein fibers are suspended. Usually clear and colorless, it has the consistency of thick syrup. Proteoglycan, which gives ground substance its viscous property, is formed by the interaction of polysaccharides and proteins secreted by fibroblasts into the extracellular fluid.

   Substances moving in and out of cells have to pass through the ground substance before they enter blood vessels. The consistency of ground substance varies from region to region. In tissue where mobility is required, the major component of ground substance is hyaluronic acid. In tissues where support is the major function, chondroitin sulfate is the major component.

   Depending on how loose or dense they appear, connective tissue proper can be classified as **loose connective tissue** or **dense connective tissue.**

   Loose connective tissue has more ground substance and less protein fibers and cells. It is the "packing material" that fills the space between organs, providing support and absorbing shock. For example, it is the presence of loose connective tissue that keeps the skin in place. At the same time, it allows the skin to be pinched up and separated to some extent from the underlying tissue. Along with the adipose tissue, this

✓ Rolfing

The techniques used by this method of manipulation have an effect on the body by exerting pressure and varied forces on the connective tissue.

layer of loose connective tissue present under the skin forms the **subcutaneous layer** or the **superficial fascia.** Adipose tissue is a special type of loose connective tissue (see Figure 1.24). It acts as a shock absorber and insulator to slowdown loss of heat.

Dense connective tissue has much more protein fiber—predominantly collagen—than loose connective tissue. The collagen fibers may be arranged regularly or irregularly, giving the tissue variable flexibility and strength. Dense connective tissue has a shiny, white appearance. Tendons, ligaments, aponeurosis, the capsule of joints, the outer layer of bones (periosteum), the outer layer of cartilage (perichondrium), are all examples of this type of tissue (see Figure 1.25).

Fluid Connective Tissue

Blood and lymph are examples of fluid connective tissue. The liquid matrix of blood is the **plasma.** Blood cells are suspended in the plasma. Proteins, nutrients, waste products, hormones, and electrolytes are dissolved in the plasma. Lymph is the fluid flowing inside lymphatic vessels, varying in composition according to the site they drain. The structure, composition, and function of blood and lymph are described in **Chapters 8 and 9**, respectively.

Supporting Connective Tissue

Supporting connective tissue provides a strong, solid framework; **cartilage** and **bone** are typical examples. Strength is provided by the presence of numerous fibers in the ground substance. In bone, in addition to the fibers, insoluble calcium salts are deposited in the ground substance. The structure of bone is described in **Chapter 3**.

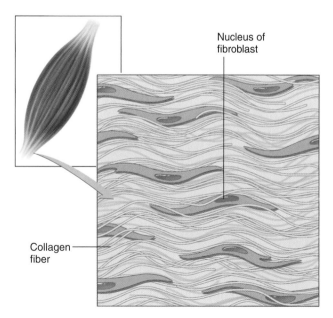

FIGURE 1.25.   Dense Connective Tissue—Tendon

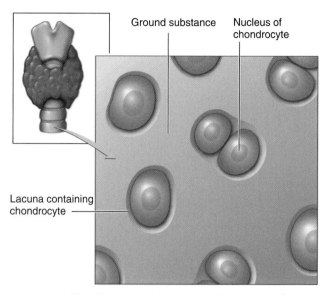

FIGURE 1.26.   Supporting Connective Tissue—Cartilage

Cartilage

Cartilage matrix (see Figure 1.26) is made up of a special polysaccharide known as **chondroitin sulfate,** which interacts with the proteins in the ground substance to form **proteoglycans.** Cartilage cells known as **chondrocytes** are found in the matrix. These cells are located in cavities known as **lacunae.** Unlike other connective tissue, cartilage does not have blood vessels and must rely on diffusion of nutrients from surrounding areas.

The property of cartilage depends on the type and proportion of protein fibers scattered in the matrix. Depending on its property, cartilage may be classified as **hyaline cartilage, elastic cartilage,** or **fibrocartilage.** Hyaline cartilage has closely packed collagen fibers, making it tough and flexible. The most common cartilage type, it is found in joints covering the ends of the bones. It is also found in the epiphyseal plate (the region where bone growth occurs). Elastic cartilage has more elastic fibers, making the cartilage more "springy." It is found in regions such as the external ear. Fibrocartilage has little ground substance and more collagen fibers, making the cartilage tough, helping it resist compression and absorb shock. It is found in the intervertebral disks (the cartilage between two vertebrae).

Connective Tissue—the Fluid Crystal

From the description of the various types of connective tissue, it can be observed that by varying the proportion of the three components—ground substance, protein fibers, and cells—the property of the tissue can be changed significantly. By having a watery ground substance, fluid connective tissue, such as blood, is formed. By introducing more protein fiber, less fluid but tougher tissue is formed. By altering the proportion of collagen, elastic, and reticular fibers, the tissue can be as tough as tendons that withstand more force or flexible (but tough) tissue, such as tissue that covers muscles. With the introduction of specialized proteins and cells, such as chondrocytes, the connective tissue is transformed into solid, flexible cartilage. With the introduction of insoluble calcium salts into the ground substance, the tissue becomes rigid—bone.

The remarkable properties of connective tissue make it comparable to fluid crystal—a type of substance that can be transformed from one state to another. As it is largely made up of nonliving material, its fluid crystal state can be manipulated to a large extent by application of heat, cold, stretch, and activity.

Connective Tissue and Thixotropic Properties

Connective tissue, such as gels, has the property of **thixotropy.** This phenomenon solidifies substances, such as gelatin, when cold or left undisturbed and liquefies substances when warmed or stirred.

Connective tissue, if not stretched and warmed by muscular activity, tends to stiffen and become less flexible. This is one of the reasons why early mobility is emphasized after injury. Stiff, less mobile joints are more common in sedentary individuals.

Massage therapy has a tremendous impact on connective tissue. The stretches, strokes, movement, and heat make connective tissue more fluid, allowing greater movement and flow, encouraging better blood flow and speedy removal of pain producing toxins from the area.

Connective Tissue and Adhesive Properties

Unfortunately, with disuse and chronic pressure, the collagen fibers of connective tissue tend to pack together by hydrogen bonding. In areas that are chronically stressed, inflamed, or that have not been used for a long time, the connective tissue layers, which separate organs, bind together, preventing easy movement and gliding of the organs over each other. This is known as **adhesions.** Nerves and blood vessels may get caught in these adhesions, causing complications. Reduced range of motion, ischemic pain, and loss of sensation and voluntary control are some of the negative outcome of adhesions.

Manipulation helps prevent adhesions in those situations or slow it down. It also helps align the collagen fibers in a way to better reduce friction and allow movement.

Membranes

Membranes, which cover and protect other structures, are formed by the combination of epithelia and connective tissue. Four such membranes exist in the body—**mucous membrane, serous membrane, cutaneous membrane,** and **synovial membrane.**

Examples of mucous membrane are the lining of digestive, respiratory, urinary, and reproductive tracts. The epithelium secretes mucous in these regions. Serous membrane lines the peritoneal, pleural, and pericardial cavities and secretes a watery fluid. The body's outer surface is covered by skin, a cutaneous membrane. The synovial membrane, which secretes the synovial fluid, lines all synovial joints.

Effects of Age on Tissue

With age, many tissue changes occur. With connective tissue, the collagen and elastic fibers change in quality, making tissue less flexible. Healing of tissue takes longer in older persons than in younger individuals.

With aging, the water content in ground substance decreases and the density of fibers increases. As a result, diffusion of substances, as well as movement of cells through the ground substance, is impaired with age. These changes impact the supply of nutrients to tissue and the rate of healing.

As tissue ages, collagen fibers increase in number and size. They also develop cross-linkages, making them less flexible. Elastic fibers undergo such changes, making them more rigid, with a tendency to fray and fragment.

As a person ages, hyaline cartilage loses water and is slowly converted to fibrocartilage. Elasticity of the cartilage is lost and certain regions, such as the articular cartilage, become thinner. The increase in fiber density encourages deposition of calcium, and calcification may be seen in cartilage and around major blood vessels. (For age-related changes: in bone, see **page 160**; nervous tissue, see **page 374**; and muscle tissue, see **page 231**).

The tissue changes reflect as loss of skin elasticity; wrinkle formation; joint stiffness; lung elastic recoil loss; costal cartilage rigidity; intervertebral disk shrinkage; height loss; heart chamber elasticity loss and less forceful contraction; valve stiffening, leading to valvular dysfunction; and less extensible blood vessels, predisposing elderly persons to hypertension.

Implications for Bodyworkers

The manual techniques used by bodyworkers have a significant effect on underlying tissue. (In this book, it is assumed that the students know the definition of terms used for various manual techniques). Strokes, such as effleurage, kneading, and petrissage, affect the fluid component of tissue by increasing blood and lymph flow and reducing edema. Friction strokes are particularly useful in the treatment of adherent connective tissue, as they help to realign collagen fibers during the remodeling phase of healing.

Connective tissue technique is a term given to those techniques that specifically affect the underlying connective tissue. **Skin rolling, friction, myofascial release,** and **direct fascial technique** are some techniques in this category.

In skin rolling techniques, the skin and the tissue overlying the deep fascia are lifted and rolled over the underlying tissue. This stroke is useful in individuals where adhesions are present between the skin and the deep fascia, as seen in burns, after healing of wounds, and surgery. Loosening such adhesions over joints may improve joint mobility. The reactive hyperemia that results also has beneficial effects. This technique is contraindicated in those persons with systemic connective tissue disorders and inflamed skin and fragile skin.

The repetitive strokes of friction produce movement between individual fibers located in dense connective tissue, reducing adhesions and promoting realignment of collagen fibers. In myofascial/fascial techniques, sustained force is applied to the superficial or deep fascia and muscle to lengthen the fascia and increase mobility. Special training is required to perform these techniques, as the effects may be both localized and generalized.

The effects of massage on organs and specific systems are discussed in the respective chapters.

✓ Make Sense of This

This was Mr. Myer's first visit to the massage clinic, and the therapist tried to take a quick history. Mr. Myer seemed knowledgeable about his medical condition and proceeded to describe all of his lifelong medical problems. He explained that his mother had **osteo**porosis and he suspects he has it too. The year before, the doctor had detected a swelling in his **bucc**al region. It turned out to be a **neuroma**. A **bi**opsy was done and surgery was advised.

Mr. Myer had to have a tracheo**stomy** while the lumpec**tomy** was performed. Unfortunately, he had **phlebitis** as a complication. He read that **phlebitis** could lead to **thromb**osis and **thromb**osis could result in **hemiplegia**. Fortunately, he recovered without many complications. "Do you notice that some of my facial muscles have **atrophied**? That's why my grin is lopsided," he said, grinning at the therapist.

Table 1.2

Anatomical Terminology

To understand health-related literature and to converse knowledgeably with other health professionals, the bodyworker must be familiar with anatomical terms. It becomes easier to learn these terms when the derivation is known. Most terms are of Greek or Latin origin; more recently, German or French. Some terms (eponyms) have been given to honor individual anatomists or physicians. Medical terms are usually comprised of two or more parts. A **root** is the essential component of the word. It may represent a disease, a procedure, or body part. A **prefix** is one or more letters attached to the beginning of a root, and a **suffix** is one or more letters attached to the end of a root. With the basic knowledge of root, prefix, and suffix and some practice, it is easy to interpret the meaning, or definition, of a term. The meaning of some of the common prefixes, suffixes and roots are given below.

Prefix/Suffix	Meaning	Example	Prefix/Suffix	Meaning	Example
A			alb-	white	albumin
a-; an-	absent, without	anesthesia	-alg	pain	myalgia
ab-	away from	abnormal	ambi-	both	ambidextrous
abdomino-	abdomen	abdominopelvic	an-	without	anencephaly
-ac; -al; -ar; -ary	pertaining to	iliac; abdominal; ocular; coronary	andr(o)-	male	androgen
acou-	relating to hearing	acoustic meatus	angi-	pertaining to blood vessels	angina
acr(o)-	extremity	acromegaly	ankylo-	crooked	ankylosing spondylitis
-acusis	hearing condition	presbycusis	ante-	in front of	antebrachial
ad-	toward	adhesion	anti-	against	antigen
aden(o)-	gland	adenocarcinoma	aque-	water	aqueous humor
adipo-	fat	adipocytes	-arche	beginning	menarche
aero-	air	aerosol	arthr-	pertaining to joint	arthritis
af-	moving towards a central point	afferent			

Table 1.2

Anatomic Terminology (Continued)

Prefix/Suffix	Meaning	Example	Prefix/Suffix	Meaning	Example
-ase	an enzyme	prot<u>ase</u>	crani(o)-	skull	<u>crani</u>osacral
-asthenia	weakness	my<u>asthenia</u> gravis	crin(o)-	secrete	endo<u>crine</u>
auto-	self	<u>auto</u>nomic	crypt-	hidden	<u>crypt</u>orchidism
B			cutane(o)-	skin	sub<u>cutane</u>ous
bi-	two	<u>bi</u>lateral	cyan-	blue	<u>cyan</u>osis
bili-	bile	<u>bili</u>rubin	cysti-	sac or bladder	<u>cysti</u>tis
bio-	life	<u>bio</u>logy	cyt(o)-	cell	<u>cyt</u>oplasm
blast-/-blast	embryonic state	erythro<u>blast</u>	**D**		
blephar(o)-	eyelid	<u>blephar</u>itis	dactyl-	digit (finger or toe)	poly<u>dactyl</u>y
brachi-	arm	<u>brachi</u>al plexus	de-	down	<u>de</u>scend
brachy-	short	<u>brachy</u>cephalic	derm-	relating to skin	<u>derm</u>atitis
brady-	slow	<u>brady</u>cardia	dextr(o)	right	<u>dextr</u>ose
bucc-	pertaining to the cheek	<u>bucc</u>inator	di-	two	<u>di</u>chotomy
C			dia-	across or through	<u>dia</u>phragm
cac-	bad	<u>cac</u>hexia	diplo-	double	<u>diplo</u>pia
calc-	stone	<u>calc</u>ulus	dips-	thirst	poly<u>dips</u>ia
capit-	pertaining to the head	<u>capit</u>ulum	dis-	apart	<u>dis</u>locate
capn-; carb-	carbon dioxide	hyper<u>capn</u>ea	dors(i)(o)-	back	latissimus <u>dorsi</u>
carcin-	cancer	<u>carcin</u>oma	duct-	conduct	<u>duct</u>us arteriosus
cardi-	heart	<u>cardi</u>ology	dur-	hard	<u>dur</u>a mater
cata-	down	<u>cata</u>bolism	dys-	bad, difficult	<u>dys</u>uria
caud-	tail	<u>caud</u>al	**E**		
cephal-	head	en<u>cephal</u>itis	e-	out	<u>e</u>pithelium
-cele	pouching or hernia	varico<u>cele</u>	-eal	pertaining to	periton<u>eal</u> dialysis
celi-	abdomen	<u>celi</u>ac artery	ecto-	outside	<u>ecto</u>pic
-centesis	puncture for aspiration	amnio<u>centesis</u>	-ectomy	removal	append<u>ectomy</u>
			ede-	swelling	<u>ede</u>ma
cerebro-	brain	<u>cerebro</u>spinal fluid	-emia	pertaining to blood	an<u>emia</u>
cervic-	neck	<u>cervic</u>x	en-	within	<u>en</u>ema
chol-	bile	<u>chol</u>ecystectomy	end-	within	<u>end</u>oscopy
chondr-	cartilage	hypo<u>chondr</u>iac region	enter(o)-	pertaining to the gut	<u>entero</u>colitis
chrom-	color	mono<u>chrom</u>atic	epi-	above	<u>epi</u>dermis
-cide	destroy	sui<u>cide</u>	erythro-	red	<u>erythro</u>cyte
circum-	around	<u>circum</u>ference	eu-	normal	<u>eu</u>thyroid
co-; con-	together	<u>co</u>enzyme; <u>con</u>joint	ex-	out of	<u>ex</u>tremity
col(i)(o)-	colon	<u>col</u>onoscopy	exo-	outside	<u>exo</u>cytosis
contra-	against	<u>contra</u>lateral	extra-	outside of	<u>extra</u>cellular
coron(o)-	crown or circle	<u>coron</u>ary artery	**F**		
corp-	body	<u>corp</u>us callosum	fasci-	band; bundle	<u>fasci</u>a
cost(o)-	rib	<u>cost</u>ochondral	febri-	fever	<u>febri</u>le

Continued

Table 1.2

Anatomic Terminology (Continued)

Prefix/Suffix	Meaning	Example	Prefix/Suffix	Meaning	Example
-ferent	carry	afferent	inter-	among	interstitial
fil-	threadlike	filament	intra-	inside	intracellular
fiss-	split	fissure	ischi(o)-	hip	ischium
for-	opening	foramen	-ism	condition	hyperthyroidism
-form	shape	cuneiform	iso-	equal	isometric
G			-ist	one who specializes in	optometrist
galact(o)-	milk	galactose	-itis	inflammation	pleuritis
gastro-	related to the stomach	gastrointestinal	**J**		
-gen	an agent which produces	fibrinogen	jejun(o)-	jejunum (empty)	jejunoplasty
-genic	originating from	osteogenic	juxta-	adjacent to; near	juxtaglomerular
gest-	carry	gestation	**K**		
gli-	glue	neuroglioma	kerat(o)-	cornea; scarred tissue	keratitis
gloss-	related to the tongue	hypoglossus	kine(t)(o)-	movement	kinesiology
glott-	opening	epiglottis	**L**		
glyco-	sugar; sweet	glycolysis	labi-	lip	labia majora
gnos(o)	knowing	diagnosis	lacri-	tears	lacrimal gland
-gram	record of	electrocardiogram	lact-	milk	lactose
gran-	particulates	granulocyte	lapar(o)-	abdomen	laparoscope
-graph	instrument for recording	polygraph	laryn(o)-	larynx	laryngectomy
gravi-	heavy	prima gravida	later-	side	lateral
gyn(o)-	woman	gynecology	-lepsy	seizure	epilepsy
H			leuk-	white	leukocyte
hema-	blood	hematology	lex(o)-	word, phrase	dyslexia
hemi-	half	hemisphere	lip-	fat	liposuction
hepat-	liver	hepatitis	lith(o)-	stone	lithotripsy
hetero-	other	heterogenicity	-logy	science of	biology
histo-	tissue	histology	lord(o)-	bent	lordosis
holo-	whole	holocrine	lymph(o)-	clear fluid	lymphocyte
homo-	same	homosexual	-lysis	dissolve	hemolysis
hydro-	water	hydrocephalus	**M**		
hyper-	excessive	hyperventilation	macro-	big	macrophage
hypo-	less	hypothyroidism	mal-	bad	malnutrition
hyster-	uterus	hysterectomy	-malacia	softening	osteomalacia
I			mamm(o)-	breast	mammogram
-ia	condition	anemia	mast(o)-	breast	mastectomy
idio-	self	idiopathic	meat(o)-	opening	meatus
ile(o)-	ileum	iliacus	medi-	middle	mediastinum
infra-	beneath	infrared	mega-	big	acromegaly
			melan(o)-	black	melanocyte

Table 1.2

Anatomic Terminology (Continued)

Prefix/Suffix	Meaning	Example	Prefix/Suffix	Meaning	Example
meno-	menstruation	menopause	**P**		
ment-	mind	mental	pachy-	thick	pachyderma
meso-	middle	mesothelium	par-	give birth to	multipara
meta-	after	metastasis	para-	near or abnormal	paraplegia
-meter	measuring device	manometer	path(o)-	disease	pathology
micro-	small	microorganism	-pathy	abnormality	encephalopathy
mio-	less, smaller	miosis	ped-	children	pediatrics
mito-	threadlike	mitochondria	-penia	lack of	neutropenia
mono-	single	monocyte	peri-	around	pericardium
morph-	shape	morphology	phag-	to eat	macrophages
multi-	many	multimedia	pharmac(o)-	medicine	pharmacology
myc(o)-	fungus	mycoplasma	pharyng(o)-	pharynx	pharyngitis
myel(o)-	marrow; spinal cord	myelitis	-phil	an affinity for	eosinophil
myo-	muscle	myometrium	phleb(o)-	vein	phlebitis
myx-	mucus	myxedema	-phobe	dread	phobia
N			phot(o)-	light	photography
narc-	numb	narcolepsy	-plasia	growth	hyperplasia
naso-	nose	nasopharyngeal	-plasty	reconstruction of	angioplasty
necro-	dead	necrosis	platy-	flat	platysma
neo-	new	neoplasm	-plegia	paralysis	hemiplegia
nephro-	kidney	nephrology	pleur(o)-	rib; side; pleura	pleural cavity
neuro-	nerve	neurology	-pnea	to breathe	dyspnea
O			pneumon(o)-	air or lung	pneumonia
oc-	against	occlusion	pod-	foot	podiatrist
ocul(o)-	eye	oculomotor	-poiesis	formation of	erythropoiesis
-oid	resembling	android	poly-	many	polymorphs
-ole	small	centriole	post-	after	postpartum
oligo-	small	oligodendrocyte	-praxia	movement	apraxia
-oma	tumor	myoma	pre-	before	prenatal
oo-	egg	oocyte	pro-	favoring; supporting	prognosis
ophthalm-	eye	ophthalmology	proct-	anus	proctology
or-	mouth	oral	prote(o)-	protein	proteolysis
orchi-	testes	orchitis	pseudo-	false	pseudostratified
ortho-	normal	orthostatic	psych(o)-	mental	psychology
-ory	pertaining to	coronory	pulmo(n)-	lung	pulmonary
-ose	full of	glucose	pyel(o)-	kidney	pyelonephritis
-osis	condition	arthrosis	py(o)-	pus	pyoderma
oste(o)-	bone	osteomyelitis	pyr(o)-	heat	pyrexia
ot(o)-	ear	otitis	**Q**		
ovo-	egg	ovary	quad-	four	quadriplegia
ox(o)-	oxygen	oxidation			

Continued

Table 1.2

Anatomic Terminology (Continued)

Prefix/Suffix	Meaning	Example	Prefix/Suffix	Meaning	Example
R			super-	above	superior
re-	again	recurrent	supra-	above	supraorbital
rect-	straight	rectus	sym-; syn-	joined	symphysis; synthesis
ren(o)-	kidney	adrenal gland	**T**		
rete-	network	reticulum	tachy-	fast	tachycardia
retro-	behind	retropharyngeal	-taxis	movement	chemotaxis
rhin-	nose	rhinitis	tele-	far	telehealth
-rrhage	excessive flow	hemorrhage	tens-	stretch	tensor
-rrhaphy	suture	herniorrhaphy	tetra-	four	tetralogy
-rrhea	flow	diarrhea	therm-	heat	thermometer
rub(r)-	red	rubor	thorac-	chest	thoracic
S			thrombo-	clot	thrombophlebitis
sarc-	flesh	sarcoma	-tomy	cut	mastectomy
sangui-	blood	serosanguinous fluid	tox-	poison	cytotoxic
schiz(o)-	split	schizophrenia	trache(o)-	trachea	tracheostomy
scler(o)-	hard	scleroderma	trans-	across	transcutaneous
scolio-	crooked	scoliosis	tri-	three	triceps
-scope	instrument to examine a part	endoscope	trich-	hair	trichosis
-sect	to cut	dissect	-tripsy	crushing	lithotripsy
semi-	partly	semipermeable	-trophy	state relating to size	hypertrophy
sensi-	feeling; perception	sensation	**U**		
sep-	decay	septicemia	-ula; -ule	small	lingula; nodule
serrate-	saw-tooth	serratus anterior	ultra-	excess	ultrasonogram
-sis	process	erythropoiesis	uni-	one	unilateral
soma-	body	somatic	-uria	urine	polyuria
somn(i) (o)	sleep	insomnia	uro-	pertaining to urine	urology
sphygm(o)-	pulse	sphygmomanometer	**V**		
spondyl(o)-	vertebra	ankylosing spondylitis	vas-	vessel	vas deferens
squam(o)-	scale	squamous epithelium	ven(i)(o)-	vein	venipuncture
-stasis	stop or stand	homeostasis	vermi-	worm	vermicularis
steat(o)-	fat	steatorrhea	vesic(o)-	bladder	vesicoureteral
steno-	narrow	stenosis	vit-	life	vitamin
stere(o)-	three dimensional	stereognosis	**Z**		
steth(o)-	chest	stethoscope	zygo-	join	zygomatic bone
-stomy	surgical opening	ileostomy			
sub-	below	sublingual			

SUGGESTED READINGS

Andrade CK, Clifford P. Outcome-Based Massage. Baltimore: Lippincott Williams & Wilkins, 2001.

Goats GCK. Connective tissue massage. Br J Sports Med 1991; 25(3):131–133.

Goats GC. Massage—the scientific basis of an ancient art: Part 1, Part 2. Br J Sports Med 1994;28(3):149–155.

Juhan D. A Handbook for Bodywork: Job's Body. New York: Station Hill Press, 1987.

Kenney RA. Physiology of Aging: A Synopsis. 2nd Ed. Chicago: Year Book Medical, 1989.

Kotzsch RE. Restructure the body with rolfing: deep massage that realigns the human form. East West Nat Health 1992;22(6):35–38.

Premkumar K. Pathology A to Z. 2nd Ed. Calgary: VanPub Books, 1999.

Sandler S. The physiology of soft tissue massage. J Bodywork Movement Ther 1999;3(2):118–122.

 # Review Questions

Multiple Choice

1. Which structure separates the thoracic cavity from the abdominopelvic cavity?
   A. Diaphragm
   B. Visceral peritoneum
   C. Liver
   D. Parietal pleura
   E. Rib cage

2. Which of the following is NOT a characteristic of a person in anatomical position?
   A. Feet together
   B. Arms at sides
   C. Body erect
   D. Eyes directed forward
   E. Palms facing posteriorly

3. To the ankle, the knee is
   A. intermediate
   B. lateral
   C. distal
   D. inferior
   E. proximal

4. Superior is to cranial as posterior is to
   A. external
   B. ventral
   C. caudal
   D. dorsal
   E. internal

5. Of the existing chemical elements, four elements make up 96% of the human body. These elements follow, EXCEPT
   A. carbon
   B. sulphur
   C. nitrogen
   D. oxygen
   E. hydrogen

Fill-in-the-Blank

1. The levels of organization from larger to smaller are:

   Organism _____ → _____ → _____ → _____ → Chemicals

2. In each situation, determine if water would move into the cell (I); out of the cell (O); or neither (N). Mark each situation with I, O, or N.

   Solute (chemical substance dissolved in water) more concentrated around the cell

   _____

   Solute less concentrated around the cell

   _____

   Solute concentration is the same as in the cell

   _____

3. Completion

   a. Within the nucleus of the atom, there are positively charged particles called _____ and uncharged particles called _____.

   b. If you subtract the atomic number from the mass number, you will identify the number of _____.

   c. In the _____ bond, a pair of electrons is shared.

   d. In the _____ type bond, a weak link between a hydrogen atom and another atom, such as oxygen or nitrogen, is formed.

   e. The ratio of hydrogen to oxygen in all carbohydrates is _____ : _____.

   f. Carbohydrates, lipids, and proteins all contain carbon, hydrogen, and oxygen. A fourth element, _____, makes up a substantial portion of protein.

   g. An increase in tissue or organ size by increase in cell size (not number) is known as _____.

4. Fill in the blanks, using the appropriate anatomical terms:

   a. The ears are _____ to the nose.

   b. The elbow is _____ to the fingers.

   c. The heart is located _____ to the vertebral column.

   d. The muscles of the abdomen are _____ to the skin over the abdominal wall.

5. Fill in the blanks with the appropriate muscle tissue type: a. cardiac muscle, b. smooth muscle, or c. skeletal muscle. (More than one type may be appropriate for certain statements.)

   a. Striations when viewed under the microscope
   _____

   b. Controlled by the autonomic nerves
   _____

   c. Intercalated disks _____

   d. Diaphragm is an example of _____

   e. The muscle found in the uterus is an example of _____

   f. Branched appearance _____

6. Fill in the blanks, using the appropriate membrane type: a. mucous, b. serous, c. cutaneous, and d. synovial.

   a. Membrane found in joints, such the knees and shoulders _____

   b. Membrane that lines the mouth _____

   c. Membrane lining of the thoracic cavity
   _____

   d. The skin is considered to be this type membrane _____

7. Below is a classification of connective tissue. Fill in the blanks with the appropriate type.

True or False

(Answer the following questions T, for true; or F, for false):
1. Diffusion, osmosis, and facilitated diffusion are all passive transport processes.
2. Plasma membranes consist of a double layer of carbohydrate molecules with proteins embedded in the bilayer.
3. Oxygen, water, NaCl and glucose are inorganic compounds.

4. There are about four different kinds of amino acids found in human proteins.
5. When the response to a stimulus results in an enhancement of the initial stimulus, it is a negative feedback mechanism.
6. Negative feedback mechanisms are more common than positive feedback mechanisms.
7. Of the three major components of the mechanisms that help to maintain homeostasis, the effectors sense the changes in the environment.
8. Mitosis is a type of cell division in which a cell divides into two new cells with the same number of chromosomes as the original cell.
9. The pH of the body is 6.5.
10. A pH of 9.0 is considered acidic.

Matching

A.

a. _____ parasagittal plane

b. _____ midsagittal plane

c. _____ transverse plane

d. _____ frontal plane

1. This plane divides the body into superior and inferior parts.
2. This plane divides the body into equal right and left portions.
3. This plane divides the body into anterior and posterior portions.
4. This plane divides the body into unequal right and left portions.

B.

a. _____ lateral

b. _____ medial

c. _____ superficial

d. _____ inferior

e. _____ anterior

1. Toward or near the surface of a structure or body.
2. Away from the midline of a structure or body.
3. Toward the front of a structure or body.
4. Toward the lower part of a structure or body.
5. Toward the midline of a structure or body.

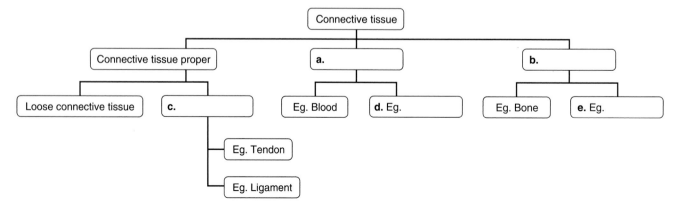

C.
a. _____ pleural cavity
b. _____ pericardial cavity
c. _____ abdominal cavity
d. _____ vertebral cavity
e. _____ pelvic cavity
f. _____ cranial cavity

1. Contains the heart.
2. Contains the spinal cord.
3. Contains the bladder and rectum.
4. Contains the lungs.
5. Contains the brain.
6. Contains the liver and stomach.

D. *Match the function (a, b, c, d, e, f, g, h, i, j, or k) to the following list of systems:*
1. _____ Cardiovascular system
2. _____ Lymphatic system
3. _____ Respiratory system
4. _____ Nervous system
5. _____ Muscular system
6. _____ Urinary system
7. _____ Skeletal system
8. _____ Digestive system
9. _____ Endocrine system
10. _____ Reproductive system
11. _____ Integumentary system

a. removes nitrogenous waste products
b. involves defense mechanisms and removal of excess fluid from the interstitial fluid compartment
c. manufactures blood cells; provides surface for muscle attachment
d. removes carbon dioxide from blood and helps maintain pH
e. propagates species
f. perceives changes in the external environment and reacts
g. helps absorb nutrients
h. helps with movement; produces heat
i. carries nutrients
j. manufactures vitamin D
k. regulates body function by secreting chemicals into the blood

E. *Match the following words with their definitions:*
1. _____ anatomy
2. _____ physiology
3. _____ embryology
4. _____ tissue
5. _____ organ

a. condition of constancy in the internal environment
b. study of the functions of the structures of the body
c. atoms that carry positive or negative charges
d. smallest unit of matter
e. collection of cells having the same function

6. _____ homeostasis
7. _____ atom
8. _____ isotope
9. _____ ion
10. _____ metabolism
11. _____ buffer

f. study of external and internal structures of the body
g. includes all the chemical reactions in the body
h. collection of different types of tissues having the same function
i. atoms of an element that have the same atomic number but different mass number
j. study of changes that occur during development in the womb
k. compounds that prevent rapid changes in pH

F. *Match the cell structure with the function mentioned:*
1. _____ ribosomes
2. _____ lysosome
3. _____ mitochondria
4. _____ microvilli
5. _____ centriole

a. plays an active part during cell division
b. manufactures proteins
c. contains destructive enzymes
d. manufactures ATP
e. increases surface area for absorption

G. *Match the word with the type of chemical reaction:*
1. _____ Exchange reaction
2. _____ Decomposition reaction
3. _____ Synthesis reaction

a. $A + B \rightarrow AB$
b. $AB + CD \rightarrow AD + CB$
c. $AB \rightarrow A + B$

H. *Match the following types of bonds with their descriptions:*
1. _____ In this type of bond, an atom looses its electrons to another atom.
2. _____ In this type of bond, the atoms share their electrons.
3. _____ In this type of bond, atoms share their electrons unequally.

a. ionic bond
b. hydrogen bond
c. covalent bond

I. *Match the following tissue types with the descriptions:*
1. _____ helps the heart pump out blood
2. _____ forms the inner lining of blood vessels

a. connective tissue
b. muscle tissue

3. _____ forms the major component of the spinal cord

   c. epithelial tissue

4. _____ forms the most abundant type of tissue in the body

   d. nervous tissue

5. _____ transmits electrochemical impulses

6. _____ forms an abundance of nonliving fibers

7. _____ forms the surface of the skin

J. Match the type of epithelium with the location.
1. _____ most of the respiratory tract lining has this type of epithelium
   a. cuboidal epithelium

2. _____ specific to the lining of the urinary bladder epithelium
   b. ciliated columnar

3. _____ lines ducts
   c. stratified squamous epithelium

4. _____ found where there is a lot of friction
   d. transitional epithelium

K. Match the following types of transport across the cell membrane with the description:
1. _____ requires the use of ATP
   a. simple diffusion

2. _____ the water moves from an area of low concentration of solutes (particles in the water) to an area of high concentration of solutes
   b. endocytosis

3. _____ transport is driven by hydrostatic pressure
   c. active transport

4. _____ large particles are taken from the exterior by indentation of the plasma membrane
   d. osmosis

5. _____ movement of the solutes is driven by the difference in concentration gradient of the solutes
   e. filtration

L. Match the following roots/suffixes/prefixes with the correct meaning:
1. _____ short   a. tachy
2. _____ bad   b. caud
3. _____ tail   c. adipo
4. _____ fat   d. brachy
5. _____ fast   e. crypt
6. _____ hidden   f. dys
7. _____ band   g. fasci

Short Answer Questions

1. Name the different systems of the body.
2. Give the functions of each system.
3. Locate, on your body, the sacral, popliteal, frontal, umbilical, and brachial regions.
4. Define the term homeostasis.
5. List the major chemicals that make up the body.
6. Name the different ways transport can occur across the cell membrane.
7. Describe the special characteristics of epithelial tissue.
8. Identify the location of squamous, cuboidal, and columnar epithelium in the body.
9. Describe the characteristics of connective tissue.
10. Explain why cartilage and dense connective tissue take longer to heal.
11. Name the positive effects of massage on connective tissue.
12. Name a few connective tissue techniques and identify the conditions where they are particularly useful.
13. Define thixotropy.

Prefixes/Suffixes/Terms

Identify the meaning of the underlined prefixes/suffixes/terms in the following text:

Mrs. Goldsmith slipped on ice and fractured her hip. Even the short period she was immobilized led to <u>atrophy</u> of her leg muscles. But this was not her only problem. Her <u>intraocular</u> pressure was high. Just a month prior to her fall, <u>en-doscopy</u> was performed to rule out gastric ulcer when she developed severe <u>epi</u>gastric pain. Later, she found out that she had <u>chole</u>lithiasis for which cholecyst<u>ectomy</u> seemed to be the only solution.

Case Study

Mrs. Simon, a 45-year-old lawyer, filed claims with her insurance agent for damages that she had incurred in an accident 6 months ago. She had been receiving treatment for whiplash from her massage therapist for more than 4 months. Mrs. Simon requests a written report of the therapist's assessment of her injury and progress with treatment.

As a health professional, what knowledge do you think a bodyworker needs to complete this report?

Coloring Exercise

A. Color each of the abdominal areas in the given diagram, using a different color and filling in the color code. Label the organism in these regions.

O lumbar regions
O umbilical region
O epigastric region
O hypogastric region
O iliac regions
O hypochondriac regions

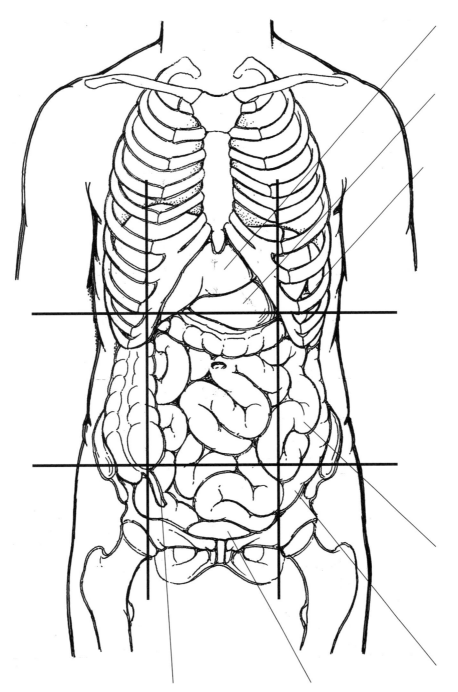

B. Color each of the labeled areas in the given diagram, using a different color and filling in the color code. Label the other body regions.

O cranial region
O pubic area
O deltoid region
O popliteal fossa
O cubital region
O crural region
O sternal region
O gluteal region

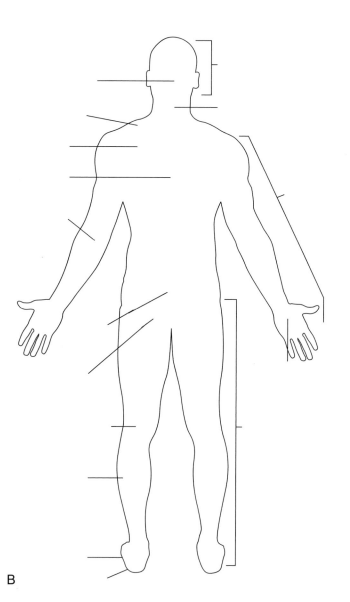

A   B

C. Color and label each of the structures in the given diagram, using a different color and filling in the color code.

O mitochondria
O nucleus
O cytoplasm
O cell membrane
O centriole
O nucleus
O endoplasmic reticulum
O Golgi apparatus

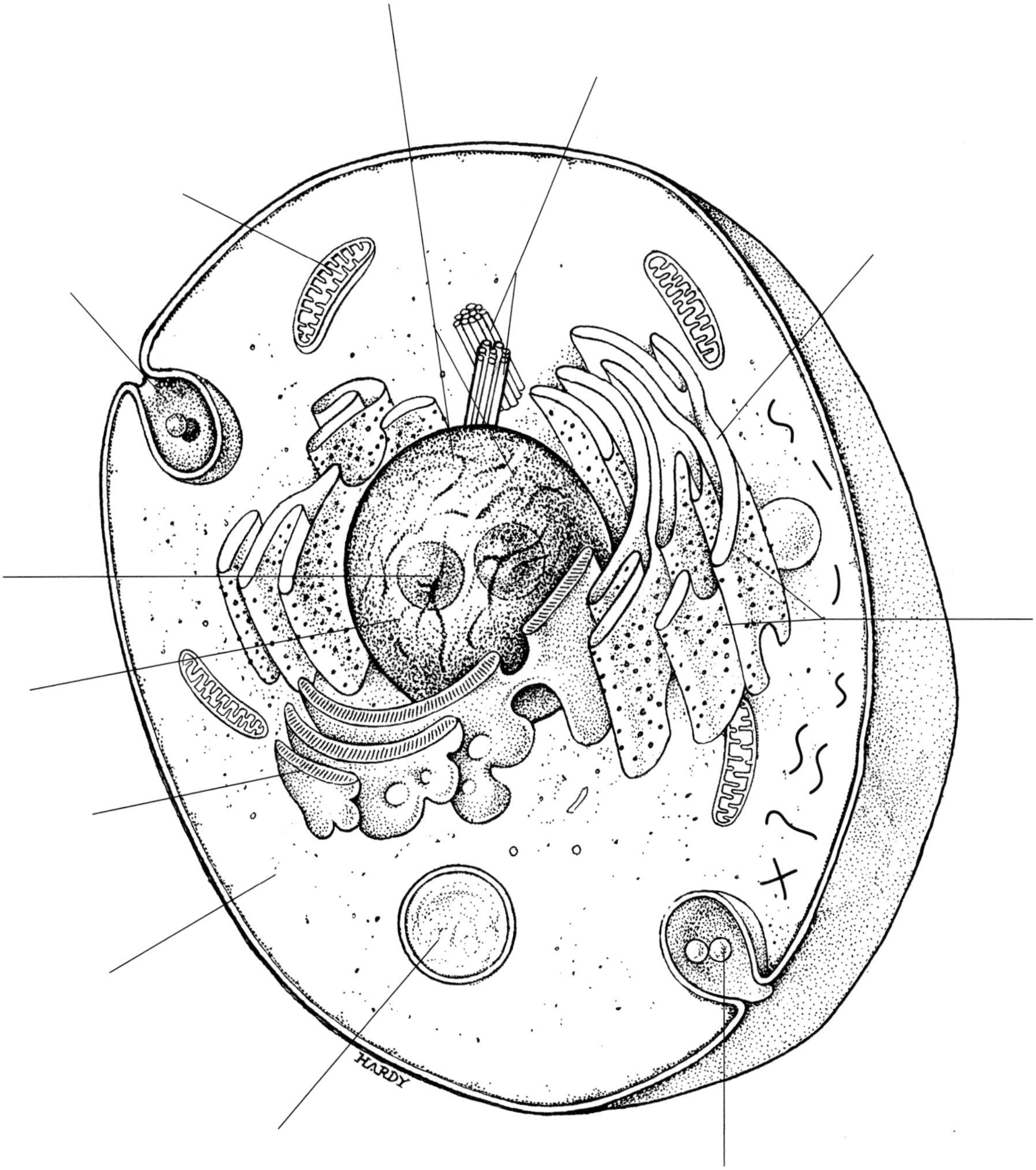

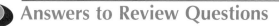 **Answers to Review Questions**

Multiple Choice

1. A; 2. E; 3. E; 4. D; 5. B

Completion

1. systems; organs; tissues; cells; chemicals
2. a. O; b. I; c. N
3. a. protons, neutrons; b. neutrons; c. covalent; d. hydrogen bond; e. 2:1; f. nitrogen; g. hypertrophy
4. a. posterior or lateral; b. proximal or superior; c. anterior or ventral; d. deep
5. a. a and c; b. a and b; c. a; d. c; e. b; f. a
6. a. d; b. a; c. b; d. c
7. a. fluid connective tissue; b. supporting connective tissue; c. dense connective tissue; d. lymph; e. cartilage

True–False

1. true
2. false, it is a phospholipid bilayer
3. false, glucose is organic
4. false, there are about 20 significant amino acids in the body
5. false, it is a positive feedback mechanism
6. true
7. false, it is the receptors, effectors produce the effect
8. true
9. false, it is 7.35–7.45
10. false, pH below 7.0 would be acidic

Matching

A. 1. c; 2. b; 3. d; 4. a
B. 1. c; 2. a; 3. e; 4. d; 5. b
C. 1. b; 2. d; 3. e; 4. a; 5. f; 6. c
D. 1. i; 2. b; 3. d; 4. f; 5. h; 6. a; 7. c; 8. g; 9. k; 10. e; 11. j
E. 1. f; 2. b; 3. j; 4. e; 5. h; 6. a; 7. d; 8. i; 9. c; 10. g; 11. k
F. 1. b; 2. c; 3. d; 4. e; 5. a
G. 1. b; 2. c; 3. a
H. 1. a; 2. c; 3. b
I. 1. b; 2. c; 3. d; 4. a; 5. d; 6. a; 7. c
J. 1. b; 2. d; 3. a; 4. c
K. 1. c; 2. d; 3. e; 4. b; 5. a
L. 1. d; 2. f; 3. b; 4. c; 5. a; 6. e; 7. g

Short-Answer Questions

1. and 2. **Integumentary**—protects body; temperature regulation; production of vitamin D; perceives sensation. **Digestive**—breaks down food; absorption of nutrients; eliminates waste. **Nervous**—detects, interprets and reacts to changes in the internal and external environment. **Respiratory**—exchange of gases, maintains pH; helps produce sound. **Cardiovascular**—carries oxygen and nutrients to tissues, removes wastes from tissues, maintains temperature; helps with defense; helps maintain the internal environment. **Endocrine**—regulates body activities by secreting hormones. **Reproductive**—helps propagate species. **Lymphatic**—returns protein and fluid to blood from the interstitial compartment; participates in defense. **Urinary**—helps eliminate nitrogenous waste; helps maintain pH. **Skeletal**—manufactures blood cells in marrow; supports body; protects organs; helps with movement; stores minerals. **Muscular**—helps with movement; generates heat.
3. Refer to Figure 1. 7.
4. It is the condition of constancy in the internal environment
5. Oxygen, carbon, hydrogen, nitrogen, calcium, and phosphorus
6. Diffusion, osmosis, filtration, carrier-mediated, vesicular transport, active transport
7. Cover surfaces; line internal passages and chambers; found in layers; are not supplied by blood vessels; multiply rapidly; form a barrier and protect; have a good nerve supply
8. Squamous epithelium can be found in the peritoneum; endothelium lining heart and blood vessels; alveoli of lungs; some parts of kidney tubules; Cuboidal epithelium can be found in glands; ducts; and some parts of kidney tubules; Columnar epithelium can be found lining the stomach; intestines; gall bladder; uterine tubes; some parts of kidney tubules
9. Connective tissue has specialized cells, protein fibers, and ground substance; the cells are scattered; they are not exposed to the exterior; most connective tissue are vascularized; most have nerve ending that respond to sensations
10. They have a poor blood supply and are mostly made up of nonliving matter (matrix)
11. The stretches, strokes, movement and heat make connective tissue more fluid, allowing greater movement and flow, encouraging blood flow, and speedy removal of pain producing toxins from the area. It can help prevent or slow adhesions; it also helps to better align collagen fibers, reducing friction and allowing movement.
12. **Skin rolling**—This stroke is useful when adhesions are present between the skin and the deep fascia, as seen in burns, after healing of wounds, and surgery; **friction**—repetitive strokes of friction produce movement between individual fibers located in dense connective tis-

sue, reducing adhesions and promoting realignment of collagen fibers; **myofascial/fascial techniques**—sustained force is applied to the superficial or deep fascia and muscle to lengthen the fascia and increase mobility.

13. It is the phenomenon that solidifies substances when cold or left undisturbed and liquefies substances when warmed or stirred.

Prefixes/Suffixes/Terms

Intraocular, inside eye; endoscopy, examination of the inside in this case stomach; epigastric, pain over the stomach region; cholelithiasis, stone in the gallbladder; cholecystectomy, removal or excision of the gallbladder.

Case Study

To begin with, an understanding of medical terminology.

CHAPTER 2

Integumentary System

Objectives On completion of this chapter, the reader should be able to:

- List the functions of the integumentary system.
- Identify the layers of the skin and the accessory structures.
- Describe the various factors that determine skin color.
- Describe the effects of ultraviolet radiation on the skin.
- Explain the role of skin in temperature control.
- Explain how different sensations, such as touch, pressure, pain, and temperature change, are "sensed" by the skin and conveyed to the central nervous system.
- Define dermatome.
- Explain the role of the accessory structures in maintaining skin functions.
- Identify the location of superficial and deep fascia.
- Identify substances that may be absorbed through the skin.
- Describe the role of microorganisms that inhabit normal skin and mucous membrane.
- Define inflammation.
- Explain the purpose of inflammation.
- List the common causes of inflammation.
- State the cardinal signs of acute inflammation and explain the underlying mechanisms.
- Explain the various ways inflammation may resolve.
- Compare and contrast acute and chronic inflammation.
- Describe the mechanisms involved in skin healing.
- Describe the effects of aging on the components of the integumentary system.
- Describe the possible effects of massage on the integumentary system.
- Compare the effects of various massage techniques on the skin.
- Describe the effects of heat application on the skin.
- Describe the effects of cold application on the skin.
- Explain the unique properties of water that make it suitable for use by bodyworkers.
- Define macule, wheal, papule, nodule, vesicle, pustule, ulcer, crust, scale, and fissure and identify the anatomic structure of skin affected by each of these skin lesions.

Although massage and other complementary therapies affect many systems, the organ system or structure that is physically handled by the therapist is the integumentary system. Therapists use their sense of touch to assess their clients' temperature, texture, and tension of soft tissue. The client perceives the manipulation by the therapist through the skin and complex mechanical, physiological, and psychological responses are produced in the deeper structures. A thorough knowledge of structure and function will help therapists treat clients more effectively. For example, some areas of the skin are more sensitive to touch than others and less pressure is sufficient. The type of technique used and the rate, vigor, and rhythm determine the effect on the client. Because *client satisfaction largely relies on the sensations evoked, knowledge of how the brain perceives sensation gains importance. Heat and cold may be used for therapy and questions, such as what effect do they have on the body.*

Manipulation of the skin often causes visible changes in color or color changes may be already present. An understanding of why this happens may be beneficial to the therapist. If clients with allergies inadvertently contact certain chemicals in the clinic, edema, itching, and redness may be produced. Knowledge of why and how this happens can help the therapist avoid these situations. In aromatherapy, essential oils are used on the skin and an understanding is needed of what can and cannot be absorbed through the skin. To understand the clinical conditions that produce skin problems and take suitable precautions, the therapist needs to know the structure of normal skin.

Chapter 2 details the functions and structure of the skin and the effects of aging and massage on the integumentary system.

The integumentary (*inte*, whole + gument, body covering) system consists of skin, together with accessory structures, such as glands, hair, nails, muscle, and nerves. Skin is made up of different types of tissue that perform specific functions and is considered an organ. The skin is the heaviest organ and has the largest surface area.

Functions of the Skin

The skin has many functions. It *protects* the underlying organs and tissues from abrasion, irradiation from sunlight, and attack by pathogens and other harmful agents. Salt, water, and certain organic wastes are lost through sweat and, thus, the skin has *excretory functions*. The skin plays an important role in *maintenance of body temperature*. It prevents loss of heat when the atmosphere is cold and facilitates loss of heat when the body gets hot. The skin *detects changes* in the surrounding environment by its ability to sense touch, pressure, pain, and temperature and relays this information to the central nervous system. The skin participates in the *synthesis of vitamin D*, which plays an important role in calcium metabolism. Its vast surface area helps *store nutrients*.

DERMATOLOGY

Dermatology is the branch of medicine concerned with the study of skin and skin diseases.

ASTOUNDING FACTS

- The skin weighs about 8 pounds (3.63 kilograms).
- The skin has approximately 640,000 sensory receptors connected to the spinal cord by more than a half million nerve fibers.
- An area of skin the size of a quarter contains about 3 million cells, 100 sweat glands, 50 nerve endings, and 3 feet of blood vessels.

The skin also serves as a *reservoir of blood*, as the volume of blood flowing in its extensive network of blood vessels can be altered according to systemic needs.

Diseases of the body are often reflected in the skin. Many internal disorders are outwardly presented as skin lesions. However, the most important function of the skin that is recognized by society is the skin's ability to *reflect emotional states*, regardless of disease. Warmth and human affection are given and received through the skin. To a large extent, human beauty is related to the structure of the skin. As society gives importance to the color, texture, and tone of skin, even slight skin imperfections evoke a variety of individual responses.

Structure of the Skin

The integument consists of the cutaneous membrane, or skin, and the accessory structures, such as hair, nails, glands, muscles, and nerves (see Figure 2.1). The skin covers an area of approximately 1.5–2 m² (59–78.7 sq in). The superficial part of the skin is the **epithelium,** or **epidermis.** Deep to the epithelium is a layer of connective tissue, the **dermis,** in which the glands, hair, and nails are located. Deep to the dermis is the **subcutaneous layer,** or **hypodermis,** which consists of loose connective tissue and adipose tissue. This layer separates the skin from the underlying muscle, bone, and other structures.

THE EPIDERMIS

The epidermis (see Figures 2.2 and 2.3) is the most superficial layer of the skin and is composed of stratified squamous epithelium. The epidermis is separated from the dermis—the deeper layer—by the basement membrane. Not having a direct blood supply, the epidermis relies on nutrients in the interstitial fluid that have diffused from the capillaries located in the dermis.

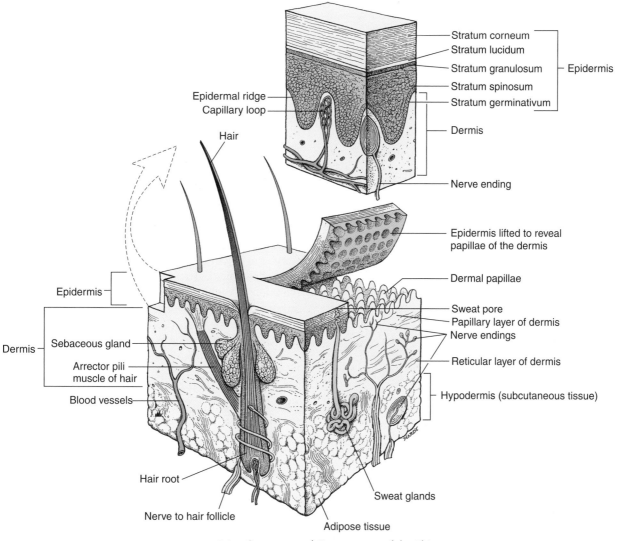

Stratum corneum
Stratum lucidum
Stratum granulosum
Stratum spinosum
Stratum germinativum

Epidermis

Epidermal ridge
Capillary loop

Dermis

Hair

Nerve ending

Epidermis lifted to reveal papillae of the dermis

Dermal papillae

Epidermis

Sweat pore
Papillary layer of dermis
Nerve endings

Dermis

Sebaceous gland

Reticular layer of dermis

Arrector pili muscle of hair

Hypodermis (subcutaneous tissue)

Blood vessels

Hair root

Sweat glands

Nerve to hair follicle

Adipose tissue

FIGURE 2.1.   Structure and Components of the Skin

There are four types of skin cells:

- **keratinocytes**
- **melanocytes**
- **Merkel cells**
- **Langerhans cells** (Figure 2.2).

Keratinocytes make up 90% of the epidermis; they lie in many distinct layers and produce a tough fibrous protein called **keratin.** Keratin helps protect the skin from heat, microorganisms, and chemicals in the environment.

The layers of the epidermis can be identified by examining a section under the microscope. Beginning with the basement membrane, which separates the epidermis from the dermis, the following layers can be identified:

- **stratum germinativum,** or **stratum basale**
- **stratum spinosum**

- **stratum granulosum**
- **stratum lucidum**
- **stratum corneum.**

In areas where skin is exposed to friction, such as the palm of the hand, sole of the foot, and fingertips, the skin is thick and consists of all five layers. In other areas, such as the eyelids, the skin is thin and stratum lucidum is absent.

The Stratum Germinativum

This single-celled layer, consisting of cuboidal or columnar epithelium, is attached to the basement membrane. It is thrown into folds known as **epidermal ridges** that extend into the dermis (Figure 2.2). The projections of the dermis adjacent to the ridges are known as the **dermal papillae.** The surface of the skin follows the ridge pattern. This pattern, referred

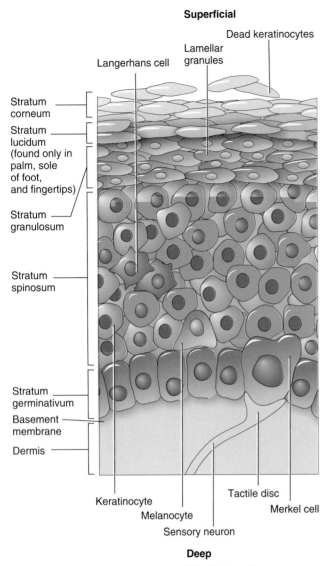

Superficial

Dead keratinocytes

Lamellar granules

Langerhans cell

Stratum corneum

Stratum lucidum (found only in palm, sole of foot, and fingertips)

Stratum granulosum

Stratum spinosum

Stratum germinativum

Basement membrane

Dermis

Keratinocyte

Melanocyte

Sensory neuron

Tactile disc

Merkel cell

Deep

FIGURE 2.2.   Layers of the Epidermis

Pigment cells, known as melanocytes, are also located in this layer and are responsible for the color of the skin. Melanocytes are scattered throughout this layer and their processes extend to the more superficial layers of the skin.

Melanocytes

Melanocytes form 8% of all skin cells and manufacture the pigment **melanin.** Melanocytes contain the enzymes required for converting the amino acid tyrosine into melanin. The melanin pigment, packaged inside the cell in small vesicles called **melanosomes,** is transferred along the processes that extend into the superficial layers of skin. In the superficial layers, the vesicles are transferred into other cells, coloring them temporarily, until they fuse with lysosomes and are then destroyed. In individuals with light skin, less transfer of melanosomes occurs among cells, and the superficial layers lose their pigments faster. In individuals with dark skin, the melanosomes are larger and transfer occurs in many of the superficial layers. Interestingly, the *number* of melanocytes per square millimeter of skin is the same for both dark- and light-skinned individuals. It is the melanin synthesis *rate* that is different. The number of melanocytes is increased in some areas of the body, such as the penis, nipples, areolae (area around the nipple), face, and limbs.

to as whorls, is especially obvious in the palms and soles. These ridges increase friction and surface area, providing a better, more secure grip of objects. The shapes of the ridges are genetically determined and unique to an individual; they do not change with time. For this reason, fingerprints can be used for identification.

As its name suggests, this layer contains germinative, or basal cells, that multiply rapidly and replace cells in the superficial layer that have been lost or shed. The keratinocytes are large and contain keratin filaments in the cytoskeleton. The keratin filaments attach the cells to each other and to the basement membrane. Areas of skin that lack hair contain specialized cells known as Merkel cells. These cells are in close contact with touch receptors and stimulate these sensory nerve endings.

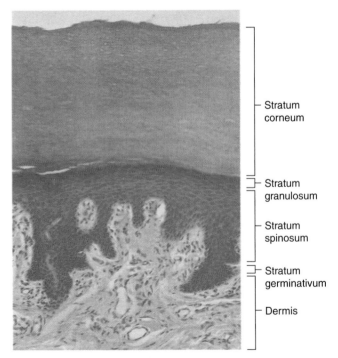

Stratum corneum

Stratum granulosum

Stratum spinosum

Stratum germinativum

Dermis

FIGURE 2.3.   A Photomicrograph of the Epidermis

Skin Cancer

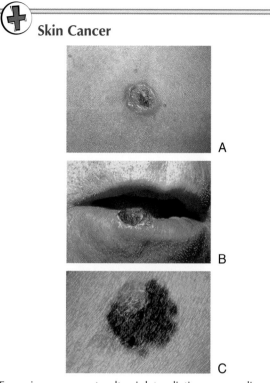

A

B

C

Excessive exposure to ultraviolet radiation can predispose a person to skin cancer. There are three common types of skin cancers: **basal cell carcinoma (A), squamous cell carcinoma (B),** and **malignant melanoma (C).** Basal cell carcinoma arises from the germinativum layer and is the most common; like squamous cell carcinoma, it does not metastasize easily. Malignant melanomas arise from melanocytes, grow rapidly, metastasize via the lymphatics, and have the poorest prognosis. Abnormal growths that are asymmetrical and have irregular borders, varying colors, and are larger than 0.5 mm may be indicative of malignant melanoma.

Albinism and Vitiligo

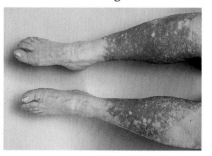

Albinism is caused by a congenital inability to synthesize melanin as a result of genetic defects in the biochemical pathway that manufactures melanin. Vitiligo is a result of melanin loss in patchy areas of the skin. It develops after birth and is progressive (brown pigment on legs is patient's normal skin color).

The melanin pigment protects the skin from the harmful effects of ultraviolet (UV) radiation. Exposure to UV rays stimulates those enzymes needed for production of melanin and produces a "tan" skin. The tan fades when the keratinocytes containing melanin are lost. Melanin production is also increased by secretion of melanocyte-stimulating hormones by the anterior pituitary gland.

Freckles

Freckles are small, pigmented spots on the skin, in which the melanocytes in the area have produced more than normal levels of melanin pigment.

Because melanin pigment is concentrated around the nucleus, it works like an umbrella, absorbing UV rays and shielding the nucleus and its high deoxyribonucleic acid (DNA) content. Melanin also protects the skin from sunburn. However, the rate of melanin synthesis is not rapid enough to provide complete protection; it is possible to get a sunburn easily, especially in the first few days of prolonged sun exposure. Mild sunburn consists of varying degrees of redness that appear 2–12 hours after exposure to the sun. Scaling and peeling follow any overexposure to sunlight. Dark skin also burns and may appear grayish or gray–black.

The cumulative effects of UV radiation exposure can damage fibroblasts located in the dermis, leading to faulty manufacture of connective tissue and wrinkling of the skin. UV rays also stimulate the production of oxygen free radicals that disrupt collagen and elastic fibers in the extracellular regions. Although a small amount of UV radiation is beneficial, larger amounts may cause alterations in the genetic material in the nucleus of cells—especially the rapidly multiplying cells in the stratum germinativum, increasing the risk of cancer. Depletion of the ozone

SUNBLOCKS

Commercial sunblocks are rated on their ability to occlude UV rays. The ratings are generally on a scale of 1–35, with 1 being least occlusive. Sunblocks with ratings of 35 are total sunblocking agents. Although UV rays are less harmful early in the morning and late in the afternoon, they have also been implicated in skin cancer. It is estimated that there would be a decrease of about 78% of skin cancers if children younger than 18 used sunscreen with a blocking agent of at least 15.

layer and overexposure to the sun may be responsible for increased incidence of skin cancer.

Synthesis of Vitamin D

Excessive exposure to sunlight is harmful; however, some exposure to sunlight is useful and needed by the body. The cells in the stratum germinativum and stratum spinosum convert the compound 7-dehydrocholesterol into a precursor of vitamin D. Vitamin D is a group of closely related steroids produced by the action of ultraviolet light on 7-dehydrocholesterol. Vitamin D synthesized in the skin is transported to the liver and then to the kidneys where it is converted into a more potent form (see Figure 2.4). Vitamin D increases calcium absorption in the intestines and is an important hormone in calcium metabolism. Lack of vitamin D can lead to improper bone mineralization and a disease called **rickets** (in children) and **osteomalacia** (in adults).

Stratum Spinosum

Stratum spinosum consists of 8–10 layers of cells located immediately above the stratum germinativum. As the cells multiply in the stratum germinativum, they are pushed upward into the stratum spinosum. Observed under the microscope, these cells have a spiny appearance, hence, their name. This layer of cells, in addition to keratinocytes, contains Langerhans cells, which are involved in defense mechanisms. Langerhans cells protect the skin from pathogens and destroy abnormal cells, such as cancer cells, that may be present.

Stratum Granulosum

Stratum granulosum consists of 3–5 layers. By the time the keratinocytes reach this layer from the layers below, they have flattened and stopped dividing. The cells have a granular appearance when viewed under the microscope and contain a granular protein known as **keratohyalin,** which organizes keratin into thicker bundles. The cells also contain **lamellar granules,** which release a lipid-rich secretion into the spaces between the cells. These lipid-rich secretions work as a sealant and slow the loss of body flu-

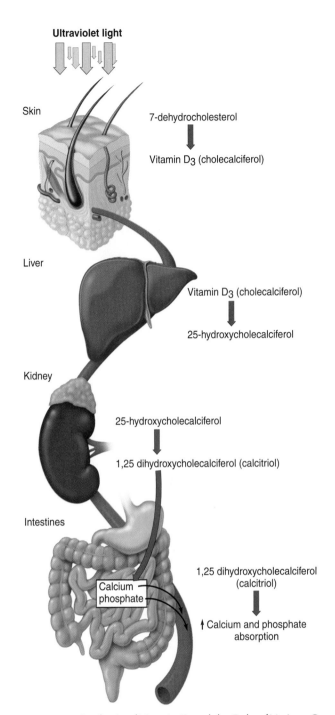

FIGURE 2.4.   Synthesis of Vitamin D and the Role of Various Organs in its Formation

ids. As the cells manufacture keratohyalin, they become flatter and thinner and the cell membranes become thicker and impermeable to water. With time, a thick layer of interlocking keratin fibers surrounded by keratohyalin may be seen within the cell membrane of the original cells, which have now lost their organelles. These structural changes provide protection against pathogens and are responsible for the impermeability of skin to water.

STRATEGY TO PREVENT VITAMIN D DEFICIENCY

The next time you buy milk in the grocery store, look at the label. Many dairy companies add cholecalciferol (identified as Vitamin D) to the milk. Cholecalciferol has drastically reduced vitamin D deficiency in the population.

Stratum Lucidum

Stratum lucidum, as its name indicates, is translucent and consists of densely packed, flat cells that are filled with keratin. This layer is more prominent in the palms of the hands and soles of the feet.

Stratum Corneum

Stratum corneum is the most superficial layer and mostly consists of dead cells and keratin. The transformation from live cells to the dead cells in this layer is known as **keratinization, or cornification** (*corne,* hard or hooflike). There are about 15–30 layers of these cells, which are periodically shed individually or in sheets. It usually takes about 15–30 days for the cells to reach this layer from the stratum germinativum. The cells then remain in the stratum corneum for about 14 days before they are shed. The dryness of this superficial layer, together with the coating of secretions from sebaceous and sweat glands, makes the skin unsuitable for growth of microorganisms. If the skin is exposed to excessive friction, the layer abnormally thickens and forms a **callus.**

Although dead cells make the skin resistant to water, it does not prevent the loss of water by evaporation from the interstitial tissue. About 500 mL of water per day is lost via the skin. This loss of water is known as **insensible perspiration,** which is different from that actively lost by sweating, called **sensible perspiration.**

Promotion of Epidermal Growth

Epidermal growth is promoted by a peptide known as **epidermal growth factor** (EGF). EGF is secreted by various tissues, such as the salivary gland and glands in the duodenum. This factor combines with receptors on the cell membrane of multiplying cells in the epidermis and promotes cell division, production of keratin, and development and repair after injury. So potent, a small sample of EGF from a person's tissue has been used outside the body to form sheets of epidermal cells to cover severe burns.

✚ Psoriasis

This condition, the cause of which is unknown, characteristically presents as scaly patches on the skin. The thickened, scaly patches are a result of the increased rate at which keratinocytes migrate from the stratum germinativum to the surface.

THE DERMIS

The dermis is the connective tissue layer that lies deep to the epidermis. It contains protein fibers and

✚ Burns and Dehydration

When the epidermis of the skin is damaged by a burn injury, water from the interstitial fluid can be more easily lost by evaporation and dehydration can quickly ensue. The loss of the protective barrier makes the person more vulnerable to invasion by pathogens. Dehydration and infection are the major complications of burn injury.

all the cells in the connective tissue proper, such as fibroblasts, macrophages, adipose cells, and mast cells. It supports the epidermis and is the primary source of its nutrients. The dermis contains loose connective tissue that lies closer to the epidermis (**papillary layer, or pars papillaris**) and dense irregular connective tissue deep to the papillary layer (**reticular layer, or pars reticularis**). Collagen and elastic fibers impart strength, elasticity, and extensibility of the skin. The dermis is vascular and contains a network of blood vessels. Lymphatic vessels are also present in abundance in this layer. Accessory structures, such as sweat glands and hair follicles, are located in the dermis. In addition, the dermis contains numerous nerve endings and nerves that convey various sensations from the skin to the central nervous system.

The consistency and texture of skin is largely determined by the water content and the collagen and elastic fibers in the dermis. The water content helps maintain the flexible and resilient properties of the skin, or the **skin turgor.** The collagen and elastic fibers are arranged in parallel bundles. The orientation of the bundles allows the skin to resist the stress placed on it during movement. While the elastic fibers stretch and come back to their original length, the collagen fibers are tough, resisting stretch but allowing twisting and bending.

Figure 2.5 shows the **lines of cleavage** of skin. This is the pattern of collagen and elastic fiber bundles established in the dermis that follow the lines of tension in the skin. The lines of cleavage are of importance, as injuries to the skin that are at right angles to these lines tend to gap because the cut elastic fibers recoil and tend to pull the wound apart. Healing is slower and there is more scarring in this type of injury compared with those injuries parallel to the lines of cleavage.

NERVE SUPPLY TO THE SKIN

The skin is supplied by autonomic nerves, which innervate the blood vessels and glands in the skin. **See page 369** for details of autonomic nerves. Briefly, autonomic nerves supply glands, blood vessels, and in-

Skin Grafts

If the stratum basale has been destroyed over a wide area of skin, as may happen in severe burns or frostbite, skin grafts may be used to speed healing and prevent infection and scarring. In a skin graft, a segment of the skin from a donor site is transplanted to the recipient site. The skin may be transplanted from another area of the body of the injured individual (autograft), taken from a donor or cadaver (allograft), or taken from another species (heterograft). At times, epidermal culturing may be used.

In epidermal culturing, a sample of the epidermis is taken from the injured individual and cultured in a controlled environment that contains growth factors and other stimulatory chemicals. This artificially produced epidermis is then used to cover the injured area. Newer procedures include use of special synthetic skin composed of a plastic "epidermis," a dermis made from collagen fibers (obtained from cow skin), and ground cartilage (obtained from sharks). These materials serve as models for dermal repair and are used as a temporary cover.

STRETCH MARKS

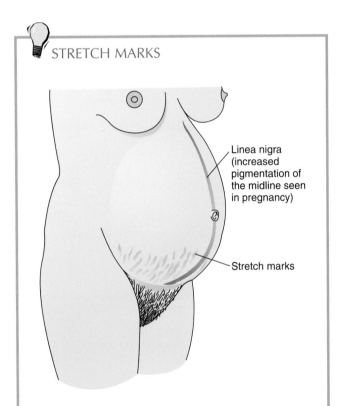

Linea nigra (increased pigmentation of the midline seen in pregnancy)

Stretch marks

Stretch marks (also called striae or lineae albicantes) are produced when the skin is stretched so much that the elastin and collagen fibers in the dermis are damaged. This prevents the skin from recoiling to its original size, with resultant creases and wrinkles commonly referred to as stretch marks. They appear as red or silver-white streaks on the surface of the skin. Stretch marks are common in the abdomen after pregnancy. They are also seen in previously obese individuals who have lost a lot of weight.

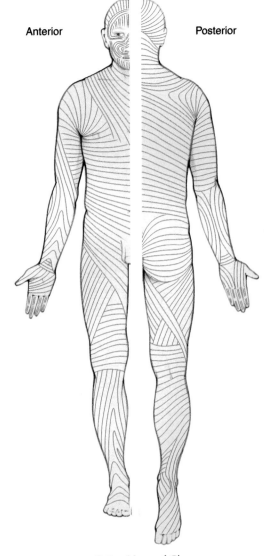

FIGURE 2.5.   Lines of Cleavage

ternal organs. There are two types: sympathetic and parasympathetic.

Sympathetic stimulation and circulating epinephrine and norepinephrine produce vasoconstriction. There are no known vasodilator fibers to the cutaneous blood vessels; dilation is caused by a decrease in the constrictor tone of the sympathetic nerves. Chemicals, such as bradykinin from sweat glands, histamine from mast cells, and vasodilator metabolites from injured cells, have a direct effect on the caliber of blood vessels.

In addition to the autonomic nerves, there are numerous sensory receptors, which respond to sensations such as touch, pressure, pain, cold, and warmth. Mild stimulations, especially if produced by something that moves across the skin, cause itching and tickling sensations (see page 317 for additional information on cutaneous receptors). Any given receptor signals or responds to only one kind of cutaneous sensation. The receptors may be free nerve endings or modified to form special structures that have a surrounding capsule or expanded tips. Some are found wound around hair follicles. The number of sensory receptors per unit area varies from region to region. More receptors are present in areas, such as the face, lips, and fingers, that are more sensitive to sensations.

Shingles

Shingles is a viral infection that infects the dorsal root ganglia; it tends to affect one or more dermatomes and produces a painful rash along its distribution. Massage is contraindicated when rashes are present.

The receptors are continuous with sensory nerves. Sensory nerves from the skin take the impulses generated in the receptors to the central nervous system. The sensory nerves from a specific area of the skin enter a particular segment of the spinal cord. The area of skin supplied by the nerves from a particular spinal segment is known as the **dermatome.** The dermatomes of the different spinal nerves throughout the surface of the body have been traced (Figure 2.6). These patterns are of clinical importance as damage to a spinal nerve results in loss of sensation in the specific dermatome.

The intimate association between the skin and the brain can be appreciated by the fact that the brain has a map, representing the entire body, in the area that perceives sensations. There is a larger representation for regions that are more sensitive than others (Figure 2.7). The pathway taken by impulses gener-

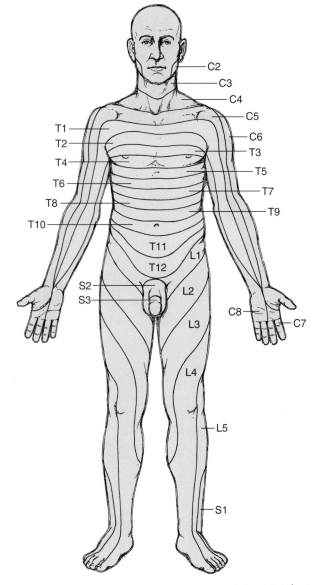
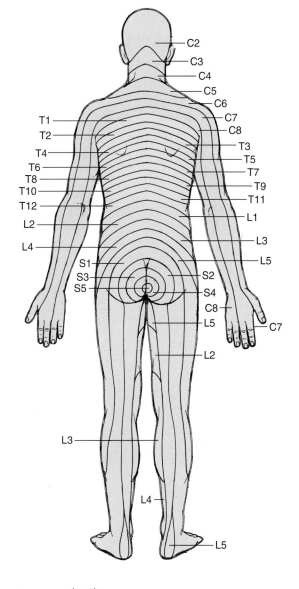

FIGURE **2.6.** Distribution of Dermatomes on the Skin

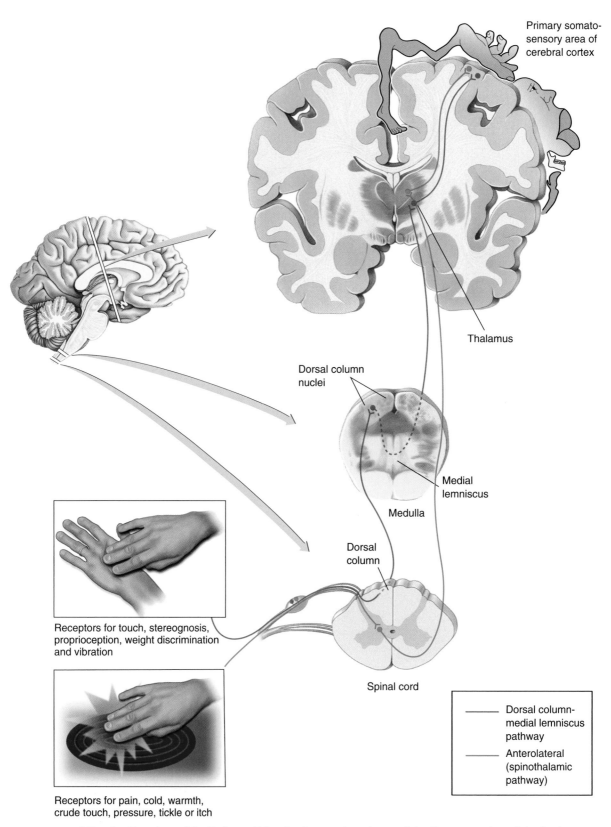

Primary somato-sensory area of cerebral cortex

Thalamus

Dorsal column nuclei

Medial lemniscus

Medulla

Dorsal column

Receptors for touch, stereognosis, proprioception, weight discrimination and vibration

Spinal cord

Receptors for pain, cold, warmth, crude touch, pressure, tickle or itch

——— Dorsal column-medial lemniscus pathway

——— Anterolateral (spinothalamic pathway)

FIGURE 2.7.   An Overview of the Pathway Taken by Sensory Impulses and the Representation of the Body in the Sensory Area of the Cerebral Cortex

ated by the sensory receptors of the skin is also very specific. This is why we are able to locate exactly—up to a few millimeters—where we have been touched on the skin. Many consider the skin an extension of the brain through which interactions between the mind and body can be made by touch. It is interesting to note that during prenatal development, both the skin and the nervous system are derived from the same embryonic layer, the ectoderm (in the embryo, all the structures of the body are derived from three layers—ectoderm, mesoderm, and endoderm).

BLOOD CIRCULATION IN THE SKIN

The skin has an extensive blood supply; 8–10% of the total blood flow in the body can be found in the skin. The heat lost from the body is regulated by altering the volume of blood flowing through the skin.

✚ Hemangiomas

As the name suggests, hemangiomas are abnormal growths of the dermal blood vessels. They may be temporary or permanent. In infants, temporary, bright, raised and rounded lesions, known as strawberry hemangiomas or capillary hemangiomas, may be seen on the skin. They tend to disappear by 5–7 years of age.

Permanent, flat, reddish-purple, disfiguring lesions are known as port-wine stains or cavernous hemangiomas. These affect the larger, deeper vessels of the dermis and are usually seen on the face. They do not disappear with age.

The arteries supplying the skin form a network at the junction of the subcutaneous layer with the dermis. This junction is known as the **cutaneous plexus.** Branches from these arteries supply the adipose tissue located in the subcutaneous layer. Other branches supply the accessory structures as they travel toward the epidermis. These branches form another network at the junction of the dermis and epidermis that follows the contours of the papilla. This junction is known as the **papillary plexus.** The capillaries at this junction join and rejoin to form venules and veins. In many regions, such as the fingers, palms, toes, and ear lobes, direct connections, known as **arteriovenous anastomoses,** link arterioles and venules. These links allow blood diversion, without it entering the superficial capillaries from which heat dissipates.

The blood vessels to the skin are well innervated by the autonomic nervous system. Blood flow can vary widely in response to changing temperatures, from as little as 1 mL to 150 mL/100 g of skin per minute. The plexuses in the skin, to some extent, serve as blood reservoirs. When blood is lost, these vessels constrict,

propelling blood into the systemic circulation to maintain blood flow to the vital organs.

Skin and Temperature Control

The normal oral temperature is 37°C (98.6°F), which is .5 degrees (0.9°F) lower than the rectal temperature representative of core body temperature. Temperatures vary at different parts of the body. In general, the extremities are cooler than the rest of the body. Body temperature must be maintained within a narrow range despite wide temperature fluctuations in the environment. The rate of chemical reactions varies with temperature and enzymes function properly only within a narrow temperature range.

The major processes by which heat is lost from the body are conduction and radiation (70%), sweat vaporization (27%), respiration (2%), and urination and defecation (1%). **Conduction** is the heat exchange between two objects in contact with each other. The amount of heat lost in this way depends on the temperature difference between the objects. Conduction is helped by convection. **Convection** is the movement of molecules away from the area of contact. For example, if the air is cool and it comes in contact with warm skin, the air around the body is warmed; this warm air rises and fresh cool air reaches the skin. Heat can be lost by convection whether the object moves through the medium (e.g., swimming in cold water) or the medium moves over the object (e.g., a cool breeze moving over the skin). **Radiation** is transfer of heat by high frequency waves from one object of a higher temperature to another. It is because of radiation that a person can feel cold in a warm room with cold walls.

Because heat is conducted from an object's surface to the surrounding environment, the amount of body heat lost is largely determined by skin temperature. The temperature of the skin, in turn, depends on the amount of blood that reaches the skin from the skin's deeper layers. Body temperature can be controlled by altering the amount of warm blood reaching the skin. Hair traps some of the heat lost from the skin to the air. When the outside environment is cold, the

---

✚ Shock

Circulatory shock is more pronounced in people with elevated temperature resulting from the dilation of cutaneous blood vessels. People in shock should, therefore, not be warmed to the extent of increasing their body temperature because this can worsen the situation.

Jaundice

In the condition jaundice, the skin has a yellowish tinge, resulting from the accumulation of bilirubin in body fluids. Bilirubin is a breakdown product of hemoglobin. Its levels increase above the normal range if there is rapid and abnormal breakdown of hemoglobin, liver dysfunction, or blockage of the bile duct.

smooth muscles attached to the individual hairs contract and make the hairs stand on end, trapping a layer of air between the hairs. This layer slows down the loss of heat. In man, clothes supplement the layer of hair. Therefore, the amount of heat lost across the clothing depends on the texture and thickness of the clothing. Dark clothing absorbs radiated heat, while light clothing reflects heat.

Transfer of heat causes another mechanism—the evaporation of sweat. Vaporization of 1 gram of water removes approximately 0.6 kcal of heat. During heavy exercise in a hot environment, sweat secretion may be as high as 1,600 mL/hour. Heat loss by vaporization can then be as high as 900 kcal/hour. The rate of vaporization depends on the humidity of the environment and the movement of air around the body.

The body's adjustment to the changing environmental temperature is largely controlled by the hypothalamus and is a result of autonomic, somatic, endocrine, and behavioral changes. Local reflex responses also contribute. For example, when cutaneous blood vessels are cooled, they become more sensitive to circulating catecholamines (e.g., epinephrine) and the arterioles and venules constrict. Other adjustments include shivering, hunger, increased voluntary activity, increased secretion of norepinephrine and epinephrine, and hair "standing on end." When hot, cutaneous vasodilation, sweating, increased respiration, anorexia, apathy, and inertia (to decrease heat production), are some of the adjustments.

The signals that activate the hypothalamus come from temperature-sensitive cells in the hypothalamus and cutaneous temperature receptors.

Variation in Skin Color

BLOOD FLOW AND SKIN COLOR CHANGES

Because blood vessels to the skin are extensive and located close to the surface, alterations in blood flow can be visually observed as changes in skin color. Color changes are better observed in those persons with light-colored skin and may not be as distinct in those persons with dark-colored skin. You can experiment on yourself or your colleagues and observe these changes. The characteristic pink color or reddish tint of the skin is a result of the oxygenated hemoglobin in the red blood cells. When blood flow is reduced temporarily, the skin becomes pale. If pressure is applied to the skin, the blood in the vessels of the skin stagnates. Oxygen in the hemoglobin is quickly used by the tissue in the area, and the hemoglobin becomes darker as a result of deoxyhemoglobin formation. When observed through the skin, this reaction gives a bluish hue, termed **cyanosis.** The bluish discoloration is more prominent in areas where the epithelium is thin, such as the lips, tongue, beneath the nails, and conjunctiva. Watch the color change when you obstruct blood flow by tying a string or rubber band around a finger.

When a person is exposed to a cold environment, the blood vessels to the skin constrict to conserve heat and the person appears pale. If the temperature is low, however, cell injury occurs in exposed areas such as the tip of the nose or ear. The metabolites liberated by the injured cells cause the smooth muscle of the blood vessel walls to dilate, producing the typical redness seen after frostbite.

During exercise, blood vessels in the skin dilate to dissipate heat, while blood vessels in most other parts of the body constrict. This is in response to the hypothalamus, which monitors temperature changes. This reflex response overrides all other reflex responses that may be triggered in the blood vessels in the skin.

White Reaction

Draw a pointed object lightly over your skin and observe what happens. The stroke line becomes pale—the **white line.** The mechanical stimulus causes the smooth muscle guarding blood flow through the capillaries, called the precapillary sphincter, to contract. As a result, blood drains out of the capillaries and small veins and the skin turns pale.

The Triple Response

Now, draw a pointed object more firmly across the skin and observe. The stroke line turns red in about 10 seconds. This is called the **red reaction.** In a few minutes, swelling (**wheal**) and diffuse redness (**flare**) occur around the stroke line. The red reaction is caused by dilation of capillaries as a result of the stroke pressure. The wheal is a result of the increase in permeability of the capillaries and movement of fluid into the interstitial tissue caused by the release of histamine from mast cells located in the region. The flare is a result of arteriolar dilation. Together, the three responses are known as the **triple response** and are part of the normal response to injury.

Reactive Hyperemia

Tie a piece of string (or you may use a rubber band) firmly around your finger. Leave it in place for one minute and then remove it and observe what happens. The skin turns fiery red soon after the occlusion is removed. This is known as **reactive hyperemia.** When blood flow to an area is restricted, the arterioles in that area dilate as a result of the release of chemicals (products of metabolism) by the oxygen-deprived cells. When blood flow is no longer restricted, blood rushes into the dilated blood vessels.

Erythema

At times, the skin appears red after injury, inflammation, or exposure to heat. This redness is a result of dilatation of capillaries in the dermis and is termed **erythema.**

PIGMENTATION OF SKIN BY CAROTENE

Carotene is an orange-yellow pigment that tends to accumulate in epidermal cells and the fat cells of the dermis. It is found in abundance in orange-colored vegetables, such as carrots and squash. Light-skinned individuals who eat a lot of these vegetables, can have an orange hue to their skin as a result of the accumulation of this pigment. In darker-skinned individuals, the hue does not show up as well. Carotene is an important pigment that can be converted to vitamin A, which plays a role in the growth and maintenance of epithelia and synthesis of light receptor pigments of the eye.

SUBCUTANEOUS LAYER, OR HYPODERMIS

The subcutaneous layer, although not actually part of the skin, is an important layer that lies deep to the dermis. It is largely composed of connective tissue,

---

⊕ Pituitary Tumors and Skin Color

Certain tumors of the pituitary gland increase secretion of melanocyte stimulating hormone (MSH) and produce darkening of the skin similar to a deep tan. Increased secretion of adrenocorticotropic hormone (ACTH), which is structurally similar to MSH, from the anterior pituitary gland may also cause similar changes in skin coloration (e.g., as in Addison disease).

💡 SUBCUTANEOUS INJECTIONS

Injections are often given in the subcutaneous layer because of its relatively scarce blood supply and distance from vital organs. Other than safety, drugs are more slowly absorbed from this layer, prolonging their duration of action.

---

which is interwoven with the connective tissue of the dermis. This layer stabilizes the skin, connecting it to underlying structures, while allowing some independent movement. At the same time, the subcutaneous tissue separates the **deep fascia** that surrounds muscles and organs from the skin. Therefore, this layer is also known as the **superficial fascia.** The subcutaneous layer has a deposit of adipose (fat) tissue and serves as an energy reservoir and insulator. The adipose tissue also protects the underlying structures by serving as shock absorbers. The distribution of fat in the subcutaneous layer changes in adulthood. In men, it tends to accumulate in the neck, arms, along the lower back, and buttocks; in women, it accumulates primarily in the breasts, buttocks, hips, and thighs.

ACCESSORY STRUCTURES

The accessory structures of the skin include the sweat glands, sebaceous glands, hair, and nails. They lie primarily in the dermis and project onto the surface through the epidermis.

Sweat Glands

The sweat glands, also known as **sudoriferous** or **eccrine glands** (see Figure 2.1), are coiled tubular glands that are surrounded by a network of capillaries. Located in the dermis, they discharge secretions directly onto the surface of the skin or the hair follicles. There are two types of sweat glands: **eccrine/merocrine** and **apocrine.** Eccrine sweat glands are located over the entire body. There are approximately 2–5 million of these glands, with the forehead, palms, and soles having the highest number.

Sweat is 99% water. The remaining 1% consists of sodium chloride (responsible for sweat's salty taste); other electrolytes; lactic acid; some nutrients, such as glucose and amino acid; and waste products, such as urea, uric acid, and ammonia. The main function of sweat is to cool the surface of the skin and, thereby, reduce the body temperature. The secretory activity of merocrine glands is controlled by the autonomic nerves and circulating hormones. When these glands are secreting at their maximal rate, such as during heavy exercise, up to a gallon (3.8 liters) of water may be lost in one hour.

The acidic pH of sweat, to some extent, deters growth of harmful microorganisms on the surface of the skin. The sweat glands may be considered to have an excretory function as water, electrolytes, and certain organic wastes such as urea are lost in sweat. Certain drugs are also excreted through sweat.

Compared with merocrine glands, there are few **apocrine** sweat glands, which are located in the armpits, around the nipples, in the bearded region (in men), and in the groin area. They start to secrete at puberty and produce a cloudy, sticky secretion, with a characteristic odor. This secretion contains lipids and proteins, in addition to the components of sweat produced by merocrine sweat glands. The apocrine glands are surrounded by myoepithelial cells, which, on contraction, discharge the apocrine secretions into hair follicles. This secretion is a potential nutrient for microorganisms and the action of bacteria on this secretion tends to intensify the odor. The apocrine glands change in size during the menstrual cycle—increasing during ovulation and shrinking at the time of menstruation.

Sebaceous Glands

The sebaceous glands are located close to the hair follicles and discharge their secretions into the hair follicles. In other areas, such as the lips, glans penis, and labia minora, they discharge directly on to the skin surface. There are no sebaceous glands in the palms and soles. The size of the glands varies from region to region. Large glands are present in the breasts, face, neck, and upper part of the chest. They secrete an oily substance and are sometimes referred to as the oil glands. The secretion, called **sebum,** is a mixture of lipids, proteins, and electrolytes. Sebum provides lubrication, protects the keratin of the hair, conditions skin, and prevents excess evaporation of water. These glands are sensitive to sex hormones, and the increase in activity at puberty makes a person more prone to acne. **Acne** is a result of blockage of the sebaceous ducts and inflammation of the sebaceous glands and surrounding area.

Other Glands of the Skin

The skin also contains other specialized glands found in specific regions. The **mammary glands** of the breast, related to the apocrine sweat glands, secrete milk. The regulation of milk secretion and ejection is complex and controlled by hormones and nerves (**see page 398** for details).

Specialized glands, known as **ceruminous glands,** are present in the external auditory canal. These glands are modified sweat glands that secrete **cerumen** or **earwax.** This sticky secretion protects the ear from foreign particles.

Hair

Hair, or **pili,** is seen in almost all parts of the body. It originates from structures known as **hair follicles,** which are found in the dermis. Hair is formed in the follicles by a specialized cornification process and is made up of soft and hard keratin, which gives it its characteristic texture and color. The deepest part of the hair follicle enlarges slightly to form the hair bulb and encloses a network of capillaries and nerves. A strip of smooth muscle, known as the **arrector pili muscle,** extends from the upper part of the dermis to connective tissue surrounding the hair. Stimulation of this muscle makes the hair stand on end (goose pimples, goose flesh, or goose bumps) and traps a layer of air next to the skin, further helping to insulate the body.

There are two types of hair. Fine, fuzzy hair is known as **vellus hair.** The heavy, deeply pigmented hair, as found in the head and eyebrow, is known as **terminal hair.** The growth of hair is greatly influenced by circulating hormones.

Hair has many functions. Scalp hair protects the head from UV rays and serves as insulation. Hair found in the nose, ears, and eyelashes helps prevent entry of larger particles and insects. The nerve plexus surrounding the follicle detects small hair movements and senses imminent injury.

Hair color reflects the pigment differences produced by melanocytes in the hair papilla. Although genetics play an important part, hormones and nutrition have an important role too. With age, as pigment production decreases, hair appears gray.

Hair grows and sheds according to a hair growth cycle. Hair in the scalp may grow for 2–5 years at the rate of about .33 mm per day. The rate varies from individual to individual. As the hair grows, the nutrients required for hair formation are absorbed from the blood. Heavy metals may also be absorbed, and hair samples can be used for identifying lead poisoning. Hair is, therefore, one of the important specimens analyzed in forensic medicine. As a hair reaches the end of the growth cycle, the attachment to the hair follicle weakens and the follicle becomes inactive. Eventually, the hair is shed and a new hair begins to form. Hair loss can be affected by such factors as drugs, diet, radiation, excess vitamin A, stress, and hormonal levels.

Nails

Nails protect the tips of the fingers and toes and limit the distortion when exposed to excess stress.

Nails are formed at the nail root, an epithelial fold deeply located near the periosteum of the bone. The body of the nail is composed of dead cells that are packed with keratin. Nail growth can be altered by body metabolism. Changes in structure, thickness, and shape can indicate different systemic conditions.

Absorption Through the Skin

Substances that are lipid-soluble can penetrate the epidermis, although rather slowly. On reaching the dermis, the substance is absorbed into the circulation. Administering a brief pulse of electricity can speed penetration. The electrical pulse creates channels in the stratum corneum by changing the position of cells.

As a result of slow absorption, drugs are often administered via the skin, producing slow and prolonged action over several days. Nicotine patches, an aid used by smokers to quit smoking, use this type of transdermal administration. By slow and continuous administration of nicotine, the craving for smoking is reduced. Gradually, the dosage of nicotine in the patch can be tapered. Dimethyl sulfoxide (DMSO) is a drug given for treatment of joint and muscle injuries. Other drugs dissolved in DMSO are easily absorbed through the skin. Estrogen, for the treatment of menopause, and vasodilator drugs, for increasing the coronary blood flow, are examples of transdermally administered drugs.

Systemic adverse effects can be produced if drugs are administered transdermally for prolonged periods. For example, corticosteroids used to treat chronic inflammation can be absorbed through the skin and produce symptoms of corticosteroid excess or Cushing's syndrome.

Microorganisms on the Skin

This chapter on the integumentary system would not be complete without considering the invisible layer of microorganisms that inhabit the surface of the skin. This huge colony of organisms is the **"normal microbial flora."** Similar to residents and tourists in a city, there are resident microorganisms (resident flora) that are regularly found in a specific area at a specific age and transient flora that inhabit the skin for hours, days, or weeks. The resident flora play an important part in maintaining health and normal function.

Resident flora prevent harmful bacteria from thriving on the skin by directly inhibiting them or competing with them for nutrients. However, resident bacteria can be infective and harmful if they are introduced in large amounts into the bloodstream, which can occur when the skin is injured or when surgery is performed without adequately cleansing the skin surface before incision. They may also be harmful in individuals whose immunity has been significantly suppressed.

It may be surprising to learn that profuse sweating, washing, and bathing cannot significantly alter normal flora. The skin must be treated with special solutions to make it sterile. This should not deter hand washing before and after treating clients, however. Potential pathogens are easily removed by water and scrubbing with soap containing disinfectants has an even greater effect.

Inflammation and Healing

Inflammation—the reaction of living tissue to injury—is easily visualized on the surface of the skin. Inflammation and healing are detailed under this system, although these processes occur throughout the body. Although inflammation produces discomfort, it is beneficial and helps the body adapt to everyday stress. Inflammation helps heal wounds and prevents and combats infection. Inflammation depends on a healthy immune system.

COMMON CAUSES OF INFLAMMATION

Some common causes of inflammation are physical (burns; extreme cold, such as frostbite; trauma); chemical (chemical poisons, such as acid or organic poisons); infection (bacteria, viruses, fungi, or parasites); and immunologic and other circumstances that lead to tissue damage, such as vascular or hormonal disturbances. It is important to note that inflammation is not always a result of infection. Conditions producing inflammation are denoted by adding the suffix, itis. For example, arthr<u>itis</u>, inflammation of the joint; burs<u>itis</u>, inflammation of the bursa; appendic<u>itis</u>, inflammation of the appendix; and neur<u>itis</u>, inflammation of the nerve.

✚ **Dermatitis and Cellulitis**

Dermatitis is an inflammation of the skin that involves the dermis. There are many forms of dermatitis, such as contact dermatitis and eczema. If the inflammation spreads along the connective tissue of the skin, it is known as cellulitis.

CARDINAL SIGNS OF INFLAMMATION

Despite the many causes of inflammation (see Figure 2.8), the sequence of physiologic changes that occur in the body are the same. If you scratch your forearm and observe the changes that occur, you will see the cardinal signs of inflammation, including redness, heat, swelling, pain, and loss of function.

These signs are caused by changes that occur at the microscopic level. When you scratch your forearm, you may notice immediate whitening of the skin. This reaction is a result of the constriction of blood vessels lying under the skin. Soon, the area appears red (hyperemia). The blood vessels in the area dilate as a result of the liberation of chemicals by the injured tissue. If touched, the area feels warm. The warmth is a result of increased blood flow. Within minutes, swelling occurs along the line of injury (exudation). This swelling is a result of the fluid leakage from the capillaries, which have become more permeable. The contents of the injured cells leak out and stimulate pain receptors in the vicinity, causing pain. The injured tissue may be unable to function properly, partly because of pain.

These signs help control the effects of the injurious agent. The fluid that leaks out and the increased blood flow dilute the toxins that are produced. The pain alerts the individual to take remedial measures. The changes that occur with injury also stimulate clotting, reducing blood loss and containing the toxins within the local area.

Role of White Blood Cells

In inflammation, together with changes in the blood vessels, the white blood cells are triggered into action. Immediately after the injury, the white blood

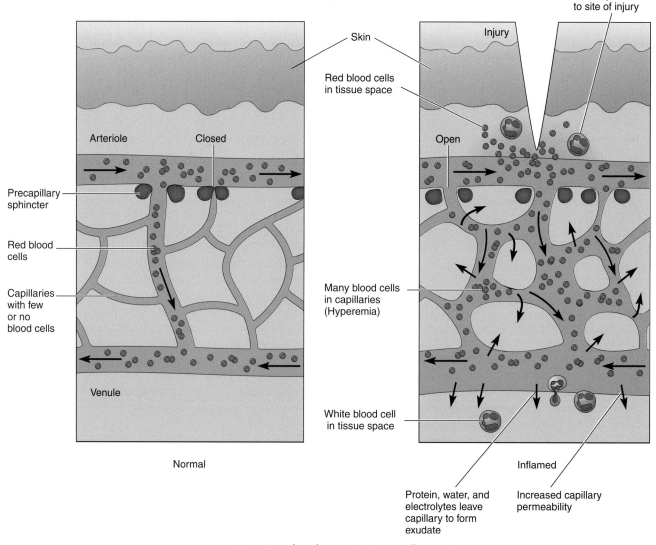

FIGURE 2.8.   Vascular Changes in Acute Inflammation

cells accumulate along the blood vessel walls, referred to as **margination** or **pavementing** of white blood cells. Attracted by the chemicals liberated by the injured tissue, they squeeze through the widened gap between the cells of the capillary wall. This stage is known as the **emigration** of white blood cells. The white cells then move to the injured region. The process by which the white cells are attracted to the tissue is called **chemotaxis.** On reaching the tissue, they destroy cells and other structures that they perceive as nonself (**see page 460**). This process is called **phagocytosis.** Of the white blood cells, neutrophils and monocytes are most capable of phagocytosis. They do so by extending two arms of the cell membrane around the foreign or dead tissue. The two extensions then fuse, engulfing the foreign tissue into the cytoplasm, forming what is called a **phagosome.** Lysosomes, vesicles containing digestive enzymes that are present in the cytoplasm of the white cell, fuse with the phagosome and kill and digest the engulfed debris.

Chemical Mediators

Although the process of inflammation is initiated by injury and death of cells, the signs and symptoms that accompany it are a result of locally liberated chemicals—the chemical mediators. These mediators are secreted in many ways. Some are secreted by white blood cells or by cells, such as mast cells, located in the connective tissue. Some of the mediators are formed by chemical reactions triggered locally by tissue injury. Some chemical mediators are histamines, prostaglandins, leukotrienes, bradykinin, tumor necrosis factor, and complement fractions (**see page 522**).

SYMPTOMS ACCOMPANYING INFLAMMATION

Whatever the cause, inflammation produces symptoms that may last for only a few hours or for days. Remember a time when you had an injury or infection. Fever, loss of appetite, lethargy, and sleepiness are some symptoms that you may have noticed. These responses are mainly a result of the chemical mediators. An increased number of white blood cells, an increased liver activity, and a decreased iron level in the blood (which results in anemia) are some unseen responses that occur during the inflammatory process. Amino acids, the building blocks of protein, are used up to make new cells and form collagen for repair. This increase in energy usage, along with loss of appetite, is responsible for weight loss often seen with inflammation.

RESOLUTION OF INFLAMMATION

Inflammation can resolve in three ways: (1) it can slowly disappear, with the tissue appearing normal or close to normal (heal); (2) it can progress, with much fluid collecting in the area (exudative inflammation); or, (3) it can become chronic.

EXUDATIVE INFLAMMATION

Inflammation invariably results in different types of fluid collecting outside the cells in the injured area. This fluid is called an **exudate.** Exudates vary in composition of protein, fluid, and cell content. For example, after a small area of your skin is burned, a blister forms. This blister is filled with a clear exudate, which indicates low protein content. This is known as **serous exudate.**

Inflammation sometimes results in a thick and sticky exudate that contains fibrous tissue. The fibers are actually a meshwork of proteins. When this type of inflammation resolves, increased adhesion and scar tissue often occurs in the area. This type of reaction is beneficial, however, as it causes the adjacent tissue to stick to each other and prevents spread of infection to surrounding areas. This exudate is known as **fibrinous exudate.**

The white fluid that collects in an inflamed area especially if it is infected, is **pus,** or **purulent exudate.** The yellowish-white color of pus is actually caused by dead tissue, white blood cells, cellular debris, and protein. Purulent exudate may collect in different ways. It may be collected within a capsule to form an **abscess.** If immunity is low, purulent exudate may spread over a large surface of tissue.

Occasionally, the fluid that collects is blood-tinged. This is **hemorrhagic exudate.** In this case, the blood vessels are injured or the tissue is crushed. Inflammation may result in a **membranous exudate,** in which a membrane or sheet is formed on tissue surface. The membrane is a result of dead tissue caught up in the fibrous secretions.

CHRONIC INFLAMMATION

An inflammation is considered **chronic** when it persists over a long period. In some cases, it may persist for months and years. As a general rule, however, a chronic inflammation is one that lasts for longer than six weeks. Medically, inflammation is considered chronic if the area is infiltrated by many lymphocytes and macrophages, if growth of new capillaries occurs, and if there is an abundance of fibroblasts in the area. Usually inflammation becomes chronic when the initial injury or irritant persists. For example, people working with asbestos can have chronic inflammation in the lungs resulting from inhaled asbestos, a condition called asbestosis. Many bacteria, fungi, viruses, and parasites can also produce chronic inflammation. For example, tubercle bacillus, engulfed by macrophages, remains alive and produces chronic inflammatory changes in the lung. Chronic inflammation may present as **fibrosis, ulcer, sinus,** or **fistula.**

Fibrosis is a reaction caused by fibroblasts that produce collagen and fibrous tissue. Fibrosis results in the formation of scar tissue and adhesions.

In some cases, chronic inflammation may lead to **ulcer** formation. An ulcer is formed when an organ or tissue surface is lost as a result of the death of cells and is replaced by inflammatory tissue. Usually, ulcers are found in the gut and the skin.

A **sinus** is another presentation of chronic inflammation. A sinus is a tract leading from a cavity to the surface. For example, sinuses may be associated with osteomyelitis, in which, as the bone cells die, they form an artificial tract leading from the bone to the surface of the skin through which the dead tissue exudes.

A **fistula** is a tract that is open at both ends and through which abnormal communication is established between two surfaces. For example, when cells die while receiving radiotherapy for treatment of cervical cancer, a fistula may develop between the bladder and the vagina.

HEALING AND REPAIR

The outcome of inflammation depends on many issues. Other than the extent of the injury to the specific tissue, repair and healing depend on the properties of the cells in the tissue. The cells of the body can be divided into three groups, based on their capacity to regenerate—**labile cells, stable cells,** and **permanent cells.**

FACTORS THAT AFFECT HEALING

One method that speeds healing is to remove foreign material by cleansing the wound. In surgery, healing is speeded by using sutures to bring the edges of the wound together. However, suture material is foreign and can deter healing when it remains in place for too long. Sutures are removed a few days after surgery or are made of absorbable materials. To prevent infection, antibiotic creams or liquids are used to cleanse wounds. If a large area has been injured, skin grafts are used to speed healing.

Cells with the capacity to regenerate throughout life quickly multiply and produce new cells to take the place of injured or dead tissue. These are known as **labile cells.** Examples are epidermal cells, genitourinary tract cells, cells lining the gut, hair follicle cells, and epithelial cells of ducts.

Another group of cells, known as **stable cells,** have a low rate of division, but are able to regenerate if injured. Examples are liver cells, pancreatic cells, fibroblasts, and endothelial cells. To regenerate, these cells require the presence of a connective tissue framework. Also, a sufficient number of live cells must be present for regeneration to occur. For example, if extensive injury occurs in the liver, the connective tissue framework is lost and the liver only heals by fibrosis, with liver failure as the outcome. However, the liver can recover fully after minimal injury.

Cells of the nervous system, cardiac muscle, and skeletal muscle are referred to as **permanent cells.** These cells cannot divide, and the injured and dead cells are replaced by fibrous tissue and scar formation.

Study of the mechanisms involved in the healing of skin wounds gives insight into healing in general. Figures 2.9 and 2.10 show the mechanism involved in the healing of deep (healing by second intention) and superficial (healing by first or primary intention) skin wounds. The role of massage in inflammation is discussed on page 75.

Effects of Aging on the Integumentary System

All components of the integumentary system are affected by aging. The skin changes that develop with age must be considered by the therapist when planning treatment for clients in an older age-group. The epidermis becomes thinner as a result of a significant decrease in the activity of the stratum germinativum, which makes older persons more prone to infection, injury, and delayed healing. The number of Langerhans cells decreases, increasing the risk of infection.

Keloids and Scars

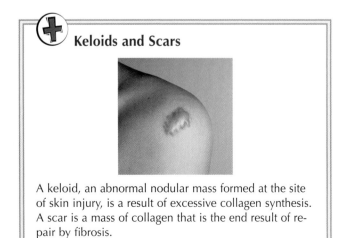

A keloid, an abnormal nodular mass formed at the site of skin injury, is a result of excessive collagen synthesis. A scar is a mass of collagen that is the end result of repair by fibrosis.

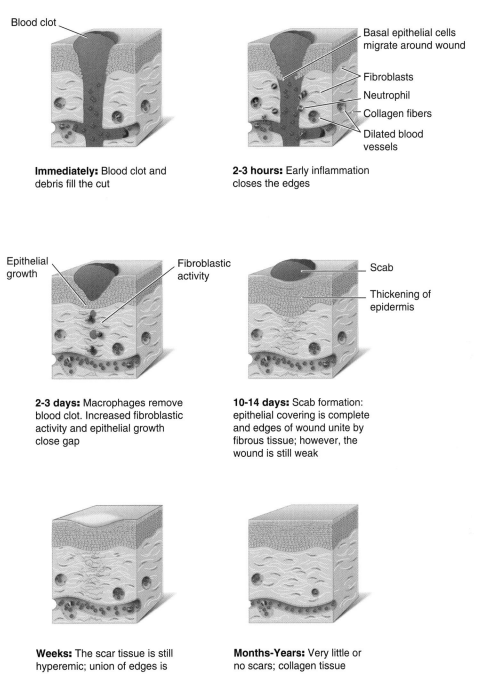

Blood clot

Immediately: Blood clot and debris fill the cut

Basal epithelial cells migrate around wound

Fibroblasts

Neutrophil

Collagen fibers

Dilated blood vessels

2-3 hours: Early inflammation closes the edges

Epithelial growth

Fibroblastic activity

2-3 days: Macrophages remove blood clot. Increased fibroblastic activity and epithelial growth close gap

Scab

Thickening of epidermis

10-14 days: Scab formation: epithelial covering is complete and edges of wound unite by fibrous tissue; however, the wound is still weak

Weeks: The scar tissue is still hyperemic; union of edges is good but not full strength

Months-Years: Very little or no scars; collagen tissue remodelled by enzymes; normal blood flow

FIGURE 2.9.   Healing of Skin Wounds by Second Intention

The decrease in the production of vitamin D_3 results in reduction in calcium and phosphate absorption from the gut, leading to fragile bones. Melanocytes decrease in number with resultant pigment changes in the skin (e.g., liver spots or senile lentigo). The skin becomes more vulnerable to injury from sun exposure.

The dermis thins and the number of elastin fibers decreases. The ground substance tends to become dehydrated. An elderly person's skin is, therefore, weaker, with a tendency to wrinkle and sag. The mechanical strength of the junction between the epidermis and dermis diminishes, which may account for the ease with which blisters form in elderly persons.

The glandular secretions decrease, resulting in dry skin that is prone to infection. The reduction in sweat production; loss of subcutaneous adipose tissue in many parts of the body, especially the limbs; and feeble skin circulation affects thermoregulation. As a result, elderly persons are more easily affected by changes in environmental temperature.

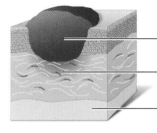

Early

— Wound filled with blood clot

— Location of acute inflammation

— Subcutaneous tissue

A few days later

— Scab

— Contraction of wound size due to action of fibroblasts

— Mitotic activity of epithelium

— New capillary loops

Approximately 1 week later

— Scab shed

— Loose connective tissue formed by fibroblasts

A few weeks later

— Epithelium covers wound site

— Scar tissue

After a month

— Collagen fibers relaid

FIGURE 2.10.   Healing of Skin Wounds by First Intention

The formation of hair slows down in the hair follicles, resulting in finer hair. Reduced melanocyte activity results in gray or white hair. Both sexes experience hair loss, with the onset at about age 30 in men and after menopause in women. Loss of axillary hair and pubic hair is slower than that of scalp hair. In men, hair growth may increase in the nostrils and ears.

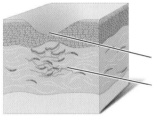

HELP FOR WRINKLES?

Tretinoin (*Retin-A* ™) is a drug in the form of a gel or cream that is derived from Vitamin A. It increases blood flow to the dermis and speeds dermal repair, decreasing the rate of wrinkle formation and reducing the appearance of already existing wrinkles. To reduce wrinkles in the skin, some persons resort to botulism toxin injection into facial muscles. By paralyzing the muscles, the pull on the skin is reduced and wrinkles disappear.

Nail growth is also slower as one ages. Changes in the nail components result in a dull, yellowish appearance. The nails tend to thicken, especially in the toes where toenails may become curved and hooked.

Age does not seem to affect the skin's ability to serve as a barrier to water vapor loss. The cutaneous nerves also do not significantly change with age.

Integumentary System and Bodyworkers

The importance of touch as an avenue for healing of the mind and body cannot be underestimated. Studies of healthy, preterm infants have shown that massage facilitates growth and development.[1] The internal state of mind directly affects the surface of the skin, evidenced by blushing when embarrassed or turning pale when frightened. Often, diseases of the mind and body present as changes in color, tone, or even abnormal lesions on the skin. Because the skin is the largest sensor that informs the mind about the external environment, it is conceivable for techniques used on the skin to affect the mind and internal organs in various ways.

It is well known that skin stimulation can trigger various reflexes.[2] Some of the therapeutic effects of massage seem to arise from altered blood flow and pain suppression in deeper structures by such reflexes. These reflexes, known as **cutaneovisceral reflexes,** involve both the autonomic nerves and the rich sensory plexuses in the skin. Some examples of cutaneovisceral reflexes are the abdominal reflex (contraction of the abdominal muscles on stroking the skin over the abdomen), the plantar reflex (contraction of the muscles of the foot on stroking the sole of the foot), and the gag reflex (emptying of the stomach on tickling the back of the throat).

Massage has the ability to mechanically change the texture and consistency of skin. For example, the skin becomes softer and suppler when massaged. With recurrent and prolonged manipulation, the skin can become more resilient, flexible, and elastic. At the superficial level, massage helps to remove dry, scaly skin. At a deeper level, important effects of massage include the ability to help realign collagen fibers in the dermis during and after the healing of deep skin wounds. Fibrous scar tissue can potentially trap nerves, blood vessels, and lymphatics. By realigning collagen fibers and facilitating the movement of skin over other superficial structures, massage can help prevent problems caused by this entrapment.

One of the physiologic effects of massage is the capacity to increase local blood and lymph flow, improving the nutritive status, facilitating the removal of toxins released by injured tissue, and quickening healing. The increase in blood and lymph flow may be a result of direct mechanical displacement, as well as reflex nervous responses of blood and lymph channels walls induced by application of pressure to cutaneous areas. In addition, release of vasodilator substances, such as histamine from mast cells, is linked to local increase in blood flow. It should be remembered that massage can quicken drug absorption in injection sites secondary to the increase in blood flow. Other physiologic effects include an increase in insensible perspiration and facilitation of sebaceous secretion.

Undoubtedly, massage can reduce the pain perceived by the brain, as explained by the gate-control mechanism (see page 342). The therapeutic effect may be a result of both a psychological and physiologic phenomenon. Even without scientific explanation, most persons automatically knead or touch or massage a painful area and find relief. Massage, in general, produces a sense of well-being and renewed vigor. Evidence also suggests that it reduces stress, anxiety, and pain perception and has a positive effect on immune function.[3,4]

INFLAMMATION AND MASSAGE

During the acute stage, massage increases comfort by relaxing unaffected areas. Lymphatic drainage techniques proximal to the site of injury help reduce swelling and pain. Passive movements of unaffected joints help maintain the health and range of motion of joints. In the chronic stage, massage helps reduce adhesions, align collagen fibers in scar tissue and maintain strength and range of motion.

MASSAGE TECHNIQUES AND THE EFFECTS ON THE BODY

The mechanical, reflex, physiological, psychological, and psychoneuroimmunologic effects of massage are related to the technique used[2]. Mechanical effects are those caused by physically moving the tissues (e.g., compression, stretch, etc.) Reflex effects are changes in function caused by the nervous system. Physio-logic effects involve changes in body processes caused by nerves, hormones, and chemicals. Psychological effects are emotional or behavioral changes. Psychoneuroimmunologic effects are those that alter hormone levels and function through stimulation of the neurohormonal system.

The techniques used in the manipulation of skin and underlying tissue can be categorized as:

- **superficial reflex techniques**
- **superficial fluid techniques**
- **neuromuscular techniques**
- **connective tissue techniques**
- **passive movement techniques.**

Superficial Reflex Techniques

When superficial reflex techniques are used, changes are brought about by reflexes. No mechanical effects are produced. Therefore, the direction of the stroke is unimportant. These techniques primarily affect the level of arousal, perception of pain, or autonomic balance and have been shown to have positive effects on the physiologic and psychological development of premature infants.[1] Examples of superficial reflex techniques include static contact, superficial stroking, and fine vibration.

Static contact is synonymous with a resting position, passive touch, superficial touch, light touch, maintained touch, or stationary hold. In this technique, minimal force is used and the therapist's hands are still. This technique produces sedative effects and reduces anxiety. It is often used at the beginning and end of massage.

Superficial stroking is also known as light stroking, feather stroking, or nerve stroking. In this technique, the therapist's hands glide over the skin with little pressure on the subcutaneous tissue. It is used to alter arousal levels and to reduce pain. Pain is reduced by stimulation of large diameter touch nerve fibers, which, in turn, reduce the transmission of pain impulses to the brain (gate control mechanism). Local reflexes triggered by the strokes reduce muscle spasm and tension.

Fine vibration, also known as vibration, cutaneous vibration, transcutaneous vibration, mechanical vibration, and vibratory stimulation, is a technique in which rapid, trembling movement with minimal pressure is produced by the therapist on the client's skin. Studies of the effects of vibration using mechanical vibration have shown that the pain threshold increases, causing reduction in pain.[5] Such an effect is produced even if the stimulation is given at different sites—proximal to, distal to, or on the site of pain or in the contralateral region. An increase in muscular tone may be seen below the site of stimulation.

Superficial Fluid Techniques

Superficial fluid techniques are those that affect structures in the dermis and subcutaneous tissue. Superficial effleurage and superficial lymph drainage techniques are in this category. In superficial effleurage—also known as effleurage—gliding, stroking, or deep stroking, gliding movements are used. In addition to producing reflex effects similar to those of superficial stroking techniques, these movements affect lymphatic and venous return in skin and deeper structures by mechanical compression. They are, therefore, particularly effective in reducing edema. These techniques also have psychological and other physiologic effects, such as reduced anxiety, increased relaxation, reduced muscle excitability, and increased intestinal movement.

The superficial lymph drainage technique uses short, rhythmic, nongliding strokes in the direction of lymph flow. The strokes result in gentle stretching of the skin and superficial fascia, together with the stimulation of contraction of lymph vessels. If performed over a large surface area of the body, it effectively increases lymph return to the veins. In addition, these techniques reduce anxiety and pain, produce sedation, and improve immune function.

Neuromuscular Techniques

Neuromuscular techniques include broad contact compression (compression, pressure, pressing), petrissage (kneading), stripping (stripping massage, deep stroking massage), and specific compression (focal compression, ischemic compression, digital compression, digital pressure, direct pressure, static friction, and deep touch)[2]. These techniques affect both superficial and deeper tissues, such as muscle. Broad contact compression has been shown to increase blood and lymph flow.[6] It may increase or decrease muscle resting tension and have a stimulating or sedative effect, depending on the rate and pressure of strokes. Hence, it is commonly used in sports massage.

In petrissage, the tissue is repetitively compressed, dragged, lifted, and released against underlying structures. These strokes relieve anxiety, improve immune function, and positively alter allergic responses. In addition, petrissage has been shown to increase mobility of connective tissue and extensibility of muscle, reduce muscle tension, enhance muscle performance, and increase joint motion.[7] These effects may be caused by cutaneovisceral reflexes and mechanical compression.

In stripping, slow, gliding strokes are applied from one attachment of muscle to the other. It may be used to reduce the activity of myofascial trigger points (points on the surface of the body that are sensitive to touch and cause pain that travels or spreads when palpated). In addition to affecting trigger points, stripping may have the same effects as petrissage. Strokes performed in the direction of the natural flow result in emptying of veins and lymphatics. For this effect to occur, the muscles must be totally relaxed and the effects of gravity must be employed (e.g., limb elevation, recumbent position). It is important for proximal muscles to be relaxed while working on distal areas. If the pressure exerted is excessive, the arterial blood flow that occurs in the opposite direction of veins and lymphatics may be impeded. Heavy pressure may also result in a protective reflex contraction of muscles.

In specific compression, pressure is applied to a specific muscle, tendon, or connective tissue in a direction perpendicular to the tissue in question. This technique is used extensively by bodyworkers, either alone or in combination with other techniques (e.g., shiatsu, acupressure, and reflexology). It may help soften adhesions and fibrosis. The fact that it is used to reduce pain and produce physiologic effects in regions far from the site of application suggests that it works by triggering complex somatovisceral reflexes.[8]

Connective Tissue Technique

Connective tissue technique uses palpation to help remodel and lengthen connective tissue. Friction (circular friction, transverse friction, deep friction, deep transverse friction, cross-fiber friction, and Cyriax friction), skin rolling (tissue rolling, rolling), myofascial release (myofascial stretching), and direct fascial techniques (connective tissue technique, bindege websmassage, myofascial massage, deep tissue massage, deep stroking, strumming, ironing, myofascial manipulation, and soft-tissue mobilization) are some of the methods used.[2] This technique is accompanied by reactive hyperemia and local increase in temperature. Hyperemia may result from release of histamine from mast cells and autonomic reflexes. It is claimed[9] that these effects may last for several hours following manipulation. Connective tissue techniques may have a powerful analgesic action that may be explained by the gate-control theory and release of natural painkillers.

Friction massage frees adherent skin, loosens scars and adhesions of deeper tissues, and reduces local edema. Repetitive, nongliding techniques are used in friction massage to produce movement between the fibers of connective tissue. In skin rolling, the tissue superficial to the deep fascia (the connective tissue layer investing muscles) is grasped and, using gliding strokes, lifted and rolled over in a wavelike motion. This stroke results in mechanical stretch of the connective tissue, releasing adhesions that may restrict

Foot Reflexology

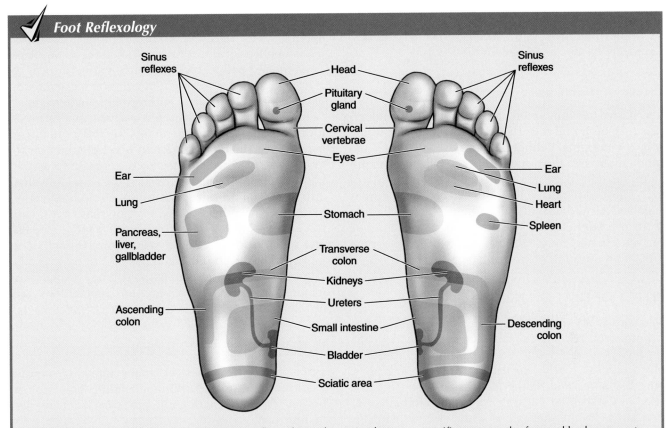

Foot reflexology is based on the belief that a reflex relationship exists between specific areas on the feet and body segments and organs. Thickening, pain, and tenderness of certain areas of the foot may reflect dysfunction of the related organ. In order to normalize the dysfunction, specific compression is applied to the reflex points on the foot. The mechanism by which this technique produces its effects is not known. General outcomes of reflexology include reduced anxiety, improved mood and energy, and increased relaxation.

Specific Compression and Acupoints

Chinese medicine believes that energy travels through the body in channels called meridians. There are 12 paired bilateral meridians and 2 median sagittal meridians. Each meridian is associated with a specific organ and its physiologic functions and has a basic quality of energy (yin or yang), which may not coincide with functions identified by Western medicine. Small points, called acupoints, have been identified along each meridian. Acupoints may be located close to the surface or deep to it and show altered sensitivity in diseased states. Stimulation of acupoints affects the related organs and physiologic functions at remote sites.

Acupoints may be stimulated by acupuncture, massage, electrical current, laser, and moxibustion (dried herbal agents, such as mugwort leaves, are formed into a cone and ignited over the acupoint). Acupressure and shiatsu use techniques such as compression to stimulate the points. Research shows that stimulating acupoints may reduce nausea and vomiting during and after surgery and may have a positive effect in sleep disorders and other disorders.

mobility. In myofascial stretching or release, nongliding traction is applied to muscle and the associated fascia. This technique, similar to direct fascial techniques, also results in mechanical lengthening of the fascia and is widely used in musculoskeletal conditions to increase mobility.

Passive Movement Techniques

Passive movement techniques use passive motion to treat various conditions. They include shaking (muscle shaking, course vibration, rolling friction, and jostling), rhythmic mobilization, and rocking (pelvic rocking, rocking vibration).[2] These techniques have

greater effects on muscles and joints. They produce sedation (possibly by stimulating vestibular reflexes) and decrease anxiety and pain perception.

Percussive Techniques

Percussive techniques alternatively deform and release tissue at varying rhythms and pressure. Clapping or cupping, tapping, hacking, pounding, and tapotement are some examples.[2] These strokes result in initial skin blanching as a result of contraction of arterioles from mechanical stimulation. Blanching is followed by redness brought about by vasodilation from overstimulation. The effects of this technique on muscle tone and alertness vary with the rate, vigor, and duration of strokes.

EFFECT OF HEAT ON SKIN

Massage is often preceded by application of heat to the involved part. Local heat can be applied in the form of poultices, hot water packs, hot water bottles, electric pads, special electric lamps, chemical pads, paraffin baths, and diathermy. General heat may be used in the form of hot water baths, steam baths, vapor baths, dry thermal cabinets, and electric blankets.

When heat is applied for a short period, it causes peripheral vasodilatation, redness of skin, general and local muscular relaxation, increase in pulse rate and respiratory rate, shallow respiration, decrease in blood pressure, and diminished heat production. Heat opens up vascular channels and softens the tissues, permitting more effective application of massage. It stimulates the circulation, speeds removal of inflammation waste products and, thereby, relieves pain, swelling, and spasm.

Dangers of Local Heat Use

- Inflammation and congestion may increase
- Severe burns, if the client is not properly monitored
- Feedback may be inadequate if there is reduced or no sensation in the region of application
- Local application of heat to ischemic parts (e.g., in those persons with peripheral vascular disease or deep vein thrombosis) may increase tissue oxygen consumption, which may worsen the underlying condition.

EFFECT OF COLD ON SKIN

The rate of skin cooling is faster than the rate of rewarming, implying that a shorter period of cold application suffices to cool the skin. The depth of cold penetration depends on the duration and the area of application. Areas of the body containing more adipose tissue take a longer time to change temperature.

If deeper structures are to be cooled, the duration of application is increased. When cold, in the form of water, is applied locally, it results in peripheral vasoconstriction and pallor. The vasoconstriction, in turn, results in a decrease in skin temperature and reduction of edema, muscle spasm, and further hemorrhage.

Analgesic effects begin when skin temperature is lowered to approximately 13.6°C (56.5°F). Analgesia is produced by the reduction in nerve conduction velocity by cold. Systemic reactions, such as increase in heart rate, respiratory rate, blood pressure, and shivering, may be produced. Soon after cold application has ended, peripheral vasodilatation may occur, with redness of skin, feeling of warmth, slowing of pulse and respiratory rates, and relaxation. This reaction may last for 20–30 minutes.

For therapeutic purposes, both types of reactions may be desirable and cold and hot applications may be alternated.

WATER AND SKIN

The special properties of water make it a good medium for heat and cold application. The application of water for therapeutic purposes is termed **hydrotherapy.**

Water is referred to as a flexible therapeutic agent because of its unique chemical and physical properties. It can be used as a liquid, solid (ice), or gas (steam). Water transports heat by convection as it easily circulates. Because many calories (the unit of quantity of heat; also expressed in joules) are required to increase temperature by even one degree, cold water absorbs a lot of heat energy when it is warmed by surrounding objects. Conversely, a lot of heat is liberated when water is cooled. Also, a number of heat calories are required for the conversion of water to steam. This prop-

Table 2.1

Arbitrary Classification of Temperatures and Adjectives Used for Describing Temperature

	TEMPERATURE	
Adjective	Centigrade	Fahrenheit
Very cold	Below 13	below 55
Cold	13–18	55–65
Cool	18–27	65–80
Tepid	27–34	80–93
Neutral or warm	34–37	93–98
Hot	37–40.5	98–105
Very Hot	40.5	105–115

Reference: Mennell JB. Physical Treatment by Movement, Manipulation and Massage. 5th Ed. London: J.& A. Churchill Ltd, 1945.

erty is advantageous as sweat evaporation from the surface of the skin cools the body effectively. Another therapeutic property of water is that of the Archimedes' principle, which states that a body wholly or partly immersed in a fluid is buoyed up by a force equal to the weight of the fluid displaced. Patients with musculoskeletal problems are able to move with considerable ease under water. Water is frequently used as a medium for applying thermal stimuli. Table 2.1 gives an arbitrary classification of temperatures and adjectives used for describing temperature.

It should be noted that the results of hydrotherapy vary with age, weight, and general physical condition. Therefore, care must be taken when treating young persons, elderly persons, those in a poor state of nutrition, and those suffering from chronic vascular diseases.

BODY WRAPS AND SKIN

Some relaxing or therapeutic treatments use herbs, clay, mud, or paraffin. They may be used to treat mus-

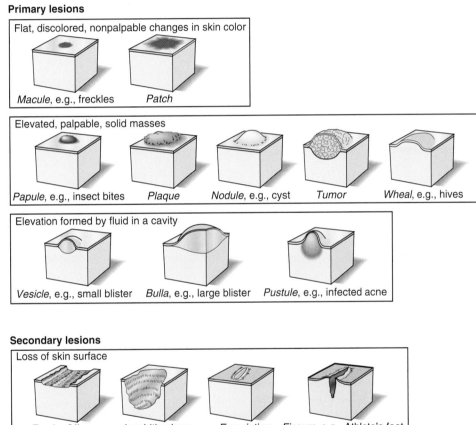

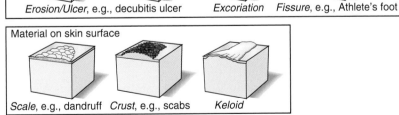

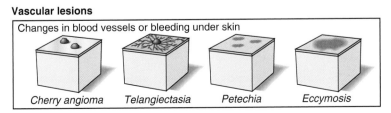

FIGURE **2.11.** Appearance of Common Skin Lesions

> ### ✓ Immersion in Sea Water and Fresh Water—the Shrink or Swell Phenomenon
>
> Note the wrinkling of the palms of your hands and soles of your feet the next time you swim in the ocean. When the body is immersed in water that has more dissolved particles than the cells (hypertonic solution), water moves out of the cells by osmosis, dehydrating the cells and making the skin appear wrinkled. Prolonged exposure to seawater can accelerate dehydration.
>
> The reverse situation occurs when the body is immersed in fresh water. Water moves into the cells (which are now hypertonic), and the cells in the epidermis can swell to 3–4 times normal volume.

cle and joint disorders, as well as to beautify and smooth the skin. Sheets, towels, or cheesecloth bags containing herbs are placed in a steaming vat and, once impregnated with the herb, drained and used to wrap the body or body part. A warm blanket and a plastic sheet are used to retain heat. In a mud wrap, the body is coated with heated mineralized mud. Muscle relaxation, increased circulation, and lymph drainage are some of the observed effects. Temporary weight loss may be observed as a result of increased loss of water by perspiration. Other beneficial wraps include a mixture of volcanic ash and paraffin and seaweed wraps.

SKIN LESIONS AND BODYWORKERS

All bodyworkers must be able to distinguish different lesions on the surface of the skin and to determine whether it is infectious. Many lesions may appear infectious but may not actually be infectious, such as some types of psoriasis, severe acne, or vitiligo. Touch therapy may be of great help to those clients who are often isolated from society because of their appearance. Areas of skin that ooze fluids or are visibly inflamed, should be avoided at all times. Although the therapist is not expected to diagnose a condition, it is vital to have enough information about those skin diseases already diagnosed by a physician to work with clients with these disorders. Figure 2.11 indicates the appearance of common skin lesions or skin signs. It is important for all bodyworkers to avoid infected, acutely inflamed, or irritable skin lesions.

REFERENCES

1. Field T. Touch. Massachusetts: MT Press, 2001.
2. Andrade CK. Clifford P. Outcome-Based Massage. Baltimore: Lippincott Williams & Wilkins, 2001.
3. de Domenico G, Wood EC. Beard's Massage. 4th Ed. Philadelphia: WB Saunders, 1997.
4. Montagu A. Touching: The Human Significance of the Skin. 3rd Ed. New York: Harper & Row, 1986.
5. Lundeberg T. Vibratory stimulation for the alleviation of pain. Am J Chinese Med 1984; 12(1–4):60–70.
6. Wakim KG. Physiologic Effects of Massage. In: Licht S, ed. Massage, Manipulation and Traction. Huntington, NY: Robert E. Keirger, 1976:38–42.
7. Fritz S. Fundamentals of Therapeutic Massage. St. Louis: Mosby-Lifeline, 1995.
8. Simons DG, Travell JG, Simons LS. Travell and Simons' Myofascial Pain and Dysfunction: The Trigger Point Manual, vol 1: Upper Half of Body. 2nd Ed. Baltimore: Williams & Wilkins, 1999.
9. Gifford J, Gifford L. Connective tissue massage. In: Wells PE, Frampton V, Bowsher D, eds. Pain: Management and Control in Physiotherapy. Chapter 14. London: Heinmemann Medical 1988.

SUGGESTED READINGS

Bale P, James H. Massage, Warm-down and rest as recuperative measures after short-term intense exercise. Physiotherapy Sport 1991;13:4–7.
Field T. Touch Therapy. Philadelphia: Churchill Livingstone, 2000.
Goats GC. Massage—The scientific basis of an ancient art: Part 1, Part 2. Brit J Sports Med 1994;28(3):149–155.
Goats GCK. Connective tissue massage. Brit J Sports Med 1991;25(3):131–133.
Mennell JB. Physical Treatment by Movement, Manipulation and Massage. 5th Ed. London: J&A Churchill Ltd, 1945.
Miller CRW. The effects of ice massage on an individual's pain tolerance level to electrical stimulation. J Orthop Sports Phys Ther 1990;12(3):105–109.

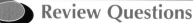

Review Questions

Multiple Choice

1. All of the following are functions of skin except one. Identify the exception:
   - A. Maintenance of body temperature
   - B. Synthesis of vitamin C
   - C. Reservoir of blood
   - D. Excretion

2. Which of the following is responsible for regeneration of the epidermis?
   - A. Stratum corneum
   - B. Stratum lucidum
   - C. Stratum granulosum
   - D. Stratum basale

3. The sensation of touch is picked up by nerve receptors located in the
   - A. stratum corneum
   - B. dermis
   - C. subcutaneous layer
   - D. stratum basale

4. Acne is a common inflammatory disorder of the
   - A. mammary glands
   - B. ceruminous glands
   - C. sebaceous glands
   - D. sudoriferous glands

5. Waterproofing of the skin is largely due to
   A. keratin
   B. carotene
   C. melanin
   D. receptors

6. The most abundant type of cells in the epidermis are
   A. adipocytes
   B. fibroblasts
   C. melanocytes
   D. keratinocytes

7. Which of the following is **not** an effect of ultraviolet radiation?
   A. Vitamin D synthesis
   B. Melanocyte activation
   C. Sunburn
   D. Vitiligo
   E. Chromosomal damage in germinative cells

8. Mammary glands are a type of
   A. sebaceous gland
   B. ceruminous gland
   C. apocrine sweat gland
   D. None of the above

9. The effects of aging on the skin include
   A. an increase in the production of Vitamin D
   B. a thickening of the epidermis
   C. an increased blood supply to the dermis
   D. a decline in the activity of sebaceous gland

10. The cardinal signs of inflammation include all of the following **except**
    A. sweating
    B. swelling
    C. redness
    D. increased temperature
    E. pain

11. The cells in the epidermis that are involved in immunity are
    A. Merkel cells
    B. melanocytes
    C. Langerhans cells
    D. keratinocytes

Fill-In-the-Blanks

1. In the condition known as _____, the skin takes on a blue color. The blue coloration is due to the pigment _____.

2. The dermis is organized into two layers. They are the _____ and the _____.

3. The muscle that causes the hair to stand on end is the _____.

True–False

(Answer the following questions T, for true; or F, for false):

1. The subcutaneous layer is primarily made up of blood vessels and nerves that respond to stimulation of skin.

2. The accessory structures are located in the dermis.

3. Lipid-soluble substances are more easily absorbed through the skin than water-soluble substances.

4. The resident flora prevent growth of harmful bacteria on the surface of the skin by competing with them for nutrients.

5. White blood cells play an important role in the healing of skin wounds.

6. Deodorants are used to mask the odor of secretions from sebaceous glands.

7. The area in the sensory cortex of brain that represents a part of the body is directly related to the number of receptors in that part of the body.

8. Stimulation of skin by massage can produce reactions in areas far removed from the site of application of massage.

9. Massage has the potential to increase insensible perspiration and facilitate sebaceous gland secretion.

Matching

A. _____ a yellow discoloration of mucous membrane as a result of liver dysfunction	1. psoriasis
B. _____ a type of skin cancer that spreads rapidly	2. cyanosis
C. _____ a condition where the cells of the epidermis migrate to the surface more rapidly than normal	3. jaundice
D. _____ a condition where there is dysfunction of melanocytes	4. melanoma
E. _____ a condition where the skin takes on a bluish tinge	5. ulcer
F. _____ a solid elevation of epidermis and dermis	6. vitiligo
G. _____ loss of epidermis	7. papule

Short Answer Questions

1. Describe the role of white blood cells in inflammatory reactions.

2. List the different ways by which inflammation may resolve.

3. Compare and contrast acute and chronic inflammation.

4. Describe the mechanical effects of massage.

5. Give examples of some reflex effects of massage.

6. Identify the manipulative techniques that primarily affect the superficial and deep fascia.

7. Explain what is meant by acupoints. How can they be stimulated?

8. Describe the effect of friction massage on skin.

9. Explain what determines the skin color of an individual.

10. Define a dermatome.

11. List four causes of inflammation.

Case Studies

1. Mrs. Brown, a 45-year-old woman, came to the massage clinic concerned about the swelling of her right upper limb following mastectomy. Surgery had been performed on her right breast a month ago. Her right axillary lymph nodes had also been removed during surgery. Mrs. Brown explained to her therapist that the swelling was quite significant and that her arm ached at the end of the day. On examination, the therapist finds no inflammation. Mild edema is present.

   The therapist positions pillows to elevate Mrs. Brown's right arm. She uses superficial effleurage and superficial lymph drainage techniques on the arm. At the end of the session, Mrs. Brown's arm felt much better. She promises to return the following week for a similar session.
   A. Why does Mrs. Brown have swelling in the right arm following surgery?
   B. What is the effect of superficial effleurage and superficial lymph drainage techniques?
   C. How are the effects produced?

2. Mr. Ronald, a 50-year-old man, woke up one morning to find that he had lost voluntary control of the right side of his body. His wife rushed him to hospital where he was diagnosed as having had a stroke. One month later, he returned home where a physiotherapist visited him on alternate days. As part of his therapy, Mr. Ronald is taken to the nearby swimming pool where he exercises in water under the watchful eye of the therapist.
   A. What are the unique characteristics of water that may be of benefit to Mr. Ronald?
   B. What physiological effects can one expect if the temperature of water was cold or hot?

3. Sheila, aged 16, loved to have a relaxation massage but was hesitant to do so because of acne that she had developed on her face and chest. A few of the lesions were inflamed.
   A. What is the skin structure affected by acne?
   B. What precautions should the massage therapist take when treating clients with acne?
   C. What special issues should the massage therapist be aware of when treating clients with acne?

4. Every summer, Kelly tried to get a perfect tan by lying naked in her secluded back yard. Her favorite time in the yard was between 10 and 12 noon when she had the house to herself and her two-year-old daughter was away at day care.
   A. What are the benefits of exposure of skin to sunlight?
   B. What are the detrimental effects of ultraviolet radiation?

5. Kristin's 75-year-old grandmother, who appears perfectly healthy for her age, complains that she is cold and wears a sweater even on balmy days.
   A. What could be the reason for her complaints?
   B. What are the effects of aging on the skin?
   C. What are the implications of age changes in skin for bodyworkers?

6. Roger thought that he kept his massage clinic warm, but clients complained that they felt cold during every session. Of course, the walls of the room were cold, but he had a heater to keep the room temperature up.
   A. What could be the reason for the clients feeling cold?
   B. How can Roger improve the situation?
   C. What physiologic changes take place in the body of the client on exposure to cold?

Answers to Review Questions

Multiple Choice

1. B, The skin helps manufacture vitamin D
2. D, Stratum basale has cells that are capable of multiplication
3. B, Most nerve receptors are located in the dermis
4. C
5. A
6. D
7. D, Vitiligo is a condition caused by reduced melanin pigmentation

8. C
9. D
10. A
11. C

Fill-In

1. Cyanosis, Deoxyhemoglobin
2. Papillary layer, or pars papillaris; reticular layer, or pars reticularis
3. Arrector pili muscle

True–False

1. False, It is the dermis
2. True
3. True
4. True
5. True
6. False, It is the sweat glands
7. True
8. True
9. True

Matching

A. 3   B. 4   C. 1   D. 6
E. 2   F. 7   G. 5

Short-Answer Questions

1. Immediately after injury, white blood cells inside the blood vessels aggregate along the walls of blood vessels, attracted to the injured site by chemicals that are released by injured tissue. They then move out of the vessels by squeezing through gaps between the cells that form the wall of capillaries. The white cells then proceed to destroy structures that are foreign or dead by engulfing them into the cytoplasm. Poisonous enzymes present in the lysosomes are used to destroy these structures.
2. Inflammation can resolve in three ways. It can slowly disappear (heal). It can progress with exudate forming in the area. It can become chronic. The exudate may be serous, fibrinous, purulent, hemorrhagic, or membranous. Chronic inflammation may present as fibrosis, ulcer, sinus, or fistula.
3. Acute inflammation lasts for a short period; chronic inflammation persists for a longer period, perhaps months or years. Medically, inflammation is considered chronic if the area is infiltrated by large numbers of lymphocytes and macrophages, if growth of new capillaries occurs, and if there is an abundance of fibroblasts in the area. Chronic inflammation may present as fibrosis, ulcer, sinus, or fistula. Acute inflammation can resolve in three ways. It can slowly

disappear (heal); it can progress with exudate forming in the area; or it can become chronic.
4. Massage can change the texture and consistency of skin. The skin becomes softer and suppler. With repeated manipulation, the skin becomes more resilient, flexible, and elastic. Massage helps remove dry, scaly skin from the surface. During and after wound healing, massage can help realign collagen fibers in the dermis and prevent complications due to entrapment. Blood and lymph flow is also increased by massage.
5. Some examples of cutaneovisceral reflexes are abdominal reflex and plantar reflex. By reflexly increasing blood and lymph flow, massage helps improve the nutritive status and removes toxins and speeds healing. The increase in blood and lymph flow is caused by direct mechanical displacement and the reflex nervous responses of the blood and lymph channels walls.
6. Neuromuscular and connective tissue techniques primarily affect the superficial and deep fascia.
7. In Chinese medicine, energy is believed to travel through the body in channels called meridians. An organ is associated with each of the meridians. The meridian is believed to have a basic quality of energy (yin and yan). Small points, known as acupoints, have been identified on the meridians. These acupoints may be located close to the surface or in deeper regions and show altered sensitivity when the body has a diseased condition. By stimulating the acupoints, the functions of the related organs are affected.
8. Friction massage frees adherent skin, loosens scars and adhesions of deeper tissues, and reduces local edema.
9. The blood flow, level of oxyhemoglobin and deoxyhemoglobin, and presence of the pigments melanin, carotene, and bilirubin are primary factors that affect skin color.
10. Sensory nerves from the skin relay impulses generated in the receptors to the central nervous system. The sensory nerves entering a particular segment of the spinal cord innervate a specific area of the skin known as the dermatome.
11. Some of the common causes of inflammation are physical, chemical, infectious, and immunologic.

Case Studies

1. A, Mrs. Brown has swelling in her right arm because the axillary lymph nodes had been removed during surgery. The lymph vessels from the upper limb drain into the axillary lymph nodes before proceeding to the right lymphatic duct and the subclavian vein. The impairment of lymph drainage, coupled with the effect of gravity, causes swelling. By ele-

vating the limb, the therapist tries to take advantage of gravity to reduce the swelling.

B, and C, Superficial effleurage and superficial lymph drainage techniques are superficial fluid techniques that have an effect on structures in the dermis and subcutaneous tissue. In superficial effleurage, gliding movements are used. These movements, in addition to producing reflex effects similar to those of superficial stroking techniques, affect lymphatic and venous return in skin and deeper structures by mechanical compression. It is, therefore, particularly effective in reducing edema. This technique also has psychological and other physiologic effects, such as reduction of anxiety, increased relaxation, reduced excitability of muscle, and increased peristalsis.

Superficial lymph drainage technique uses short, rhythmic, nongliding strokes in the direction of lymph flow. The strokes result in gentle stretching of the skin and superficial fascia together with the stimulation of contraction of lymph vessels. If performed over a large surface area of the body, it effectively increases lymph return to the veins. In addition, these techniques reduce anxiety, produce sedation, reduce pain, and improve immune function.

2. A, Water is referred to as a "flexible therapeutic agent" because of its unique chemical and physical properties. Because a body wholly or partly immersed in a fluid is buoyed up by a force equal to the weight of the fluid displaced, patients with musculoskeletal problems are able to move with considerable ease under water. This is why Mr. Ronald may benefit from treatment in water. Water may also be used as a medium for applying thermal stimuli.

B, Cold water would result in peripheral vasoconstriction and pallor. Reduction of edema and muscle spasm are other effects. Due to a reduction in the rate of nerve conduction, pain perception would be diminished. An increase in heart rate, blood pressure, and shivering may be expected.

Hot water would result in peripheral vasodilatation, redness of skin, muscle relaxation, decrease in blood pressure, increase in heart rate, and shallow, rapid breathing. Heat, by stimulating circulation speeds removal of waste products from inflammatory sites, thereby relieving pain, swelling, and spasm.

3. A, Acne produces inflammation of the sebaceous glands.

B, Acne is not contagious and it cannot be spread from one region of the body to another by touch. Infection can be introduced by unclean, oily hands; hands should be washed thoroughly before touching the area of acne. The inflamed areas should be avoided. Judgment should be made on an individual basis, as some clients may like light massage of the affected area without oil. Ointments and lotions that may clog the opening of the sebaceous glands should not be used. Friction and deep tissue pressure should not be used.

C, Sheila may be self-conscious because of her appearance. The therapist should be particularly sensitive to such issues.

4. A, Exposure to ultraviolet (UV) rays stimulates enzymes that produce melanin and a tan is produced. The melanin pigment protects the skin from the harmful effects of the UV radiation. By concentrating around the nucleus, the melanin pigment works like an umbrella, absorbing the UV rays and shielding the nucleus and its high deoxyribonucleic acid (DNA) content. Some exposure to sunlight is useful and needed by the body as the cells in the stratum germinativum and stratum spinosum convert a compound 7-dehydrocholesterol into a precursor of vitamin D.

Melanin also protects the skin from developing sunburn. However, the melanin synthesis rate is not rapid enough to provide complete protection and it is possible to get a sunburn easily, especially in the first few days of prolonged sun exposure.

B, The cumulative effects of UV radiation exposure can damage fibroblasts located in the dermis, leading to faulty manufacture of connective tissue and wrinkling of the skin. UV rays also stimulate the production of oxygen free radicals that disrupt collagen and elastic fibers in the extracellular regions. UV rays can cause alterations in the genetic material in the nucleus of cells, especially the rapidly multiplying cells in the stratum germinativum, increasing the chances of cancer.

5. A, Adipose tissue in the subcutaneous layer serves as insulation. In elderly persons, subcutaneous adipose tissue is lost in many parts of the body, especially the limbs, and the feeble skin circulation also affects thermoregulation.

B, All components of the integumentary system are affected by aging. The epidermis becomes thinner with the activity of the stratum germinativum decreasing significantly, making older persons more prone to infection, injury, and delayed healing. The Langerhans cells reduce in number, increasing the susceptibility of the elderly to infection. The decrease in the production of Vitamin D₃ results in reduction in the absorption of calcium and phosphate from the gut, leading to fragile bones. The melanocytes decrease in number, and the skin becomes more vulnerable to injury by exposure to the sun.

The ground substance tends to become dehydrated. The skin of the elderly is, therefore, weaker, with a tendency to wrinkle and sag. The mechanical strength of the junction between the epidermis and dermis diminishes, which may account for the ease with which blisters form in the elderly. The glandular secretions diminish, resulting in dry skin. Hair loss, changes in the appearance of nails, and loss of subcutaneous fat are other changes seen in elderly persons.

C, The skin changes in the elderly make them more prone to infection and injury. Therefore, only gentle pressure should be used. The therapist should be aware that healing is slower. As thermoregulation is affected, the temperature of the room and heat/cold applications should be carefully monitored.

6. A, Although Roger keeps the room temperature high, the cold walls could affect the clients by convection and radiation.

B, Roger could improve the situation by investigating why his walls are cold and correcting the problem, if possible.

C, When the body is exposed to cold, systemic reactions, such as an increase in heart rate, respiratory rate, blood pressure, and shivering, may be produced to maintain the core temperature. The hair stands on end and the air trapped between the skin and hair provide additional insulation.

When cold is applied locally, it results in peripheral vasoconstriction and pallor. The vasoconstriction, in turn, results in a decrease in skin temperature and reduction of edema, muscle spasm and further hemorrhage. Analgesic effects are seen when the temperature is lowered to about 13.6°C. Analgesia is incurred by the reduction in nerve conduction velocity by cold. Soon after a cold application has ended, there may be peripheral vasodilatation, with redness of skin, feeling of warmth, slowing of pulse and respiratory rates, and relaxation. This reaction may last for 20-30 minutes.

Coloring Exercise

Structure and components of the skin. Label and color those structures indicated by arrows.

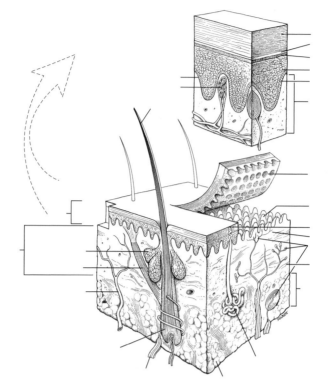

Distribution of dermatomes on the skin. Identify the area of the skin related to the cervical (pink); thoracic (green); lumbar (red); and sacral (blue) spinal segments.

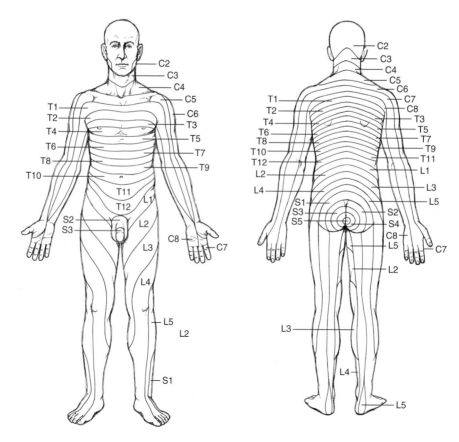

CHAPTER 3

Skeletal System and Joints

Objectives
Skeletal System

On completion of this chapter, the reader should be able to:

- Give the functions of bone.
- Describe the microscopic structure of bone.
- Describe the role of calcium in bone formation and explain how calcium is regulated.
- List the different types of bones and give examples.
- Identify the parts of a long bone.
- Identify the two divisions of the skeleton.
- Identify the subdivisions of the axial skeleton.
- Identify the bones of the skull and the face.
- Identify the sutures and fontanels of the skull.
- Identify the various regions of the vertebral column.
- Identify the subdivisions of the appendicular skeleton.
- List the bony components of the pectoral and pelvic girdles and upper and lower limbs.
- Identify the major bony landmarks in the bones of the body.

Joints

- List the various joint types and classify the different joints of the body by these types.
- Describe the structure of a typical synovial joint.
- List the different types of synovial joints and discuss how the range of motion in each type is related to the structure.
- Describe the articulation between the vertebrae.
- Describe the structure, range of motion, and muscles that move the various joints of the body.
- Describe age-related changes to bones and joints.
- Describe the possible effects of massage on the skeletal system and joints.

The therapist is mostly called on to deal with conditions related to muscles and joints. To understand the problem and manage it effectively, the therapist must assess movement and range of motion. The following treatment invariably requires stretching, passive and active motions. To do a professional job, the therapist should have an understanding of joint structure, be able to identify bony landmarks, know the possible range of motion of each joint, and know the muscles that produce various movements. Knowledge of the origin and insertions of muscles and direction of fibers is also essential.

This chapter describes the bones of the body, bone formation, anatomic landmarks, and major joints.

Common ailments of these joints are also addressed. The student is encouraged to use the numerous figures included, as well as their own bodies, while learning the names and locations of the various structures.

The Skeletal System

BONE FUNCTIONS

The primary function of bone is to be a supporting framework for the rest of the body. It is often compared to the steel girders that support buildings. But, unlike steel girders, bone is one of the most metabolically active tissues; remaining active throughout life and having the capacity to change shape and density according to mechanical demands. Bone contributes to the shape and positioning of the various structures of the body. Together, some bones protect important organs. The heart and lungs, for example, lie securely in the bony thoracic cage. The brain lies in the protective cranial cavity made up of many bones.

The bones, with their joints, act as levers that are manipulated by the muscles attached to them and positioned across the joints. Bones are the main reservoir for minerals, such as calcium and phosphorus. Calcium is an important mineral required for conduction of impulses in nerves, muscle contraction, and clotting of blood. It is vital for the body to maintain the blood levels of calcium within a narrow range, and bone serves as a reservoir when the blood levels of calcium fluctuate. Bone is also a factory where blood cells are manufactured. Bone may also be considered as one of the sites where fat is stored because yellow bone marrow is primarily adipose tissue.

STRUCTURE AND FORMATION OF BONE

Bone is a special form of connective tissue. Similar to other connective tissue, it has ground substance with collagen fibers and cells (**see page 34–35**). However, the ground substance in bone has a large deposition of calcium and phosphorus that makes the tissue hard and rigid. The minerals are in the form of **hydroxyapatite crystals** (calcium carbonate and calcium phosphate mineral salts). Minerals account for 60% to 70% of the dry weight of bone; water accounts for 5% to 8%; and organic matter, of which collagen is main, the remaining weight. The collagen fibers are arranged in various directions, with the arrangement being altered according to lines of stress and tension created by the weight and activity of the body. The presence of collagen fiber gives bone its flexibility and resilience (tensile strength). Collagen fibers and minerals combined make the bone flexible, compressible, and able to withstand considerable shear forces. The gel-like ground substance that surrounds the collagen fibers is made up of large, complex molecules called **proteoglycans.** Proteoglycans are mucopolysaccharides bound to protein chains.

Like all tissue, bone requires its own supply of blood and nerves. Unlike other softer tissue, bone is solid and must grow around blood vessels and nerves in a more complex process. To better understand this complex process, bone formation in the fetus must be examined. The process of bone formation is known as **ossification,** or **osteogenesis,** (Figure 3.1). Ossification may occur in two ways. In **intramembranous ossification,** bone is formed within or on fibrous connective tissue membranes. Flat bones of the skull and the mandible are formed by intramembranous ossification. In **endochondral ossification,** the more common type of ossification, bone is formed within hyaline cartilage.

In the fetus, special cells known as **chondroblasts** appear in areas where bone must be present. Chondroblast secretions result in the formation of cartilage, which eventually takes the precise shape of bone in that area. In this way, cartilage forms a mold in which minerals can be deposited to form bone. The connective tissue around the cartilage forms a highly vascular membrane around the mold. Nerves are also incorporated in the membrane. The membrane has many chondroblasts, which help cartilaginous growth on the surface of the model. This membrane is known as the **perichondrium.**

At a later stage, chondroblasts undergo transformation and begin to secrete the chemicals that precipitate deposition of minerals around them. Nutri-

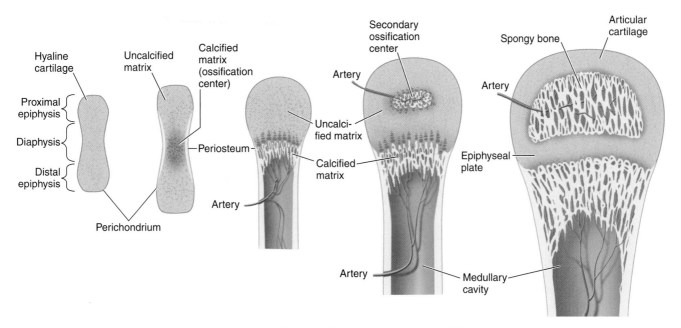

FIGURE **3.1.**   Ossification of Bone—Enchondral Ossification

ent arteries grow into the cartilage, stimulating os-teogenic cells to transform into **osteoblasts.**

The chondroblasts in the membrane are also trans-formed and bone begins to form both inside and on the surface of the cartilage model.

The beginning and rate of ossification varies from bone to bone. In each bone, ossification begin at dif-ferent sites known as **ossification centers.** Ossifica-tion continues until the cartilage model has been re-placed by bone. The bone has the potential to grow in length as long as adjacent ossification centers have not fused together. Once fused, the bone can only be-come thicker.

A typical bone has a hard outer shell, with a blood and nerve supply, known as the **periosteum.** The pe-riosteum is actually ossified perichondrium. Because the blood and nerve supply are located here, the pe-riosteum is an important component of bone. It also houses the **osteogenic cells** (cells that divide to form osteoblasts) and osteoblasts that are required for new bone formation on the surface, according to stresses and strains placed on the bone. The fusion of bones

that occur in some regions of the body is also a result of the presence of periosteum. In addition, ligaments that cross joints are fused with the periosteum of ad-jacent bones, adding to joint stability. Tendons of muscles also blend with the collagen fibers of the periosteum at the point of attachment.

BONE REMODELING

For bone to grow and rearrange collagen fibers and minerals in lines of stress, two processes—one that builds and another that removes—must be in place. While osteoblasts help with bone formation, another group of cells (**osteoclasts**) reabsorb bone. In this way, the bone retains its shape and grows without be-coming thicker.

Normally, the outer layer of bone is dense and is known as **compact,** or **cortical bone.** Internally, the bone is less dense, with bone spicules surrounded by spaces filled with red marrow. This is the **spongy, can-cellous,** or **trabecular bone.** Spongy bone is found in larger amounts in short, flat, and irregularly shaped bones. A **bone marrow cavity,** or **medullary cavity,**

ECTOPIC BONE FORMATION

It is possible for bone to develop in unusual places. Physi-cal or chemical events can stimulate the development of osteoblasts in normal connective tissue.

Sesamoid bones develop within tendons near points of friction and pressure; bone may also appear within a blood clot at an injury site or within the dermis subjected to chronic abuse. Bone may be deposited around skeletal muscle; this condition is called *myositis ossificans.*

BONE MARROW

In people with severe anemia, platelet deficiency, or white blood cell disorders, a sample of bone marrow may be taken with a needle for investigation. Bone marrow is also used for transplanting into a person with low blood cells count. In adults, bone marrow is aspirated from flat bones, such as the sternum, for this purpose.

may be found at the center of the bone. Cortical bone always surrounds cancellous bone, but the quantity of each type varies. About 75% of the bones in the body are compact. Because compact bone is solid, blood vessels that supply the cells with nutrients and nerves are contained in canals. The canals that run transversely from the periosteum are the **perforating,** or **Volkmann's canals.** These canals connect with **haversian canals,** canals that run longitudinally through the compact bone. The collagen fibers are arranged in **lamellae,** concentric layers around the canals forming cylinders called **osteons** or **haversian systems.** The osteoblasts surrounded by calcified matrix in the compact bone become mature bone cells called the **osteocytes.** They are located in small cavities known as **lacunae.** The lacunae communicate with other adjacent lacunae by tiny canals (**canaliculi**) that ramify throughout the bone connecting adjacent cells (see Figure 3.2) and the haversian canals. The osteocytes, therefore, obtain nutrients from the blood vessels in the haversian canals.

PARTS OF A LONG BONE

The activity of osteoclasts and osteoblasts is particularly rapid at the ends of long bones that extend in length. The region (see Figure 3.3) at the ends of bones is the **epiphysis** (plural, epiphyses). New cartilage is constantly being formed here to increase the length. This new cartilage is a thin region known as the **epiphyseal plate,** where the osteoblasts constantly turn cartilage into bone. As more cartilage is formed, the epiphyseal plate advances, leaving bone behind it. Thus, bone is remodeled by cellular activity. **Diaphysis** is the region of bone between the epiphysis. The diaphysis forms the middle, cylindrical part of the bone. The **metaphysis** is the region of bone that lies between the diaphysis and the epiphysis, and it includes the epiphyseal plate.

The ends of long bones, adjacent to the joint, are covered with hyaline cartilage—**articular cartilage.** The articular cartilage absorbs shock and reduces friction in joints. The inner region of long bones houses the medullary or marrow cavity. In children this cavity is

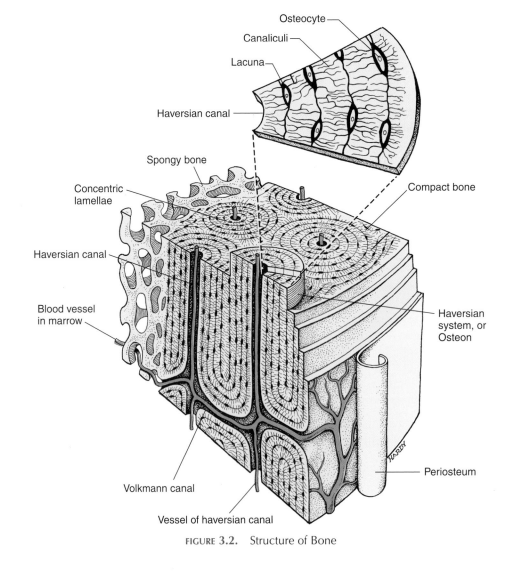

FIGURE 3.2. Structure of Bone

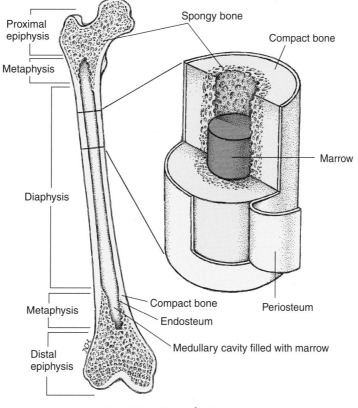

FIGURE **3.3.**   Parts of a Long Bone

filled with **red bone marrow** (where blood cells are formed). In older individuals, the red bone marrow is replaced by **yellow marrow** that is largely made up of adipose tissue. The medullary cavity is lined by a membrane known as the **endosteum**. It contains bone-forming cells (osteogenic cells, osteoblasts and osteoclasts).

Bone continues to lengthen rapidly during puberty and stops in adulthood. However, bone deposition and resorption continues throughout life and is modified by diet and endocrine, mechanical, chemical, and psychological factors.

Effect of Diet on Bone

For proper bone formation, there must be adequate protein, calcium, and phosphorus, among others, especially at rapid growth phases such as childhood, adolescence, pregnancy, and lactation. Because bone is also a calcium reservoir, if demands are increased, calcium is removed from the bones to meet those needs and the bones can get weaker. Small quantities of fluoride, magnesium, manganese, and iron are also needed. Vitamin C is needed for proper collagen fiber development. Other vitamins, such as vitamin A, B_{12}, and K, are needed for protein synthesis and osteoblastic activity.

Effect of Hormones on Bone

Three hormones are important in maintaining blood levels of calcium. This implies that they affect the mineralization of bone in the process. Parathormone, from the parathyroid gland (**page 402**) and vitamin D (**page 60**) increase the blood levels of calcium while the hormone calcitonin, from the thyroid gland, decreases the levels. In bone, parathormone and vitamin D increase osteoclastic activity and resorption of bone and decrease excretion of calcium by the kidneys and increase absorption in the gut. Calcitonin does the opposite; if dietary calcium is inadequate, bone resorption occurs.

In addition to these hormones, growth hormone, thyroid hormone, insulin, and sex hormones are all required for proper bone formation.

Effect of Mechanical Factors on Bone

The plasticity of bone can be illustrated in many ways. Bones of athletes are stronger and denser as compared with sedentary individuals. Similar to other tissue that atrophy with disuse, bone becomes weaker and less dense when not stressed. Conversely, excessive stress placed on one or more bones makes those bones alone stronger and denser. Hence, posture,

BONE FRACTURES

A fracture is a partial or complete break in the continuity of the bone that usually occurs under mechanical stress. It may be caused by trauma or in conditions that weaken bone.

- An *open* or *compound fracture* is one where broken bone projects through the skin.
- A *closed* or *simple fracture* does not produce a break in the skin.
- A *complete fracture* involves a complete break in the entire section of bone, while in an *incomplete fracture* there is some continuity.
- *Stress fractures* are usually seen in the leg. This occurs as a result of repetitive mechanical stress on the microtrabecular structure of bone caused by jarring on impact. The metatarsals, fibula, and tibia are commonly affected. Running on hard surfaces, high impact aerobic exercises, osteoporosis, and obesity are some predisposing factors.

Bone Healing After Fracture

The process of bone remodeling is used for healing of fractures. The basic mechanisms involved in the healing of bone are similar to what occurs in the skin or any other tissue (see **page 72, 73**). The healing process of bone in relation to time after injury is shown below. If the time taken for the broken bones to join together is more than normal, it is referred to as **delayed union.** If the ends of the broken bones are not aligned properly, then the union is abnormal. This is known as **malunion.** Rarely, the broken ends are not joined together even after the normal time taken for healing. This is known as **nonunion.**

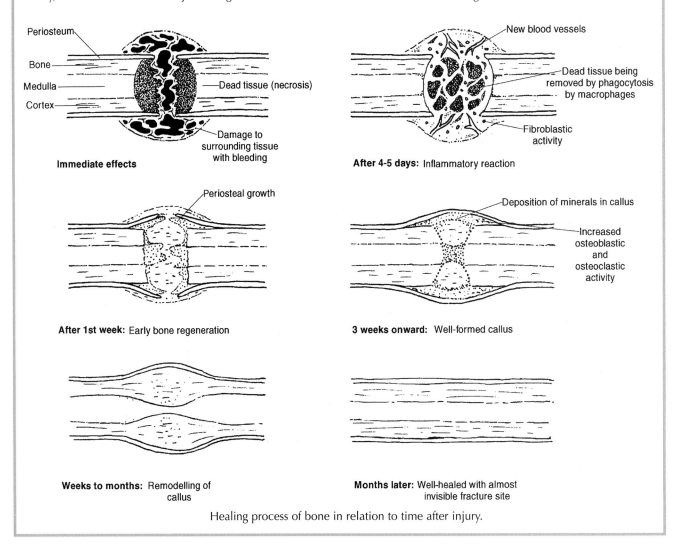

Immediate effects

After 4-5 days: Inflammatory reaction

After 1st week: Early bone regeneration

3 weeks onward: Well-formed callus

Weeks to months: Remodelling of callus

Months later: Well-healed with almost invisible fracture site

Healing process of bone in relation to time after injury.

muscle tone, and weight can all affect the remodeling process.

TYPES OF BONES

The bones of the body are classified, according to shape, as **long bones, short bones, flat bones,** and **irregular bones** (see Figure 3.4). **Long bones,** as the name suggests, are long, with the length being greater than the width. The femur or thighbone, the humerus of the arm, metacarpals, metatarsals, and phalanges are a few examples.

Short bones are almost equal in length, width, and height. Most of the carpals—the small bones located in the wrist (except pisiform, sesamoid bone)—and most of the tarsals—the small bones in the ankle region (except calcaneus, irregular bone)—are good examples of short bones.

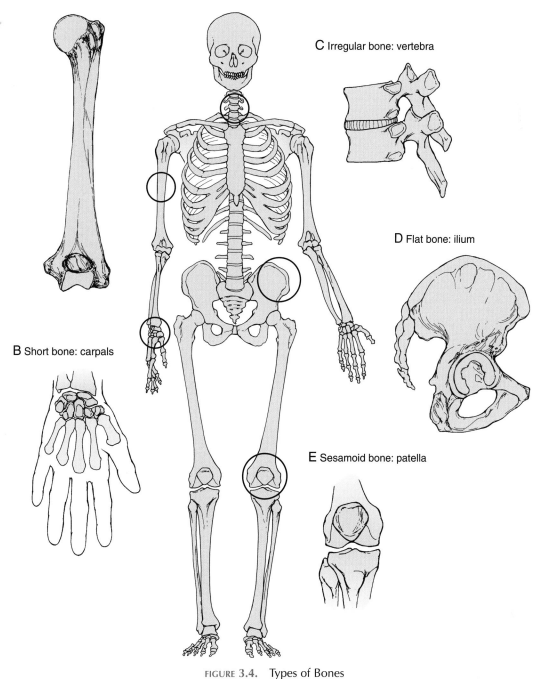

A Long bone: humerus

C Irregular bone: vertebra

D Flat bone: ilium

B Short bone: carpals

E Sesamoid bone: patella

FIGURE **3.4.** Types of Bones

Table 3.1

Anatomic Terms and Descriptions. The Bony Landmarks of Individual Bones are Named Based on Some Common Skeletal Terminology. Familiarity With these Terms will Make it Easier to Remember the Landmarks

Anatomic Term	Description
Condyle	smooth, rounded end that articulates with another bone
Crest	prominent ridge
Facet	small, flat surface that articulates with another bone
Fissure	long cleft
Fossa	shallow depression
Foramen	small, round passage through which nerves/blood vessels pass in and out or through the bone
Head	expanded end
Line	low ridge
Meatus	canal leading through the substance of a bone
Neck	narrowed part closely related to an expanded end
Process	projection or bump
Ramus	extension of a bone that makes an angle to the rest of the structure
Sinus	chamber within the bone, usually filled with air
Spine	pointed process
Sulcus	narrow groove
Trochanter	large, rough projection
Trochlea	pulleylike end of bone that is smooth and grooved
Tuberosity	smaller, rough projection

Flat bones are broad and thin with a flattened and/or curved surface. The shoulder blade (scapula), some of the skull bones, ribs, and breastbone (sternum), are all examples of flat bone. Their thin, broad area helps protect inner organs and/or provide surface area for muscle attachment. Flat bones contain the red bone marrow in which blood cells are manufactured.

Irregular bones are those in various shapes and sizes. The facial bones and vertebrae are all examples of this type. Small, irregularly shaped bones, called **sutural** or **wormian bones,** are found where two or more other bones meet in the skull. The number, size, and shape vary by individual.

Rarely, small, flat, round bones develop inside tendons. These bones are called **sesamoid bones.** The patella is a sesamoid bone found in all individuals. Other sesamoid bones are often found around the knee joint or the joints of the hands or feet. Sesamoid bones help reduce friction and stress on tendons and may also help to change the direction of tension placed on the tendon.

To examine joints and learn about muscles and the movements they produce, the names of the bones of the body and the anatomic landmarks of each bone must be looked at in greater detail (see Table 3.1).

The Human Skeleton

The human skeleton (see Figures 3.5 and 3.6) can be considered to have two main divisions—the **axial** and the **appendicular skeleton.** The axial portion is made of bones in the central or longitudinal axis; the

BONES OF THE AXIAL SKELETON

Skull (22 bones)
Cranial bones (8)
Facial bones (14)
Bones associated with the skull (7 bones)
Auditory ossicles (6)
Hyoid bone (1)
Vertebral column (26 bones)
Vertebrae (24)
Sacrum (1)
Coccyx (1)
Thoracic cage (25 bones)
Ribs (24)
Sternum (1)

BONES OF THE APPENDICULAR SKELETON

Pectoral girdles (4 bones)
Clavicle (2)
Scapula (2)
Upper limbs (60 bones)
Humerus (2)
Radius (2)
Ulna (2)
Carpals (16)
Metacarpals (10)
Phalanges (28)
Pelvic girdles (2 bones)
Coxa or Hip (2)
Lower limbs (60 bones)
Femur (2)
Patella (2)
Tibia (2)
Fibula (2)
Tarsals (14)
Metatarsals (10)
Phalanges (28)

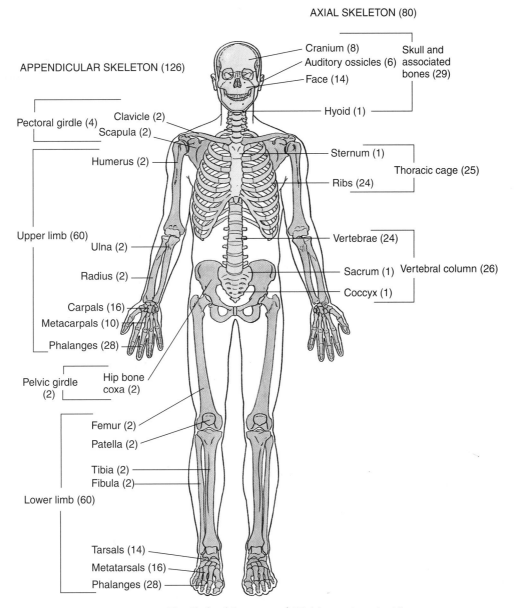

FIGURE 3.5. The Skeletal System and Divisions—Anterior View

skull, vertebrae, ribs, and **sternum.** Tiny bones (**ossicles**) located in the middle ear and the **hyoid bone,** located in the neck, are also part of this division. The appendicular skeleton is made up of bones that form the appendices—the limbs—and includes the bones that attach the limb to the axial skeleton: the **bones of the shoulder** and **pelvic girdle** and the **bones of the upper** and **lower limb.**

The skeletal system consists of 206 bones, of which approximately 40% (80 bones) is part of the axial skeleton. The axial skeleton creates a framework that supports and protects delicate organs of the body and provides a large surface area for the attachment of muscles. Muscles that alter the position of the head, neck, and trunk; those that perform respiratory

movements; and muscles that stabilize the position of the limbs when they move are all attached to the axial skeleton. The joints between the bones of the axial skeleton are strong and allow only limited movement.

The Axial Skeleton

THE SKULL

The bones of the skull (see Figures 3.7–3.15) protect the brain and guard the entrances to the digestive and respiratory systems. The bones that cover the brain form the **cranium** while the others are associated with the face (**facial bones**). The tiny **ossicles** of

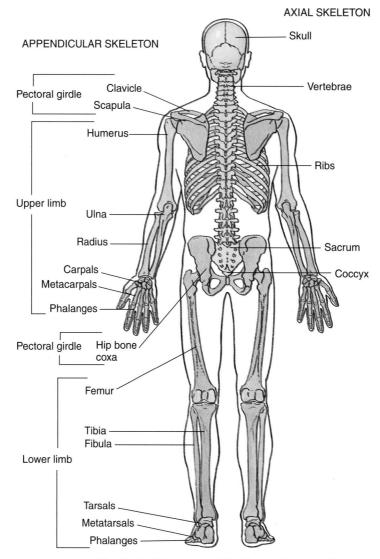

AXIAL SKELETON

APPENDICULAR SKELETON

Skull

Vertebrae

Pectoral girdle

Clavicle

Scapula

Humerus

Ribs

Upper limb

Ulna

Radius

Sacrum

Carpals

Coccyx

Metacarpals

Phalanges

Pectoral girdle

Hip bone coxa

Femur

Tibia

Fibula

Lower limb

Tarsals

Metatarsals

Phalanges

FIGURE 3.6. The Skeletal System and Divisions—Posterior View

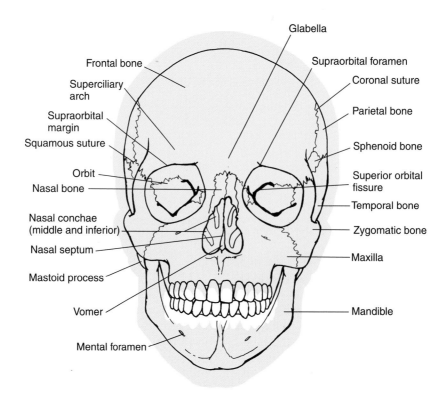

Glabella

Frontal bone

Supraorbital foramen

Superciliary arch

Coronal suture

Supraorbital margin

Parietal bone

Squamous suture

Sphenoid bone

Orbit

Superior orbital fissure

Nasal bone

Nasal conchae (middle and inferior)

Temporal bone

Nasal septum

Zygomatic bone

Mastoid process

Maxilla

Vomer

Mandible

Mental foramen

FIGURE 3.7. Adult Skull—Anterior View

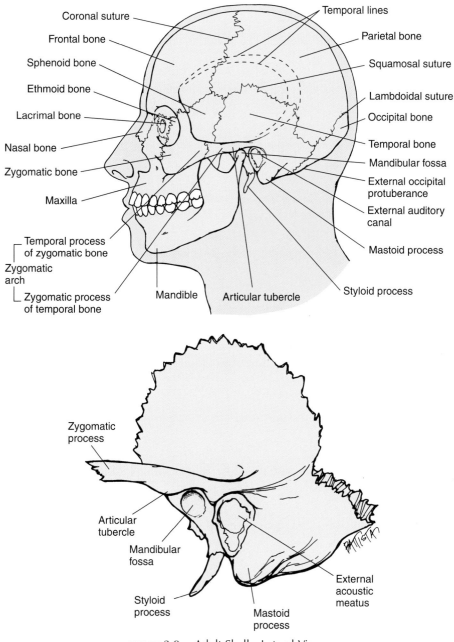

Coronal suture
Frontal bone
Sphenoid bone
Ethmoid bone
Lacrimal bone
Nasal bone
Zygomatic bone
Maxilla
Temporal process
of zygomatic bone
Zygomatic
arch
Zygomatic process
of temporal bone
Mandible
Articular tubercle

Temporal lines
Parietal bone
Squamosal suture
Lambdoidal suture
Occipital bone
Temporal bone
Mandibular fossa
External occipital
protuberance
External auditory
canal
Mastoid process
Styloid process

Zygomatic
process
Articular
tubercle
Mandibular
fossa
Styloid
process
Mastoid
process
External
acoustic
meatus

FIGURE 3.8. Adult Skull—Lateral View

the middle ear and the **hyoid** bone, attached to the lower jaw by ligaments, are also part of the skull.

The Cranium

The cranium consists of the **frontal** (1), **parietal** (2), **occipital** (1), **temporal** (2), **sphenoid** (1), and **ethmoid** (1) bones. These bones form the **cranial cavity,** which contains the brain, blood vessels, and nerves cushioned by fluid. The suture is a joint where two or more of these bones meet. The suture between the parietal bones is the **sagittal suture;** the suture between

BONES OF THE SKULL (22 BONES)

Cranium (8)	**Face** (14)	**Associated bones** (7)
Occipital (1)	Nasal (2)	Auditory ossicles (6)
Parietal (2)	Zygomatics (2)	Hyoid (1)
Frontal (1)	Maxillae (2)	
Temporal (2)	Palatines (2)	
Sphenoid (1)	Lacrimals (2)	
Ethmoid (1)	Inferior	
	conchae (2)	
	Vomer (1)	
	Mandible (1)	

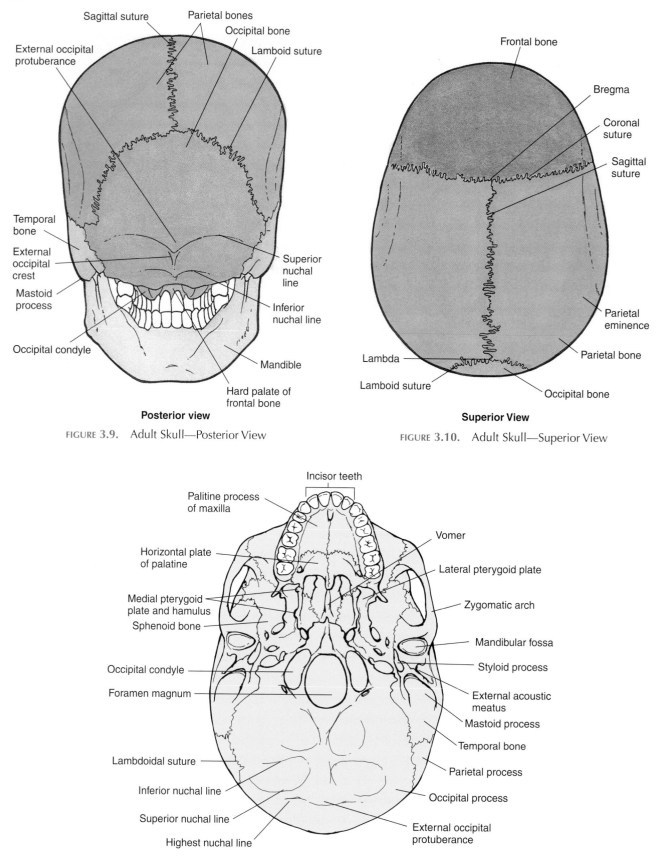

Posterior view

FIGURE **3.9.** Adult Skull—Posterior View

Superior View

FIGURE **3.10.** Adult Skull—Superior View

Inferior View

FIGURE **3.11.** Adult Skull—Inferior View

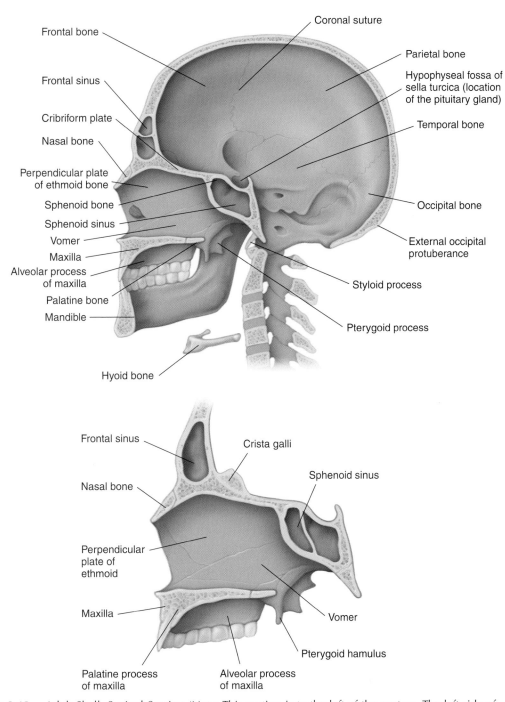

FIGURE **3.12.** Adult Skull. Sagittal Section (Note: This section is to the left of the septum. The left side of the septum is seen)

the two parietal and occipital bone is the **lambdoidal suture.** The **squamosal suture** joins the parietal to the temporal bone. The frontal bone and the parietal bones are joined at the **coronal suture.** The outer surface of the cranium provides surface area for attachment of the muscles of the face. The inner surface provides attachment for the meninges, the thick, connective tissue membranes that surround the brain. The cranial bones also protect the special sensory organs, the eye, hearing, equilibrium, taste, and smell. Many depressions and grooves can be seen on the inside surface of the cranial cavity. These grooves are for venous sinuses and for meningeal arteries. The joint between the first vertebra and the occipital bone allows head movement.

The important landmarks of the skull are shown in Figures 3.7–3.15.

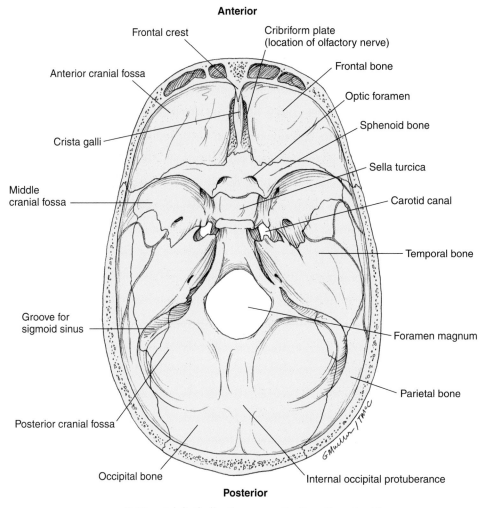

Anterior

Frontal crest

Cribriform plate
(location of olfactory nerve)

Anterior cranial fossa

Frontal bone

Optic foramen

Crista galli

Sphenoid bone

Sella turcica

Middle
cranial fossa

Carotid canal

Temporal bone

Groove for
sigmoid sinus

Foramen magnum

Parietal bone

Posterior cranial fossa

Occipital bone

Internal occipital protuberance

Posterior

FIGURE 3.13. Adult Skull—Transverse Section, Superior View

Facial Bones

The facial bones (14) mainly protect the opening of the digestive and respiratory systems. The superficial bones are the **lacrimal** (2), **nasal** (2), **maxilla** (2), **zygomatic** (2), **palatine** (2), **inferior nasal conchae** (2), **vomer** (1), and **mandible** (1). The muscles that control the facial expressions and those that help manipulate the food in the mouth are attached to these bones.

Paranasal Sinuses

Some bones of the skull contain air-filled chambers called **sinuses.** The sinuses make the bone much lighter than it would be otherwise. They also contribute

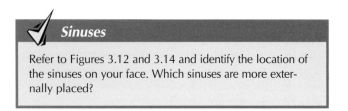

✓ *Sinuses*

Refer to Figures 3.12 and 3.14 and identify the location of the sinuses on your face. Which sinuses are more externally placed?

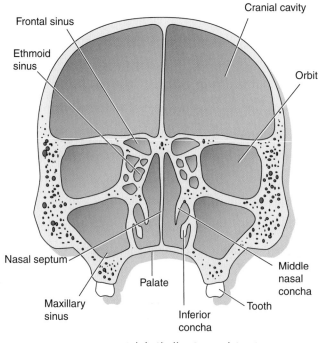

Cranial cavity

Frontal sinus

Ethmoid
sinus

Orbit

Nasal septum

Middle
nasal
concha

Palate

Tooth

Maxillary
sinus

Inferior
concha

FIGURE 3.14. Adult Skull—Coronal Section

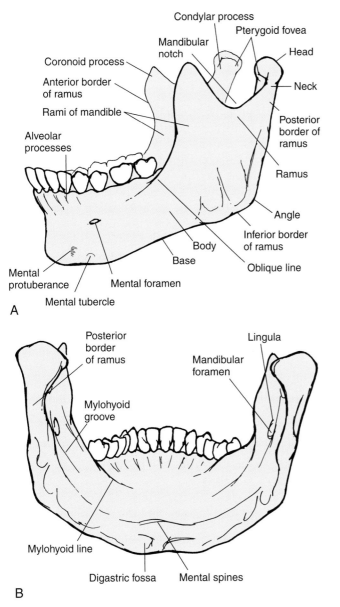

FIGURE **3.15.** Mandible. **A,** Lateral View; **B,** Posterior View

Important Surface Markings of Individual Bones

The surface markings of individual bones must be studied using the diagrams, as well as the information given, as only some of them are highlighted here. Also see the figures in chapter 4 for the location of attachment of muscles.

The **occipital bone** covers the back of the head. When you run your hand over the back of the head, you can feel a bump—the **external occipital protuberance.** Three ridges run horizontally, close to this crest. These are the **inferior, superior,** and **supreme** or **highest nuchal lines.** Some muscles and ligaments of the neck are attached to these lines. A large opening is seen in the inferior surface of the occipital bone, the **foramen magnum.** It connects the cranial cavity with the spinal cavity formed by the vertebral column. Two rounded protuberances on either side of the foramen (**occipital condyles**) articulate with the first cervical vertebra (**atlanto-occipital joint**). Many openings are present in the bones of the skull, which are passages for blood vessels and nerves entering and leaving the cranial cavity. The details of these openings are beyond the scope of this book.

On the **parietal bone,** horizontal ridges (**temporal lines** [superior and inferior temporal lines]) can be felt superior to the ears. The temporalis muscle attaches to this ridge. This is the muscle that can be felt above the ear, on the side of your face. The contraction of this muscle can be felt if the lower jaw is moved.

The **frontal bone** forms the forehead and roof of the eye socket (**orbit**). The frontal sinuses are located in this bone at the center of the forehead. The most prominent part of the frontal bone, superior to the root of nose and anterior to the frontal sinus, is the **glabella.**

The **temporal bone** contributes to part of the cheekbone—the **zygomatic arch. The temporal process of the zygomatic bone** and the **zygomatic process of the temporal bone** combined, form the zygomatic arch. This bone articulates with the mandible at the **mandibular fossa** to form the **temporomandibular joint.** The anterior aspect of the mandibular fossa is bound by the **articular tubercle.** The head of the mandible moves on to this tubercle when the mouth is fully opened. The temporomandibular joint is described in greater detail on **page 131.**

Close to the mandibular fossa, posteriorly, is the opening of the ear—the **external auditory meatus** or **external acoustic meatus**—that leads into the **external auditory canal.** Feel the prominent bulge behind the ear. This is the **mastoid process.** The sternocleidomastoid muscle (the prominent muscle seen in the front of the neck when you turn your head) is attached to the mastoid process. The mastoid process

to the resonance of the voice. The sinuses are lined by a vascular membrane that produces mucus, which helps to warm and moisten the air that is breathed before it reaches the lungs. All the sinuses are adjacent to the nose and communicate with the nasal cavity, hence, the name. The frontal, temporal, sphenoid, and ethmoid bones of the cranium and the maxillary bone of the face contain sinuses.

Orbits

The **orbits** are two, pyramid-shaped depressions containing the eyeballs. The orbits are formed by seven bones. The nerves and blood vessels that supply the eyeballs and muscles that move the eyes enter and leave through openings located in the orbit.

contains air-filled compartments, the **mastoid sinus** or **mastoid air cells.** These sinuses communicate with the middle ear. Another process, the **styloid process,** protrudes close to the mastoid process. The styloid process gives attachment to ligaments that keep the hyoid bone in place. Some muscles of the tongue are also attached. Close to the styloid process, is the **stylomastoid foramen** through which the nerve that controls the facial muscles (the facial nerve) passes.

The **eustachian tube,** or **pharyngotympanic tube,** is part of the temporal bone. This tube, filled with air, connects the pharynx and the middle ear. By opening and closing the tube, the air pressure between the external ear canal and middle ear canal are equalized. This is important for producing oscillations of the auditory ossicles in the middle ear and normal hearing.

The **sphenoid bone** is butterfly-shaped, with two wings (**greater** and **lesser**), and serves as a bridge between the cranium and the facial bones. Important structures of the brain are closely related to this bone. Superiorly, the center of this bone has a depression called the **hypophyseal fossa.** The bony enclosure that forms this fossa is called the **sella turcica,** so called as it resembles the Turkish saddle. The hypophyseal fossa houses the pituitary gland (a major endocrine gland). Close to the hypophyseal fossa anteriorly is the opening for the optic nerve—the **optic foramen.** The **sphenoid sinuses** are located in the middle of the sphenoid bone. Between the two wings is the **superior orbital fissure,** through which blood vessels and nerves pass in and out of the cranial cavity into the orbit. On the inferior surface of the skull (Figure 3.11), two processes (**medial** and **lateral plate of pterygoid**) protrude from the sphenoid bone. Certain muscles that move the mandible are attached to these processes.

The irregularly shaped **ethmoid bone** is located in the middle of the skull. It forms part of the orbit wall, the roof of the nasal cavity, and part of the nasal septum. The **perpendicular plate** of the ethmoid forms part of the nasal septum (Figure 3.12). An important part of the ethmoid is the **cribriform plate** (Figures 3.12 and 3.13). The olfactory nerves, responsible for the sense of smell, pass through small holes in this plate, from the roof of the nasal cavity into the cranial cavity. A sharp triangular process (**crista galli**) projects upward from the cribriform plate, giving attachment to the meninges. Another important part of this bone is the **ethmoidal sinus,** or air cells. These are 3–18 air-filled cavities that open into the nasal cavity. Part of the ethmoids form the **superior** and **middle conchae**—bones that project into the cavity of the nose (see Fig. 3.14). The conchae make the air flowing through the nose turbulent, swirling particles in the air against the sticky mucus on the sides. It also slows the airflow, allowing time for the air to be saturated

with water and warmed to body temperature. In addition, the conchae help direct the air toward the roof of the nasal cavity where the olfactory nerves are located.

BONES OF THE FACE

The bones of the face include the **maxillae, palatines, nasals, mandible, zygomatics, lacrimals, inferior conchae,** and **vomer.**

The right and the left **maxillae** are large facial bones that form the upper jaw. This bone articulates with all the facial bones except the mandible. An important part of this bone is the air-filled cavities, the **maxillary sinuses,** that open into the nasal cavity. The inferior part of the maxilla forms the **alveolar process** (Figure 3.12), which contains the **alveoli** (sockets) for teeth. A horizontal projection, the **palatine process** (Figure 3.11), forms the anterior two-thirds of the hard palate (hard part of the roof of mouth).

The **palatine bones** are L-shaped and form the posterior part of the hard palate. The small **nasal bones** support the superior portion of the bridge of the nose. The flexible, cartilaginous portion of the nose is attached to the nasal bone (see Figure 3.7). The **vomer** is a small bone that forms the inferior portion of the

---

✚ Ailments of the Skull

Sinusitis is an inflammation of one or more sinuses. Sinuses tend to get inflamed when there is an upper respiratory tract infection. While the fluid that collects in most of the sinuses drains relatively well into the nose, there is difficulty in draining the maxillary sinus. This is because the opening into the nose is close to the roof of the sinus, similar to having the door of a room closer to the roof rather than the floor. That is why maxillary sinusitis is more common and persists longer. The nerve, taking sensations from the mouth, lies very close to this sinus. Sinusitis may, therefore, present as a toothache as a result of irritation of this nerve. Inflammation of the mastoid sinus (mastoiditis) can cause severe ear pain, fever, and swelling behind the ear.

Pituitary Tumor is an abnormal growth of the pituitary. With a pituitary tumor, there is no scope for the tumor to expand in the confined bony space except to grow upward. One symptom is change in vision as a result of the pressure of the tumor on the optic nerve lying directly above. Because the sphenoid sinus lies just inferior to the hypophyseal fossa, surgeons find it easier to reach the pituitary through the nose/pharynx via this sinus.

Hydrocephalus. Rarely, the pressure of the cerebrospinal fluid increases inside the skull in infants and results in bulging of the fontanels. If the increase in pressure persists, the skull of the infant enlarges abnormally. This condition is called hydrocephalus. In infants who are dehydrated, the fontanels are depressed.

Head and Neck—Surface Landmarks

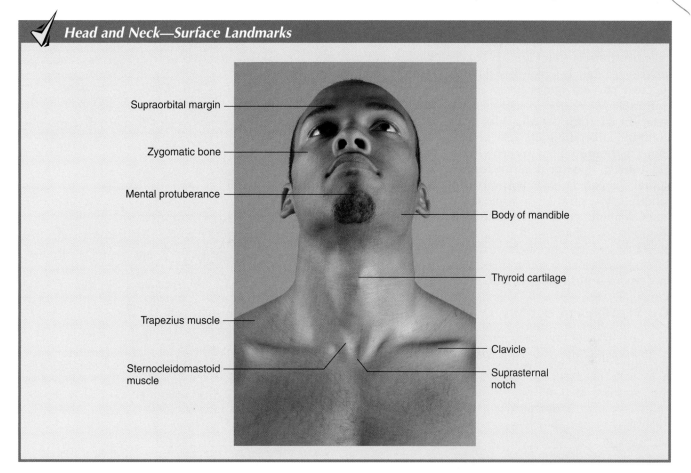

Supraorbital margin

Zygomatic bone

Mental protuberance

Body of mandible

Thyroid cartilage

Trapezius muscle

Clavicle

Sternocleidomastoid muscle

Suprasternal notch

nasal septum (Figure 3.7). The **inferior nasal conchae** (Figures 3.7 and 3.14) are the lowermost bony projections into the nasal cavity. They have the same function as the middle and superior conchae.

The **zygomatic** bones, or cheekbones (Figure 3.8), articulates with the frontal, maxilla, sphenoid, and temporal bones. The **temporal process** articulates with the zygomatic process of the temporal bone, the **frontal process** with the frontal bone, and the **maxillary process** with the maxillary bone. This bone forms part of the lateral wall of the orbital cavity. The **lacrimal** bones (Figure 3.8), the smallest facial bones, are located close to the medial part of the orbital cavity. They have a **lacrimal canal**—a small passage that surrounds the tear duct, through which the tears flow from the eye into the nasal cavity. This is why you blow your nose every time you cry.

THE MANDIBLE

The **mandible** (Figure 3.15) forms the lower jaw and is the strongest and largest facial bone. It is the most movable bone in the skull (excluding the auditory ossicles, which vibrate with sound). It is divided into the horizontal portion (**body**) and the ascending portion (**ramus**) (plural, rami). The point where the

body and the ramus meet is the **angle.** The posterior projection of the ramus (**condylar process**) articulates with the mandibular fossa and articular tubercle of the temporal bone to form the temporomandibular joint. The temporomandibular joint is described on **page 131.** The condylar process has a **head** and a **neck.** The anterior projection (**coronoid process**) of the ramus is the location where the temporalis muscle inserts. This is the muscle that can be felt or seen moving in your temples when you move your jaw. The dent between the two processes is known as the **mandibular notch.** On the superior surface of the body, the **alveolar processes** with the **alveoli** (depressions) give attachment to the teeth of the lower jaw. Nerves and blood vessels pass through the bone through special foramina. The **mental foramen** is located inferior to the location of the premolars, and the **mandibular foramen** is located on the inner surface of the ramus. Dentists often anesthetize the nerves passing through these foramina.

The **hyoid bone** (see Figure 3.12), a small, U-shaped bone located in front of the neck, is held in place by ligaments. The hyoid bone serves as a base for the attachment of several muscles that are concerned with the movement of the tongue and larynx.

The bones in an infant's skull are not fused. Instead, there are fibrous areas between the bones called **fontanels** (see Figure 3.16). The largest is the anterior fontanel, which lies where the frontal and the two parietal bones meet. There is a **posterior fontanel** where the occipital and parietal bones meet. In addition, there are fontanels in the side of the skull, along the squamosal and lambdoid sutures, called **sphenoidal** or **anterolateral fontanels** and **mastoid** or **posterolateral fontanels.** The sphenoidal, mastoid, and posterior fontanels fuse a month or two after birth, while the anterior fontanel fuses at about age two. The fontanels allow the skull to modify its shape as it passes through the pelvic outlet of the mother, without damage to the brain. The time of closure of sutures is variable and slight movement is possible even into adulthood.

THE VERTEBRAL COLUMN

The vertebral column (see Figures 3.17–3.19) consists of 26 bones—24 **vertebrae,** 1 **sacrum,** and 1 **coccyx.** Together, they protect the spinal cord, maintain an

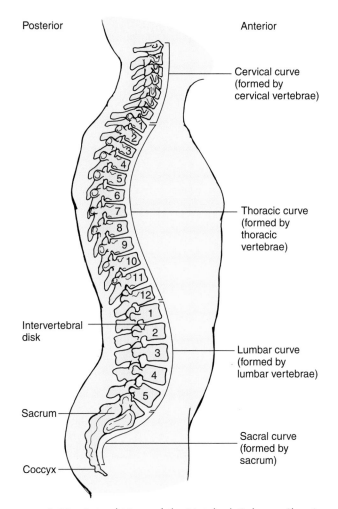

FIGURE **3.17.** Lateral View of the Vertebral Column, Showing the Four Normal Curves and Regions

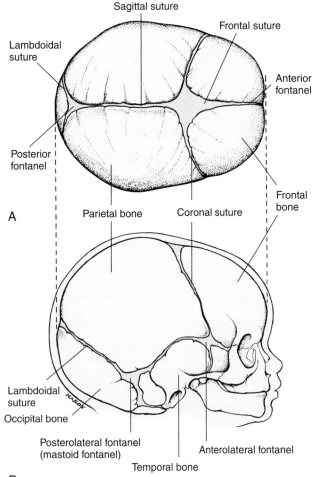

FIGURE **3.16.** Infant Skull. **A,** Lateral View, Fontanels; **B,** Superior View

upright body position, and provide support to the head, neck, and trunk. They also transmit the weight of the body to the legs and provide a surface for attachment of muscles of the trunk.

Vertebral Regions and Spinal Curvatures

The vertebral column is subdivided into the **cervical** (7 vertebrae), **thoracic** (12 vertebrae), **lumbar** (5 vertebrae), **sacral** (1 vertebra), and **coccygeal** (1 vertebra) **regions.** Although the cervical, thoracic, and lumbar consist of individual vertebrae, the sacrum is formed by the fusion of 5 individual vertebrae and the coccyx is formed by the fusion of 3–5 vertebrae. For ease, the vertebrae are labeled according to the position in individual regions e.g., the 7th cervical vertebra is labeled C7; 2nd thoracic vertebra as T2; and so on.

The individual vertebra of the vertebral column are aligned to form four spinal curves (see Figure 3.17)—the **cervical, thoracic, lumbar,** and **sacral curvature.** The thoracic and sacral curvatures have the concavity of the curve facing forward.

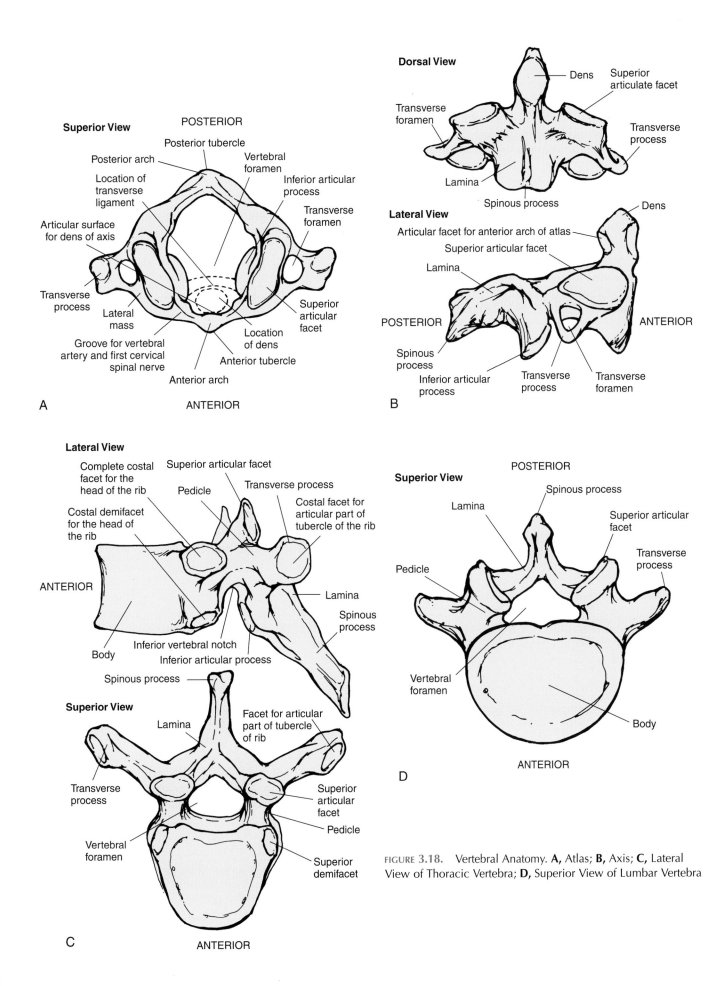

Superior View

POSTERIOR

Posterior tubercle

Posterior arch

Vertebral foramen

Location of transverse ligament

Inferior articular process

Articular surface for dens of axis

Transverse foramen

Transverse process

Lateral mass

Superior articular facet

Groove for vertebral artery and first cervical spinal nerve

Location of dens

Anterior tubercle

Anterior arch

A

ANTERIOR

Dorsal View

Dens

Superior articulate facet

Transverse foramen

Transverse process

Lamina

Spinous process

Lateral View

Dens

Articular facet for anterior arch of atlas

Superior articular facet

Lamina

POSTERIOR

ANTERIOR

Spinous process

Inferior articular process

Transverse process

Transverse foramen

B

Lateral View

Complete costal facet for the head of the rib

Superior articular facet

Pedicle

Transverse process

Costal facet for articular part of tubercle of the rib

Costal demifacet for the head of the rib

ANTERIOR

Lamina

Spinous process

Body

Inferior vertebral notch

Inferior articular process

Spinous process

Superior View

Lamina

Facet for articular part of tubercle of rib

Transverse process

Superior articular facet

Vertebral foramen

Pedicle

Superior demifacet

C

ANTERIOR

Superior View

POSTERIOR

Spinous process

Lamina

Superior articular facet

Pedicle

Transverse process

Vertebral foramen

Body

D

ANTERIOR

FIGURE 3.18. Vertebral Anatomy. **A,** Atlas; **B,** Axis; **C,** Lateral View of Thoracic Vertebra; **D,** Superior View of Lumbar Vertebra

Each vertebra consists of three parts: the **body, vertebral arch,** and **articular processes** (see Figure 3.18). The body is thick, disk-shaped, and located anteriorly. The bodies are interconnected by ligaments. Interspersed between each vertebra are fibrocartilage pads called **intervertebral disks.** Two **vertebral arches** lead off posterolaterally from the body. The two, short, thick processes leading off from the body are known as **pedicles.** The pedicles have depressions on the superior and inferior surfaces (**vertebral notches**). The pedicles join the **laminae,** the flat, posterior part of the arch. These arches meet posteriorly to enclose an opening called the **vertebral foramen.** Because the vertebrae lie on top of each other, the successive vertebral foramina form a **vertebral canal.** The spinal cord lies in the vertebral canal. Laterally, a small foramen is formed where the notches on the pedicles of successive vertebrae align. This is the **intervertebral foramen.** The spinal nerves exit the vertebral canal through these foramina. Posteriorly, each vertebra has a projection called the **spinous process.** This forms the bumps that are seen in the middle of the back in a lean individual. The most prominent of these bumps at the base of the neck indicates the location of the C7 spinous process. C7 is, therefore, called the **vertebra prominens** (see p. 111).

A large elastic ligament, the **ligamentum nuchae,** is attached to the spinous process of C7. From here, it continues upward, attached to the spinous processes of the other cervical vertebrae before it reaches the prominent ridge on the occipital bone, the **external occipital crest** (see Figure 3.9). This ligament maintains the cervical curvature, even without the help of muscular contraction. If the head is bent forward, this elastic ligament helps bring the head to an upright position.

Transverse processes project laterally on both sides. The processes are sites for muscle attachment. Each vertebra has articular processes that project inferiorly (**inferior articular process**) and superiorly (**superior articular process**). This is the area where adjacent vertebrae articulate. The superior articular processes of the lower vertebra articulate with the inferior articular processes of the vertebra located above. The articulating surface of the processes are known as **facets.**

Characteristics of Vertebrae in Different Regions

The characteristics of the vertebrae in different regions vary according to major function. For example, the cervical vertebra have a large vertebral foramen because all the nerves ascending and descending from the brain form the spinal cord here. As the lower regions are approached, the vertebral foramen become smaller. This is because of the exit of spinal nerves according to the region they supply. As the spinal cord descends, more and more nerves leave; hence, the tapering appearance of the spinal cord. The cervical vertebrae are also smaller in size as they have to bear only the weight of the head. The vertebrae in the other regions become sturdier, the lumbar being the largest (Figure 3.18D) because they have to bear more weight. The thoracic vertebrae have extra facets on the transverse processes and the body that articulate with the ribs (Figure 3.18C). The transverse processes of the cervical vertebrae have a foramen (**transverse foramen**), through which the vertebral artery, vein, and a plexus of sympathetic nerves pass. The spinous processes of the cervical vertebrae C2–C6 are often bifid.

The first cervical vertebra is called the **atlas** (Figure 3.18A) as it bears the weight of the head. It articulates with the occipital condyles of the skull. This joint—the atlanto-occipital joint—permits the nodding of the head. The atlas does not have a body and spinous process, instead it has anterior and posterior arches and a thick, lateral mass. The second vertebra is called the **axis** (Figure 3.18B). It has a projection (**dens,** or **odontoid process**) that projects superiorly from the region of the body of the vertebra. This process is held in place against the inner surface of the atlas by a transverse ligament. This joint allows the head to rotate and pivot on the neck. The dens is actually the fusion of the body of the atlas with that of the axis.

Because the position of the head on the cervical vertebrae resembles a bowl being balanced on a small rod, contraction of small muscles attached to the base of the head can initiate marked changes in head position. However, these muscles, being weak, cannot fully support the head if it is jolted violently, as in a car crash. Such a jolt can result in dislocation of the cervical vertebrae and injury to the spinal cord, ligaments, and muscles of the neck. The movement of the head in this situation resembles the lashing of a whip; hence, the name **whiplash** for this kind of injury.

The Sacrum

The sacral vertebrae (see Figure 3.19) begin to fuse with each other at puberty. They are completely fused between 25–30 years of age. The fused sacrum is triangular with the **base** located superiorly and the **apex** pointing downward. The lateral part of the sacrum has articulating surfaces for the pelvic girdle. Large muscles of the thigh are attached to its large surface. The sacrum also protects the lower end of the digestive tract and organs of reproduction and excretion. The upper end of the sacrum articulates with the last lumbar vertebra. Internally, the **sacral canal** is a continuation of the vertebral canal. The nerves from the spinal cord, along with the membranes, continue along the length of the sacral canal and enter and leave the canal through the foramina in the sacrum.

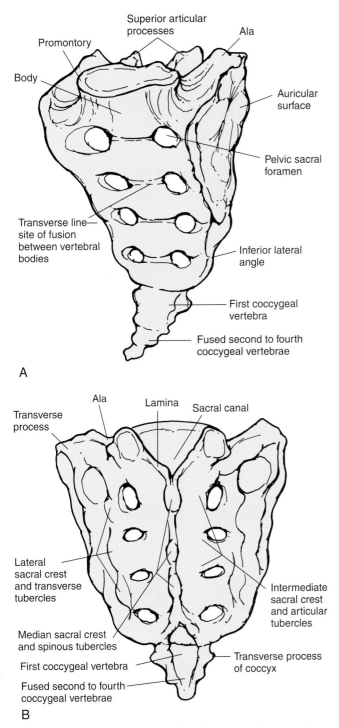

Superior articular
processes

Ala

Promontory

Body

Auricular
surface

Pelvic sacral
foramen

Transverse line—
site of fusion
between vertebral
bodies

Inferior lateral
angle

First coccygeal
vertebra

Fused second to fourth
coccygeal vertebrae

A

Ala

Lamina

Sacral canal

Transverse
process

Lateral
sacral crest
and transverse
tubercles

Intermediate
sacral crest
and articular
tubercles

Median sacral crest
and spinous tubercles

First coccygeal vertebra

Transverse process
of coccyx

Fused second to fourth
coccygeal vertebrae

B

FIGURE 3.19. Sacrum. **A,** Anterolateral View; **B,** Posterior View

The coccyx also consists of vertebrae, which begin to fuse by about age 26. It provides attachment to ligaments and anal muscles.

Intervertebral Disks

From the axis to the sacrum, the vertebral bodies are separated from each other by fibrocartilage called **intervertebral disks.** Each disk-shaped structure is made of a tough outer layer, the **annulus fibrosus.** The collagen fibers of this layer attach adjacent bodies of the vertebrae. The annulus fibrosus encloses a gelatinous, elastic and soft core called the **nucleus pulposus.** Seventy-five percent of this core is water, with scattered strands of elastic and reticular fibers. The disks serve as shock absorbers. They also allow the vertebrae to glide over each other slightly, without losing alignment. Because the disks contribute to one-fourth of the length of the vertebral column, the height of the individual diminishes as the disks loose water and become narrower with age.

Disks can be compressed beyond normal limits. This can happen during a hard fall or whiplash injury or even when lifting heavy weights. If this happens, the nucleus pulposus distorts the annulus fibrosus and forces it into the vertebral canal or the intervertebral foramen. Sometimes it is the nucleus pulposus that protrudes into the canal or foramen in a condition called **slipped disk, disk prolapse,** or **herniated disk.** The distorted disk can compress the spinal cord (in the canal) or the spinal nerves (in the foramina), leading to loss of function in areas supplied by the compressed nerves. It presents as severe backache or burning or tingling sensations in the region supplied by the nerves. Depending on the extent, control of skeletal muscle may also be lost. Some common regions where disks may prolapse are between C5–C6, L4–L5, and L5–S1.

THE THORAX

The bones that form the **thoracic cage** are the **sternum, ribs,** and **vertebrae.** The thoracic cage protects the heart, lungs, and other organs. It provides attachment to muscles that stabilize the vertebral column and the pectoral girdle. Muscles that produce respiratory movements are also attached. The thorax is narrower superiorly and is flattened anteroposteriorly. **Costal** (hyaline) **cartilage,** present anteriorly, connects the ribs to the sternum.

The Sternum

The sternum, or breastbone (see Figures 3.20A and B), lies in the anterior aspect of the thoracic cage, in the midline. The broader, upper part, the **manubrium,** articulates with the clavicles, first and second ribs. A shallow depression in its most superior part is the **suprasternal,** or **jugular notch.** On the lateral aspect of the manubrium, the **clavicular notches** are depressions that articulate with the clavicles to form the sterno-clavicular joint. The first two ribs articulate with the manubrium to form the sternocostal joints at the **costal notches.**

The **body** (**corpus**) of the sternum is attached to the inferior surface of the manubrium. A slight elevation that can be felt at this junction is referred to as

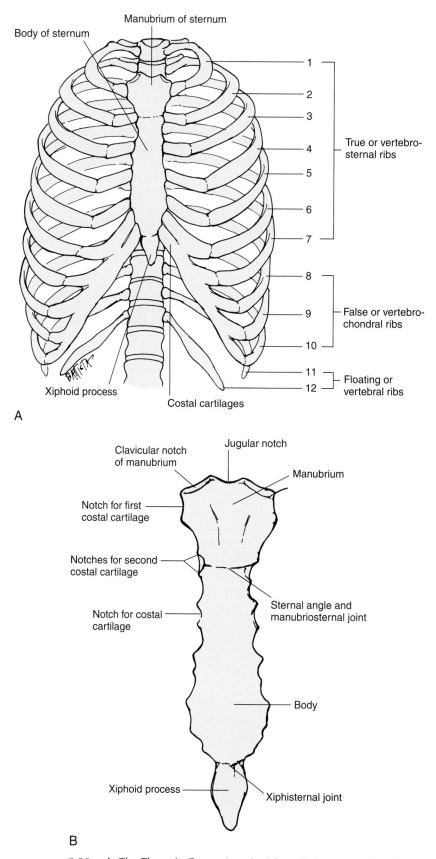

FIGURE 3.20.   **A,** The Thoracic Cage—Anterior View; **B,** Sternum—Anterior View

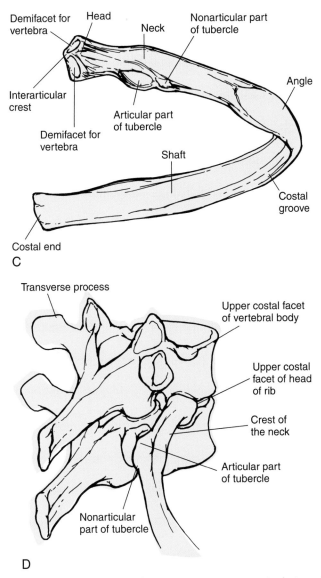

FIGURE 3.20., cont'd **C,** Rib—Posterior View; **D,** Articulation of Rib With Vertebra—Superior View

the **sternal angle.** The body articulates with the costal cartilages of ribs 2–7 at the **costal notches.** The most inferior part of the sternum is the **xiphoid process,** to which the diaphragm and the rectus abdominus muscles are attached. The sternal angle is an important landmark because the second costal cartilage is attached to the sternum at this point. The ribs and intercostal spaces below this point can easily be counted from here. It also indicates the location where the trachea divides into the two primary bronchi. The sounds made by the closing of the aortic and pulmonary valves (second heart sound) are best heard in the second intercostal spaces.

The Ribs

The ribs (Figure 3.20 A and C) are long, flat, and curved. They extend from the thoracic vertebrae to the middle of the thoracic cavity. The ribs are connected to the sternum by **costal cartilages.** The first seven pairs are known as **true ribs** or **vertebrosternal ribs** because each of these ribs have individual costal cartilages that connect them to the sternum. Ribs 8–12 are known as **false ribs** or **vertebrochondral ribs** because they are not connected to the sternum individually, instead the costal cartilages of the ribs 8–10 are fused together before they reach the sternum. Ribs 11 and 12 are not attached to the sternum; they are only attached to the vertebrae. These ribs are called **floating,** or **vertebral ribs.**

Typically, the posterior end of the rib has a **head** with two **facets** that articulate with the facets on the bodies of the vertebrae to form the **vertebrocostal joint.** Lateral to the head is the constricted portion called the **neck.** On the posterior aspect of the neck, there is a short projection, the **tubercle.** The articular part of the tubercle articulates with the facet on the transverse process of the lower of the two thoracic vertebrae (to which the head articulates). The neck continues on as the **body,** or **shaft.** The shaft curves anteriorly and medially beyond the tubercle, forming the **costal angle.** The superior and inferior surfaces of the ribs give attachment to the intercostal muscles. The space between any two ribs is known as the **intercostal space.** The intercostal muscles, blood vessels, and nerves are located here.

There is a groove on the internal aspect of the rib, the **costal groove,** in which the intercostal nerves and blood vessels lie.

The positioning of the ribs resembles that of a bucket handle (see Figure 3.21). If the ribs are pushed down, the transverse diameter of the thorax is decreased. It also results in the sternum being pulled inward, decreasing the anteroposterior diameter. If the ribs are pulled upward, there is an increase in the transverse and anteroposterior diameter. This is how the thoracic capacity is altered during respiration. The presence of the costal cartilages makes the thoracic cavity flexible and able to withstand sudden impact; however, severe blows can fracture the ribs.

The Appendicular Skeleton

PECTORAL GIRDLE AND THE UPPER LIMBS

The upper arm articulates with the trunk at the **shoulder,** or **pectoral girdle.** The pectoral girdle consists of the clavicle (collarbone) and the scapula (shoulder blade). Amazingly, the only joint between the pectoral girdle and the trunk is where the clavicle articulates with the manubrium of the sternum. The scapula is held against the thorax by muscle. This architecture allows for increased mobility but de-

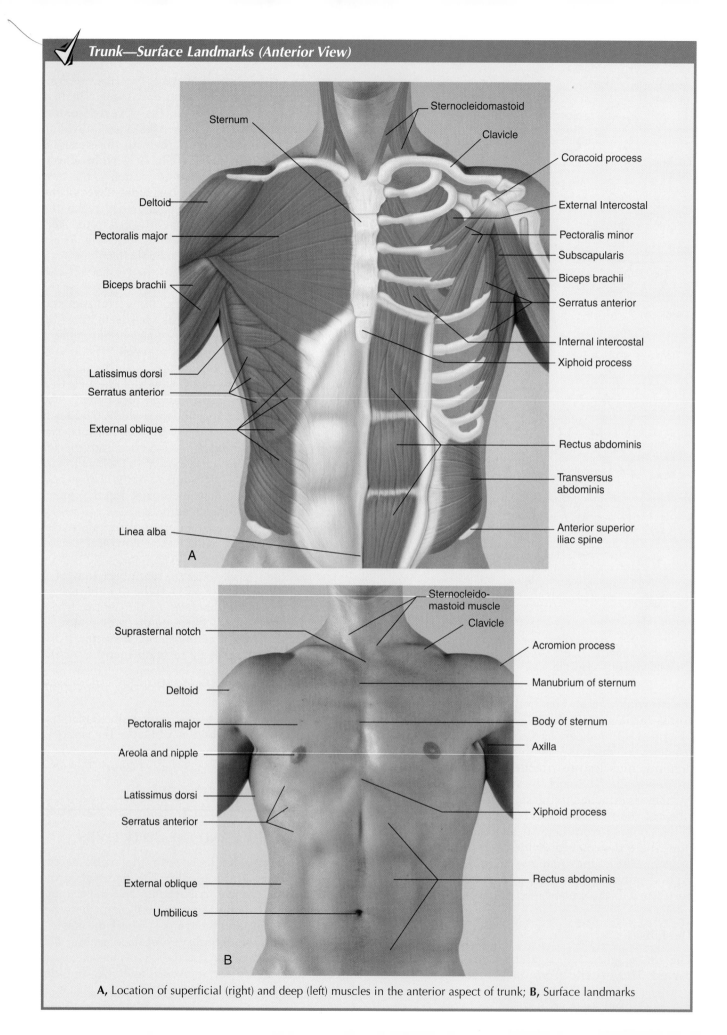

A, Location of superficial (right) and deep (left) muscles in the anterior aspect of trunk; **B,** Surface landmarks

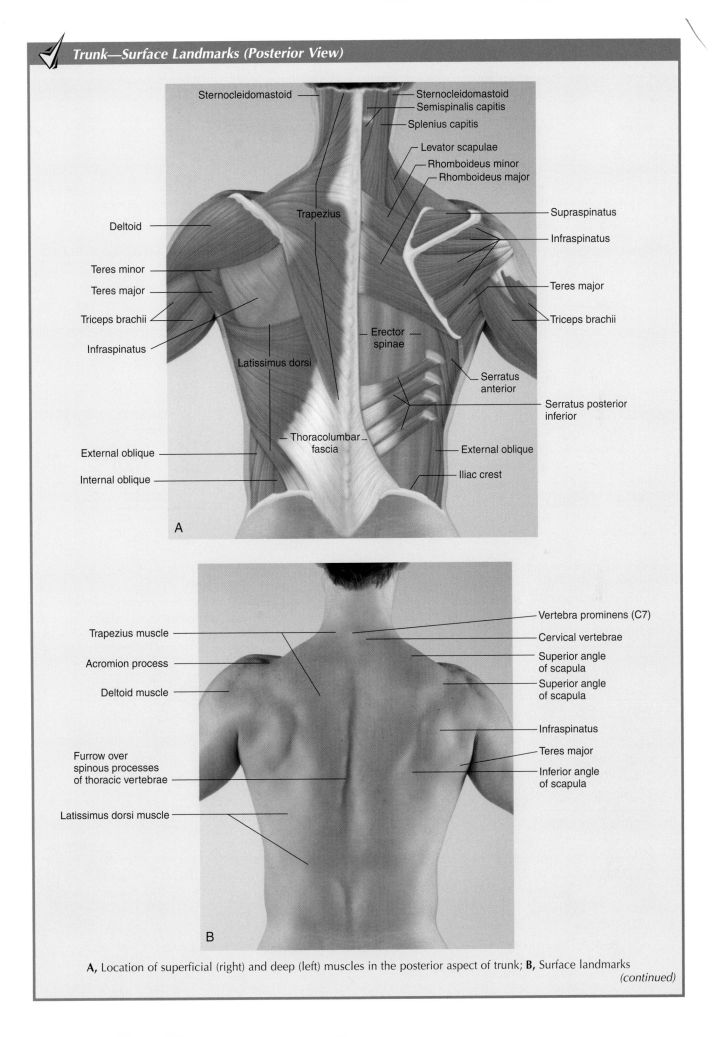

Sternocleidomastoid

Sternocleidomastoid
Semispinalis capitis
Splenius capitis

Levator scapulae
Rhomboideus minor
Rhomboideus major

Trapezius

Supraspinatus

Deltoid

Infraspinatus

Teres minor
Teres major

Teres major

Triceps brachii

Triceps brachii

Infraspinatus

Erector
spinae

Latissimus dorsi

Serratus
anterior

Serratus posterior
inferior

External oblique

Thoracolumbar
fascia

External oblique

Internal oblique

Iliac crest

A

Trapezius muscle

Vertebra prominens (C7)

Acromion process

Cervical vertebrae

Superior angle
of scapula

Deltoid muscle

Superior angle
of scapula

Infraspinatus

Furrow over
spinous processes
of thoracic vertebrae

Teres major

Inferior angle
of scapula

Latissimus dorsi muscle

B

A, Location of superficial (right) and deep (left) muscles in the posterior aspect of trunk; **B,** Surface landmarks

(continued)

Trunk—Surface Landmarks (Posterior View)—cont'd

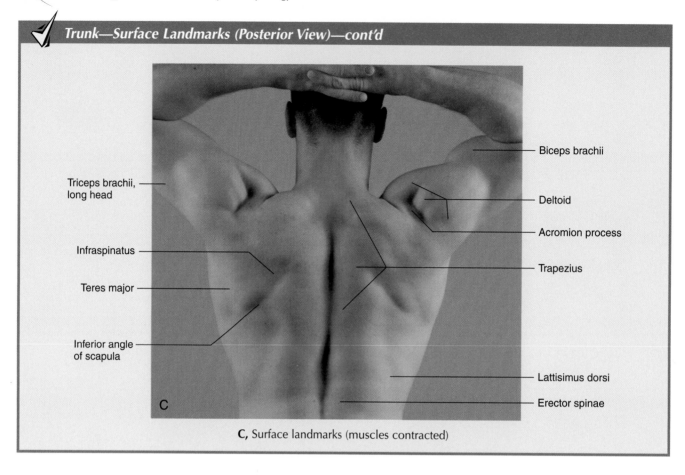

Triceps brachii, long head

Infraspinatus

Teres major

Inferior angle of scapula

Biceps brachii

Deltoid

Acromion process

Trapezius

Lattisimus dorsi

Erector spinae

C

C, Surface landmarks (muscles contracted)

creased strength. The muscles attached to the pectoral girdle stabilize the shoulder while upper limb movements are produced. Ridges and thickened areas are seen in regions of the scapula and clavicle where these powerful muscles are attached.

The Clavicle

The clavicle (see Figure 3.22) is the S-shaped bone seen or felt below the neck, along the front of the shoulder. The medial part of the clavicle is convex anteriorly and extends laterally and somewhat horizontally from the manubrium of the sternum to the tip of the shoulder.

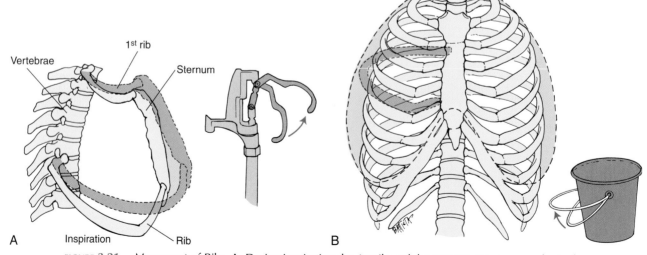

Vertebrae

1st rib

Sternum

A   Inspiration   Rib   B

FIGURE 3.21. Movement of Ribs. **A,** During inspiration the 1st rib and the sternum move upwards similar to a pump handle; **B,** The ribs move upward and outward during inspiration and downward and inward during expiration similar to a bucket handle.

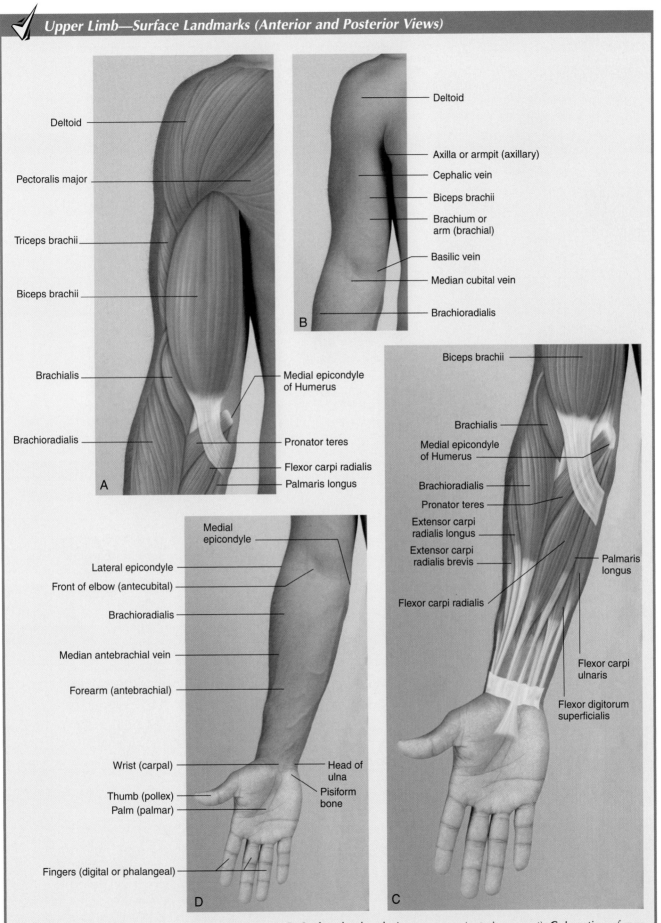

Deltoid

Pectoralis major

Triceps brachii

Biceps brachii

Brachialis

Brachioradialis

Medial epicondyle of Humerus

Pronator teres

Flexor carpi radialis

Palmaris longus

A

Deltoid

Axilla or armpit (axillary)

Cephalic vein

Biceps brachii

Brachium or arm (brachial)

Basilic vein

Median cubital vein

Brachioradialis

B

Biceps brachii

Brachialis

Medial epicondyle of Humerus

Brachioradialis

Pronator teres

Extensor carpi radialis longus

Extensor carpi radialis brevis

Flexor carpi radialis

Palmaris longus

Flexor carpi ulnaris

Flexor digitorum superficialis

C

Medial epicondyle

Lateral epicondyle

Front of elbow (antecubital)

Brachioradialis

Median antebrachial vein

Forearm (antebrachial)

Wrist (carpal)

Head of ulna

Pisiform bone

Thumb (pollex)

Palm (palmar)

Fingers (digital or phalangeal)

D

A, Location of muscles in upper arm (anterior aspect); **B,** Surface landmarks in upper arm (anterior aspect); **C,** Location of muscles in forearm (anterior aspect); **D,** Surface landmarks in forearm and hand (anterior aspect)

(continued)

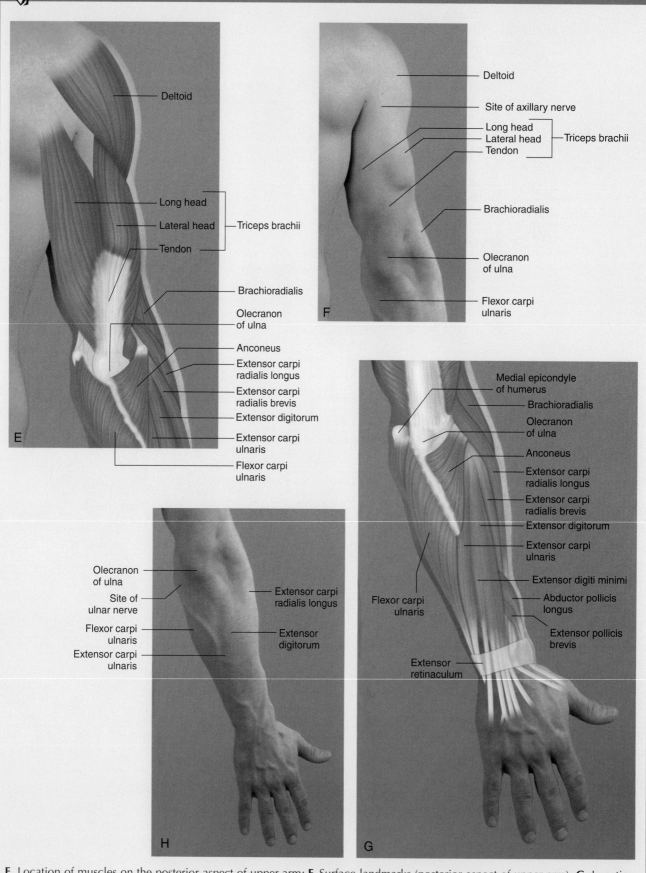

E, Location of muscles on the posterior aspect of upper arm; **F,** Surface landmarks (posterior aspect of upper arm); **G,** Location of muscles on the posterior aspect of forearm; **H,** Surface landmarks (posterior aspect of forearm)

SURFACE ANATOMY—SHOULDER

Run your index and middle finger over the clavicle and the upper surface of the acromion and backward along the spine of the scapula. What muscles are related to these bony surfaces? Can you feel the tip of the coracoid process below the lateral part of the clavicle? It can be felt upward and laterally below the lower border of the deltoid.

The end closest to the sternum is the **sternal end,** and it articulates with the manubrium of the sternum (sternoclavicular joint). The other end is the **acromial end;** it articulates with the acromion of the scapula (acromioclavicular joint). The clavicle is the most frequently fractured bone in the body. Fractures of the clavicle often occur after a fall on the outstretched hand. The fracture tends to be in the midregion where the two curves of the clavicle meet. Most clavicular fractures do not require a cast because they heal rapidly.

The Scapula

The scapula (see Figures 3.22 and 3.23), or the shoulder blade, is a triangular bone with some projections on the upper lateral angle of the triangle. It extends over the second and seventh ribs on the posterior and

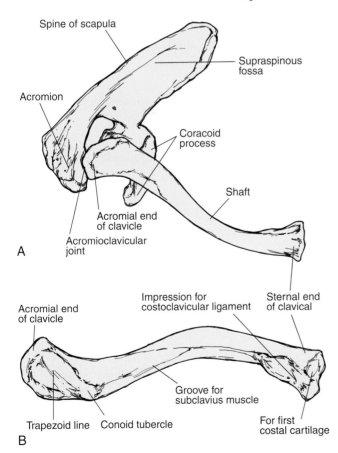

FIGURE 3.22.   The Clavicle—**A,** Superior View; **B,** Inferior View

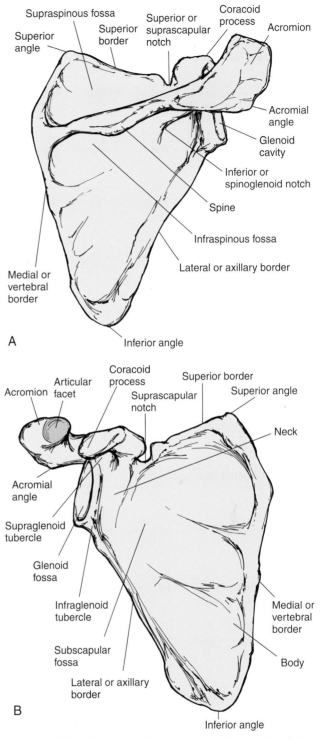

FIGURE 3.23.   Scapula. **A,** Posterior View; **B,** Anterior View

superior aspect of the thorax. The three sides of the triangle are the **superior border; medial,** or **vertebral border;** and the **lateral,** or **axillary border.** The angles of the triangle are the **superior angle, inferior angle,** and **lateral angle.** The lateral angle is thickened and rounded—the **neck,** before it widens to form the cup-shaped **glenoid fossa.** The glenoid fossa articulates with the upper end of the humerus at the scapulohumeral joint or shoulder joint. A rough surface on the superior aspect of the fossa (**supraglenoid tubercle**), denotes the location of the attachment of the long head of the biceps. A rough surface on the inferior aspect of the fossa (**infraglenoid tubercle**) gives the location of attachment of the long tendon of the triceps. Two prominent extensions extend over the superior aspect of the glenoid fossa. The smaller, anterior extension is the **coracoid process.** The larger, posterior prominence is the **acromion process.** The acromion articulates with the lateral end of the clavicle at the acromioclavicular joint. Both processes are sites of attachment of ligaments and tendons of muscles.

Medially, the acromion is continuous with a ridge on the posterior aspect of the scapula called the **scapular spine.** There is a depression superior to the scapular spine called the **supraspinous** or **supraspinatus fossa.** The depression inferior to the spine is called the **infraspinous** or **infraspinatus fossa.** The muscles

supraspinatus and infraspinatus are attached to these areas respectively. The depression on the anterior aspect of the scapula that faces the ribs is called the **subscapular fossa.** The muscle subscapularis is attached here.

The Humerus

The humerus (see Figure 3.24) is a bone of the upper limb. The bones of the upper limb include those of the arm, forearm, wrist, and hand. The humerus extends from the shoulder to the elbow. It is a long bone with a rounded upper end called the **head,** a long **shaft,** and a widened, lower end that articulates with the ulna and radius (bones of the forearm). The head articulates with the glenoid fossa of the scapula. There are two prominences on the lateral surface of the head known as the **greater** and **lesser tubercles.** If you run your hand lateral to the tip of the acromion process, you will feel the greater tubercle as a bump anterior and inferior to the process.

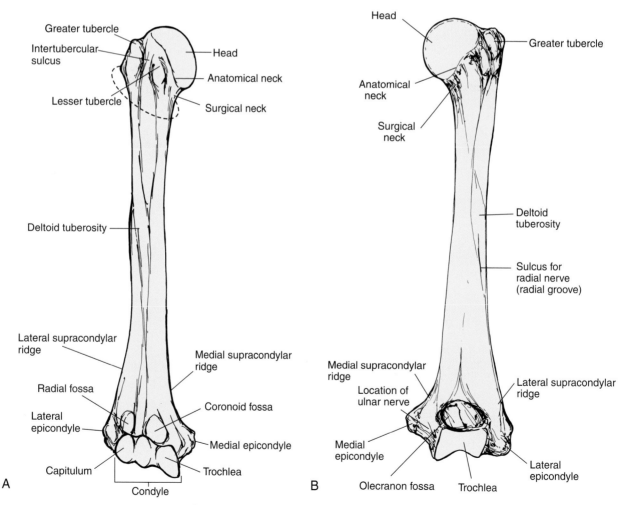

FIGURE 3.24.   Humerus. **A,** Anterior View; **B,** Posterior View

The **intertubercular groove,** or the **intertubercular sulcus,** runs between the two tubercles. The tendon of the biceps runs in this groove to attach to the supraglenoid tubercle of the scapula. As previously explained, the bumps and ridges in bones are locations where muscles are attached. The head of the humerus narrows a little between the tubercles and the articular surface (the smooth area on the head). This is the **anatomical neck.** The capsule that surrounds the shoulder joint ends at the anatomical neck; however, what actually looks like a neck, is the narrowing inferior to the tubercles. This narrowed area is called the **surgical neck** because this is the region where fractures are common.

A bump is located on the lateral surface of the shaft, near the halfway point; this is the **deltoid tuberosity.** The deltoid muscle (the muscle that gives the rounded effect to the shoulder) is attached at this point. A depression in the posterior surface of the shaft—the **radial/spiral groove**—indicates the path taken by the radial nerve as it runs down the arm.

The lower end of the humerus is widened or expanded from side to side. Two ridges—**lateral** and **medial supracondylar ridges/crests**—continue on to two projections, the **medial** and **lateral epicondyle** on the medial and lateral aspects of the lower end. The ulnar nerve passes posterior to the medial epicondyle. The epicondyles are sites of attachment of most muscles of the forearm.

Pressure on the ulnar nerve, which is relatively superficial posterior to the medial epicondyle, is responsible for the tingling felt when an individual accidentally hits an elbow against an object.

The posterior aspect of the lower end of the humerus has one depression. This is the **olecranon fossa,** where the olecranon process of the ulna is accommodated when the elbow is extended. On the anterior aspect, there are two depressions. The lateral depression is the **radial fossa,** where a projection from the radius is accommodated. Medially, there is another depression known as the **coronoid fossa.** This, too, accommodates a process, the coronoid process of the ulna when the elbow is flexed.

The widened part of the lower end of the humerus is the **condyle.** Inferior to the fossa, anteriorly and medially, the inferior end of the humerus is shaped like a pulley—the **trochlea.** This articulates with the ulna. On the anterior aspect, inferior to the radial fossa, is the rounded **capitulum.** The capitulum articulates with the head of the radius.

The Ulna

The ulna (see Figure 3.25), together with the radius, forms the bones of the forearm. The ulna is located medially. The proximal end of the ulna has two processes, the **olecranon process** that forms the superior and posterior portion and the **coronoid process** that forms the anterior and inferior process. The depression between the two processes is the **trochlear notch.** This is the part of the ulna that articulates with the trochlea of the humerus. This joint is known as the **olecranon joint** or the **humeroulnar joint.** Just inferior to the coronoid process, is the **ulnar tuberosity.** A slight depression on the lateral side of the ulna indicates the surface that articulates with the radius, the **radial notch.** This is the **radioulnar joint.** Other than the joint, the radius and ulna are held together by a thick sheet of connective tissue that runs from the lateral border of the ulna (**interosseous border**) to the radius. This is the **interosseous membrane.** The lower end of the ulna has a rounded **head** and a small projection on the posterior aspect called the **styloid process.**

The Radius

The rounded, upper end of the radius (Figure 3.25) is called the **head.** Note that the head of the ulna is distal and that of the radius is proximal. The head articulates with the capitulum of the humerus and the radial notch of the ulna (proximal radioulnar joint). It narrows to form a **neck** and continues on to a prominence, the **radial/bicipital tuberosity.** The biceps are inserted to this region. The radius also has an **interosseous border** to which the interosseous membrane is attached. A slight, roughened area on the middle of the convex lateral aspect of the shaft of the radius is the **pronator tuberosity,** to which the pronator teres (muscle) is attached.

The distal end of the radius is widened. This surface articulates with the bones of the wrist: lunate, scaphoid, and the triquetrum (radiocarpal joint). A small projection in the lateral aspect is the **styloid process** of the radius. A depression in the medial surface of the lower end, the **ulnar notch,** indicates the location of articulation with the ulnar head (distal radioulnar joint). When the palm is turned back—*pronation* (Remember the anatomical position?), the ulnar notch of the radius glides over the head of the ulna. In this position, the lower end of the radius is located medially; hence, the importance of having an anatomical position. When the palm faces forward—*supination,* the radius and ulna lie side by side.

The Carpals

The eight carpal bones are lined up in two rows: four proximal and four distal. The proximal carpals, lateral to medial, are **scaphoid, lunate, triangular** or **triquetrum,** and **pisiform.** The distal carpals are the **trapezium, trapezoid, capitate,** and **hamate.**

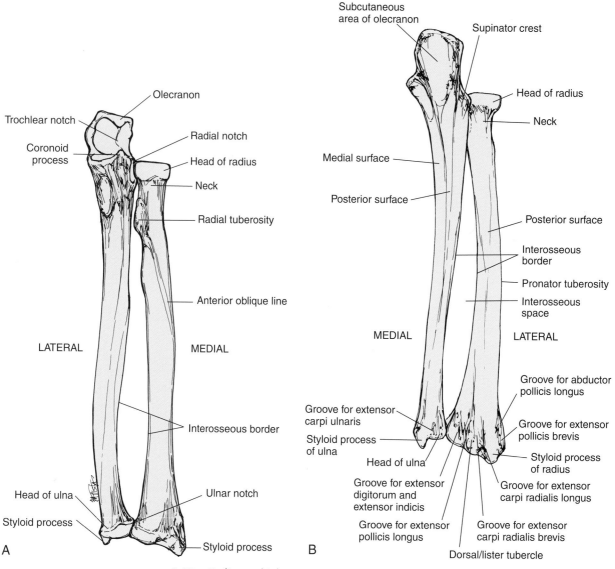

FIGURE **3.25.**   Radius and Ulna. **A,** Anterior View; **B,** Posterior View

The carpals are held together by ligaments. They articulate with each other at intercarpal joints that allow some gliding and twisting. Anteriorly, the **flexor retinaculum** ligament runs across the carpals from side to side, enclosing a tunnel through which tendons of muscles going to the hand, along with nerves and blood vessels, pass. This is the **carpal tunnel** (see Common Wrist Ailments). The compression of the median nerve located in this tunnel is responsible for the various symptoms of **carpal tunnel syndrome.**

SURFACE ANATOMY—WRIST

Do you realize that your wristwatch goes around the lower end of the ulna and radius and not the carpal bones? Feel the lower end of the radius and ulna. Note that the styloid process of the radius is lower than that of the ulna bone.

The skin crease at the wrist corresponds to the upper border of the flexor retinaculum. The retinaculum is the size of a postage stamp, with its long axis transverse. The flexor retinaculum is attached laterally to the tubercle of the scaphoid and tubercle of the trapezium and medially to the pisiform and the hook (hamulus) of hamate. The median nerve lies deep to the tendon that becomes prominent in the middle of the skin crease, when you flex your wrist. The tendon is that of palmaris longus muscle. The pulse felt in the lateral part of the wrist is that of the radial artery. Can you feel it? The pisiform bone can be felt as a prominence in the medial part of the wrist.

In your palm, compare the location of the metacarpal bones in relation to the skin creases.

The Hand

The carpals articulate with five **metacarpals,** the bones that support the palm. The metacarpals are labeled I to V, with the thumb being I (see Figure 3.26). The metacarpals articulate with the **phalanges.** Each finger—except the thumb—have three phalanges. The thumb has two. The phalanges are **proximal** (the one closer to the metacarpal), **middle,** and **distal phalanx,** according to the position.

THE PELVIC GIRDLE AND LOWER LIMBS

The **pelvic girdle** consists of two bones, the fused **coxae** or **innominate bones.** Anteriorly, the two hipbones are connected by fibrocartilage at the **pubic symphysis.** Posteriorly, they are joined to the sacrum and coccyx of the axial skeleton at the sacroiliac joint. The pubic symphysis, the two hipbones, and the sacrum and coccyx combined form a basin-like **bony pelvis.**

The bones of the pelvic girdle and lower limbs are larger because they incur greater stress. The lower limb consists of the **femur, tibia, fibula, tarsals, metatarsals,** and **phalanges.**

THE PELVIC GIRDLE

Each coxa, or hipbone (see Figure 3.27), is made of three bones that have fused together, the **ilium, ischium,** and the **pubis.** The ilium articulates with the sacrum posteriorly and medially. On the lateral surface of the coxa, there is a rounded depression called the **acetabulum.** The femur articulates with the hipbone at the acetabulum. The three bones (ilium, ischium, and pubis) meet inside the **acetabular fossa** (the depression formed by the walls of the acetabulum).

Ilium

The ilium (see Figure 3.28) is the largest of the three bones and provides an extensive surface for attachment of muscles and tendons. It is in the form of a ridge superiorly, the **iliac crest.** Anteriorly, the iliac crest forms a prominence called the **anterior superior iliac spine.** Posteriorly, the crest ends at the **posterior superior iliac spine.** Posteriorly and inferiorly, there is a deep notch called the **greater sciatic notch.** The medial surface of the ilium has a shallow depression called the **iliac fossa.** Other important landmarks on the ilium are shown in Figure 3.28.

Ischium

One important landmark on the ischium is the **ischial spine**—a projection just inferior to the greater sciatic notch. The **ischial tuberosity** is the roughened projection inferior to the ischial spine. This is the bone in your buttock that bears your weight when you sit. The ischium has a projection called the **ischial ramus,** which continues with the projection **inferior ramus** of the pubis. Together with the **superior ramus** of the pubis, the rami enclose an opening called the **obturator foramen.** In the body, this foramen is lined by connective tissue that provides a base for attachment of muscles both on the interior and exterior surfaces.

The pelvis is divided into the **true (lesser)** and the **false (greater) pelvis.** The true pelvis is the region below an imaginary line that runs from the superior aspect of the sacrum to the superior margin of the pubic symphysis. The upper bony edge of the true

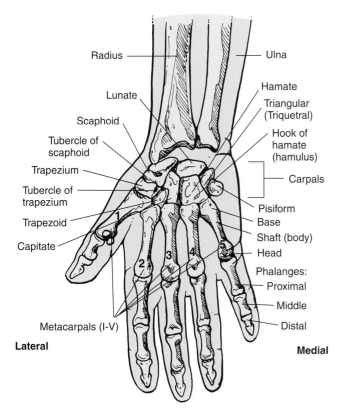

FIGURE **3.26.**   Bones of the Wrist and Hand—Anterior View

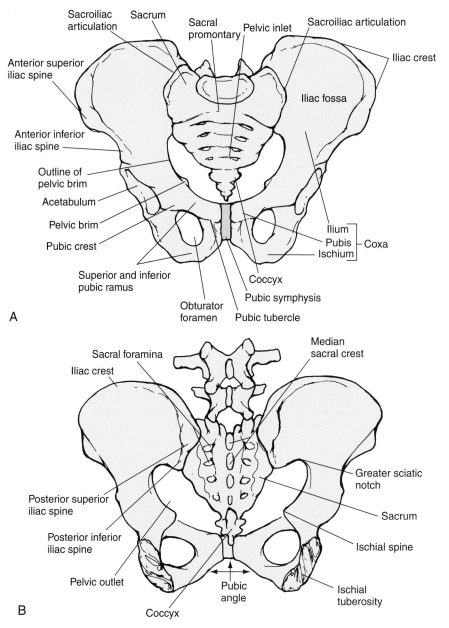

FIGURE 3.27.   The Pelvis. **A,** Anterior View; **B,** Posterior View

pelvis is the **pelvic brim** and the opening is the **pelvic inlet.** When an obstetrician says that the head of the baby is fixed, it indicates that the head has entered the pelvic inlet.

The **pelvic outlet** is the opening bound by the inferior edges of the pelvis. This body region is called the **perineum** and is bound by the coccyx, the ischial tuberosities, and the inferior border of the pubic symphysis. Strong perineal muscles support the organs in the pelvic cavity.

Differences Between the Male and Female Pelves

The male and female pelvis differs in shape and size. In females, the pelvis is lighter and smoother, with less prominent markings. The entire pelvis is low and broad. To facilitate childbearing, both the pelvic inlet and outlet are larger and wider in females. The arch made by the inferior rami of the pubis (pubic arch) is wider and the sacrum and coccyx are less curved, widening the pelvic outlet. Hormones secreted at pregnancy soften and loosen the ligaments and cartilage in the pelvis, enabling the pelvis to widen further, if necessary, at delivery.

In females, the acetabulum is small and faces anteriorly compared with that of males, where it is larger and faces laterally. This is partly responsible for the difference in gait between men and women. The shape of the obturator foramen is also different, being oval in females and round in males.

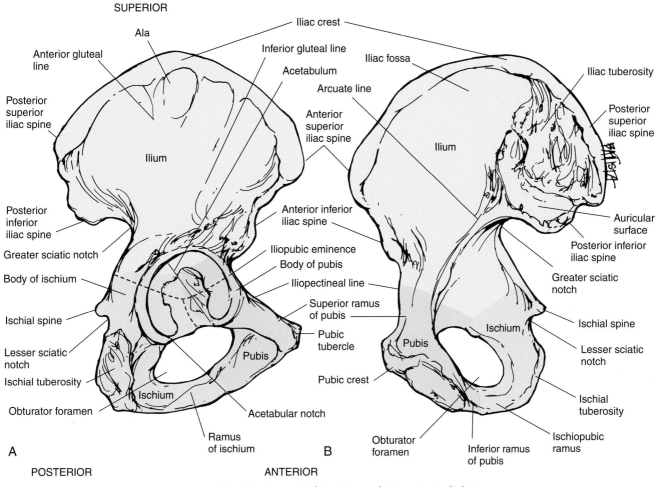

FIGURE **3.28.** Hip Bone (Right). **A,** Lateral View; **B,** Medial View

The Femur

The femur (see Figure 3.29) is the longest and heaviest bone in the body. Proximally, it articulates with the pelvis and distally with the tibia and patella at the knee joint. The superior aspect of the femur is rounded to form a **head.** The head narrows into a distinct **neck** that, in turn, joins with the **shaft** at an angle of about 125°. At the junction of the neck and shaft, a projection is seen laterally. This is the **greater trochanter.** On the posteromedial surface, inferior to the greater trochanter, is the **lesser trochanter.** Anteriorly, a raised surface that runs between the greater and lesser trochanter, the **intertrochanteric line,** marks the point where the articular capsule of the hip joint is attached.

Along the posterior aspect of the shaft of the femur, the **linea aspera** ridge runs down the center. Distally, the linea aspera divides into two ridges: the **medial** and the **lateral supracondylar ridge.** The lower end of the femur widens into the **medial** and **lateral condyles.** The medial and lateral supra-condylar ridges end at roughened projections, the **medial** and **lateral epicondyles,** located on the medial and lateral condyles, respectively. A prominence just superior to the medial epicondyle, the **adductor tubercle,** is where the tendon of the adductor magnus attaches. A deep depression, the **intercondylar fossa,** is seen between the condyles on the posterior surface of the lower end of the femur. Anteriorly, there is a smooth surface between the condyles. This is the surface that articulates with the patella, the **patellar surface, or trochlear femoris.**

The Patella

The patella (Figure 3.29C) is a large, triangular (with the apex pointing inferiorly) sesamoid bone, which is formed within the tendon of the quadriceps femoris muscle. The anterior, superior, and inferior surfaces are rough, indicating the regions that are attached to the ligaments and tendons. The anterior and inferior surface is attached to the patellar ligament, which connects the patella to the tibia. The anterior and superior

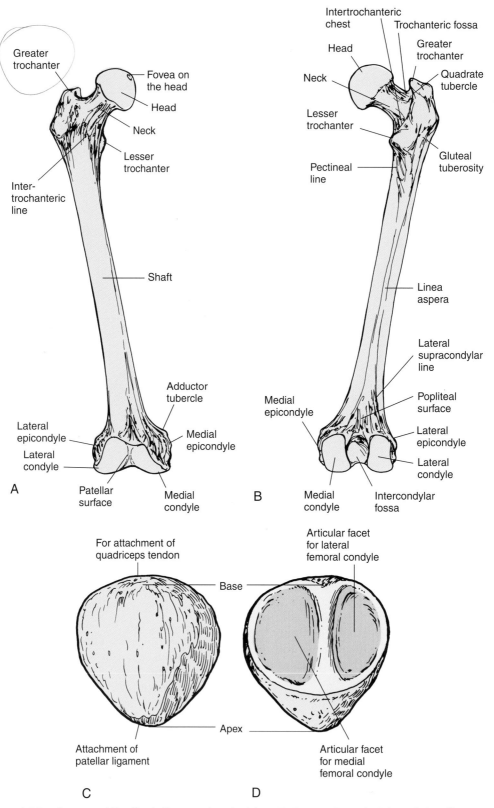

FIGURE 3.29.   Femur and Patella. **A,** Femur—Anterior View; **B,** Femur—Posterior View; **C,** Patella—Anterior View; **D,** Patella—Posterior View

surface is attached to the quadriceps tendon. The posterior surface is smooth, with a medial and lateral facet that articulates with the medial and lateral condyles of the femur.

The Tibia

The tibia (see Figure 3.30) is a large bone located medial to the fibula. The proximal end articulates with the condyles of the femur and the proximal end of the fibula. The distal end articulates with the tarsal bone—talus and the distal end of the fibula (laterally). The tibia and fibula, similar to the radius and ulna of the upper limb, are connected to each other by an interosseous membrane. The proximal, or upper end, is widened into a **medial** and **lateral tibial condyle.** A smaller projection, the **intercondylar eminence,** separates the two condyles in the superior aspect of this widened end. The superior aspect that articulates with the condyles of the femur has a **medial** and **lateral articular surface.** Anteriorly, the proximal end has a roughened area, the **tibial tuberosity.** This is where the patellar ligament is attached. The **anterior crest,** or **border,** of the tibia is a ridge that runs inferiorly, down the center of the tibia. This is the ridge that can be felt on the anterior aspect of the lower leg. Distally, too, the tibia widens to form projections. The large projection, the **medial malleolus,** is the bony prominence seen on the medial aspect of the ankle. It articulates with the talus. In the lateral aspect, the distal end of the tibia articulates with the distal end of the fibula at the **fibular notch.**

The Fibula

The fibula (Figure 3.30) is slender and is located lateral to the tibia. The proximal end is widened into the **head.** The head of the fibula articulates with the tibia, just inferior to the lateral condyle of the tibia. Along the shaft, a thin ridge, the **interosseous crest,** marks the surface that gives attachment to the strong connective tissue **interosseous membrane.** The interosseous membrane bridges the gap between the tibia and the fibula along the two shafts, stabilizing the bones and increasing the anterior and posterior surface area for attachment of muscles. The lower end of the fibula widens to form a prominence called the **lateral malleolus.** The bony projection on the lateral aspect of the ankle is the lateral malleolus that articulates with the talus bone. Although the upper

end of the fibula does not participate in the knee joint, the lower end is an important component of the ankle joint.

The Ankle

The ankle (tarsus) (see Figure 3.31) consists of the seven tarsal bones: the **talus, calcaneus, cuboid, navicular,** and the three **cuneiforms.**

The talus (Figure 3.31C) is the second largest of the tarsals and articulates with the lower end of the tibia and fibula. The superior, lateral, and medial surface of the talus appears smooth, as they are part of the ankle joint. The lateral surface has roughened surfaces that indicate the attachment of strong ligaments that stabilize the joint.

The heel bone, or the calcaneus, is the largest tarsal. The posterior surface of the calcaneus is roughened where the tendo calcaneus, or the Achilles tendon, of the calf muscles is attached. Anteriorly and superiorly, it is smooth where it articulates with the

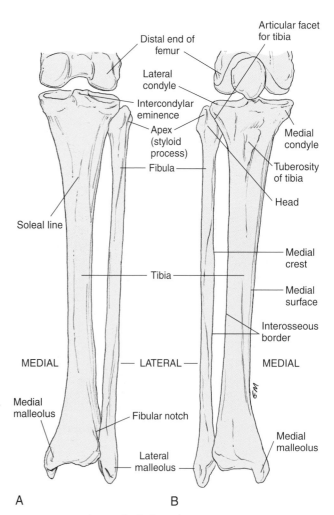

FIGURE 3.30. Tibia and Fibula (right). **A,** Posterior View; **B,** Anterior View

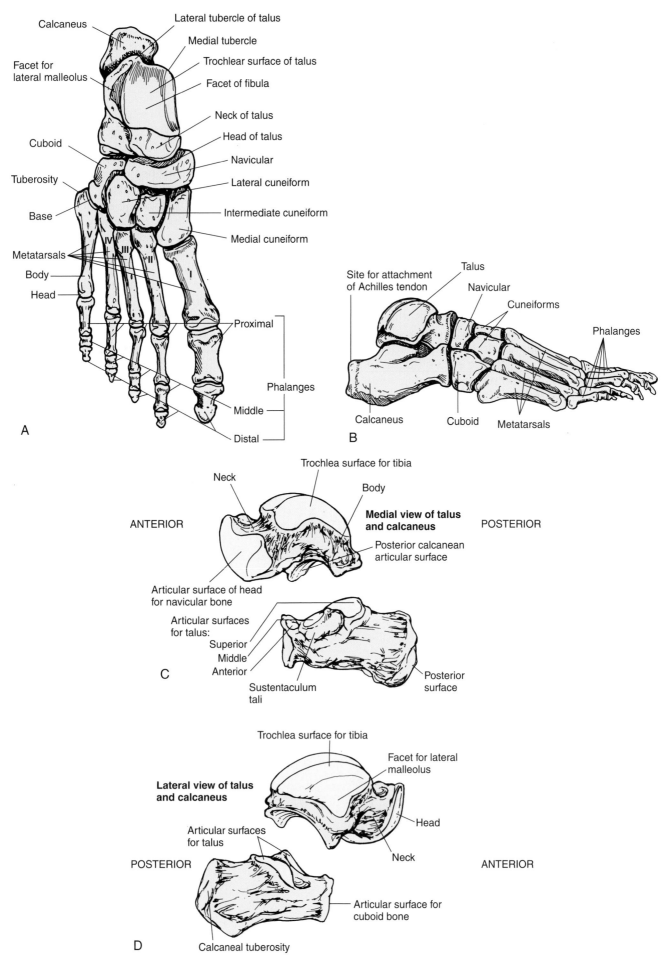

A — Calcaneus
Facet for lateral malleolus
Cuboid
Tuberosity
Base
Metatarsals
Body
Head
Lateral tubercle of talus
Medial tubercle
Trochlear surface of talus
Facet of fibula
Neck of talus
Head of talus
Navicular
Lateral cuneiform
Intermediate cuneiform
Medial cuneiform
V IV III II
Proximal
Phalanges
Middle
Distal

B — Site for attachment of Achilles tendon
Talus
Navicular
Cuneiforms
Phalanges
Calcaneus
Cuboid
Metatarsals

C — Neck
Trochlea surface for tibia
Body
ANTERIOR
Medial view of talus and calcaneus
POSTERIOR
Posterior calcanean articular surface
Articular surface of head for navicular bone
Articular surfaces for talus:
Superior
Middle
Anterior
Sustentaculum tali
Posterior surface

D — Trochlea surface for tibia
Facet for lateral malleolus
Lateral view of talus and calcaneus
Articular surfaces for talus
POSTERIOR
Head
Neck
ANTERIOR
Articular surface for cuboid bone
Calcaneal tuberosity

FIGURE **3.31.** Ankle and Foot. **A,** Superior View; **B,** Lateral View; **C,** Talus and Calcaneus—Medial View; **D,** Talus and Calcaneus—Lateral View

other tarsal bones. The cuboid and the cuneiforms articulate with the five **metatarsals.**

The five metatarsals form the bones of the sole of the foot. They are labeled I to V, proceeding medial to lateral (opposite that of the palm). Each metatarsal, like the metacarpals, has a base, body, and head. Distally, the metatarsals articulate with the **proximal phalanges.** There are 14 phalanges—each toe has three, except for the great toe (hallux), which has two. As in the hand, the phalanges are named proximal, middle, and distal phalanges, according to the position.

Joints

Although the bones provide the solid structure to which muscles are attached, it is the presence of **joints,** or **articulations,** which enable the body to move. The way two or more bones join with each other determines the type of movement and the range of motion.

To understand the possible movements of a joint, the joints have been classified in many ways.

JOINT CLASSIFICATIONS

Joints are classified according to the structure and function (i.e., how much movement they allow). Structurally, they are classified as **fibrous** (has fibrous connective tissue between the bones), **cartilaginous** (has cartilage between bones), and **synovial** (has a cavity with fluid separating the bones). Functionally, they are classified as **synarthrosis** (immovable joint), **amphiarthrosis** (slightly movable joint), and **diarthrosis** (freely movable joint). The *functional* classification is described below. Note that the fibrous and cartilaginous joint types fall under synarthrosis and amphiarthrosis and synovial joint type falls under diarthrosis of the functional classification. A joint in singular form is spelled with –*is,* and with –*es* in plural form (e.g., synarthrosis [singular]; synarthroses [plural]).

Synarthroses

In some parts of the body, joints exist where the movement is minimal or not possible. This type of joint is known as **synarthrosis** (synonym, together) or **immovable joint.** The region where the two bones meet may have fibrous tissue or cartilage. An example of an immovable joint is where the different bones of the skull meet. The location of the joint can be identified in infants before the skull bones fuse. The subtype of joint seen in the skull is known as *suture.* Synarthrosis is also seen in the jaw, where the

tooth is embedded into the socket or alveolus. Dense fibrous tissue, as in the skull, connects the tooth to the socket. This subtype of joint is *gomphosis.*

Another category of joint under synarthrosis is seen between parts of a single bone—between the epiphysis and diaphysis separated by the cartilaginous epiphysial plate, before the ossification centers fuse. Another example is found between the ribs and the sternum. The type of synarthrosis with cartilage in the joint area is known as *synchondrosis.*

The bones in some parts of the body, as in certain bones of the skull, fuse, with no trace of the joint. This type of joint is known as *synostosis.* An example of synostosis is the fusion of the two sides of the frontal bone in infancy.

Amphiarthroses

Certain joints allow slight movement. These are known as **amphiarthroses,** or **slightly movable joints.** These joints, while allowing some slight movement, are stronger than those joints that allow free movement. In one subtype, *syndesmosis,* the two bones are connected by ligaments. For example, the tibia and the fibula of the leg and the ulna and radius of the arm are joined together by the tough interosseous ligament. In another subtype, *symphysis,* the two bones covered with hyaline cartilage is joined by a pad of fibrocartilage. The joint between the two pubic bones (pubic symphysis), the joint between the body of the vertebrae (bones separated by the intervertebral disks), and the joint between the manubrium and body of sternum are examples of symphysis. Note that the symphyses are present in the midline of the body.

Diarthroses

Most joints of the body are freely movable. These are known as **diarthroses,** or **freely movable joints.**

Because the articular surfaces of the joints are separated by **synovial fluid** and **synovial membrane** lines the articular cavity, these joints are also known as **synovial joints.**

Structure of a Typical Synovial Joint

The structure of a typical synovial joint is shown in Figure 3.32. The synovial joint is surrounded by a thick connective tissue **joint** or **articular capsule.** The capsule runs across the bones that articulate with each other and becomes continuous with the periosteum. The capsule may be described as having two layers—the **external fibrous layer** and the **internal synovial layer,** also referred to as the **synovial membrane.** The fibrous layer is made of dense, irregular connective tissue that is flexible enough to allow movement and strong enough to prevent dislocation

Common Joint Ailments

Joint disorders may occur as a result of the aging process (e.g., osteoporosis), autoimmune diseases (e.g., rheumatoid arthritis), trauma (e.g., dislocations, fractures), infection (e.g., rheumatic fever), and genetic abnormalities (e.g., gout).

Arthritis includes all inflammatory conditions that affect synovial joints. Invariably, arthritis produces damage to the articular cartilage with resultant pain and stiffness.

Bursitis is a condition in which there is inflammation of the bursa. Typically, pain is increased when the ligament or tendon is moved. Bursae can get inflamed if there is excessive friction as a result of repetitive motion or pressure over the joint or when the joint gets infected or injured.

Locking is a result of a loose body becoming trapped between joint surfaces, causing momentary or prolonged mechanical jamming.

Sprain is damage to the ligaments that occurs when the ligament is stretched beyond its normal limits, tearing the collagen fibers. The ligaments are strong and sometimes break part of the bone to which they are attached before they tear. Because ligament is connective tissue made up of thick collagen fibers, with a limited blood supply, it takes longer to heal than other tissue.

Synovitis. The synovial membrane responds to injury by becoming acutely inflamed, with resultant swelling and increased fluid production. There is a rubbery feeling to the enlarged joint.

of the bones. This layer is penetrated by blood vessels and nerves. In some joints the capsule may be thickened along lines of stress or reinforced with separate thick connective tissue called **ligaments.**

The **synovial membrane** is present along the inner surface of the capsule, forming a closed sac called the **joint** or **synovial cavity.** Its inner layer consists of specialized squamous or cuboidal cells that help manufacture the **synovial fluid** present in the cavity. This innermost layer is surrounded by a network of connective tissue that contains blood vessels, nerves, and, in some joints, fat. The accumulation of adipose tissue is known as **articular fat pads.** The synovial membrane covers tendons that pass through certain joints. For example, it covers the popliteal tendon in the knee and it covers the tendon of the long head of the biceps in the shoulder. It does not cover that part of the joint where cartilage is present.

The surfaces of the bones that form the joint do not come in direct contact with each other because they are lined by the **articular cartilage.** This hyaline cartilage is smooth, following the contours of the bone surface. It does not have a blood supply, nor is it innervated. It is nourished by synovial fluid and diffusion from small blood vessels that supply the bone. The cartilage, along with the synovial fluid, helps reduce friction between

the moving surfaces. Damage to the articular cartilage can reduce easy movement of the surfaces over each other and limit the range of motion.

The **synovial fluid** in the joint cavity resembles the interstitial fluid but contains proteoglycans secreted by the fibroblasts of the synovial membrane. The fluid is, therefore, thick and viscous. Synovial joints have about 3 mL (0.1 oz) of fluid in the cavity. The synovial fluid serves to (a) *lubricate the joint*—the fluid reduces the friction between the moving surfaces of the joint; (b) *distribute nutrients and remove wastes*—the articular cartilage, having no direct blood supply, derives most of its nutrients from the synovial fluid and disposes its waste products into it. The synovial fluid is constantly circulating in the joint as it moves, and its composition is maintained by exchange between the fluid and the blood flowing in the capillaries that supply the joint. The production of synovial fluid is facilitated by the movement of joints; (c) *absorb shock*—as the joints move, the articular surfaces are compressed and the fluid helps distribute the pressure evenly across the articular surfaces; and (d) *defense*—the synovial fluid contains a few white blood cells that remove debris and prevent entry of microorganisms.

The synovial joint may have other **accessory structures** that further strengthen and stabilize the joints. These may be in the form of additional pads of **cartilage, fat, ligaments, tendons,** or **bursae.**

Some joints, such as the knee joints, have additional **fibrocartilage** interspersed between the artic-

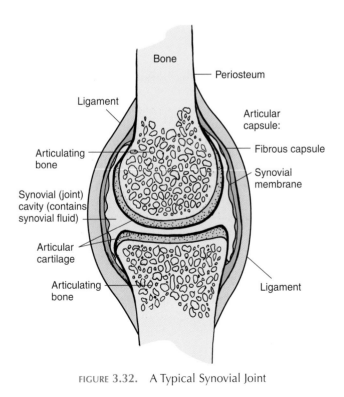

FIGURE **3.32.** A Typical Synovial Joint

ular surfaces inside the synovial cavity. These moon-shaped disks, known as **articular disks** or **meniscus** (plural, menisci), alter the shape of the articulating surfaces and/or help channel the synovial fluid.

Some joints have **fat pads** lined by synovial membrane. They protect the articular cartilage and fill the spaces in the joint cavity as the joint moves, akin to packing material.

Ligaments are thick, connective tissue bands that help stabilize moving surfaces. Some are thickenings of the joint capsule and known as **accessory ligaments.** Accessory ligaments strengthen the joint capsule and reduce rotation at the joint. Others are thick bands that lie outside the joint capsule, providing additional support to the joint and known as **extracapsular ligaments.** Others lie inside the synovial joint, preventing movements that may damage the joint and are known as **intracapsular ligaments.**

Tendons—the thick connective tissue that connects muscle to bone—although not part of the joint, help stabilize, support, and limit the range of motion of the joint as they pass across it. Some tendons have connective tissue sheaths filled with synovial fluid and lined with synovial membrane, surrounding them where they lie directly over bone. The sheaths help reduce friction as the tendons go through bony or fibrous tunnels. These sheaths are known as **synovial tendon sheaths.**

Many joints are surrounded by pockets of synovial fluid-filled cavities in the connective tissue surrounding them. These cavities, lined by synovial membrane, are **bursae** (singular, bursa). Bursa may be separate from the joint or connected to the joint cavity. The bursae serve as shock absorbers and also reduce friction between moving structures near the joint. Bursae may be found near tendons, joint capsules, ligaments, muscle, bone, or skin (Figures 3.40 and 3.46).

All joints are supplied by branches of **nerves** that innervate skeletal muscles close to the joint. Sensory nerves supplying the joint respond to stretch, pain, and degree of movement and convey the information to the spinal cord and brain for a suitable response. The receptors are located in the articular capsule and ligaments.

The joints receive their blood supply from surrounding arteries. The articular cartilage does not have a blood supply. Instead, it gets nutrients from the synovial fluid. Waste products are removed from the joints by veins.

STABILITY OF SYNOVIAL JOINTS

Synovial joints allow a wide range of motion and have to be protected from movements beyond the normal range that can damage the joint. They are protected by:

- the collagen fibers of the capsule
- intracapsular and extracapsular ligaments
- the tendons that surround the joint
- the shape of the articular surface and the bones
- muscles and other structures that surround the joint.

The structures that stabilize the joint may vary from one joint to another. For example, the hip joint is extensively supported by intracapsular as well as extracapsular ligaments. The articular surface of the femur is rounded, providing further stability. The thick muscles around the hip make it strong and stable. The elbow, however, is stabilized more by the bones that tend to interlock with each other as the elbow moves.

MOVEMENT ACROSS THE JOINTS

The type of movement possible across a joint depends on the shape of the articulating surfaces, the ligaments, structures around the joint, and the muscles that cross the joint (see Figure 3.33).

If the articular surfaces are relatively flat, one possible movement is **gliding** (i.e., the articulating surfaces can move forward and backward or from side to side), similar to moving a book over the surface of the table without lifting the book.

Now, do a small experiment to explore all the other movements possible. Place the pencil or pen in front of you vertically on the table and try these movements: Keeping the point of the pencil or pen in contact with one point on the table, move the pencil or pen forward and backward. In this movement, the pen moves only in one axis and is similar to the movement of the door in its hinges. Some joints allow this kind of **monaxial movement.**

Next, with the point of the pencil still in contact with one point on the table, move the other end in a circle. This type of movement is known as **circumduction.** This is the kind of movement your arm makes when you pitch a ball.

Try this: Keeping the point on the table, move the pencil so that the part of the pencil that originally faced you faces the opposite side (i.e., rotate it as in using a screwdriver). This movement is known as **rotation.** If the anterior surface of the bone rotates towards the midline of the body, it is known as **medial, internal,** or **inward rotation.** If the rotating movement is away from the midline of the body, it is known as **lateral, external,** or **outward rotation.**

These various, experimental movements have been named according to the direction of movement in relation to the anatomical position. The range of motion possible in each joint is described in relation to these terms.

Flexion is the movement in the anterior/posterior plane that *reduces* the angle between the articulating

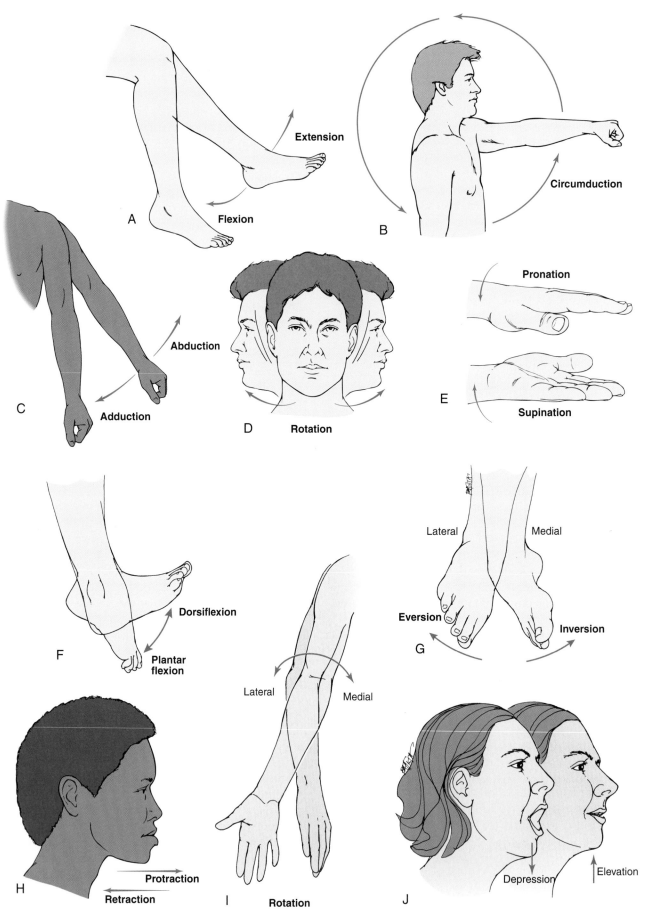

FIGURE 3.33. Joint Movements. **A,** Flexion and Extension (Knee joint); **B,** Circumduction (Shoulder joint); **C,** Abduction and Adduction (Shoulder joint); **D,** Rotation (Atlanto-axial joint); **E,** Pronation and Supination (Elbow joint); **F,** Dorsiflexion and Plantar Flexion (Ankle joint); **G,** Inversion and Eversion (Ankle joint); **H,** Protraction and Retraction (Temporomandibular joint); **I,** Medial and Lateral Rotation (Shoulder joint); **J,** Depression and Elevation (Temporomandibular joint)

bones. For example, keep your arm straight beside you and bend your elbow so that your fingers touch your shoulder. This is flexion at the elbow. Now stand in the anatomical position and reduce the angle between the articulating surfaces of all the joints possible. What is your final position? You should be curled into a ball, with your fingers clenched and toes curled.

Extension is the opposite movement of flexion, in which the angle between the articulating bones is *increased* in the anterior/posterior plane. Extension at the elbow will be bringing your arm to the side of your body after scratching the tip of your shoulder with your fingers. When you stand in the anatomical position, all your joints are extended. In some joints, it is possible to extend the articulating bones beyond the anatomical position. This is known as **hyperextension.** When you move the head to look at the ceiling, you hyperextend your neck.

When the articulating bone moves along the frontal/coronal plane, away from the longitudinal axis of the body, the movement is known as **abduction.** Try this. Stand about two feet away from the wall at right angles (i.e., with your side facing the wall). Then put your arm out to touch the wall. Your arm is now abducted at the shoulder. In abduction at the shoulder, the humerus has moved away from the midline along the coronal plane.

The opposite of abduction is **adduction,** in which the bone moves *toward* the longitudinal axis. Not all joints can adduct and abduct. Determine all the joints where adduction and abduction is possible. In the hand, the movement of the fingers away from the middle finger (i.e., spreading the fingers) is abduction. Bringing the fingers toward the middle finger is adduction. In the foot, moving away from the second toe is considered as abduction. Because the thumb articulates in a plane at right angles to the other fingers, adduction of the thumb moves the thumb toward the palm in the sagittal plane.

Rotation, as described above, can be medial or lateral. At the elbow, the rotatory movements of the radius over the ulna bone are termed **pronation** and **supination.** When the elbow is moved to have the palm of the hand facing the back, it is known as pronation. When the elbow is moved back to the anatomical position—facing the front—it is known as supination.

The flexion and extension of the foot have confusing terms. According to the terms, you are flexing your foot when you both move the foot up and down, such as in standing on your toes and then lowering yourself to stand on your heel. However, when you stand on your toes, the movement *at the ankle* is referred to as **plantar flexion.** When you stand on your heel, it is known as **dorsiflexion.**

There are other movements with specific names. **Inversion** is the movement in which the foot is

TEST YOURSELF

Sit on the floor with your legs crossed and your hands on your knees. What is the position of every joint in your body? To start you off; the knees are flexed, the ankles are. . .

moved with the sole of the foot facing inward. **Eversion** is the opposite movement, in which the foot is moved so that the sole faces outward.

A special type of movement is possible in humans because of the unique articulation of the thumb. This movement, which allows us to grasp tiny objects such as holding a pen or picking up a needle from the floor, is known as **opposition,** in which the thumb is able to touch or oppose each of the other fingers.

The movement in which you jut your jaw out—moving the bone anteriorly in the horizontal plane—is known as **protraction. Retraction** is the opposite of protraction. When the bone moves in a superior/inferior direction, it is known as **elevation** and **depression,** respectively. When you open your mouth, your mandible is depressed and when you close the mouth, the mandible is elevated.

The movement in which the trunk is turned to the side, as in bending sideways, is known as **lateral flexion.**

CLASSIFICATION OF SYNOVIAL JOINTS

The synovial joints are classified according to the shapes of the articulating surfaces and the types of movements and range of motion they permit (see

KNOW THE JOINTS BETTER

Before studying each joint:
- look at the bones that are involved
- study the origins and insertions of muscles around the joint, to logically deduce the movements possible and the actions of each muscle
- identify the location of the bony prominences in and around the joint on your own body or that of your colleague
- identify the approximate location of each muscle involved and watch them move as you or your colleague executes the movement
- look at the direction of the muscle fibers of each muscle involved, to help you direct your massage strokes and pressure in the most efficient and useful manner when treating clients
- if bursae are present around the joint, identify the approximate location on the surface of the body
- finally, learn the skills of assessing the joint systematically by inspection, palpation, and checking the range of motion passively and actively

Figure 3.34). The different subtypes of joints are **ball and socket, hinge, pivot, ellipsoidal or condyloid, saddle,** and **gliding** or **planar.** These joints may also be classified as **nonaxial, monaxial, biaxial,** and **multiaxial** (or **polyaxial**) **joints,** according to the movements allowed along no axel, one axel, or two or more axels. In nonaxial joints, the movement allowed is not around any axis; in monaxial, the movement is along one axis; in biaxial, along two axes; and in multiaxial, the movement occurs along three or more axes and in directions between these axes.

Ball-and-Socket Joint

In a ball-and-socket joint, one of the articulating surfaces is rounded like a ball and the other surface has a depression to fit the ball. These are multiaxial, the most mobile of joints, allowing all types of move-ments—angular and rotational. Therefore, flexion, extension, abduction, adduction, medial and lateral rotation, and circumduction are all possible (e.g., hip joint, shoulder joint).

Hinge Joint

The articulating surfaces are somewhat curved in a hinge joint, allowing movement in one plane (monaxial) similar to the movement of a door. Here, flexion and extension is possible (e.g., elbow joint, knee joint, ankle joint, interphalangeal joint, and joint between the occipital bone and the atlas of the vertebra).

Pivot Joint

Here, too, the articulating surfaces permit monaxial movement like the hinge joint, but only rotation is

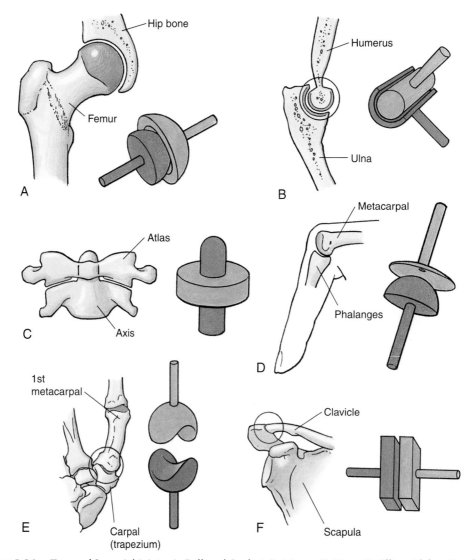

FIGURE **3.34.**   Types of Synovial Joints. **A,** Ball-and-Socket; **B,** Hinge; **C,** Pivot; **D,** Ellipsoidal or Condyloid; **E,** Saddle; **F,** Gliding or Planar

possible (e.g., the joint between the first and second vertebra—the atlas and the axis, and the rotation of the head of radius over the shaft of the ulna proximally).

Ellipsoidal or Condyloid Joint

In this biaxial joint, one of the articulating surfaces is oval and fits into a depression in the other articulating surface. Here, movement is possible in two planes. Flexion, extension, adduction, abduction, including circumduction is possible, but rotation is not (e.g., the articulation between the distal end of radius with the carpal bones, phalanges with the metacarpal bones, and phalanges with the metatarsal bones).

Saddle Joint

In this biaxial joint, the articulating surfaces resemble a saddle, being concave in one axis and convex in another. It is a modified condyloid joint that allows freer movement. The saddle joint allows angular movements but prevents rotation. Therefore, flexion, extension, adduction, abduction, circumduction, and opposition are possible in this joint (e.g., articulation between the carpal bone and metacarpal bone of the thumb).

Gliding Joint

The articulating surfaces are flattened or slightly curved and allow sliding movements. These are non-axial joints. The range of motion is slight and rotational movements, although possible, are restricted by bones, ligaments and tendons around the joint (e.g., at the ends of clavicle, between carpal bones, between tarsal bones, and between the articulating facets of spinal vertebrae).

Individual Joints

Many of the aches and pain exhibited by clients in a massage clinic originate from injury and damage to joints and their accessory structures. Those working as part of the health care team treating athletes, deal with ailments related to joints and muscles. Thorough knowledge of the structure of each joint, the range of motion possible, and the muscles that make these movements possible is important to treat such clients. In addition, a scheme for assessing each joint systematically is vital.

Each major joint in the body is described in this section in terms of the articular surfaces, type of joint, ligaments, movements possible, range of motion, list of muscles producing movements, an overview of physical assessment, and common ailments. (The information provided below may be more than what is required by some schools of massage therapy. The student is advised to consult the curriculum or their instructors regarding requirements.)

TEMPOROMANDIBULAR JOINT (TMJ)

The temporomandibular joint (see Figure 3.35) is affected by dysfunction and disease in more than 20% of the population at sometime in their life. It is a complex joint; its function is affected by multiple structures such as the bones of the skull; mandible; maxilla; hyoid; clavicle; sternum; the joint between the teeth and the alveolar cavities; muscle and soft tissue of the head and neck; and muscles of the cheeks, lips, and tongue. It is affected by the posture of the head and neck and cervical curvature. The joint is used almost continuously for chewing, swallowing, respiration, and speech. Imbalance relating to any of the associated structures can affect this joint. Conversely, problems relating to the joint can reflect as dysfunction of any of the associated structures. Hence, dysfunction of this joint is difficult to diagnose and manage.

Articulating Surfaces and Type of Joint

The mandibular condyle articulates with the mandibular fossa of the temporal bone in this joint (see Figure 3.36). The surface of the fossa is concave posteriorly and convex anteriorly because of the articular eminence. The presence of an interarticular disk/cartilage/meniscus, compensates for the difference in the shapes of the two articular surfaces (the condyle has a convex surface). The disk also divides the joint into a superior and inferior cavity and, because of it, the articular surfaces of the bones are not in direct contact with each other. The outer edges of the disk are connected to the capsule. The joint is strengthened by ligaments (Figure 3.35B and C). This joint is a combination of a plane and a hinge joint.

Ligaments

The articular capsule, or **capsular ligament,** is a sleeve of thin, loose fibrous connective tissue that surrounds the joint. The **lateral ligament (temporomandibular ligament)** is a thickening of the capsule laterally, positioned in the lateral side of the capsule under the parotid glands. It stabilizes the joint laterally and prevents extensive anterior, posterior, and lateral displacement of the mandibular condyle. The **stylomandibular ligament,** not directly related to the joint, extends from the styloid process to the posterior border of the ramus of the mandible. It prevents the mandible from moving forward extensively as when

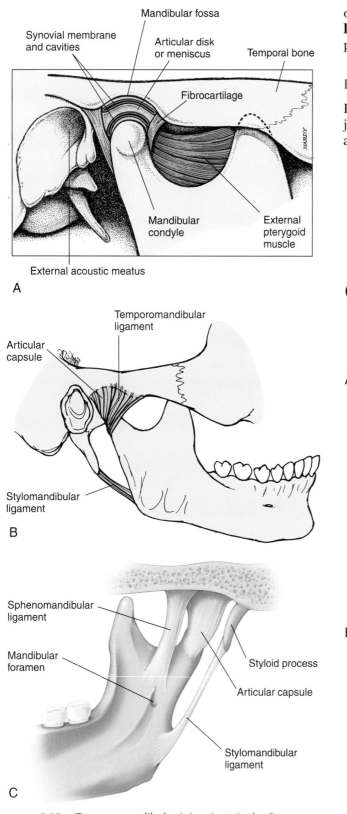

opening the mouth wide. The **sphenomandibular ligament** stabilizes the joint medially and helps suspend the mandible when the mouth is opened wide.

Possible Movements

Depression and elevation of the mandible (hinge joint) and protraction and retraction (gliding joint) are possible. The mandible can also be moved later-

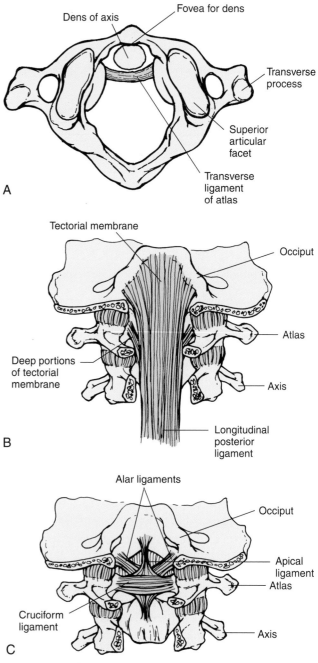

FIGURE **3.35.** Temporomandibular Joint. **A,** Articular Structures; **B,** Ligaments. Temporomandibular Ligament—lateral view; **C,** Sphenomandibular and Stylomandibular Ligaments—Medial View

FIGURE **3.36.** The Ligaments Associated With the Atlas, Axis, and Occiput. **A,** Superior View; **B,** Posterior View Showing Superficial Ligaments; **C,** Posterior View Showing Deep Ligaments

ally as a result of the presence of the articular cartilage. The movement of the mandible is a result of the action of both cervical and mandibular muscles.

Range of Motion

Normally, the jaw can be depressed low enough to allow three fingers to be inserted into the mouth between the incisor teeth.

Muscles

Muscles that open (depress) the jaw:
Primary depressors
    External (lateral) pterygoid muscle
    Anterior head of the digastric
Secondary depressors
    Gravity
    Muscles attached to the hyoid bone (suprahyoid muscles—digastric, stylohyoid, mylohyoid, geniohyoid—and infrahyoid muscles—sternohyoid, thyrohyoid, omohyoid)
Muscles that close (elevate) the jaw:
Primary elevators
    Masseter
    Temporalis
Secondary elevators
    Internal (medial) pterygoid
    (Superior head of the lateral pterygoid stabilizes the disk and condylar head during elevation)
Muscles that retract the jaw:
    Posterior fibers of the temporalis
    Deep fibers of the masseter
    Digastric
    Suprahyoids
Muscles that protract the jaw:
    Medial pterygoid
    Superficial fibers of the masseter
Lateral movement:
    Lateral and medial pterygoid on one side and contralateral temporalis muscle assisted by digastric, geniohyoid, and mylohyoid

Physical Assessment

A complete history of problems relating to the joint, including when it started, how it occurred, and previous management is important. History of habitual protrusion and muscular tension is important. Difficulty opening and closing the mouth, frequent headaches, and abnormal sounds from joints are some symptoms associated with the joint dysfunction.

The posture of the person should be examined. Typically, the shoulders are elevated, with the head forward, a stiff neck and back, and shallow, restricted breathing. The area around the joint should be inspected carefully. The movement of the jaw must be noted to ensure continuous, symmetrical movements. The alignment of the teeth should also be examined.

The movements of the condyle of the mandible can be palpated by placing the finger inside the external auditory canal. Clicking sounds may be present if the articular disk is damaged or if there is swelling. The pterygoid muscles can be palpated through the inside of the mouth (disposable gloves should be worn for this procedure). The range of motion—both active and passive—should be checked together with palpation of all relevant muscles for tender points (Refer to books on musculoskeletal assessment for more details).

INTERVERTEBRAL ARTICULATION

Articulating Surfaces and Type of Joint

Adjacent vertebrae articulate with each other via articular facets located inferiorly and superiorly. This joint is known as the **zygapophyseal joints, interarticular,**

Common Temporomandibular Joint Ailments

Hypermobility of the temporomandibular joint is a result of laxity of the articular ligaments. Nail biting, gum chewing, prolonged pacifier use, prolonged bottle feeding, mouth breathing, and habitual teeth grinding are risk factors. Muscle retraining is important in the management process.

Temporomandibular joint dysfunction syndrome is a common ailment affecting this joint. About 10.5 million adults in a general population sample are affected by this problem. The actual cause of the syndrome is still not clear and many factors have been attributed to it. Trauma, organic diseases, trigger points, and psychological problems are all risk factors. It is most often misdiagnosed. Often, pain from other areas, like a tooth, may be referred to the joint and mistaken for this syndrome. The criteria for diagnosis are muscle pain and tenderness in one or more muscles of mastication, clicking or popping noises in the joint, and restricted mandibular range (<35 mm).

Trauma, direct or indirect, as in whiplash injuries, can affect joint function.

Osteoarthritis and **rheumatoid arthritis** are other ailments that may affect this joint.

Soft tissue mobilization techniques are an important component in the treatment of dysfunction relating to this joint. It includes deep friction massage to the capsule of the joint, kneading and stroking techniques applied intraorally to the pterygoids and insertion of temporalis, deep pressure joint massage, connective tissue massage, stretching techniques, myofascial release, passive and active exercises (refer to books on management of common musculoskeletal disorders for details of techniques).

or **facet joints** (Figure 3.18). The bodies of the vertebrae also articulate with each other, with most vertebral bodies, excluding the first and occiput, first and second cervical, and vertebrae of the sacrum and coccyx, being separated from each other by the **intervertebral disks.**

The articular surfaces of the vertebral processes are gliding joints, allowing some rotation and flexion. The articulation between the vertebral bodies is a symphyseal joint. The joint between the first cervical vertebra (atlas) and the second vertebra (axis) (**atlantoaxial joint**) is a pivot joint.

The atlas has neither vertebral body nor intervertebral disk. The axis that projects into the atlas in the region where the vertebral body would be, if present, permits rotation of the ringlike atlas around it, forming a pivot joint. Hence, there are two atlantoaxial joints. The medial atlantoaxial joint is between the facet for dens on the atlas and the odontoid process of the axis. The lateral atlantoaxial joint is between the inferior facets of the lateral masses of the atlas and the superior facets of the axis. The superior facet of the lateral masses of the first cervical vertebra—atlas, articulates with the occipital condyles as the **atlanto-occipital joint.** The atlanto-occipital joint allows for flexion, extension, and lateral bending; the atlantoaxial joints allow flexion, extension, and rotation.

Ligaments

The bones are held in place by various ligaments. Figure 3.36 shows the various superficial and deep ligaments related to the atlas, axis, and occiput. The transverse ligament, alar ligament, cruciate, and apical ligaments stabilize the upper cervical spine and prevent damage to the brain stem by dislocation of the dens.

Certain ligaments (see Figure 3.37) run between the vertebral bodies and processes to help stabilize the vertebral column. The **anterior longitudinal ligament** connects the bodies of adjacent vertebra anteriorly, while the **posterior longitudinal ligament** does the same posteriorly. The **ligamentum flavum** connects the lamina of adjacent vertebrae. Other ligaments, known as the **interspinous ligaments,** connect adjacent spinous processes. The **supraspinous ligament** connects the spinous processes from C7 to the sacrum. The **intertransverse ligament** connects adjacent transverse processes.

Possible Movements

The vertebrae are capable of bending forward (flexion), bending backward (hyperextension), and sideways (lateral flexion and rotation).

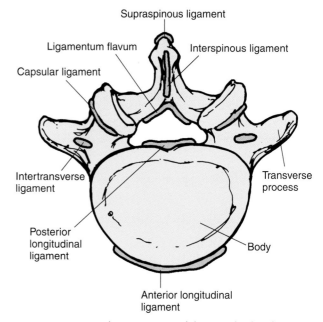

FIGURE **3.37.** The Ligaments of the Vertebral Column

Range of Motion

Range of motion depends on the angle and size of the articulating surfaces and the resistance offered by the intervertebral disk. It also depends on the muscles and ligaments around the spine. For proper movement, remembered that, when one group of muscles (agonists) contract in a direction, the muscles that bring about the opposite movement (antagonists) have to relax. Similarly, the ligaments lying in the opposite side of the movement have to stretch.

The greatest motion possible in the spine is in the lower lumbar region—between L5 and S1, where the joint surfaces are largest and disks the thickest. Conversely, there is more chance of damage, inflammation (arthritis), and herniation of disks in this region.
Cervical region
    Flexion, 45°
    Extension, 55°
    Lateral bending, 40°
    Rotation, 70°
Lumbar region
    Flexion, 75°
    Hyperextension, 30°
    Lateral and medial bending, 35°

Muscles

The erector spinae muscles (**page 207**) and the abdominal muscles (**page 208**) help with the various spinal movements. The trapezius, scalenes, sternocleidomastoid, and other neck muscles help with movements in the cervical region.

The muscles of the cervical spine can be divided into four functional groups: superficial posterior, deep posterior, superficial anterior, and deep anterior. The trapezius is a major superficial posterior muscle. The levator scapulae, splenius capitis, and splenius cervicis are other large superficial muscle groups that extend the head and neck.

The multifidi and suboccipital muscles belong to the deep posterior muscle group. The multifidi, which have their origin on the transverse processes and insert into the spinous process above, extend the neck when contracted together and bend the neck to the same side when acting unilaterally.

The sternocleidomastoid is the largest and strongest anterior muscle that flexes the neck. Other neck flexors are the scalenus muscles. The deep anterior neck muscles are the longus coli and longus capitis.

Physical Assessment of the Spine—Cervical Region

Inspection

The neck, the upper limb, and the upper body should be exposed to examine this region. The position of the head and movement should be noted.

Palpation

Bone and cartilage: The bone and cartilage that can be easily palpated are the hyoid bone (superior to the thyroid cartilage), the thyroid cartilage (in men, it forms the Adam's apple), and the mastoid processes and the spinous processes of the cervical vertebrae. The C2 spinous process is the first one that can be palpated as you run your hand down from the occiput.

Muscles: The sternocleidomastoid, extending from the sternoclavicular joint to the mastoid process that helps to turn the head from side to side and to flex it, is a common site of injury. Other muscles, such as the trapezius, can be palpated from origin to insertion. The superior nuchal ligament that extends from the occiput to the C7 spinous process can be easily palpated as well. Both active and passive range of movement of the neck should be tested.

Other structures: The cervical chain of lymph nodes may be palpable if enlarged. The parotid gland can also be felt as a boggy, soft swelling over the angle of the mandible if enlarged. The pulsation of the carotid arteries can be easily felt on either side of the trachea.

Because the nerves to the upper limb rise from the C5 to T1 spinal cord level, it is important to examine the functioning of the nerves. The function of the nerve can be tested by examining the sensations in the

Blood Vessels and Cervical Manipulations

The subclavian arteries that pass between the scalenus anticus and scalenus medius may be compressed, producing symptoms such as edema, discoloration, pallor, or venous congestion in the arms.

The other important arteries of interest to therapists are the vertebral arteries. These arteries pass through the lateral foramina of the cervical vertebrae before they enter the cranial cavity through the foramen magnum. At the point where the atlas meets the occiput, the artery is a little lax, to allow full rotation of the atlas. The vertebral arteries are partially occluded when the cervical spine is extended and rotated. In conditions where the blood flow through the carotid arteries (which is responsible for the major part of blood supply to brain) is not normal, occlusion of the vertebral arteries can cause a reduction of blood flow to the brain stem and cerebellum, resulting in symptoms such as dizziness; slurring of speech; rapid, involuntary movement of the eyeball; and loss of consciousness.

Strokes and deaths resulting from vasospasm or thrombosis of the vertebral arteries as a result of manipulation of the upper cervical spine are not uncommon. It is important to test the vertebral arteries before using traction or mobilization techniques. Each vertebral artery can be tested individually by placing the neck in full rotation, extension, and lateral flexion and holding for approximately 1 minute. If the patient complains of dizziness, blurred vision, slurring of speech, traction or mobilization is contraindicated.

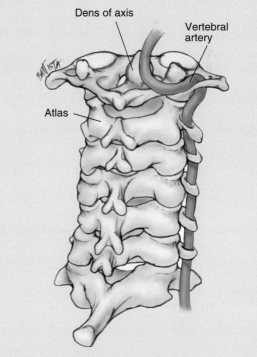

Posterior View of the Upper Cervical Spine Showing the Path of a Vertebral Artery. Note the Lax Artery just Superior to the Atlas.

shoulder and the upper limb, as well as the strength of the muscles in the region.

Special tests (requiring specific training) test the ligaments of the upper cervical spine.

Physical Assessment of the Spine—Lumbar Region

Inspection

Watch for unnatural or awkward movement of the spine or signs of pain when the person exposes the spine when disrobing or walking.

Look at the skin for swelling, redness, etc. in the region of the spine and identify abnormal curvatures of the spine.

Palpation

Bony prominences and ligaments: Posteriorly, feel the spinous processes, posterior superior iliac spine, sacrum, coccyx, iliac crests, ischial tuberosity, and greater trochanter, identifying painful areas.

Muscles: Palpate the muscles on either side of the spine and the abdominal muscles. Note tenderness, spasm, or differences in size between the right and left side.

Nerve: The sciatic nerve is an important nerve that may get compressed by spinal deformities. Palpate for tenderness in the midpoint between the ischial tuberosity and greater trochanter with the hip flexed.

Range of motion: Check flexion by asking the client to lean forward and try to touch the toes without bending the knee. Check extension by asking the client to bend backward with your hand on the posterior superior iliac spine. Check lateral bending by asking the client to lean to the right and the left as far as possible. Rotation is checked by turning the trunk to the right and left with the pelvis stabilized.

RIB CAGE ARTICULATIONS

Articulating Surface, Type of Joints, and Ligaments

The ends of the true ribs (1–7) join the costal cartilage anteriorly at **costochondral (sternocostal) joints.** The true ribs are attached to the sternum by individual cartilages; the false ribs (8–10) have a common junction with the sternum. The first rib is joined to the manubrium by a cartilaginous joint and movement is limited. The second rib articulates with a demifacet on the manubrium and body through a synovial plane joint. The cartilages of the third to sev-

---

✓ Common Spine Ailments

Abnormal spinal curvatures. At times, the spinal curvatures are abnormal. An exaggerated thoracic curvature is called **kyphosis** (hump back). An abnormal anterior lumbar curvature is termed **lordosis.** If the vertebrae have abnormal lateral curves, **scoliosis.**

Ankylosing spondylitis is a condition in which stiffening, ossification, and calcification of the spine occur progressively, with loss of movement of the spine.

Low back pain. Low back pain is a term used to describe subjective feelings of pain and tenderness felt in the lumbar spine. It is a syndrome (with a number of symptoms) not a disease. It occurs as a result of chronic overuse of the lumbosacral area. It is a common condition because the strain placed on the lumbar spine is great and varies with positions. For example, the strain placed on lying on the back with leg extended = 25 kg (55 lb); standing = 100 kg (221 lb); bending forward with knee extended = 200 kg (441 lb); sitting = 145 kg (320 lb).

Osteoporosis is a disorder in which bone resorption is greater than the rate of replacement. As in other bone, osteoporosis can occur in the vertebral column, increasing the risk of fracture of vertebra.

Prolapsed disk is a condition associated with neurologic problems (see page 107).

Sacroiliac joint pain is a dull pain felt over the back of the joint and the buttock. Referred pain may be felt in the groin, back of leg, lower abdomen, or pelvic region. Pain is increased on changes in position. Transmission of abnormal forces or forces due to asymmetry to the lumbar region or hip region can result in such pain. Pain in this region is often experienced by pregnant women. This is a result of the relaxation of the ligaments and joints under the influence of the hormone relaxin, secreted during pregnancy.

Shaken baby. In children, the fusion between the dens and the axis is incomplete. Severe shaking or impact can cause the dens to dislocate and damage the spinal cord.

Spina bifida is a condition in which there is a defect in the fusion of the right and left half of one or more vertebrae during the development of the fetus, resulting in malformation of the spine. The spinal cord and meninges may or may not protrude through the gap.

Whiplash is the term given to the injury that occurs when the neck is thrown forward, backward, or laterally suddenly and forcefully, as in a car crash. The muscles and nerves, including the cervical spinal cord and other structures of the neck, can be injured according to the severity.

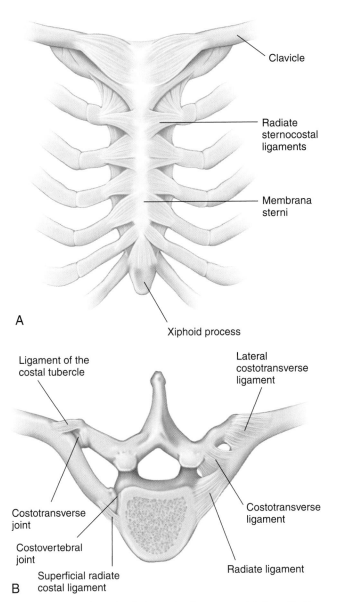

A

Clavicle

Radiate sternocostal ligaments

Membrana sterni

Xiphoid process

Ligament of the costal tubercle

Lateral costotransverse ligament

Costotransverse joint

Costotransverse ligament

Costovertebral joint

Superficial radiate costal ligament

B

Radiate ligament

FIGURE 3.38. Rib Articulations. **A,** Costosternal Joints; **B,** Costovertebral Joints

The joints between the manubrium and body or sternum—**sternomanubrial joint**—and the body of sternum and xiphoid process—**xiphisternal joint**—allow little movement.

Movements, Range of Motion, and Muscles

Each rib has its own range and direction of movement that differs a little from the others. The first ribs, with their firm attachment to the manubrium, move forward and upward as a unit. The movement occurs at the head of the ribs, with resultant elevation of the manubrium. The other ribs have a typical bucket-handle movement (**see page 109**). The false ribs, in addition to elevation of the anterior end, have a caliperlike movement in which the anterior ends are moved laterally and posteriorly to increase the transverse diameter of the thoracic cage.

The sidebending and rotation of the thoracic spine is limited by the rib cage and little movement is possible at the costovertebral, costotransverse, and costochondral joints. The rib on the side to which the thoracic vertebra rotates becomes more convex while the opposite rib becomes flattened posteriorly.

Joints of the Pectoral Girdle and Upper Limb

The bones involved in the function of the shoulder girdle include the upper thoracic vertebrae, the first and second ribs, manubrium of the sternum, the scapula, the clavicle, and the humerus. For example, to elevate the arm fully, the scapula needs to rotate, the clavicle must elevate, and the thoracic vertebrae extend along with elevation of the humerus. The scapula serves as a

enth ribs have small synovial joints that attach to the body of the sternum. The cartilages of the adjacent false ribs are attached to each other at the **interchondral joints.**

The ribs and the vertebrae articulate at two locations (Figure 3.38). The head of each rib articulates with the bodies of two adjacent vertebrae at the costal demifacet present at the junction of the body and posterior arch of the thoracic vertebrae (Figure 3.18C). The bones are held in place by the **radiate ligament.** A cartilage disk separates the two articulating surfaces. This synovial joint is known as the **costovertebral joint.** The rib tubercle articulates with the corresponding vertebral transverse process at the synovial joint (**costotransverse joint**). Costotransverse ligaments hold this joint in place.

ATYPICAL RIBS

Cervical ribs: Sometimes, one or more extra ribs that articulate with a cervical vertebra (usually the seventh) may be present. This is the cause of the **cervical rib syndrome,** in which the rib may apply pressure on the subclavian artery (arterial thoracic outlet syndrome) or adjacent nerves (true neurogenic thoracic outlet syndrome).

Bicipital rib: Where the first thoracic rib is fused with the cervical vertebra.

Bifid rib: Where the body of the rib is bifurcated.

Lumbar rib: Occasionally, a rib articulating with the first lumbar vertebra may be present.

Slipping rib: This is a term for the condition in which there is a partial dislocation between the rib and the costal cartilage.

THE AXILLA

The axilla is pyramid-shaped, with the apex located superiorly. It lies inferomedial to the shoulder joint and is the space between the arm and the thorax, which enables vessels and nerves to pass between the neck and the upper limb. The apex of the axilla is formed by the clavicle anteriorly, scapula posteriorly, and the outer border of the first rib medially. The base is covered with fascia. The pectoralis major forms part of the anterior wall and the subscapularis, teres major, and the tendon of the latissimus dorsi the posterior.

platform on which movements of the humerus are based. The clavicle holds the scapula and humerus away from the body to provide more freedom of movement of the arm. Little movement of the humerus is possible without associated actions of the scapula.

The movement of the shoulder is facilitated by three joints:

- the sternoclavicular joint
- the acromioclavicular joint
- the shoulder, glenohumeral or scapulohumeral joint and the contact between the scapula and the thoracic cage (this is not a joint)

THE STERNOCLAVICULAR JOINT

Articulating Surface and Type of Joint

It is formed by the sternal end of the clavicle and the upper lateral part of the manubrium and the superior surface of the medial aspect of the cartilage of the first rib (see Figure 3.39). It is a gliding joint, which has a fairly wide range of movement because of the presence of an articular disk within the capsule. The articular disk helps prevent medial dislocation of the clavicle. It

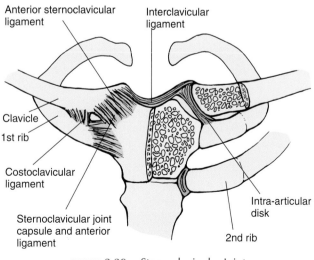

FIGURE 3.39.   Sternoclavicular Joint

is more common for the clavicle to break or the acromioclavicular joint to dislocate even before a medial dislocation at this joint could occur.

Ligaments

Four ligaments—the **anterior sternoclavicular, posterior sternoclavicular, interclavicular,** and **costoclavicular**—support the joint. The attachment of the ligaments is self-explanatory.

Movements, Range of Motion, and Muscles

A wide range of gliding movements is possible. The movements are initiated in conjunction with the shoulder movement. The muscles that move the shoulder also move this joint.

ACROMIOCLAVICULAR JOINT

Articulating Surface and Type of Joint

This joint is formed by the lateral end of the clavicle and the acromion of the scapula. It is a planar joint.

Ligaments

The major ligaments are the **superior** and **inferior acromioclavicular ligaments** and the **coracoclavicular ligaments** (conoid and trapezoid) (see Figure 3.40). The latter, although situated away from the joint, provides joint stability. The trapezoid and conoid ligaments are important for preventing excessive lateral and superior movements of the clavicle. They also help suspend the scapula from the clavicle.

Movements, Range of Motion, and Muscles

Little movement takes place in this joint.

GLENOHUMERAL JOINT

Articulating Surface and Type of Joint

This joint is formed by the head of the humerus and the glenoid fossa of the scapula. It is a ball-and-socket

PROTECTIVE ARCH OVER THE SHOULDER

The acromion, the coracoacromial ligament, and the coracoid process form a protective arch over the glenohumeral joint, preventing the humeral head from dislocating superiorly. However, when there are abnormal joint mechanics, this could be the site of impingement on the greater tubercle, supraspinatus tendon, and the subdeltoid bursa.

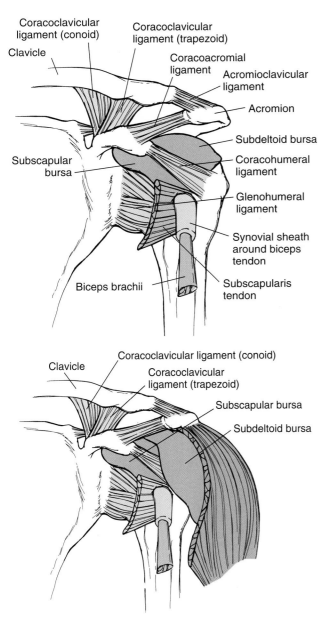

Coracoclavicular ligament (conoid)
Coracoclavicular ligament (trapezoid)
Clavicle
Coracoacromial ligament
Acromioclavicular ligament
Acromion
Subdeltoid bursa
Coracohumeral ligament
Subscapular bursa
Glenohumeral ligament
Synovial sheath around biceps tendon
Biceps brachii
Subscapularis tendon

Clavicle
Coracoclavicular ligament (conoid)
Coracoclavicular ligament (trapezoid)
Subscapular bursa
Subdeltoid bursa

FIGURE **3.40.** Shoulder Region. Ligaments and bursae of the Shoulder Region—Anterior View

joint and the most freely movable joint in the body. The shallow glenoid fossa is deepened by the presence of a circular band of fibrocartilage, the **glenoid labrum.** The head of the humerus is prevented to some extent from upward displacement by the presence of the acromion and coracoid processes of the scapula and the lateral end of the clavicle. A number of ligaments (Figure 3.40A) help stabilize this joint further.

Ligaments

The **glenohumeral ligament** consists of three thickened sets of fibers on the anterior side of the capsule and extends from the humerus to the margin of the glenoid cavity. It prevents excess lateral rotation and stabilizes the joint anteriorly and inferiorly.

The **coracohumeral ligament** extends from the coracoid process to the neck of the humerus and strengthens the superior part of the capsule.

The **coracoacromial ligament** extends from the coracoid process to the acromion process.

The **coracoclavicular** and **acromioclavicular ligaments** extend to the clavicle from the coracoid process and acromion, respectively.

The **transverse humeral ligament** extends across the lesser and greater tubercle, holding the tendon of the long head of the biceps in place.

Bursae

Two major and two minor bursae (Figure 3.40) are associated with the shoulder joint. The **subdeltoid bursa** is located between the deltoid muscle and the joint capsule. The **subacromial bursa** and the **subcoracoid bursa,** as the names suggest, are located between the joint capsule and the acromion and coracoid processes, respectively. A small **subscapular bursa** is located between the tendon of the subscapularis muscle and the capsule.

Possible Movements

Flexion, extension, adduction, abduction, circumduction, and medial and lateral rotation are all possible in this joint, and many muscles located around the joint help with movement. In addition, the shoulders can be elevated, depressed, retracted (scapula pulled together), and protracted (scapula pushed apart as in reaching forward with both arms).

For movements to occur at the shoulder, the functions of many joints and tissue must be optimal. Some contributing factors are the acromioclavicular joint, sternoclavicular joint, the contact between the scapula and the thorax, and the joints of the lower cervical and upper thoracic vertebrae. For example, the first 15–30° during abduction is a result of the glenohumeral joint. Beyond this, the scapula begins to contribute by moving forward, elevating and rotating upwards, partly a result of movement at the sternoclavicular and acromioclavicular joints. For every 3° of abduction, 1° occurs at the scapulothoracic articulation and the other 2° occur at the glenohumeral joint. Abduction using only the glenohumeral joint is possible up to 90°.

As the humerus elevates to 120°, the tension developed in the joint capsule laterally rotates the humerus and prevents the greater tubercle from impinging on the acromion. At this point, the subdeltoid bursal tissue is gathered below the acromion. (If the bursa is swollen, it can result in restricted movement and/or injury to the tissue). Abduction beyond 160° occurs as a result of movement (extension) at the lower cervical and upper thoracic vertebrae. In unilateral abduction, the spine also rotates in the opposite direction of the moving arm.

Range of Motion

Flexion, 90°
Extension, 45°
Abduction, 180°
Adduction, 45°
Internal rotation, 55°
External rotation, 40–45°

Muscles

Many muscles participate in shoulder movement. Of these, the tendons of four muscles provide stability to the joint and are known as the **rotator,** or **musculotendinous cuff.** The four muscles involved are the supraspinatus, infraspinatus, teres minor, and subscapularis (you can remember it by the acronym SITS). The tendons of these muscles blend with the joint capsule. When the arm is hanging at the side, the tension of the superior aspect of the joint capsule is sufficient to keep the two articulating surfaces in contact. When the arm is moved from the side, the rotator cuff muscles must contract to keep the head of the humerus in position.

Muscles that help with flexion:
Primary flexors
    Deltoid (anterior portion)
    Coracobrachialis
Secondary flexors
    Pectoralis major
    Biceps brachii
Muscles that help with extension:
Primary extensors
    Latissimus dorsi
    Teres major
Secondary extensors
    Teres minor
    Triceps (long head)
The muscles that help with abduction:
Primary abductors
    Deltoid (middle portion)
    Supraspinatus
Secondary abductors
    Serratus anterior
    Deltoid (anterior and posterior portions)
The muscles that help with adduction:
Primary adductors
    Pectoralis major
    Latissimus dorsi

Secondary adductors
    Teres major
    Deltoid (anterior portion)
Muscles that help with internal rotation:
Primary internal rotators
    Subscapularis
    Pectoralis major
    Latissimus dorsi
    Teres major
Secondary internal rotator
    Deltoid (anterior portion)
Muscles that help with external rotation:
Primary external rotators
    Infraspinatus
    Teres minor
Secondary external rotator
    Deltoid (posterior portion)
Muscles that help elevate the shoulder:
Primary elevators
    Trapezius
    Levator scapulae
Secondary elevators
    Rhomboid major
    Rhomboid minor
Muscles that help with scapular retraction (as in the position of attention or bracing the shoulder):
Primary retractors
    Rhomboid major
    Rhomboid minor
Secondary retractor
    Trapezius
Muscles that help with scapular protraction:
Primary protractor
    Serratus anterior

Physical Assessment

It must be remembered that pain in the shoulder and arm could be referred pain from the myocardium, neck, and diaphragm.

After inspecting the skin and area around the joint for abnormal swelling, wasting of muscles, or discoloration of the skin, the bony prominences and the muscles should be palpated for tender points. Then the range of motion should be tested both actively and passively.

If a person is unable to move his shoulder joint actively through the normal range of motion, it could be a result of muscle weakness, tightening of the fibrous tissue of the capsule or ligaments, or abnormal bony growths. Limitations as a result of muscle weakness can be ruled out if full range of movement is achieved by moving the joint passively. If the limitation persists even when moving the joint passively, the problem is probably a result of ligaments, capsule, or bony growths.

THE ELBOW JOINT

Articulating Surfaces and Type of Joint

The elbow joint (see Figure 3.41) is a hinge joint with three components. The **humeroulnar joint** is where the trochlea of the humerus articulates with the trochlear notch of the ulna. The **humeroradial joint** is formed by the capitulum of the humerus and the head of the radius, and the **proximal radioulnar joint** is the articulation between the head of the radius and the radial notch of the ulna. The latter is not part of the hinge but is a pivot joint. The capsule and joint cavity are continuous for all three joints. The elbow joint is relatively stable because it is well supported by bone and ligaments.

Ligaments

Two major ligaments—the **ulnar (medial) collateral ligament** and the **radial (lateral) collateral ligament**—support the joint on either side and rise from the medial and lateral epicondyle of the humerus, respectively. The head of the radius is held in the radial notch of the ulna by the **annular ligament.**

Bursa

An **olecranon bursa** is located posteriorly over the olecranon process.

Possible Movements

The elbow joint allows flexion and extension. Forearm supination and pronation are also possible and a result of the articulation between the radius and ulna proximally and distally.

Range of Motion

Flexion, 135°
Extension, 0–5°
Supination, 90°
Pronation, 90°

Muscles

Muscles that flex the elbow:
Primary flexors
    Brachialis
    Biceps brachii
Secondary flexors
    Brachioradialis
    Supinator

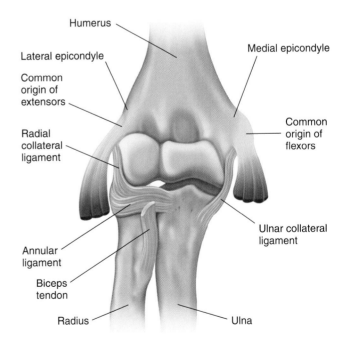

FIGURE **3.41.** Right Elbow Joint, Radius, and Ulna—Anterior View, Showing the Ligaments

Muscles that help with extension:

Primary extensor
Triceps

Secondary extensor
Anconeus

Muscles that help with supination:

Primary supinators
Biceps
Supinator

Secondary supinator
Brachioradialis

Muscles that help with pronation:

Primary pronators
Pronator teres
Pronator quadratus

Secondary pronator
Flexor carpi radialis

Physical Assessment

Inspection

Note the angle made by the forearm with the upper arm—the **carrying angle.** Normally, it is about 5° in men and 10–15° in women. Swelling, scars, and skin discolorations should be recorded.

Palpation

The bony prominences that can be easily felt at the elbow are the medial epicondyle, the olecranon, the olecranon fossa of the humerus into which the olecranon fits, the ulnar border, the lateral epicondyle, and the head of the radius.

Medially, the ulnar nerve can be easily located in the sulcus between the medial epicondyle and the olecranon process. If the olecranon bursa is inflamed, it can be felt as a thick and boggy structure over the olecranon. Tenderness over the lateral collateral ligament and the annular ligament can be identified.

The shallow depression in front of the forearm is the cubital fossa. The biceps tendon and the pulsation of the brachial artery can be felt here.

In addition, the various muscles, active and passive range of motion should be checked.

DISTAL (INFERIOR) RADIOULNAR JOINT

This pivot joint anchors the distal radius and ulna and participates in supination and pronation. It has a joint capsule independent of the wrist joint. See above for muscles that help with supination and pronation.

MIDDLE RADIOULNAR JOINT

This is syndesmosis and includes the interosseous membrane and the oblique cord (fibrous tissue) that runs between the interosseous border of the radius and ulna. The oblique cord which is a flattened band

---

Common Elbow Ailments

Cubital tunnel syndrome is a collection of signs and symptoms produced as a result of constriction by the aponeurosis of the flexor carpi ulnaris on the medial aspect of the elbow, with resultant pressure on the ulnar nerve.

Humeral epicondylitis includes inflammation in the region of the medial and/or lateral epicondyle.

Lateral epicondylitis is commonly referred to as **tennis elbow** or **lateral tennis elbow.** Because many muscles originate and insert into the elbow region, it is a common site for inflammation and pain. In this condition, the common origin of the extensors from the lateral epicondyle is strained and inflamed as a result of repeated extension of the wrist against some force.

Medial epicondylitis has a variety of names: **epitrochleitis, javelin thrower's elbow, medial tennis elbow, golfer's elbow,** and **pitcher's elbow.** Here, the origin of the flexors from the medial epicondyle is inflamed. Rarely, the triceps tendon is inflamed. This is known as the **posterior tendinitis.**

Myositis ossificans is a condition in which there is calcification in a muscle. The brachialis muscle is a common site for such ossification because it gets damaged in a supracondylar fracture of the humerus and posterior dislocation of the elbow.

Olecranon bursitis (miner's elbow) is an inflammation of the olecranon bursa as a result of repeated trauma, such as jerky extension in dart throwing or repeated falling on the elbow in contact sports.

---

that runs between the superior part of the ulna to the radius, prevents displacement of the radius when the arm is pulled. The interosseus membrane serves to stabilize the elbow and radioulnar joints, helps transmit forces from the hand, and increases the surface available for muscle attachment.

JOINTS OF THE WRIST AND HAND

Many joints are present in the region of the wrist and hand (see Figure 3.42). These include the distal radioulnar joint, radiocarpal joint (wrist joint), intercarpal joints, midcarpal joint, carpometacarpal joints, intermetacarpal joints, metacarpophalangeal joints, and interphalangeal joints.

THE WRIST JOINT (RADIOCARPAL JOINT)

Articulating Surfaces and Type of Joint

The wrist is a condyloid joint formed by the articulation between three carpal bones (scaphoid, lunate, and triquetrum) with the distal end of the radius and an articular disk. The articular disk separates the ulna from the carpals, making the distal radioulnar joint distinct from the radiocarpal joint.

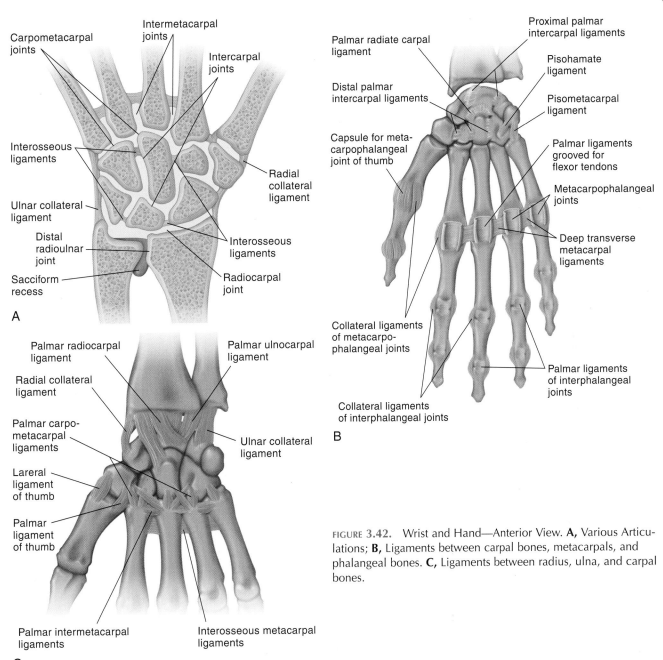

FIGURE **3.42.** Wrist and Hand—Anterior View. **A,** Various Articulations; **B,** Ligaments between carpal bones, metacarpals, and phalangeal bones. **C,** Ligaments between radius, ulna, and carpal bones.

Ligaments

Many ligaments (Figure 3.42B), such as the **palmar** and **dorsal ulnocarpal** and **radiocarpal ligaments, radial collateral ligaments,** and **ulnar collateral ligaments,** stabilize the joint and the carpal bones in this region. They also ensure that the carpals follow the radius during pronation and supination.

An important ligament in the hand complex is the **transverse carpal ligament,** or the **flexor retinaculum.** The transverse carpal ligament forms the roof of the palmar arch formed by the carpals (see Figure 3.43). The hook of the hamate and the pisiform form the ulnar side of the arch and the trapezium and the

radial side of the scaphoid form the radial side. The tendons of the flexor digitorum superficialis and flexor digitorum profundus, surrounded by a common synovial sheath, pass through the carpal tunnel. The tendon of the flexor carpi radialis, the tendon of flexor pollicis longus, and the median nerve also pass through the tunnel.

Possible Movements

The wrist allows flexion, extension, abduction (radial deviation), adduction (ulnar deviation), and circumduction of the hand.

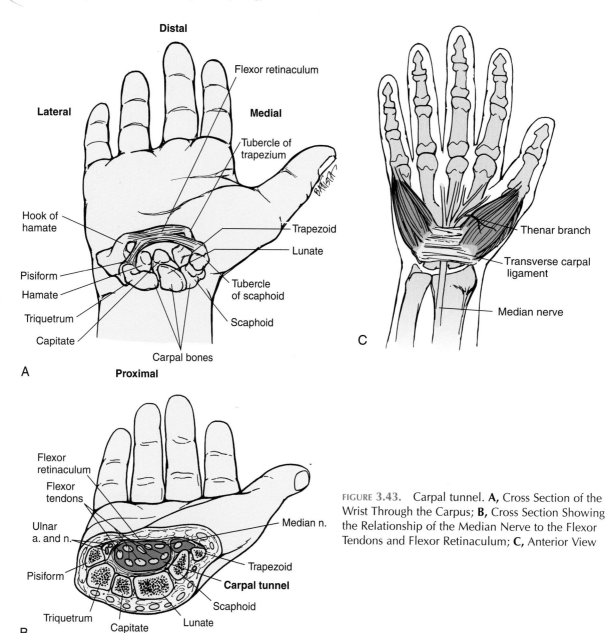

FIGURE **3.43.**   Carpal tunnel. **A,** Cross Section of the Wrist Through the Carpus; **B,** Cross Section Showing the Relationship of the Median Nerve to the Flexor Tendons and Flexor Retinaculum; **C,** Anterior View

Range of Motion

Ulnar deviation, 30°
Radial deviation, 20°
Flexion, 80°
Extension, 70°

Muscles

The muscles that move the hand pass over the wrist joint and help move it. There are 6 flexors and 2 pronators on the anterior or flexor surface of the forearm and a total of 12 muscles on the extensor surface of the forearm. The abductor pollicis longus and the flexor and extensor carpi radialis longus and

brevis help with radial deviation. The flexor and extensor carpi ulnaris help with ulnar deviation.

OTHER JOINTS OF THE HANDS

There are many joints in the region of the hand (Figure 3.42) as there is articulation between the various carpal bones. These are gliding joints.

A saddle joint is present between the proximal end of the first metacarpal and the trapezium that allows all the movements of the thumb. The carpometacarpal joint (between hamate and metacarpal bone) of the little finger is also a saddle joint. The carpometacarpal joints of the remaining fingers are plane joints that permit little or no movement. The function of the carpometacarpal joints is primarily to allow cupping of the hand around the shape of objects.

The joints between the metacarpal bones and the phalanges—the metacarpophalangeal joints—are of the condyloid type, allowing flexion, extension, abduction, adduction, and some axial rotation. Flexion and extension is more extensive. Some hyperextension is also possible at these joints. The joints between the phalanges—interphalangeal joints—are of the hinge type, allowing flexion and extension. The joint between the phalanges of the thumb also allow some axial rotation.

Range of Motion

Flexion and extension at the various joints are different.

Metacarpophalangeal joints: flexion, 90°; extension, 30–45°

Proximal interphalangeal joint: flexion, 100°; extension, 10°

Distal interphalangeal joint: flexion, 90°; extension, 10°

Adduction and abduction of fingers: 20°

Because the thumb articulates at right angles to the rest of the fingers the movements of the thumb is different. The carpometacarpal joint (trapezium-thumb metacarpal joint) of the thumb is a saddle joint that is mobile and allows all movements, including circumduction.

Metacarpophalangeal joint of thumb: adduction, 50°; flexion, 90°; extension, 20°; abduction, 70°. It is also possible to oppose the thumb. Minimal axial rotation is also possible at this joint.

Physical Assessment

Inspection

The dorsal and palmar surfaces should be examined and the way the hand is held should be noted. Normally, the fingers are held parallel to each other in a slightly flexed position. Damage to nerves supplying the hand produces typical deformities.

GRIPS

Precision grips of the hand involve griping of small objects using the pads of the digits. Here, there is rotation at the carpometacarpal joint of the thumb and at the metacarpophalangeal joints of the thumb and fingers. Mostly, the small muscles of the hand are used.

In *power grips,* in which considerable force is required, the hand comes into action. The long flexors and extensors work strongly to fix the wrist and to grip the object.

ARCHITECTURE OF THE HAND

The skeletal composition of the hand can be divided into fixed and mobile units. The distal row of carpal bones and the metacarpals of the index and long fingers are fixed and are firmly attached to each other.

The mobile units are the thumb; the phalanges of the index finger; the phalanges of the long, ring, and small fingers; and the fourth and fifth metacarpals. The mobile units move around the fixed units of the hand.

Palpation

The various bones can be easily felt through the skin and may be palpated for tender points. Both active and passive range of motion should also be tested.

Joints of the Pelvic Girdle and Lower Limbs

The joints of the pelvic girdle (see Figure 3.44) must be considered in conjunction with the joints of the lower lumbar region and hips because dysfunction of any one structure can affect the function of all others. For example, fusion of the lower lumbar vertebrae, differences in leg length, and stiffening of any of these joints can result in pain and stress on other structures.

Therefore, the structures of this region are often referred to as the lumbopelvic complex, which includes the fourth and fifth lumbar joints, the sacroiliac joints, sacrococcygeal joint (symphysis), the hip joints, and the pubic symphysis.

A major function of the pelvic girdle is to transmit the weight of the upper body to the lower limbs and

Common Wrist Ailments

Carpal tunnel syndrome is a common ailment in the wrist region. Occasionally, as a result of inflammation and swelling, etc., the structures passing through the carpal tunnel become compressed, including the median nerve. This results in the sensations in the skin and the control of muscles supplied by this nerve being affected. This condition is known as carpal tunnel syndrome. Pain, tingling, and loss of wrist mobility are some of the common symptoms.

Gymnast's wrist, or dorsal radiocarpal impingement syndrome, occurs as a result of repetitive wrist dorsiflexion, especially when performed with an extra load or force such as in gymnastics during beam exercises, floor exercises, or jumping. Impingement occurs in the dorsal aspect of the radiocarpal joint in this condition and there is pain over the wrist.

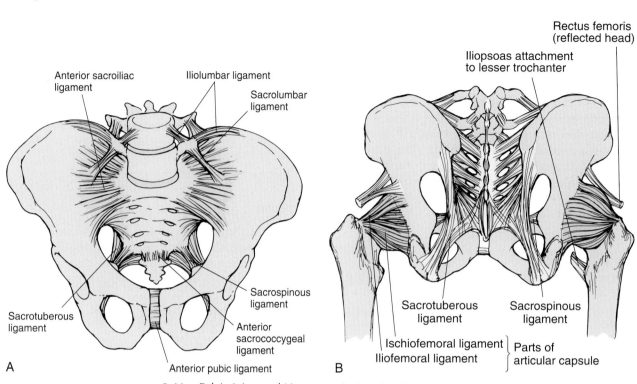

FIGURE 3.44. Pelvic Joints and Ligaments. **A,** Anterior View; **B,** Posterior View

forces from the lower limb to the upper body. The sacroiliac joints are important for walking by absorbing forces from the leg and protecting the disks.

SACROILIAC JOINT

In osteopathic medicine, the sacroiliac joint is considered as two joints—the sacroiliac joint (where the sacrum moves in relation to the ilium) and iliosacral joint (where the ilium moves in relation to the sacrum). This is so because the sacrum is associated with the spine and helps transmit forces from above to the pelvis, and the ilium is closely associated with the lower limb and transmits forces upwards.

Articulating Surfaces and Type of Joint

The two synovial joints between the medial surface of the ilium and the lateral aspect of the upper sacral

vertebrae are L-shaped when viewed laterally (see Figures 3.19A and 3.28B). The articular surfaces are covered with cartilage and marked by elevations and depressions that fit each other and make the joint stronger. It is a gliding joint.

Ligaments

The ligaments that bind the sacrum to the ilium withstand the major forces through the sacroiliac joints. They form a network of fibrous bands. Many ligaments—**iliolumbar, sacrolumbar, sacroiliac** (anterior and posterior), **sacrotuberous** (sacrum to ischial tuberosity), and **sacrospinous**—are found around the joints (Figure 3.44). Of these, the iliolumbar, which extends from the transverse process of the 5th vertebrae to the posterior iliac crest, is the most important as it stabilizes the 5th vertebrae on the sacrum. In addition, the muscles adjacent to the joint—gluteus maximus, gluteus minimus, piriformis, latissimus dorsi, quadratus lumborum, and iliacus—have fibrous attachments that blend with the ligaments and make the joints even stronger.

Possible Movements and Range of Motion

The movements of this joint are limited, but even this limited movement is important. The main function of this joint is to serve as a shock absorber. The movement of the sacrum is described as flexion (nutation) and extension (counter-nutation). During flexion the

COMPARISON OF THE SHOULDER AND PELVIC GIRDLES

	Shoulder Girdle	Pelvic Girdle
Articulation with vertebral column	via muscles	via sacroiliac joint
Sockets for joint	shallow	deep
Mobility	more	less
Strength	less	more
Risk of dislocation	more	less

sacral promontory moves anteriorly and inferiorly with the apex moving posteriorly, while the iliac bones approximate and the ischial tuberosities move apart. Such a movement occurs when walking and when bending forward (flexion) and backward (extension). During walking, the movement of the sacrum is determined by the forces from above, while the movement of the ilium is determined by the femur.

Muscles

Though this joint is surrounded by strong muscles, none play a direct part in moving the sacrum. Sacral movement is a result of the pull of forces through ligaments and gravity. By pulling on the ilia, the muscles in the vicinity have an indirect effect on the sacrum.

There are 35 muscles attached to the sacrum or hipbones and, together with the ligaments and fascia, they help coordinate movement of the trunk and lower limbs. Problems associated with any of them can result in alteration of the mechanics of the pelvis. The quadratus lumborum, erector spinae, abdominal muscles, rectus femoris, iliopsoas, tensor fascia latae, piriformis, short hip adductors, hamstrings, gluteus maximus, medius and minimus, vastus medialis and lateralis, the pelvic floor muscles are important muscles that must be considered in a client with low back pain.

Physical Assessment

When assessing this joint, it is important to take a good history that includes history of trauma and abnormal stress to the region. Typically, the pain arising from this joint is unilateral, increased by walking, getting off the bed, and climbing stairs, etc. Examination of this joint should be done in conjunction with the hip joint and lumbar spine as the pain may be referred to this joint from those areas. Description of individual tests used for assessing this joint is beyond the scope of the book. The gait, posture, alignment of bony structures, difference in leg length, and passive and active movements should be tested, and treatment aimed at normalizing the stresses on the lumbopelvic complex should be based on the findings.

THE HIP JOINT

Articulating Surfaces and Type of Joint

The hip joint, also referred to as the **acetabulofemoral** or **iliofemoral joint,** is one of the most stable joints because the articular surfaces of the rounded head of the femur and the acetabulum of the pelvis fit well into each other. The acetabulum is further deepened by the fibrocartilage (**acetabular labrum**) located in the acetabulum. In addition to shape of the articular surface, the hip joint, similar to the shoulder, has supporting ligaments (see Figure 3.45). It is a ball and socket joint.

Ligaments and Bursa

The thick capsule is reinforced by strong ligaments. The **iliofemoral ligament** is a thick band that runs between the anterior inferior iliac spine and the intertrochanteric line of the femur. This ligament prevents excessive internal and external rotation. When standing, this ligament is twisted and pulled taut and results in "locking" of the joint, allowing the person to stand with little muscle action. The **pubofemoral ligament** extends from the pubic portion of the acetabular rim to the inferior portion of the neck of the femur. The **ischiofemoral ligament** runs between

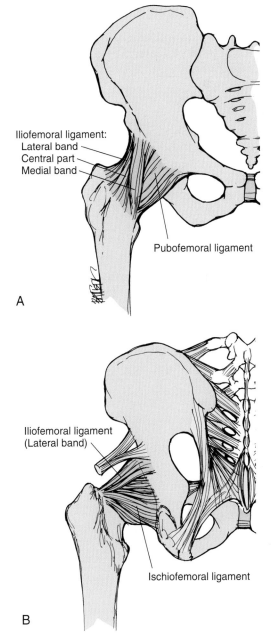

FIGURE 3.45. Hip Joint Ligaments **A,** Anterior View; **B,** Posterior View

the ischial acetabular rim and the superior portion of the femoral neck. The **transverse acetabular ligament** runs between the gap in the inferior margin of the acetabular labrum. Another ligament, the **ligamentum teres,** is located inside the joint capsule and runs between the acetabular notch and a small depression (fovea capitis) located in the femoral head.

A few bursae surround the hip joint. The **iliopectineal bursa** lies on the anterior aspect of the hip joint, deep to the iliopsoas muscle, as it crosses the joint. It may communicate with the joint cavity of the hip joint. The **trochanteric bursae** lie over the greater trochanter, deep to the gluteus maximus, reducing friction between the bone and muscle.

Possible Movements

The hip permits flexion, extension, adduction, abduction, medial rotation, lateral rotation, and some circumduction.

Range of Motion

Abduction, 45–50°
Adduction, 20–30°
External/lateral rotation, 45°
Internal/medial rotation, 35°
Flexion, 135°
Extension, 30°

Muscles

The action of most muscles around the hip can be determined from the location. The flexor muscles are located in the anterior quadrant, the extensors in the posterior quadrant, the adductors in the medial, and the abductors in the lateral quadrant.
Muscles that flex the hip:
Primary flexor
  Iliopsoas
Secondary flexors
  Rectus femoris
  Sartorius
Muscles that extend the hip:
Primary extensor
  Gluteus maximus
Secondary extensor
  Hamstrings
Muscles that abduct the hip:
Primary abductor
  Gluteus medius
Secondary abductors
  Gluteus minimus
  Tensor fascia lata
Muscles that adduct the hip:
Primary adductor
  Adductor longus

Secondary adductors
  Adductor brevis
  Adductor magnus
  Pectineus
  Gracilis
Muscles that rotate the hip laterally:
  Gluteus maximus
  Gluteus medius and minimus (posterior fibers)
  Iliopsoas
Muscles that rotate the hip medially:
  Adductor magnus, longus, brevis
  Gluteus medius and minimus (anterior fibers)

Physical Assessment

Inspection

The gait should be observed as the person enters the room. It is preferable to have the patient's body exposed waist down. When standing normally, the anterior superior iliac spine should be level with a slight anterior curvature of the lumbar spine. Absence of the lumbar lordosis may indicate spasm of the muscles. Weakness of the abdominal muscles may exhibit an abnormally increased lordosis. Look for muscle wasting and body asymmetry.

Palpation

Bony prominences: Various bony prominences can be easily palpated. These are the anterior superior iliac spines, iliac crest, greater trochanter, and pubic tubercles anteriorly. Posteriorly, the posterior superior iliac spine and the ischial tuberosity can be palpated.

Other structures: The inguinal ligament, which runs between the anterior superior iliac spine and the pubic tubercle, marks part of the route taken by the male testis as it descends into the scrotum. Bulges in this region may indicate an inguinal hernia. The femoral artery pulsation can be felt just inferior to the inguinal ligament. The femoral vein lies just medial to the artery. Tenderness over the sciatic nerve as it emerges from the sacral region can be palpated.

The active and passive range of motion of the hip should be tested as well, together with discrepancies between the two legs.

THE KNEE JOINT

Articulating Surfaces and Type of Joint

The knee joint, or tibiofemoral joint, (see Figure 3.46) is one of the largest, most complex, and most frequently injured joints in the body and a thorough knowledge of its anatomy is important. It is a hinge joint. The fibula does not articulate with the femur and comes in contact only with the lateral surface of the tibia.

The lower end of the femur, with its condyles and deep fossa between them, articulates with the flat upper surface of the tibia. Numerous ligaments, cartilages, and tendons help stabilize this joint. The articulating surface is deepened by the presence of two half-moon–shaped fibrocartilage disks—the **medial** and **lateral meniscus**—located on the tibia (Figure 3.46E). The menisci also serve as shock absorbers, spreading the stress on the joint over a larger joint surface and helping lubricate the joint and reduce friction.

Ligaments

The knee joint has ligaments located inside and outside the joint capsule. Inside the joint, there are two ligaments that run anteroposteriorly, preventing excessive forward and backward movement. The **anterior cruciate ligament** runs from the anterior part of the tibia to the medial side of the lateral femoral condyle. It prevents excessive forward movement (hyperextension) of the tibia. The **posterior cruciate ligament** extends superiorly and anteriorly from the posterior aspect of the tibia to the lateral side of the medial condyle. It prevents the tibia from slipping backward and, with the popliteus muscle, it prevents the femur from sliding anteriorly over the tibia in a squatting position.

The **patellar tendon**—a thick, fibrous band that extends from the patella to the tibial tuberosity—is actually an extension of the quadriceps tendon that stabilizes the joint anteriorly. Thin fibrous bands—**patellar retinaculum**—extend from the side of the patella to the tibial condyles. Posteriorly, the capsule

is thickened to form the **oblique popliteal ligament,** an extension of the semimembranous tendon. Another thickening—the **arcuate popliteal ligament**—runs from the posterior fibular head to the capsule.

Medially, the **medial collateral ligament,** or the **tibial collateral ligament,** runs from the medial epicondyle of the femur to the medial surface of the tibia. This ligament helps stabilize the joint medially and prevents anterior displacement of the tibia on the femur.

Another ligament—**lateral collateral ligament,** or the **fibular collateral ligament,** runs from the lateral epicondyle of the femur to the head of the fibula, stabilizing the joint laterally. Other small ligaments exist. The **coronary ligament** attaches the menisci to the tibial condyle, the **transverse ligament** connects the anterior portions of the medial and lateral menisci, and the **meniscofemoral ligament** runs posteriorly, joining the lateral menisci to the medial condyle of the femur.

In addition to the support provided by the ligaments, the joint is stabilized medially by the **pes anserinus tendons** (semitendinosus, gracilis, and sartorius) and the semimembranosus tendon. The posterolateral region is supported by the biceps femoris tendon, and the posterior aspect is reinforced by the origins of the gastrocnemius muscles and the popliteus muscles.

Bursae

The knee joint is surrounded by numerous bursae. The largest is the **suprapatellar bursa,** or **quadriceps bursa,** an extension of the joint capsule that allows movement of the thigh muscles over the lower end of the femur. Subcutaneous bursae—the **subcutaneous** or **superficial prepatellar** and **infrapatellar bursa** and the **deep infrapatellar bursa**—surround the patella. A large fat pad, the infrapatellar fat pad, exists deep to the patella tendon. The fat pad is lined on the deep surface by synovial membrane and is thought to help lubricate the joint as it deforms during flexion and extension of the knee.

In addition to the above, bursae exist in the popliteal fossa—**popliteal bursa**—and near the gastrocnemius—the **gastrocnemius bursa.** The **semimembranous bursa,** which lies deep to the semimembranosus tendon and the medial origin of the gastrocnemius muscle, often communicates with the joint. Other bursae may exist between the pes anserinus and the iliotibial band.

Possible Movements

The knee joint allows flexion (with an associated glide), extension (with an associated glide), and internal and external rotation. Active rotation of the knee occurs only when the knee is flexed.

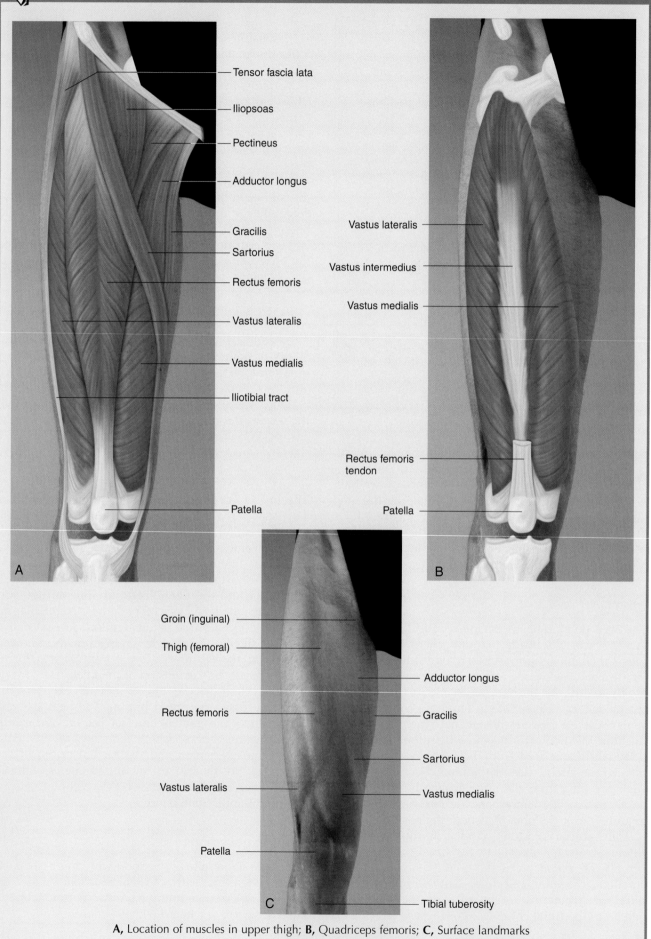

Tensor fascia lata

Iliopsoas

Pectineus

Adductor longus

Gracilis

Sartorius

Rectus femoris

Vastus lateralis

Vastus medialis

Iliotibial tract

Patella

A

Vastus lateralis

Vastus intermedius

Vastus medialis

Rectus femoris tendon

Patella

B

Groin (inguinal)

Thigh (femoral)

Rectus femoris

Vastus lateralis

Patella

Adductor longus

Gracilis

Sartorius

Vastus medialis

Tibial tuberosity

C

A, Location of muscles in upper thigh; **B,** Quadriceps femoris; **C,** Surface landmarks

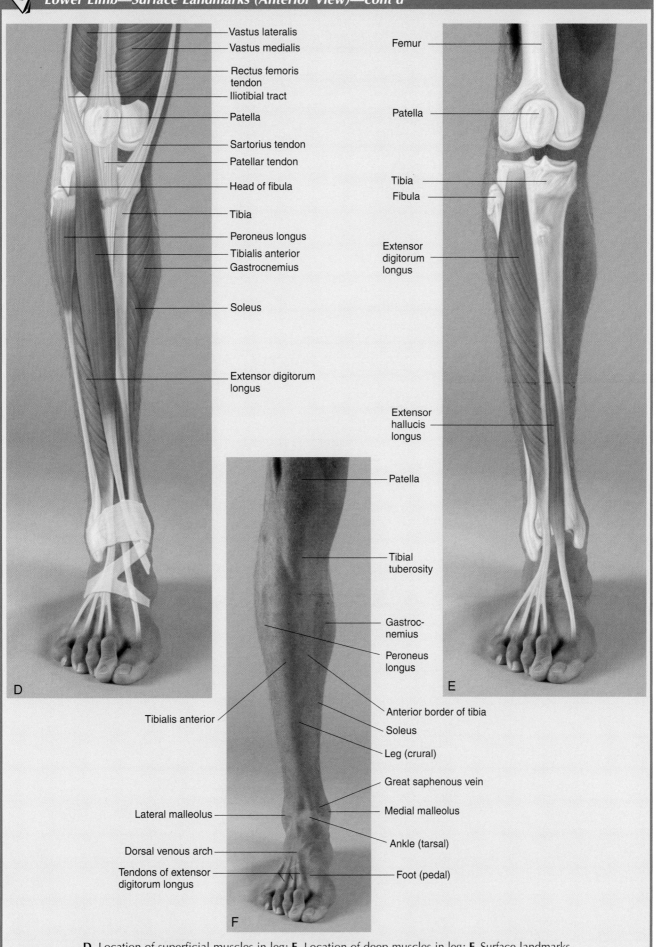

Vastus lateralis
Vastus medialis
Rectus femoris tendon
Iliotibial tract
Patella
Sartorius tendon
Patellar tendon
Head of fibula
Tibia
Peroneus longus
Tibialis anterior
Gastrocnemius
Soleus
Extensor digitorum longus

D

Femur
Patella
Tibia
Fibula
Extensor digitorum longus
Extensor hallucis longus
Patella
Tibial tuberosity
Gastroc-nemius
Peroneus longus

E

Patella
Tibial tuberosity
Gastroc-nemius
Peroneus longus
Tibialis anterior
Anterior border of tibia
Soleus
Leg (crural)
Great saphenous vein
Lateral malleolus
Medial malleolus
Dorsal venous arch
Ankle (tarsal)
Tendons of extensor digitorum longus
Foot (pedal)

F

D, Location of superficial muscles in leg; **E,** Location of deep muscles in leg; **F,** Surface landmarks

Lower Limb—Surface Landmarks (Posterior View)

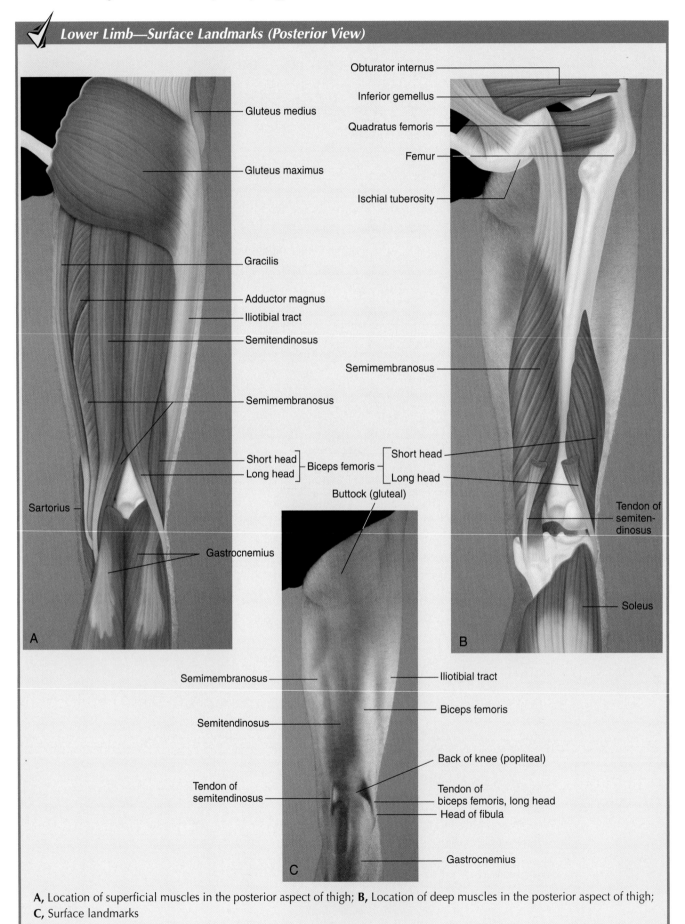

Obturator internus
Inferior gemellus
Quadratus femoris
Femur
Ischial tuberosity

Gluteus medius
Gluteus maximus

Gracilis
Adductor magnus
Iliotibial tract
Semitendinosus

Semimembranosus

Semimembranosus

Short head ⎤
Long head ⎦ Biceps femoris

Short head ⎤
Long head ⎦ Biceps femoris

Sartorius

Tendon of semitendinosus

Gastrocnemius

Soleus

A

B

Buttock (gluteal)

Semimembranosus
Semitendinosus

Iliotibial tract
Biceps femoris

Back of knee (popliteal)

Tendon of semitendinosus

Tendon of biceps femoris, long head
Head of fibula

Gastrocnemius

C

A, Location of superficial muscles in the posterior aspect of thigh; **B,** Location of deep muscles in the posterior aspect of thigh;
C, Surface landmarks

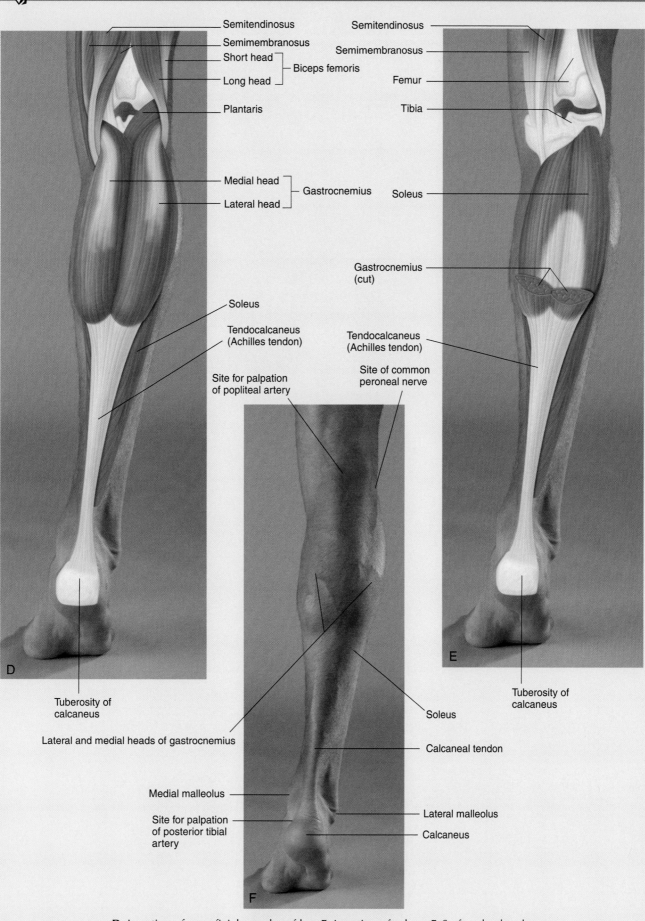

Semitendinosus

Semimembranosus

Short head ⎤
　　　　　　⎬ Biceps femoris
Long head ⎦

Plantaris

Medial head ⎤
　　　　　　⎬ Gastrocnemius
Lateral head ⎦

Soleus

Tendocalcaneus
(Achilles tendon)

Site for palpation
of popliteal artery

Tuberosity of
calcaneus

Lateral and medial heads of gastrocnemius

Medial malleolus

Site for palpation
of posterior tibial
artery

Semitendinosus

Semimembranosus

Femur

Tibia

Soleus

Gastrocnemius
(cut)

Tendocalcaneus
(Achilles tendon)

Site of common
peroneal nerve

Tuberosity of
calcaneus

Soleus

Calcaneal tendon

Lateral malleolus

Calcaneus

D

E

F

D, Location of superficial muscles of leg; **E,** Location of soleus; **F,** Surface landmarks

Lower Limb—Surface Landmarks (Posterior View)—cont'd

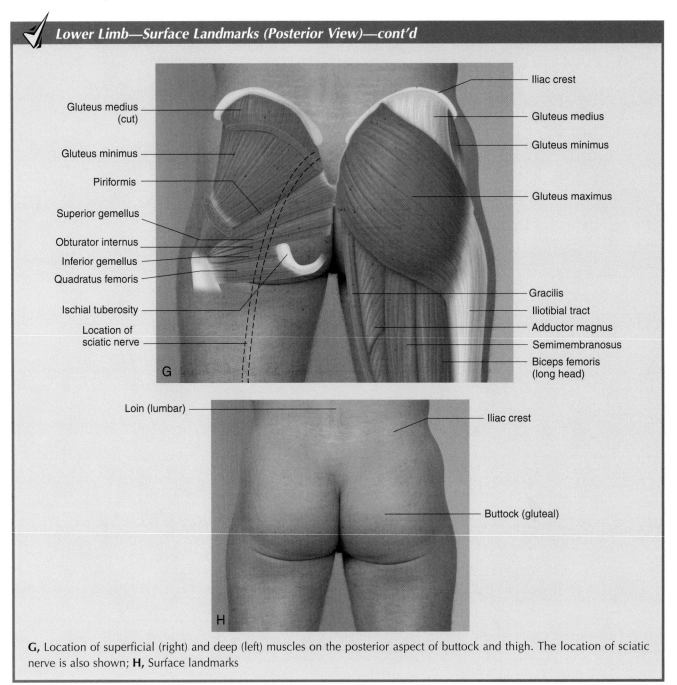

G, Location of superficial (right) and deep (left) muscles on the posterior aspect of buttock and thigh. The location of sciatic nerve is also shown; **H,** Surface landmarks

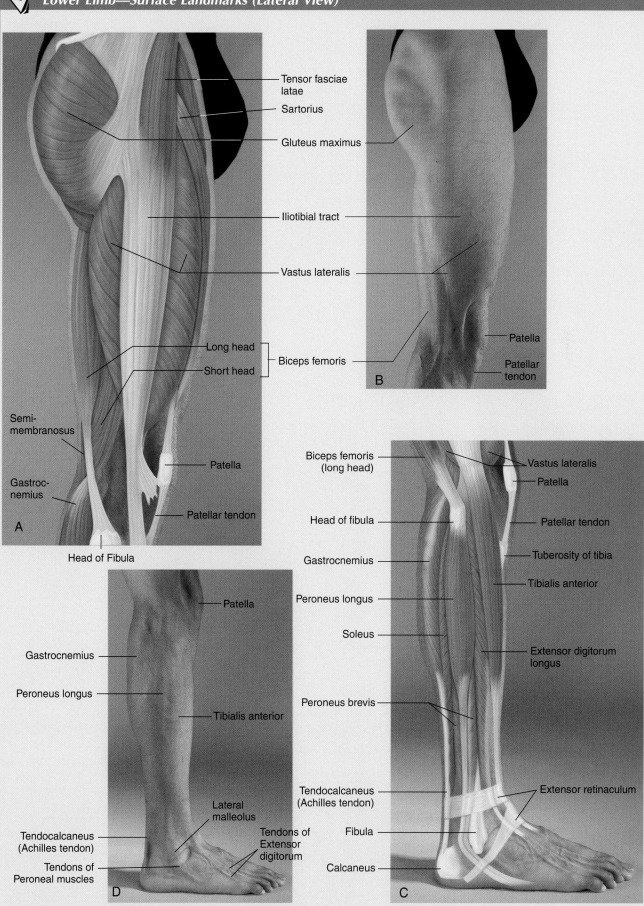

Tensor fasciae latae

Sartorius

Gluteus maximus

Iliotibial tract

Vastus lateralis

Long head
Short head
} Biceps femoris

Semi-membranosus

Gastroc-nemius

Patella

Patellar tendon

A

Head of Fibula

Patella

Patellar tendon

B

Biceps femoris (long head)

Head of fibula

Gastrocnemius

Peroneus longus

Soleus

Peroneus brevis

Tendocalcaneus (Achilles tendon)

Fibula

Calcaneus

Vastus lateralis

Patella

Patellar tendon

Tuberosity of tibia

Tibialis anterior

Extensor digitorum longus

Extensor retinaculum

C

Patella

Gastrocnemius

Peroneus longus

Tibialis anterior

Lateral malleolus

Tendons of Extensor digitorum

Tendocalcaneus (Achilles tendon)

Tendons of Peroneal muscles

D

A, Location of muscles in the lateral aspect of thigh; **B,** Surface landmarks (thigh - lateral aspect); **C,** Location of muscles in the lateral aspect of leg; **D,** Surface landmarks (leg - lateral aspect)

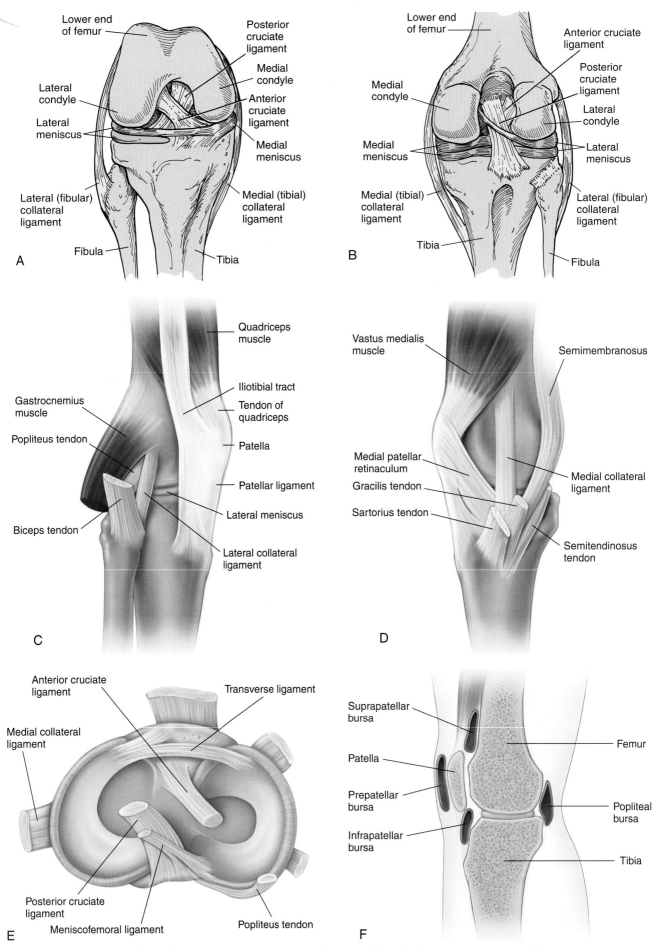

FIGURE 3.46. Knee Joint; **A,** Anterior View – Joint Flexed and Patella Removed; **B,** Posterior View – Joint Extended; **C,** Lateral View; **D,** Medial View; **E,** Superior Aspect of the Tibia showing the Location of Ligaments; **F,** Medial Aspect of the Knee showing the location of Bursae.

Range of Motion

Flexion, 135°
Extension, 0°
Internal rotation, 10°
External rotation, 10°

Muscles

Muscles that flex the knee:
  Hamstrings: semimembranosus, semitendinosus, biceps femoris
Muscle that extends the knee:
Primary extensor
  Quadriceps
Muscles that rotate the knee medially:
  Semitendinosus
  Semimembranosus
Muscle that rotates the knee laterally:
  Biceps femoris

Physical Assessment

Inspection

The gait of the individual must be closely watched. Identify abnormal swellings and asymmetry of muscles. The knee should be fully extended while standing.

Palpation

Many parts of the bones can be easily palpated in and around the knee. The medial and lateral femoral condyle, the head of the fibula and the patella, and others may be palpated. The muscles and tendons in and around the joint should be palpated for tenderness. Enlarged bursae (a common ailment) can be felt as a boggy, soft swelling. Tenderness in the joint margins may be a result of tears in the medial and lateral meniscus. The medial and lateral collateral ligaments are also easily palpated. The insertion of the tendons of the sartorius, gracilis, and semitendinosus can be palpated on the medial aspect of the joint. The iliotibial tract, a thick fibrous band, runs on the lateral aspect of the knee joint.

In the popliteal fossa, the pulsation of the popliteal artery can be felt.

The stability of the joint must be tested by checking the collateral and cruciate ligaments. The range of motion should also be tested actively and passively.

TIBIOFIBULAR JOINT (PROXIMAL AND DISTAL)

The superior or proximal tibiofibular joint is a plane synovial joint formed by the head of the fibula and the posterolateral surface of the tibia (Figure 3.47).

✚ Common Knee Ailments

Arthritis, inflammation of the joint, is common to all joints, including the knee joint.

Housemaid's knee is an abnormal enlargement of the prepatellar bursa. Inflammation is a result of pressure over it as when kneeling. It is common in carpet layers and roofers.

Iliotibial tract friction (snapping band). In this condition, the iliotibial band moves backwards and forwards across the knee when the knee is extended and flexed. Running long distances may cause friction, with thickening and swelling of the iliotibial tract, pain, and a snapping sensation in the lateral aspect of the knee.

Injury. This joint is most easily injured in sports. The medial collateral ligament can get torn by a lateral blow to the knee (as in a tackle in football). Rarely, a medial blow to the knee can result in tearing of the lateral collateral ligament. The anterior and posterior cruciate can be torn if force is applied in the anteroposterior or posteroanterior directions. Injury to the meniscus in the form of a tear may occur in athletes. When the joint is injured, excessive production of synovial fluid can cause the joint to swell (joint effusion) and bleeding into the joint (**hemarthrosis**) may occur.

Patellar tendinitis (jumper's knee) is an overuse injury (resulting from repetitive jumping), characterized by pathologic changes in the quadriceps and the patellar tendon. It is more common in players of volleyball, basketball, and sports that involve jumping. It presents as pain and tenderness in the anterior aspect of the knee.

Patellar tracking dysfunction (chondromalacia patellae) is a condition in which the articular cartilage on the deeper surface of the patella (patellofemoral joint) is softened and worn.

The synovial cavity is often continuous with the knee joint, allowing slight superior and inferior glide and anteroposterior glide and rotation of the fibula.

The tibia and fibula are bound together by the interosseous membrane that separates the leg into anterior and posterior compartments.

The inferior tibiofibular joint is a syndesmosis formed by the articulation of the fibula with the lateral aspect of the distal end of the tibia. The joint is reinforced by the anterior and posterior tibiofibular ligaments.

THE ANKLE JOINT AND JOINTS OF THE FOOT

Articulating Surfaces and Type of Joint

The ankle joint (Figure 3.48) is formed by the distal end of the tibia, fibula, and the superior surface of the talus. This joint is also known as the **talocrural joint.**

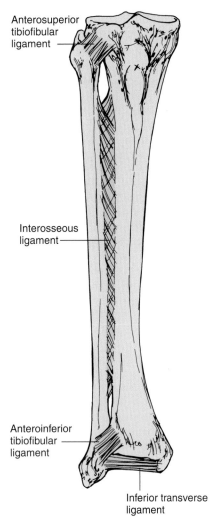

Anterosuperior tibiofibular ligament

Interosseous ligament

Anteroinferior tibiofibular ligament

Inferior transverse ligament

FIGURE 3.47.   Tibiofibular Joints.

joint. It is a hinge joint with the lateral and medial aspect of the capsule thickened to form ligaments.

Other articulations (see Figure 3.49) occur between the talus and calcaneus (**subtalar joint**); between the tarsal bones (**midtarsal joints**—talocalcaneonavicular and calcaneocuboid joints); between the anterior tarsals (**anterior tarsal joints**—cubonavicular, cuneonavicular, cuneocuboid, and intercuneiform joints); between the tarsals and the metatarsals (**tarsometatarsal joints**); between the metatarsal and phalanges (**metatarsophalangeal joint**); and between the phalanges (the **proximal** and **distal interphalangeal joints**).

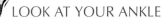

CENTER OF GRAVITY

The center of gravity lies slightly behind and about the same level as the hip joint. Its projection passes anterior to the knee and ankle joints.

LOOK AT YOUR ANKLE

Examine your own ankle or use a skeleton and note which malleolus is longer than the other. Keeping this in mind, visualize the joint in an inversion and eversion sprain. In which of the two sprains will the tarsal bones come in contact with the malleolus earlier? Which of the two sprains do you think occur more commonly?

Ligaments

The **medial ligament,** or the **deltoid ligament,** is a thickening of the medial fibrous capsule that attaches the medial malleolus to the navicular, calcaneus, and talus bones. The **calcaneofibular ligament** extends from the lateral malleolus to the calcaneus. Anteriorly and posteriorly, ligaments extend from the lateral malleolus to the talus to form the **anterior talofibular** (most frequently injured) and **posterior talofibular ligaments.** The various ligaments prevent tilt and rotation of the talus and forward and backward movement of the leg over the talus.

Possible Movements

The ankle allows dorsiflexion and plantar flexion. However, the subtalar joint and tarsal joints allow further movement. Eversion and inversion is possible at the subtalar joint. The foot can be adducted and abducted at the midtarsal joints. The metatarsophalangeal joints and interphalangeal joints are hinge joints, allowing flexion and extension of the toes.

Range of Motion

Dorsiflexion, 20°
Plantar flexion, 50°
Inversion and eversion, 5°
Adduction, 20°
Abduction, 10°
Flexion (toes), 45°
Extension, 70–90°

Muscles

Muscles that cause plantar flexion:
Primary plantar flexors
   Gastrocnemius
   Soleus
Secondary plantar flexors
   Tibialis posterior
   Flexors of the toes
   Peroneus longus and brevis
Muscles that cause dorsiflexion:
   Tibialis anterior

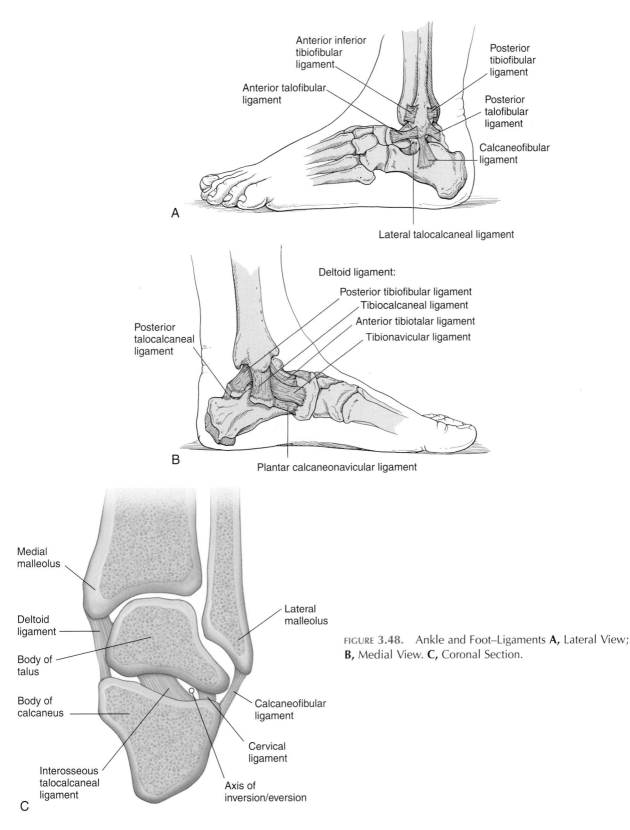

Anterior inferior tibiofibular ligament

Anterior talofibular ligament

Posterior tibiofibular ligament

Posterior talofibular ligament

Calcaneofibular ligament

Lateral talocalcaneal ligament

A

Deltoid ligament:
Posterior tibiofibular ligament
Tibiocalcaneal ligament
Anterior tibiotalar ligament
Tibionavicular ligament

Posterior talocalcaneal ligament

Plantar calcaneonavicular ligament

B

Medial malleolus

Deltoid ligament

Body of talus

Body of calcaneus

Interosseous talocalcaneal ligament

Lateral malleolus

Calcaneofibular ligament

Cervical ligament

Axis of inversion/eversion

C

FIGURE **3.48.** Ankle and Foot–Ligaments **A,** Lateral View; **B,** Medial View. **C,** Coronal Section.

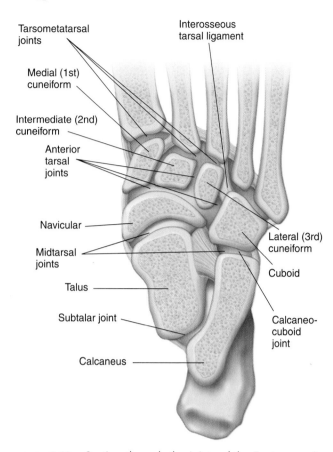

FIGURE **3.49.** Section through the Joints of the Foot—superior view.

Peroneus tertius
Extensors of the toes
Muscles that invert the foot:
    Tibialis anterior and posterior
    Muscles that evert the foot:
    Peroneus longus, brevis, and tertius

Physical Assessment

Inspection

The external appearance of the shoe and foot should provide information. The alignment of the toes and the shape of the foot and arches should be inspected. The color of the skin and presence of swelling should also be noted.

Palpation

The bones of the foot and ankle are easily palpated. Some bony prominences that can be located are the malleoli, talus, calcaneus, and the metatarsal and phalanges. The deltoid ligament is also palpable inferior to the medial malleolus. The long saphenous vein, if dilated may be visible just anterior to the medial malleolus. Both active and passive range of motion should be tested at the various joints.

ARCHES OF THE FOOT

The foot has three major arches that help distribute the weight of the body between the heel and the ball of the foot during standing and walking. Two longitudinal—the **medial** and the **lateral longitudinal arch**—and one transverse—the **transverse arch**—exist. The shape of the arch is maintained by ligaments, the tendons attached to the foot, and the configuration of the bones. The medial arch is formed by the calcaneus, talus, navicular, cuneiforms and the medial three metatarsal bones. The lateral arch is formed by the calcaneus, cuboid, and the two lateral metatarsals. The transverse arch is formed by the cuboid and cuneiform bones.

Age-Related Changes on the Skeletal System and Joints

The slower movement, weakness, and altered physical appearance are a result of changes in the musculoskeletal system.

With age, there is a decrease in height as a result of the shortening of the vertebral column. The intervertebral disks and the vertebrae decrease in height. The continued growth of nose and ear cartilage makes them larger. Subcutaneous fat tends to be redistributed with more in the abdomen and hips and less in the extremities. This redistribution makes the bony landmarks more prominent with deepening hollows in the axilla, shoulders, ribs, and around the eyes.

The ground substance, in relation to the collagen fibers, is reduced in the tissue, resulting in stiffness, less ability to deform to stress, and reduced nutri-

 Common Leg Ailments

Flatfoot is when there is a failure of the foot to form the arches (especially medial).

Injury is common in the ankle and usually results from forcible inversion or eversion, tearing the ligaments. This is known as ankle sprain. The anterior talofibular ligament is usually affected.

Plantar fasciitis is an overuse injury that causes pain in the medial tubercle of the calcaneus and/or along the medial arch of the foot as a result of inflammation of the plantar fascia. It results from continued stretching of the fascia, such as in long distance running.

Shinsplint is a term used interchangeably for many different conditions involving the lower leg, thus, causing confusion. Typically it is used to describe the inflammation caused by repeated stress on the musculotendinous structures arising from the lower part of the tibia.

TENDONS AND VESSELS ON THE DORSUM OF FOOT

Using the diagram, identify the tendons on the dorsum of your foot.

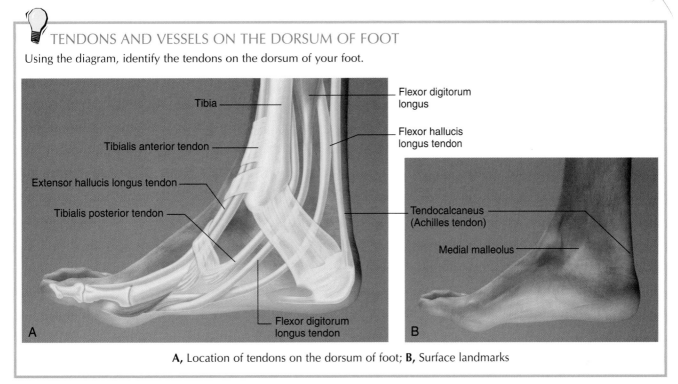

A, Location of tendons on the dorsum of foot; **B,** Surface landmarks

tional status. Changes in the vertebral column, stiffening of the ligaments and joints, and hardening of the tendons result in mild flexion of the vertebrae, hips, knees, elbows, wrists, and neck.

With age, bone formation is slowed in relation to absorption. This results in loss of bone mass and weakening of the structure (**osteoporosis**). Certain changes that occur are also a result of disuse. The loss is greater in women as the estrogen levels drop. Trabecular bone (the network found in the medullary cavity) loss is greater than cortical bone and areas with a higher ratio of trabecular bone, such as the head of femur, radius, and vertebral bodies, are more prone for fractures.

The production of synovial fluid in the joints decreases with age. The articular cartilages become thinner. Because joints are also affected by genetic makeup and wear and tear, the changes observed with age vary individually. Osteoarthritis is associated with increasing age.

VULNERABLE SITES

There are a few sites that need to be palpated gently as a result of the superficial location of vessels and nerves. If excessive pressure is applied, there is potential for damage to these structures as they are pressed against the hard bone. In the upper arm, the ulnar nerve lies over the medial epicondyle of the humerus and the radial nerve is close to the lateral epicondyle. In the neck, large vessels and nerves are located in the anterior part. The popliteal artery and vein lies superficially in the popliteal fossa.

The Skeletal System, Joints, and Massage

In general, massage therapy is not used extensively to correct bony deformities. However, problems related to tendons, bursae, and muscles around joints can be addressed. Also, the psychological benefits of touch should not be forgotten.

When joints are immobilized, the connective tissue elements, such as capsules, ligaments, and surrounding tendons, tend to lose their elasticity because of the release of water from the ground substance that allows connective tissue fibers to come in closer contact and form abnormal cross-linkages between them. By manipulation of joints (including joint replacements), a massage therapist can facilitate breakage of cross-linkages and increase range of motion. Range of motion can also be improved by regular passive and active exercises, use of special techniques to prevent adhesions, and by reducing spasm of surrounding muscles. Chiropractors and physiotherapists specialize in the use of techniques that help mobilize joints.

ATHLETE'S FOOT

This does not indicate the strong foot you would expect to see in an athlete! It is a fungal infection and commonly occurs between the toes.

Massage has been shown to be of benefit to those suffering from joint-related disorders such as arthritis.[1] It reduces stiffness and swelling, increases blood flow, relieves pain and muscle spasm, and mobilizes fibrous tissue.[2] By improving muscle action, it induces a state of general relaxation. Ice massage or immersion, applied using specific techniques, are especially helpful in pain relief and, thereby, introduction of early mobilization exercises.[3] Massage prior to mobilization is also very useful.

Massage has been shown to benefit those with some types of low back pain by decreasing pain and associated depression and anxiety and by increasing range of motion.[4-9] However, a 1999 review[6] of studies in which massage was used for low back pain concluded that there is inadequate evidence; that massage has some potential as a therapy, but more reliable studies are needed. Some studies published after this review have shown improvements in range of motion.[7-10]

Massage has also been shown to improve the range of motion and performance of university dancers[11] and the elderly.[12] A study of patients with spinal cord injuries[13] showed improvement in range of motion and muscle function in these patients.

Massage may lessen the fibrosis that usually develops after injury. Friction massage has been used on muscles, ligaments, tendons, and tendon sheaths for prevention and treatment of scar tissue formation.[14] Deep transverse friction massage has been found to be particularly beneficial in conditions such as chronic tendinitis and bursitis. This technique breaks down scar tissue, increases extensibility and mobility of the structure, promotes normal orientation of collagen fibers, increases blood flow (thereby, speeding healing), reduces stress levels, and allows healing to take place.[14] Although friction massage is beneficial to the underlying structures as stated above, it should be avoided if the nutritional status of the skin is compromised in the area.

Before massaging a client with musculoskeletal disorders, a therapist should obtain a thorough history. Massage is contraindicated locally and generally in many musculoskeletal conditions. Acute arthritis of any type, fractures, dislocation, ruptured ligaments, and recent trauma (e.g., whiplash) are some conditions that are locally contraindicated. Severe osteoporosis, and prolapse of intervertebral disk with nerve dysfunction are just a few of the conditions with general contraindications.

REFERENCES

1. Field T, Hernandez-Reif M, Seligman S, et al. Juvenile rheumatoid arthritis benefits from massage therapy. J Pediatr Psychol 1997;22:607–617.
2. Goats GC. Massage—the scientific basis of an ancient art: Part 2. Physiological and therapeutic effects. [Review]. Br J Sports Med1994;28:153–156.
3. Yurtkuran M, Kocagil T. TENS, electropuncture and ice massage: Comparison of treatment for osteoarthritis of the knee. Am J Acupunct 1999;27:133–140.
4. Hernandez-Reif M, Field T, Krasnegor J, Theakston T. Low back pain is reduced and range of motion increased after massage therapy. Int J Neurosci 2001;106:131–145.
5. Pope MH, Phillips RB, Haugh LD, et al. A prospective randomized three-week trial of spinal manipulation, transcutaneous muscle stimulation, massage and corset in the treatment of subacute low back pain. Spine 1994;19:2571–2577.
6. Ernst, E. Massage therapy for low back pain: a systematic review. J Pain Symptom Manage 1999;17:65–69.
7. Cherkin DC, Eisenberg D, et al. Randomized trial comparing traditional Chinese medical acupuncture, therapeutic massage, and self-care education for chronic low back pain. Arch Intern Med 2001;161(8):1081–1088.
8. Preyde M. Effectiveness of massage therapy for subacute low-back pain: A randomized controlled trial. CMAJ 2000;162(13): 1815–1820.
9. Kalauokalani D, Cherkin DC, Sherman KJ, et al. Lessons from a trial of acupuncture and massage for low back pain: patient expectations and treatment effects. Spine 2001;26:1418–1424.
10. Kolich M, Taboun SM, Mohamed AI. Low back muscle activity in an automobile seat with a lumbar massage system. Int J Occupational Safety Ergonomics 2000;6:113–128.
11. Leivadi S, Hernandez-Reif M, Field T, et al. Massage therapy and relaxation effects on university dance students. J Dance Med Sci 1999;3:108–112.
12. Hartshorn K, Delage J, Field T, et al. Senior citizens benefit from movement therapy. J Bodywork Movement Ther 2001:5:1–5.
13. Diego M, Hernandez-Reif M, Field T, et al. Spinal cord injury benefits from massage therapy. Int J Neurosci 112 (2):133–142, 2002 Feb.
14. Andrade CK, Clifford P. Outcome-Based Massage. Baltimore: Lippincott Williams & Wilkins, 2001.

SUGGESTED READINGS

Bobsall AP. Flash Anatomy. Flash Anatomy Inc, 1989. Bryan Edward Publications, Anaheim, CA.

Braverman DL. Schulman R.A. Massage techniques in rehabilitation medicine. Phy Med Rehabil. 10(3):631–649, 1999 Aug.

Bray R. Massage: Exploring the benefits. Elderly Care 1999;11(5): 15–16.

Clemente CD. Gray's Anatomy. 30th Ed. Baltimore: Williams & Wilkins, 1985.

Corbett M. The use and abuse of massage and exercise. Practitioner 1972;208:136–139.

Crosman LJ, Chateauvert SR, Weisberg J. The effects of massage to the hamstring muscle group on range of motion. J Orthop Sports Phys Ther 1984;6(3):168–172.

Field T. Massage therapy effects. Am Psychol Assoc 1998;53: 1270–1281.

Fraser J. Psychophysiological effects of back massage on elderly institutionalized patients. J Adv Nurs 1993;18:238–245.

Ginsberg F, Famaey JP. A double-blind study of topical massage with Rado-Salil ointment in mechanical low-back pain. J Int Med Res 1987;15:148–153.

Grant AE. Massage with ice (cryokinetics) in the treatment of painful conditions of the musculoskeletal system. Arch Phys Med 1964;45:233–238.

Hammer WI. The use of transverse friction massage in the management of chronic bursitis of the hip or shoulder. J Manipulative Physiol Therap 1993;16(2):107–111.

Hertling D, Kessler RM. Management of Common Musculoskeletal Disorders: Physical Therapy Principles and Methods. Baltimore: Lippincott Williams & Wilkins, 2002.

Hyde TE, Gengenback MS (eds). Conservative Management of Sports Injuries. Baltimore: Lippincott Williams & Wilkins, 1997.

Juhan D. A Handbook for Bodywork—Job's Body. New York: Station Hill Press, 1987.

Mein EA, Richards DG, McMillin DL, McPartland JM. Physiological regulation through manual therapy. Phys Med Rehabil: A State of the Art Review 2000;14(1):27–42.

Melzack R, Jeans ME, Stratford JG, Monks RC. Ice massage and transcutaneous electrical stimulation: comparison of treatment for low back pain. Pain 1980;9:209–917.

Nordin M, Frankel VH. Basic Biomechanics of the Musculoskeletal System. Baltimore: Lippincott Williams & Wilkins, 2001.

Premkumar K. Pathology A to Z. A Handbook for Massage Therapists. 2nd Ed. Calgary: VanPub Books, 1999.

Schmitt, H, Zhao JQ, Brocai DR, Kaps HP. Acupuncture treatment of low back pain. Schmerz 2001;15:33–37.

Scull CW. Massage-physiological basis. Arch Phys Med 1945;26:159–167.

Stamford B. Massage for athletes. Phys Sports Med 1985;13:176.

Stoll ST, Simmons SL. Inpatient rehabilitation and manual medicine. Phys Med Rehabil: State of the Art Review 2000;14(1):85–106.

Tixa S. Atlas of Palpatory Anatomy of the Lower Extremities. New York: McGraw-Hill, 1999.

Tortora GJ, Grabowski SR. Principles of Anatomy and Physiology. 9th Ed. New York: John Wiley & Sons, 2002.

Wakim KG. Physiologic effects of massage. In: Licht S, ed. Massage, Manipulation and Traction. Huntington, NY: Robert E. Keirger, 1976:38–42.

Yang Z, Hong J. Investigation on analgesic mechanism of acupuncture finger-pressure massage on lumbago. J Trad Chinese Med 1994;14(1):35–40.

Ylinen J, Cash M. Sports Massage. London: Stanley Paul, 1988.

Review Questions

For the massage therapist, all aspects of this chapter are important as it lays the foundation for the study of the origin, insertion, and action of muscles. Also, most clients who seek help have problems relating to the musculoskeletal system. The student is encouraged to look at the objectives and ensure that all the objectives have been satisfactorily achieved. A few sample questions are given below to help you begin.

Multiple Choice

1. Cells involved in the resorption of bone are called
   A. osteoclasts.
   B. osteoblasts.
   C. osteocytes.
   D. osteogenic cells.

2. Which bone is not a part of the cranium?
   A. Ethmoid
   B. Parietal
   C. Hyoid
   D. Occipital

3. Which bone does not contain a paranasal sinus?
   A. Ethmoid
   B. Sphenoid
   C. Occipital
   D. Frontal

4. The function of the skeletal system is to
   A. protect the internal organs.
   B. produce blood cells.
   C. support.
   D. all of the above.

5. The shaft of the long bone is known as the
   A. diaphysis.
   B. epiphysis.
   C. metaphysis.
   D. epiphyseal plate.

6. Factor(s) affecting bone growth include
   A. growth hormone.
   B. thyroid hormone.
   C. mechanical stress.
   D. calcium levels in blood.
   E. all of the above.

7. The movement at the elbow when the fingers touch the shoulder is called
   A. extension.
   B. flexion.
   C. adduction.
   D. abduction.

8. All of the following is true about the articulation of the knee joint EXCEPT:
   The knee joint consists of joints between the
   A. femur and the patella.
   B. femur and the tibia.
   C. femur and the fibula.

9. The talocrural joint is capable of
   A. dorsiflexion.
   B. plantar flexion.
   C. inversion.
   D. A and B.

10. A movement away from the midline is known as
    A. flexion.
    B. inversion.
    C. adduction.
    D. abduction.

11. Of the following hormones, all are involved with calcium regulation EXCEPT
    A. thyroid hormone.
    B. parathormone.
    C. vitamin D.
    D. calcitonin.

Matching

1. The different types of bones are given below. Match the bone with the correct type. The types may be used more than once.

1. _____ patella
2. _____ femur
3. _____ scapula
4. _____ vertebra
5. _____ carpals
6. _____ sternum
7. _____ maxilla
8. _____ tibia

a. long bone
b. short bone
c. flat bone
d. irregular bone
e. sesamoid bone

2. Write next to each of the following bones:
   a. if part of the appendicular skeleton; and
   b. if part of the axial skeleton.

1. _____ sacrum
2. _____ scapula
3. _____ sternum
4. _____ hyoid
5. _____ hip bone
6. _____ phalanges

3. Match the subtypes of synovial joints with their examples.

1. _____ joint between carpal bones
2. _____ atlantoaxial joint
3. _____ interphalangeal joint
4. _____ shoulder joint
5. _____ distal end of radius with the carpals
6. _____ hip joint
7. _____ rotation of the head of radius over the shaft of ulna proximally

a. ball-and-socket
b. hinge
c. condyloid
d. pivot
e. gliding

Fill-In

Complete the following:

1. In the table given below, fill in the appropriate cells. One row is filled in as an example. Use the following key for the possible movements: f = flexion; ex = extension; ab = abduction; ad = adduction; cir = circumduction; r = rotation

Joint	Bones that Articulate	Joint Type	Possible Movements
Shoulder	Glenoid fossa of scapula; head of humerus	Ball-and-socket	f, ex, ab, ad, cir
Elbow			
Ankle			
Knee			
Atlantoaxial			
Hip			

Short-Answer Questions

1. Describe the effects of aging on the joints.

Case Studies

1. One problem that Kate faced every day was to gauge the amount of pressure that could be safely used when treating older clients. She had heard a rumor of one therapist breaking the ribs of an elderly client while trying to help the client off the table! She was not sure if that was true, but could it happen? She had heard of osteoporosis—a bone problem. But what really happens to the bones? Who is more prone to osteoporosis? Does calcium help in any way?
   A. How is bone formed?
   B. What is the structure of bone?
   C. What are the factors that affect the density of bone?
   D. How is calcium regulated in the body?
   E. What are the effects of aging on bone and joints?
   F. What precautions should be taken while massaging a client with osteoporosis?

2. Mr. Hamilton was a regular client. One week ago, he fell off a ladder trying to clean ice off his roof. He fractured the neck of the humerus and was now in a plaster cast. He was coming to the clinic later that day for his monthly, scheduled massage.
   A. Is it safe to massage over the exposed part of limb?
   B. How long does the bone take to heal?
   C. How does it heal?
   D. What are the factors that affect the healing of bone?
   E. What is the "neck" of the humerus?
   F. What are the muscles related to the proximal part of the humerus?

3. Mrs. Dixon is an elderly lady who loves to be massaged. She was diagnosed with rheumatoid arthritis 5 years ago. When the therapist first met her, the joints of both hands were red and swollen, and Mrs. Dixon was in pain. Now, 5 years later, despite taking medicine, her hands are disfigured, and Mrs. Dixon has difficulty holding a cup, writing, and doing many other activities with her hands that one takes for granted. Her doctor had explained that the cartilage in her joints had been affected by the condition.
   A. Is cartilage different from bone?
   B. Does it heal the same way as bone?
   C. What is the structure of a synovial joint?
   D. What are the precautions that should be taken by a massage therapist while dealing with clients with A. acute inflammation? B. chronic inflammation?

4. June was a 19-year-old girl who had been referred to the therapist by a friend. June had been suffering from temporomandibular joint syndrome for over 6 months and was willing to try any form of treatment to relieve the constant ache in the right side of her face. She complained of crackling sounds every time she opened her mouth.
   A. What is the structure of the temporomandibular joint?
   B. What are the possible movements?
   C. What are the muscles that move the joint?

Answers to Review Questions

Multiple Choice

1. A
2. C
3. C
4. D
5. A
6. E
7. B
8. C
9. D
10. D
11. A

Matching

1.
1. e
2. a
3. c
4. d
5. b
6. c
7. d
8. a

2.
1. b
2. a
3. b
4. b
5. a
6. a

3.
1. e
2. d
3. b
4. a
5. c
6. a
7. d

Fill-In

Refer to **pages 133–160** under individual joints.

Case Studies

Case 1. This is an important topic for bodyworkers. See **page 88** for formation of bone; **page 402** for the role of parathyroid gland; vitamin D (**page 60**); calcitonin (**page 402**); and estrogen (**page 434**) on calcium metabolism; **page 160** for age-related changes in musculoskeletal system; and **page 442** for menopause.

Case 2. See **page 116** for the anatomy of the humerus; **page 215, 216** for the muscles attached to this region; and **page 92** for different types of fractures and healing of fracture.

Case 3. See **page 125** for the structure of a typical synovial joint; and **page 142** for the various joints of the wrist and hand. The student is encouraged to do further research on rheumatoid arthritis—the signs, symptoms, and treatment and the joints commonly affected.

Case 4. See **page 103** for the structure of the mandible; and **page 131** for the structure of the temporomandibular joint.

Coloring Exercise

1. In the diagram of a long bone, label the region of diaphysis and color it blue. Label the epiphysis and color it green. Identify the region of the epiphysial plate and the articular cartilage and color it yellow. Color the region of the medullary cavity red.

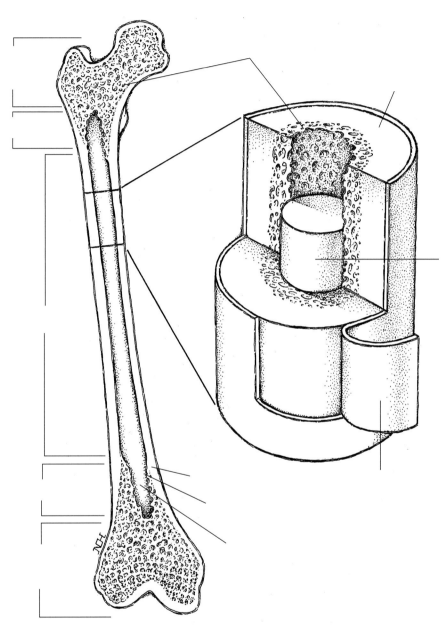

2. In the diagram of microscopic bone structure: A. label the central canal with blood vessels and color it red; B. label the periosteum and color it yellow. C. shade the region of the compact bone orange and the region of the spongy bone pink. D. outline all the blood vessels in red. E. label the region of compact bone; region of spongy bone; osteon; in the enlarged part, label the osteocyte, lacuna, and canaliculi.

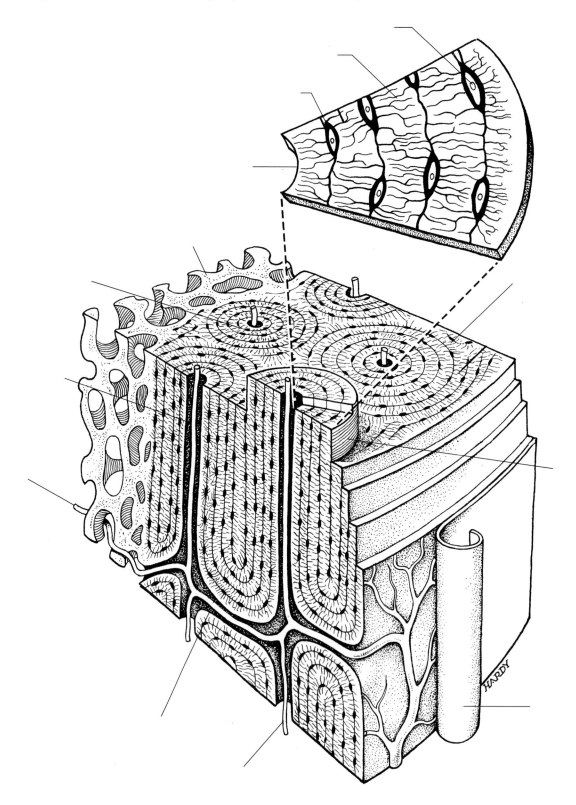

3. In the diagram of the skull (lateral view), label the following bones: frontal, parietal, ethmoid, lacrimal, nasal, temporal, mandible, zygomatic, occipital, and maxilla. Use a different color for each bone. Label the coronal, squamosal, and lambdoidal sutures; external auditory canal; and mastoid process and styloid process.

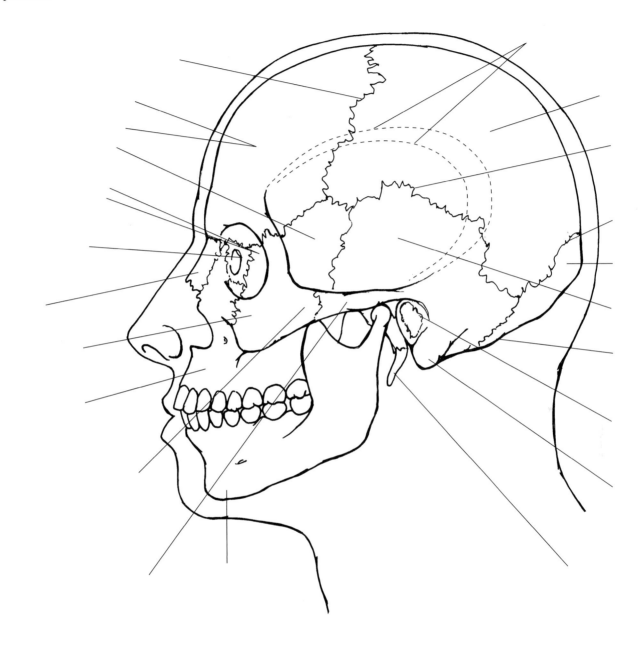

4. Color the scapula (posterior view) yellow. Outline the spine of the scapula in orange. Label all the parts indicated. Using Figure 4.28D, mark the origins of the following muscles in red: supraspinatus, infraspinatus, teres major, deltoid, and rhomboideus major and minor and the insertion of the trapezius in blue.

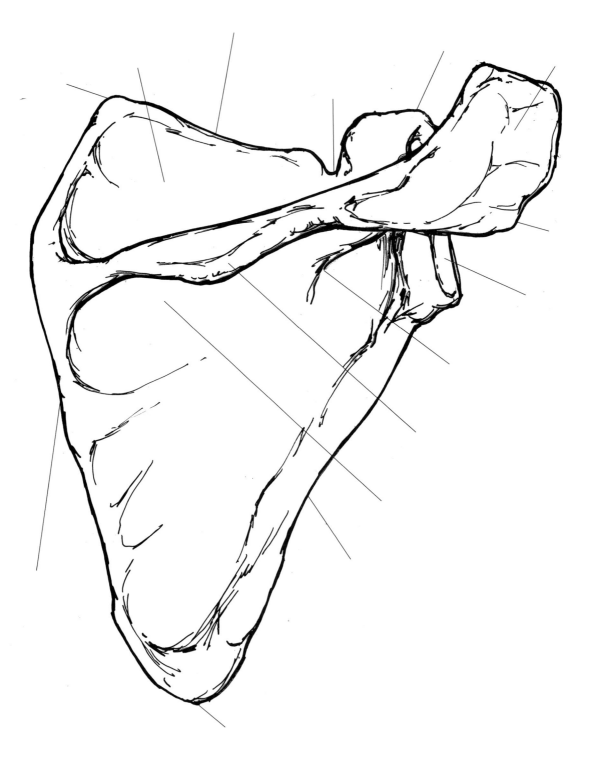

5. Color the anterior view of the humerus yellow and label the different parts. Using the Figure 4.28D, color and label the origins of muscles in red and insertions in blue.

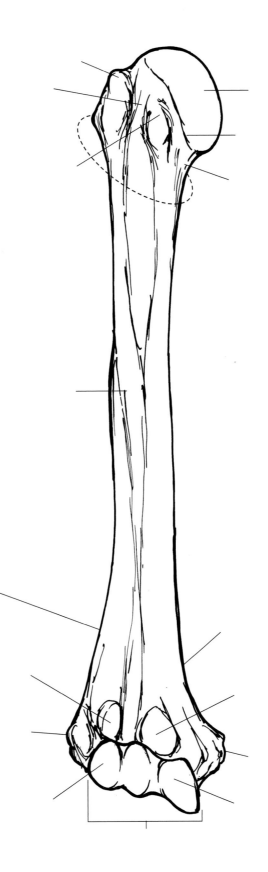

6. Color the anterior view of the tibia and fibula yellow and label the parts. Using Figure 4.35E, color and label the origins of muscles in red and insertions in blue.

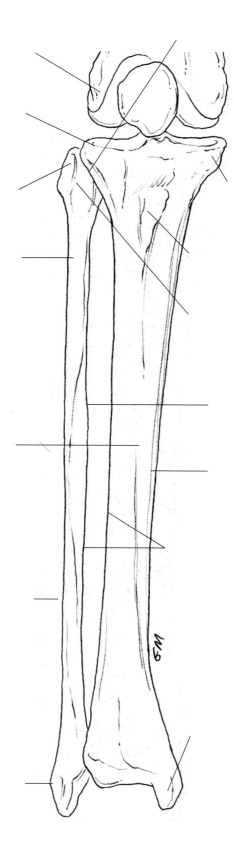

7. In the diagram of a typical synovial joint, color each part a different color.

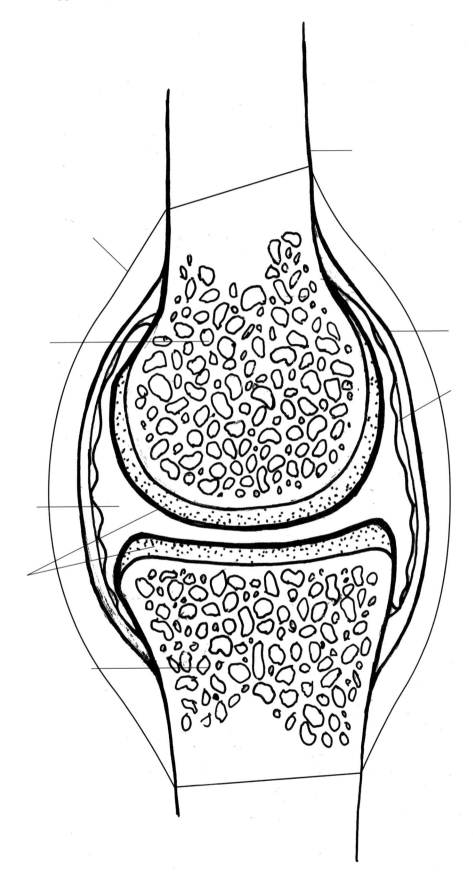

8. In the diagram of the knee joint (anterior view), label the parts and color the femur yellow, the tibia pink, the fibula red, the ligaments brown, and the meniscus orange.

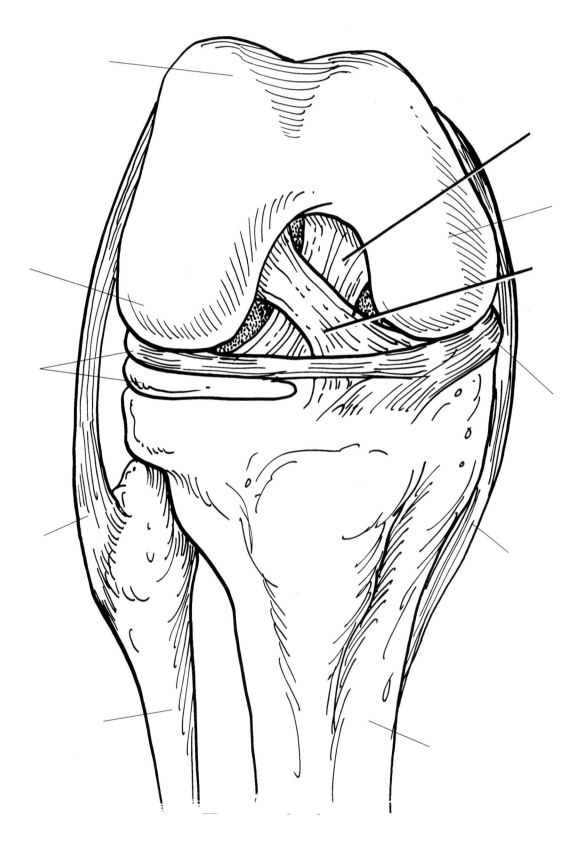

CHAPTER 4

Muscular System

Objectives **On completion of this chapter, the reader should be able to:**

- List the functions of muscle tissue.
- Describe the microscopic structure of skeletal muscle fiber.
- Outline the steps involved in the process of muscle contraction.
- Describe the structure of the myoneural junction.
- Describe the arrangement of muscle fibers.
- Describe the factors that affect the speed, direction, and force of muscle contractions.
- Explain how muscle fiber arrangement alters the force and direction of contractions.
- Describe the structure and function of a motor unit.
- Explain the role of muscle spindle in muscle contraction.
- Explain the mechanisms by which energy is obtained for the contraction process.
- Compare aerobic and anaerobic metabolism and relate it to muscular performance.
- Differentiate between slow twitch and fast twitch fibers.
- Describe the effects of physical training on muscle function.
- Compare and contrast skeletal, cardiac, and smooth muscle tissue.
- Describe the different types of smooth muscle.
- Explain the different ways muscle nomenclature is derived.
- Explain how muscles interact to produce and oppose movements.
- Identify the location and direction of fibers of the major muscles on the body surface.
- Identify and give the origin, insertion, and actions of major muscles related to the axial skeleton.
- Identify and give the origin, insertion, and actions of major muscles related to the appendicular skeleton.
- Group the muscles according to the movements they produce in the shoulder, elbow, wrist, hip, knee, ankle joints, and spine.
- Describe the effects of aging on the muscular system.
- Describe the effects of massage on the muscular system.

The demand for massage therapy and therapists in sports and in other areas is on the rise and is likely to stay that way. Almost all professional sports teams have health professionals on call, and the massage therapist plays a key role before, during, and certainly after a game. Other than sports, massage is sought by clients with myofascial pain or chronic pain of musculoskeletal origin, and by many others for the beneficial effects of massage.

Although all the effects of massage on the body have not been fully explained scientifically, there is no doubt that the outcome is positive. The growing clientele with musculoskeletal problems reiterates the importance of a therapist having a thorough understanding of the anatomy and physiology of the muscular system.

This chapter describes the physiology of muscle contraction and the origin, insertion, action, and innerva-

tion of major muscles of the body and the commonly related ailments. Students are encouraged to use all visual aids available, such as the Figures, the photographs, and certainly their own bodies when studying this chapter.

Muscle Tissue and Physiology of Muscle Contraction

All body functions involving movement require muscle activity. Muscle activity is required for skeletal movement, heart contraction, food moving through the gut, urination, and breathing, among many others. Certain muscles, even when not producing movement, remain contracted to maintain posture and oppose the effects of gravity.

To perform these varied activities, three types of muscle are present in the body: **skeletal, cardiac,** and **smooth.** The skeletal muscles constitute about 40% to 50% of body weight. They are attached to the skeleton and are responsible for skeletal movement and stabilizing body position. Cardiac muscle is located in the heart; smooth muscle is present in the gut, around the bronchi in the lungs, urinary tract, reproductive organs, and blood vessels. Cardiac muscle helps move blood throughout the body, and smooth muscle helps move fluid and food matter. Smooth muscle also helps regulate flow out of certain organs (e.g., a ringlike arrangement of smooth muscle at the lower end of the urinary bladder regulates outflow of urine). Although the contractile mechanism is the same in the three muscle types, the types vary in microscopic appearance, strength of contraction, duration of contraction, control by the nervous system, and in other ways—all adaptations according to the job performed.

Muscles produce heat during activity, and this heat is used to maintain the core body temperature.

This section addresses the structure of skeletal muscle and the process of muscle contraction.

STRUCTURE OF SKELETAL MUSCLE

Macroscopic Structure of Muscle   ● = wrapper

Skeletal muscle, as we know it (e.g., biceps brachii), is a collection of muscle cells, nerves, connective tissue, and blood vessels. Each muscle *cell* is known as a **muscle fiber.** Muscle fibers are cylindrical, arranged parallel to each other, and at times may run through the entire length of the muscle. The fibers are held in place by connective tissue, which surround individual fibers, bundles of muscle fibers and, finally, the entire muscle. It is the connective tissue that attaches muscle to the periosteum of bones and

conveys the force generated by the muscle to the bone, across one or more joints. Other than the connective tissue surrounding individual fibers, bundles of fibers, and the entire muscle, connective tissue (**fascia**) separates muscle from the skin (**superficial fascia** or **subcutaneous layer**) and holds groups of muscles with similar functions together (**deep fascia**).

The connective tissue that surrounds an individual fiber is the **endomysium** (see Figure 4.1). **Fascicles** are bundles of muscle fibers surrounded by additional connective tissue, the **perimysium.** The perimysium attaches adjacent fascicles together in addition to carrying blood vessels and nerves to the muscle fibers. The whole muscle is surrounded by connective tissue called the **epimysium.** This connective tissue (part of the deep fascia) separates muscles from each other and the surrounding organs. The epimysium, in turn, is continuous, with a rope-like connective tissue—the **tendon** or connective tissue sheet—**aponeurosis.** The tendon or aponeurosis ultimately weaves intimately with the periosteum of bone, attaching the muscle. By this interconnection of connective tissue, the power generated by the contraction of individual muscle fibers is conveyed to the bone. The fleshy part of the muscle that lies between the connective tissue that attaches it to both ends of the bone is known as the **belly** of the muscle.

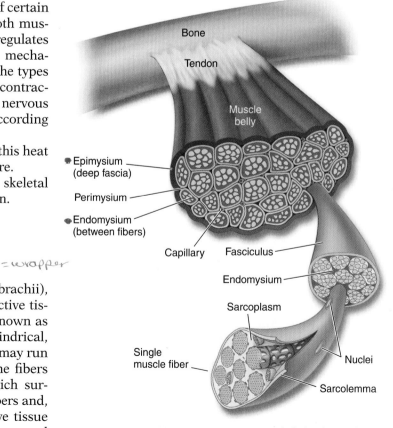

FIGURE **4.1.** Macroscopic Structure of Skeletal Muscle

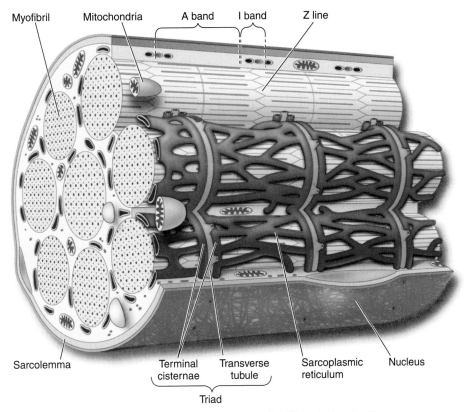

Myofibril   Mitochondria   A band   I band   Z line

Sarcolemma   Terminal cisternae   Transverse tubule   Sarcoplasmic reticulum   Nucleus

Triad

FIGURE **4.2.** Microscopic Structure of a Skeletal Muscle Fiber.

Microscopic Structure of Individual Muscle Fibers

Knowledge of the microscopic structure (see Figure 4.2) is required to understand the contractile process of muscle. The shape of the muscle fiber is cylindrical, and each fiber may extend through the length of the muscle.

Each fiber appears striated under a microscope (i.e., having dark and light bands); it is referred to as **striated muscle** (the cause of the striated appearance is explained later). The muscle fiber, like all other cells, has many cell organelles. The cytoplasm, known here as **sarcoplasm,** is enclosed in a cell membrane called the **sarcolemma.** The skeletal muscle fiber is multinucleated and has hundreds of nuclei located just below the cell membrane. It is believed that the number of nuclei denotes the number of embryonic muscle cells (**myoblasts**) that have fused to form one cell fiber. Certain myoblasts (**satellite cells**) do not fuse and are seen as individual cells between the muscle fibers. The satellite cells may enlarge, divide, and fuse with damaged muscle fibers, assisting in the regeneration of tissue. However, regeneration of muscle tissue is minimal and cells cannot divide.

Muscle fiber has numerous tubes, known as **T tubules** or **transverse tubules,** that run transversely into the sarcoplasm. The tubules are continuous with the sarcolemma and transmit impulses generated by a nerve into the cell. Inside the sarcoplasm, the T tubules encircle the **myofibrils,** long cylindrical structures that extend the entire length of the muscle fiber. Hundreds of myofibrils are seen in each muscle fiber. Each myofibril is actually a collection of specialized proteins called **myofilaments.** The activity of the myofilaments produce contraction and relaxation of the muscle.

Other than the transverse tubules, which are actually invaginations of the sarcolemma into the sar-

✓ Toothpick Analogy

For those who found the preceding paragraph confusing here is an analogy. The muscle fiber can be thought of as a container of toothpicks. The container is equivalent to the sarcolemma or cell membrane; the toothpicks are equivalent to the myofibrils packed into each muscle fiber. If the toothpicks were made up of two different materials, each would be equivalent to the two specialized proteins called myofilaments. Now imagine many *containers* of toothpicks, bundled and wrapped together. This will be equivalent to the muscle fascicles surrounded by perimysium. If many of the fascicles, in turn, are wrapped together, this will be equivalent to the whole muscle, such as the biceps, surrounded by epimysium.

coplasm, there is another network of tubules (**sarcoplasmic reticulum [SR]**) in the sarcoplasm. SR is equivalent to the endoplasmic reticulum of other cells; it surrounds individual myofibrils on each side of the T tubules. Close to the T tubules, SR is enlarged to form an expanded chamber called the **terminal cisternae.** SR contains a high concentration of calcium ions that is required for muscle contraction.

Sarcoplasm also contains glycogen—storage forms of glucose that can be broken down during metabolism. In addition, sarcoplasm contains a red, hemoglobinlike protein called **myoglobin.** Myoglobin, similar to hemoglobin, is capable of binding oxygen. This oxygen is used by the mitochondria for adenosine triphosphate (ATP) production.

THE MYOFILAMENT: THE SPECIALIZED PROTEINS OF MYOFIBRILS

Each myofibril is made up of **myofilaments,** which are regular arrangements of protein filaments (Figure 4.3). Myofilaments, unlike the myofibrils, do not run the entire length of the muscle fiber, but are arranged in smaller sections called **sarcomeres.** The sarcomere is the functional unit (the smallest structure(s) of an organ that can perform the function) of the muscle, and it is the activity at the level of the sarcomere that causes muscle to contract.

Myofilaments consist of two types of protein, **actin** and **myosin.** Because of size, actin is known as the **thin filament,** and myosin is known as the **thick filament.** The thick and thin filaments are arranged in a specific manner to facilitate muscle contraction. The filaments are arranged parallel, with bundles of thick filaments alternating with bundles of thin. When the muscle is viewed under the microscope, the thick and the thin filament arrangements allow light to pass through differently, and the muscle looks as if it has alternating dark (thick filaments) and light bands (thin filaments).

Arrangement of Thick and Thin Filaments

The thin actin filaments are arranged in such a way that they can slide between the myosin filaments (see Figure 4.3). The actin filaments are held in place by

---

Muscular Dystrophies

Abnormalities may be seen at the level of the myofilaments or at the sarcolemmal level. This results in muscle weakness and progressive deterioration of the muscle. These conditions are called **muscular dystrophies.** There are various types of muscular dystrophies; these disorders are inherited from the parent(s).

---

protein fibers running at right angles to the myofibril. This is known as the **Z line,** or **Z disk** (Z is an abbreviation for zigzag). The Z disk separates one sarcomere from another. The myosin filaments are held in place by protein fibers that, like the Z line, run at right angles to the direction of the myofibril. This is the **M line** (M for middle—it is in the middle of the sarcomere). The width of myofibril, occupied by the actin filaments (on either side of the Z line), is the **I band,** and the width of myofibril, occupied by the myosin filaments, is the **A band.** The myosin and actin filaments do not overlap at the center of the A band—the A band appears lighter and this is known as the **H zone.**

Structure of Thin (Actin) Filaments

The thin, actin filament consists of three types of proteins that play a key role in muscle contraction (Figure 4.3).

Actin is actually twisted strands of globular proteins. An analogy would be two strings of pearls twisted together. Each globular molecule has a site that has an affinity for myosin filament. These sites (**active sites** or **myosin-binding sites**) are covered by **tropomyosin,** another strand of protein. Tropomyosin in this position prevents actin-myosin interaction.

A third type of protein (**troponin**) is located at regular intervals on the tropomyosin. Troponin holds the tropomyosin in position. It also carries a site; however, this site has an affinity for calcium.

Structure of Thick (Myosin) Filaments

Each thick filament consists of many (approximately 300) myosin molecules. Each myosin molecule resembles two hockey sticks that have the shafts wound together, with a long arm (**tail**) and an angulated base (**head**). The myosin molecules are arranged with all the heads directed outward. Therefore, the heads project toward adjacent actin molecules. All tails face the M line, so that there are some heads to the right and some to the left of the M line.

The heads of the myosin molecules have a site that has an affinity for actin. Because the heads interact with the actin during contraction, they are also known as **crossbridges.** The head has the ability to move forward and backward on the tail, as if there was a hinge at the junction of the head and the tail. It is the movement of the heads that results in reduction in muscle size during contraction.

Other than actin and myosin, many other proteins help secure the myofilaments in place and provide the elasticity and extensibility of myofibrils.

To understand this section, familiarity with the detailed structure of the muscle fiber is crucial. If necessary, review the details and the Figures.

The actual process of muscle contraction can be explained by the **sliding filament theory.**

SLIDING FILAMENT MECHANISM

The sliding filament mechanism explains the process of muscle contraction at the molecular level. This process is initiated by impulses from the nerve that innervates the muscle fiber.

Muscle-Nerve Communication

Skeletal muscle only contracts when stimulated by the communicating nerve. Each muscle fiber is in contact with a nerve ending. The cell body of the nerve fiber (a single neuron) is located in the spinal cord, brainstem, or brain, according to where the skeletal muscle is located and to where it originated in the embryonic stage. The axons of these neurons

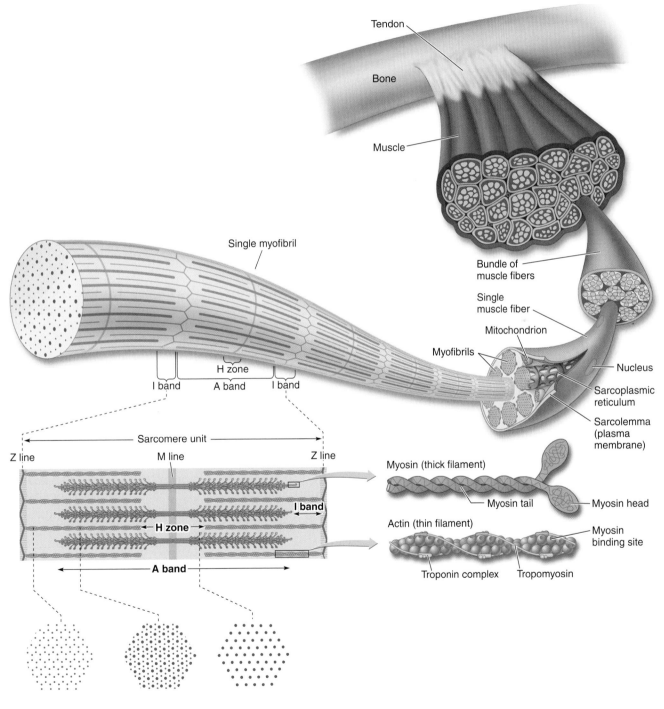

FIGURE **4.3.** Structure of Myofibril and Myofilaments

RIGOR MORTIS

The body becomes rigid a few hours after death. This state is called **rigor mortis.** Calcium from the sarcoplasmic reticulum leaks into the sarcoplasm and causes actin-myosin interaction. Because the blood supply has stopped and there is no production and supply of ATP, the bound actin and myosin are unable to detach from each other. The body becomes "stiff as a board." With time—15 to 25 hours later—the enzymes from the lysosomes of the cells break down the myofilaments, and the body becomes soft.

extend from the cell bodies to individual muscles. For example, when we say that the ulnar nerve supplies the adductor muscle of the thumb, we are indicating the bundles of axons of motor neurons that go together as the ulna nerve before they split to supply the individual muscle fibers of the adductor muscle that moves the thumb.

The axons branch when they reach the muscles they supply, and each axon communicates with one or more muscle fibers. Thus, if a neuron is stimulated, all of the muscle fibers it communicates with will contract. The axon, its branches, and all the muscle fibers it supplies are known as a **motor unit** (see Figure 4.4). A motor neuron innervates an average of 150 muscle fibers. However, in muscles that require precise control, a neuron may innervate only two or three fibers.

At the point where they come in close contact with the muscle fiber, each nerve ending is modified. The region where the nerve and the muscle communicates is the **myoneural junction** or **neuromuscular junction** (see Figure 4.5). The nerve ending expands here to form a **synaptic knob.** The cytoplasm of the nerve ending has vesicles containing molecules of **acetylcholine** (ACh). A small gap—**synaptic cleft**—exists between the synaptic knob and the sarcolemma of the muscle fiber. The portion of the sarcolemma directly under the synaptic knob is the **motor endplate.** The sarcolemma underlying the synaptic knob has pro-

Tetanus

Tetanus is a bacterial infection that makes motor neurons hypersensitive to stimulus. The bacteria are found everywhere and enter the body through any skin wound. Because the bacteria thrive in tissue with low oxygen levels, unclean, deep wounds are more likely to result in tetanus. The toxin produced by the bacteria is responsible for violent muscle spasms. The disease is also known as lockjaw because the muscles of the jaw eventually spasm. The disease has a high death rate; however, it can be prevented by immunization (tetanus shots).

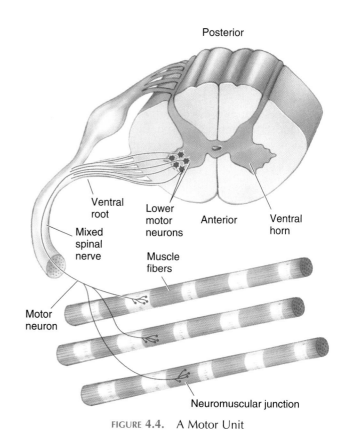

FIGURE **4.4.**   A Motor Unit

teins (**receptors**) on its surface that have an affinity for ACh. The receptors are actually ion channels that are regulated by ACh. The connective tissue matrix in the synaptic cleft has **acetylcholinesterase** enzymes that can destroy ACh.

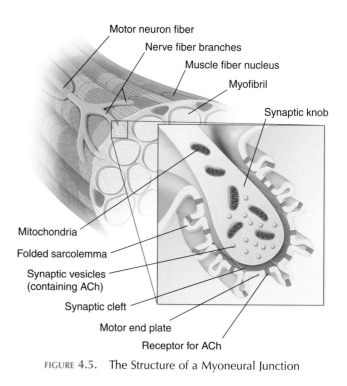

FIGURE **4.5.**   The Structure of a Myoneural Junction

> ### ✓ *A Summary of the Steps Involved in Muscle Contraction*
>
> - action potentials or impulses from the central nervous system come down the nerve axon of the motor nerve when movement must occur
> - the impulse, on arriving at the myoneural junction, causes the ACh vesicles to fuse with the nerve cell membrane and release its contents into the synaptic cleft
> - ACh binds to the ACh receptors on the sarcolemma, opening sodium channels
> - The rush of sodium into the sarcoplasm causes the inside of the cell to become positive as compared with the outside
> - This potential change is communicated directly into the sarcoplasm via the T tubules
> - The sarcoplasmic reticulum releases calcium into the sarcoplasm as a result of the potential change
> - Calcium binds to troponin
> - Binding of calcium to troponin causes troponin to shift tropomyosin and uncover the active site for myosin on the actin
> - Myosin binds to the uncovered active site on actin
> - ATP provides the energy for the bound myosin head to pivot toward the M line
> - ADP and P are released when the myosin head pivots
> - Attachment of another ATP to the bound myosin head causes it to release from the actin and bind to another molecule of actin
> - The cycle continues and the muscle fiber shortens as long as calcium is bound to troponin.

Nerve Impulse and Activity in the Myoneural Junction

When a specific muscle is moved, nerve impulses or action potentials (see **page 309** for details of action potentials) pass down the nerve axon until the myoneural junction is reached. This triggers opening of calcium channels in the nerve axon, with resultant movement of calcium into the axon. The calcium movement triggers vesicles containing ACh to fuse with the nerve cell membrane and release ACh into the synaptic cleft. ACh attaches to the ACh receptors on the motor endplate, resulting in opening of the ion channels in the sarcolemma. The changes produced by ACh only last for a short time because the acetylcholinesterase located in the synaptic cleft begins to break down ACh. The sarcolemmal properties reach that of the resting stage when all ACh is destroyed.

Excitation-Contraction Coupling

When ACh binds to the receptor, the change that occurs is the opening of sodium channels on the sarcolemma. This results in sodium (which is of a higher concentration outside the cell than inside) rushing

into the sarcoplasm of the muscle fiber. At rest, the inside of the muscle fiber is electrically negative compared to the outside. When positively charged sodium enters the cell, the inside becomes positive. This change in potential triggers a series of reactions inside the muscle fiber at the molecular level that produces muscle contraction (see Figure 4.6). The link between the potential change in the sarcolemma and the contraction of the muscle is known as **excitation-contraction coupling.**

The potential change at the sarcolemma continues down into the T tubules, directly into the muscle fiber where it triggers the sarcoplasmic reticulum to release calcium into the sarcoplasm. The calcium binds to the calcium site on the troponin (the protein on the actin). This binding causes the troponin to shift the tropomyosin, exposing the active site for myosin located on actin. When exposed by the movement of tropomyosin, the myosin heads attach to the active site.

The myosin head moves toward the M line in a hingelike action, deriving energy from breaking down ATP (adenosine triphosphate).

$$ATP \rightarrow ADP \text{ (adenosine diphosphate)} + phosphate$$

ADP and phosphate, the breakdown products, move away and another ATP binds to the myosin head to provide energy. The attachment of the next ATP to the myosin head causes the myosin to detach from the actin site, move back into its original posi-

DRUGS, TOXINS, ANTIBODIES, AND MYONEURAL JUNCTION

During surgery, muscles are made to relax by administering drugs (muscle relaxants) that block ACh receptors at the myoneural junction. These drugs are similar to curare, a plant poison originally used by native Indians on arrowheads.

In certain cases of food poisoning, such as botulism, the toxin produced by the microorganism blocks the release of ACh at the myoneural junction, resulting in respiratory paralysis and death. Small quantities of toxin (Botox) are used in medicine to reduce muscle spasms. Botox is also used in cosmetic surgery to reduce wrinkles.

Myasthenia gravis is a chronic autoimmune disease characterized by muscle weakness (especially in the face and throat), in which the immune system attacks muscle cells at the neuromuscular junction. Drugs that reduce the activity of cholinesterase (anticholinesterase agents) are used to prolong the effects of ACh in patients with this disease.

Many pesticides work by affecting the myoneural junction. To prevent complications, proper precautions should be taken when handling these pesticides.

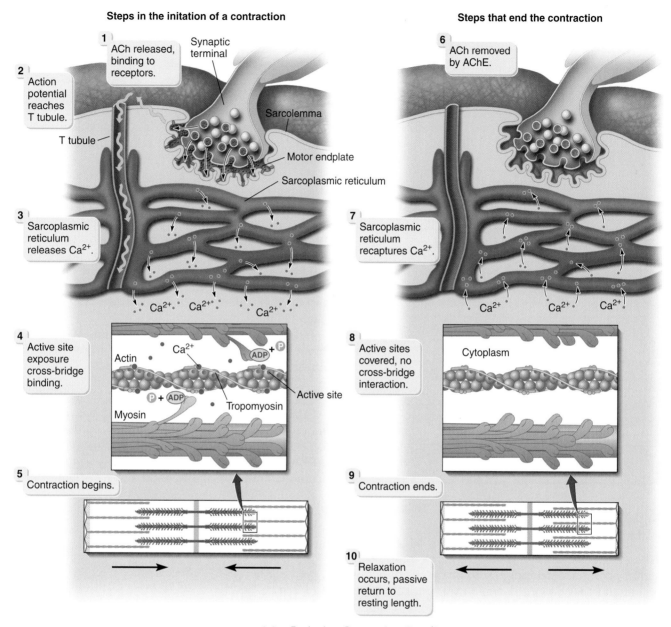

Steps in the initation of a contraction

1 ACh released, binding to receptors.

Synaptic terminal

2 Action potential reaches T tubule.

T tubule

Sarcolemma

Motor endplate

Sarcoplasmic reticulum

3 Sarcoplasmic reticulum releases Ca^{2+}.

Ca^{2+} Ca^{2+} Ca^{2+}

4 Active site exposure cross-bridge binding.

Actin Ca^{2+} (ADP) + (P)

(P) + (ADP)

Active site

Myosin Tropomyosin

5 Contraction begins.

Steps that end the contraction

6 ACh removed by AChE.

7 Sarcoplasmic reticulum recaptures Ca^{2+}.

Ca^{2+} Ca^{2+} Ca^{2+}

8 Active sites covered, no cross-bridge interaction.

Cytoplasm

9 Contraction ends.

10 Relaxation occurs, passive return to resting length.

FIGURE 4.6. Excitation-Contraction Coupling

tion, and attach to another active site on the actin. Thus, the actin is moved closer to the M line, with the myosin attaching and detaching from the active sites on subsequent actin molecules. This process contin-

ues for as long as calcium ions are present in the sarcoplasm and ATP is available for energy. Thus, the actin filament slides between the myosin filaments, shortening the muscle fiber.

Relaxation of Muscle Fiber

Soon after the impulse arrives, the sarcoplasmic reticulum that released its calcium content into the sarcoplasm starts pumping the calcium back, using ATP as energy. If no other impulse arrives, the calcium continues to be pumped back from the sarcoplasm until the resting levels of calcium are reached. When the calcium level drops in the sar-

ATP REQUIREMENTS

Even a small muscle has muscle fibers that run into thousands. A single muscle fiber may have 15 billion thick filaments. When active, each thick filament breaks down approximately 2,500 ATP molecules. Approximately how many ATP molecules would a single muscle fiber use up?

coplasm, the troponin loses calcium from its binding site and the tropomyosin returns to its original position, blocking the active sites in the actin and ending the actin-myosin interaction. This results in relaxation of the muscle.

As long as action potential/impulses arrive at the myoneural junction, ACh continues to be released. As mentioned, ACh is broken down by acetylcholinesterase. If impulses stop, no additional ACh is released, and the remaining ACh in the synaptic cleft is removed by acetylcholinesterase. The sodium channels that were opened by ACh binding to receptors close, and the potential inside the sarcoplasm is brought back to its resting state. (The details of how the potential is brought back are not elaborated here).

Analogy of Tug-of-War

The movement of myosin head and actin can be compared with a tug-of-war game, in which individuals (myosin heads) on the winning side grip the rope (actin filament), pull (pivotal action of the head), release (myosin detachment), and grip the rope further down (the next actin molecule), pull, release, and so on.

Time Lapse Between Nerve Impulse and Contraction

The **latent period** is the short duration of time that elapses when a muscle responds to a single impulse before the muscle begins to shorten. This includes the time taken for the impulse to travel down the nerve, release ACh, and all the reactions that take place within the sarcoplasm before sliding of the filaments occurs. In addition, it includes the time for the tendon and other connective tissue (e.g., perimysium, epimysium) to be stretched before the force can be transmitted to the bone. Because the muscle is attached to the bone via the connective tissue tendon, the tendon (with its elastic fibers) must be stretched

for the force produced by the muscle to reach the bone. This is similar to lifting a ball tied to an elastic band. Before the ball can be lifted off the ground, the elastic band must be tautly stretched. In the muscle, the first few impulses produce enough muscle contraction to stretch the tendon. If impulses continue to come down the nerve, the tension is transmitted to the bone more effectively.

The **contraction period** is the duration of muscle contraction in response to a nerve impulse, and the **relaxation period** is the duration taken by the fiber to relax after a contraction (see Figure 4.7). The recording of the response of the muscle to a single nerve impulse is known as a **muscle twitch.** For a short time after the first impulse arrives, the muscle is unable to respond to a second stimuli. This period is known as the **refractory period.** The refractory period in skeletal muscle is short, about 5 milliseconds (ms). As a result of the short refractory period, another impulse arriving just after 5 ms can produce a muscle response. Note that this impulse would arrive during the contraction period of the first muscle twitch. Therefore, it is possible for the response to the second impulse to fuse with that of the first to produce a sustained contraction (see **page 186**, Recruitment of Motor Units).

Fortunately, the refractory period in cardiac muscle is long, about 300 ms. This prevents sustained contractions of the heart—a situation that would stop circulation of blood.

CHARACTERISTICS OF WHOLE MUSCLE CONTRACTION

Although the contractile mechanism is the same, muscle characteristics are modified in many ways to enable the body to adjust force and speed of contraction and direction and range of motion. At the microscopic level, variations in contraction duration exist between muscles. Macroscopically, variations in fascicle arrangement and size of motor units are present. Together, structural and functional variations allow us to execute both crude and intricate, movements.

MUSCLE-NERVE PREPARATION

The characteristics of whole muscle contraction have been studied in isolated muscle-nerve preparations from lower animals. Using electrodes, the nerve can be stimulated at varying frequencies and the tension that develops in the muscle can be studied (**A**). Alternately, the initial length of the muscle can be varied and the tension studied by stimulating the nerve (**B**). Using such muscle-nerve preparations, the relationship between tension and time after muscle stimulation has been recorded.

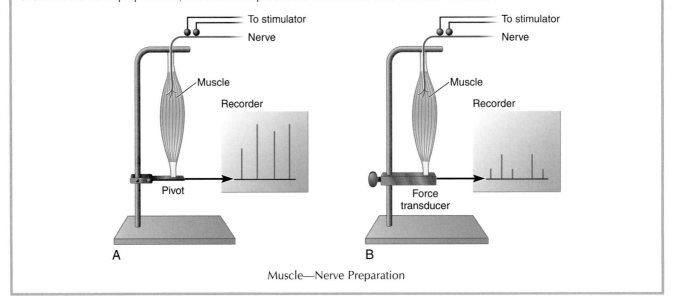

Muscle—Nerve Preparation

The ultimate force transmitted to bone across joints depends, to a large extent, on the way muscle fibers are organized (e.g., the direction of fiber arrangement, where the muscle originates and inserts—closer or further from the joint—and in which direction they pull). Of course, the range of motion in a joint also depends on the *articular surface,* the *pliability of structures around the joint,* such as ligaments and tendons, and the *relaxation of muscles that oppose the movement.* The therapist must keep all these factors in mind when caring for a client with reduced mobility.

Some factors that affect the speed, direction, and force of contraction of muscle are:

- Variation in contraction duration
- The initial length of the muscle fiber
- Recruitment of motor units
- The frequency of stimulation
- Arrangement of muscle fascicles
- Effective use of the lever system
- Type of muscle fiber (see **page 194**)
- Availability of nutrients and oxygen.

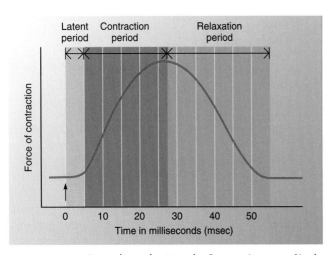

FIGURE **4.7.** A Recording of a Muscle Contraction to a Single Nerve Impulse—Muscle Twitch

Muscles and Nerve Activity

In postural muscles, when sustained contraction is required over long periods, the body stimulates motor units asynchronously. When one group of motor units is stimulated, the others relax. Then another group of motor units is stimulated while the previous group relaxes. In this manner, sustained, continuous, and nonjerky contractions are produced over long periods without the muscle becoming fatigued.

Because each muscle has many motor units, stimulating some or all of the motor units achieves gradation in the power generated by the muscle. For example, only a few motor units must be stimulated to achieve enough power to lift a 1-kilogram weight. Many more motor units of the muscle must be stimulated to lift a 10-kilogram weight.

Intrinsic Variation in Contraction Duration in Muscles

The **contraction phase** is the period when the tension rises to a peak as the crossbridges react with the active sites of the actin filaments (Figure 4.7). The **relaxation phase** is the period when the crossbridges detach and the muscle reaches its original state. The duration of the muscle twitch, produced by a single impulse, varies individually according to function. For example, eye muscles have a short twitch (perhaps 10 ms). This is important because fast eye movements must occur for the eyes to be able to follow an object. However, the twitch of muscles such as the soleus lasts for about 100 ms.

Role of Initial Length of Muscle on Tension Developed

In the game of tug-of-war, the tension produced on one side is proportional to the number of people pulling on the rope. Similarly, the tension produced in individual muscle fibers is proportional to the number of myosin heads interacting with the actin in *all* the sarcomeres in *all* of the myofibrils in the muscle fiber. The interaction largely depends on the amount of *overlap* between myosin and actin myofilaments before contraction begins.

When a muscle is stimulated, only the myosin heads within the zone of overlap can bind to active sites on actin and produce tension. If the sarcomere is as short as possible, the myosin heads are jammed into the adjacent Z lines, pivoting cannot occur and

> ### ✓ *Excursion Ratio of a Muscle*
>
> The ratio of stretched length to contracted length of a muscle is known as the **excursion ratio.** A ratio of 2:1 is considered average and seems to be adequate to allow joints to move through their full ranges. If a muscle crosses many joints, the excursion ratio may not be adequate to allow simultaneous extension or flexion of the various joints involved.

no tension is produced. Also, the actin (thin) filaments on each side of the sarcomere slide over and cover each other, reducing the active sites exposed to myosin. In this situation, only a little tension is produced when the muscle fiber is stimulated.

The highest tension is produced when the maximum number of myosin-actin interactions can occur (see Figure 4.8). If the sarcomere length is increased even further, the overlap between actin and myosin decreases and tension is reduced. If the length is increased until there is no overlap at all, no tension can be produced. In the body, the length of the resting muscle is close to its optimal length. It is prevented from stretching too much by ligaments, other muscles, and surrounding organs. When this muscle is stimulated, maximal tension can be produced. For example, the biceps brachii is close to its optimal length when the elbow is extended. Maximal tension, therefore, can be achieved when it is stimulated in this state. Of course, force of movement will be affected by the state of the joint across which the mus-

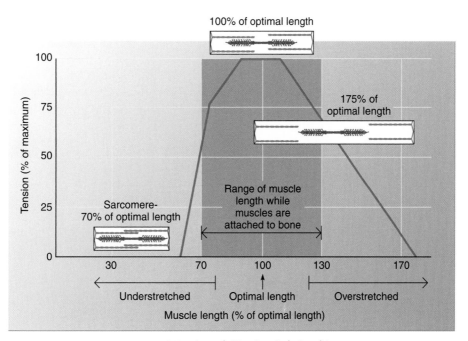

FIGURE **4.8.** Length-Tension Relationship

cle acts and also the manner in which the contracting muscle is attached to the bone (Refer to the lever action of muscle, discussed later on page 187).

Recruitment of Motor Units

A muscle (e.g., biceps brachii) is made up of numerous muscle fibers, and small groups of muscle fibers are innervated by a single motor neuron (Figure 4.4). Therefore, the muscle biceps is innervated by many neurons; in other words, it has many motor units. The body alters tension produced by adjusting the number of motor units stimulated. If *low tension* is required, only a few motor units are stimulated. If *higher tension* is required, more motor units are recruited. *Maximal tension* is produced if all motor units are stimulated. Only some motor units are activated in one muscle at any given time and others are inactive. By asynchronously recruiting motor units, muscle fatigue is avoided.

Frequency of Stimulation

The body also alters tension by altering the frequency of stimulation sent down the nerve. It has been shown that the force of muscle contraction increases up to a point if the frequency of stimulation is increased. This has been explained by the availability of calcium in the sarcoplasm. In each muscle fiber, the calcium released from the sarcoplasmic reticulum during the first impulse is still available in the sarcoplasm if the next impulse arrives soon after. That is, the next impulse arrives before calcium can be pumped back into the reticulum.

Wave summation is the increase in tension seen in successive contractions. Because the muscle tension increases in a steplike manner (and, if recorded, appears like stairs), it is called the **treppe,** or **staircase phenomenon.** If the impulse frequency is rapid, the contraction phase of subsequent contractions fuse and the muscle exhibits sustained contraction known as **tetanization** or **tetanus** (see Figure 4.9).

Organization of the Muscle Fibers

Muscle fiber arrangement and direction are important in the tension produced, direction of movement, and range of motion across joints.

The muscle fibers are bundled together as fascicles. The arrangement of fascicles in relation to each other and to the tendon where they are attached varies from one muscle to another. Five different fascicular arrangement patterns have been identified—**parallel, convergent (triangular), pennate, fusiform,** and **circular** (see Figure 4.10).

Parallel Muscles

These muscles have fibers that run parallel to each other along the long axis of the muscle. Most muscles of the body are parallel, some flat and some cylindrical with tendons on one or both ends. In muscles with tendons on both ends, the muscle appears spindle-shaped, with a central body, **gaster** or **belly** (*gaster,* meaning stomach). The biceps brachii, the muscle which produces the bulge in front of the upper arm, is a typical example of a muscle with a belly. When parallel muscles contract, the entire muscle shortens equally, as all the muscle fibers are parallel. The force of contraction, of course, will depend upon the number of muscle fibers that have been stimulated. An example of parallel muscle fiber is the stylohyoid muscle.

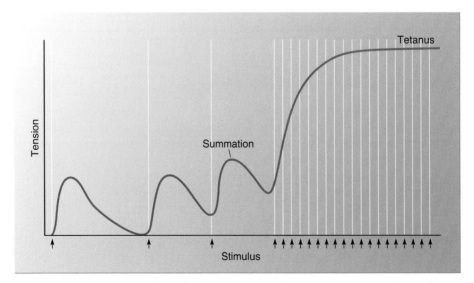

FIGURE **4.9.**   Recordings of Muscle Contractions With Varying Frequency of Stimulation

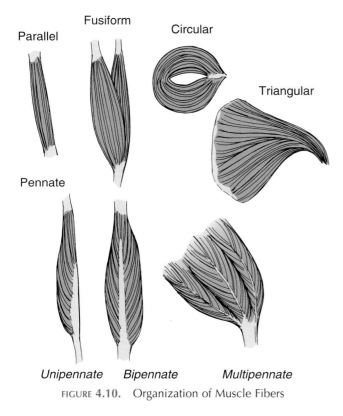

Parallel · Fusiform · Circular · Triangular · Pennate · Unipennate · Bipennate · Multipennate

FIGURE **4.10.** Organization of Muscle Fibers

Convergent or Triangular Muscles

The convergent muscles have a broad base but attach at a common site. The muscle fibers are arranged like a fan. The muscle may pull at a tendon or a connective tissue sheet. A typical example is the pectoralis muscle located in the front of the upper chest. Because the fibers are not parallel, convergent muscles can be manipulated to pull at different directions by stimulating specific groups of cell fibers at any given moment. If all the fibers contract at the same time, however, the force exerted is not as high as that of the parallel muscle with equivalent number of muscle fibers because, in convergent muscles, muscle fibers pulling on opposite sides of the tendon are pulling in different directions.

Pennate Muscles

These muscles are feather-shaped (*penna,* meaning feather*).* The fascicles are arranged obliquely, forming a common angle with a central tendon that may extend along almost the entire length of the muscle. Because the fascicles pull on the tendon at an angle, they do not move the tendon as far as a parallel muscle with equivalent muscle fibers. However, this arrangement facilitates the accommodation of more muscle fibers in a unit area compared with a parallel muscle, making it possible for a pennate muscle to exert more force than a parallel muscle of equal size. If all of the fascicles are on the same side of the tendon, the muscle is termed **unipennate.** An example of unipennate muscle is the

extensor digitorum, a muscle that extends the fingers. If fascicles are on both sides, the muscle is **bipennate.** An example of bipennate muscle is the extensor of the knee, rectus femoris. If the tendon branches, with fascicles arranged obliquely in each branch, the muscle is **multipennate.** The deltoid muscle, the muscle giving the rounded appearance to the shoulder, is an example of multipennate muscle.

Fusiform Muscles

Here, fascicles that are almost parallel, end in flat tendons. The digastric muscle is an example.

Circular Muscles, or Sphincters

In circular muscles, the fibers are arranged in a circle around an opening. Contraction of a circular muscle, therefore, closes or reduces the size of the opening and relaxation opens it or makes the opening wider. These muscles guard entrances and exits of internal passages. The muscles around the mouth (orbicularis oris) and the anus (sphincter ani) are typical examples.

Lever System

The force, speed, and distance of movement are modified by the site of muscle connection to the bone, the **lever.** A lever is a rigid structure that moves on a fixed point, the **fulcrum.** A good example of a lever system is a seesaw. The seesaw moves on a central, fixed point—the fulcrum. To move one end of the seesaw—the **resistance**—power must be exerted on the other side—the **effort,** or force.

In the body, the bone is the lever and the joint is the fulcrum; effort, or force, is provided by the contraction of the muscle (see Figure 4.11). The presence of the lever can change the direction of the applied force, the distance and speed of movement of the applied force, and the effective strength of the force.

Look at the three types of levers we use in everyday life to make our jobs easier. Our bodies do the same thing.

The **first-class lever** (Figure 4.11A) has the fulcrum in the center, and the effort and resistance are located on either side. There are not many muscles attached this way in the body. The muscles of the neck are examples in which the head balances on the cervical vertebrae (the fulcrum), and the muscles in the back of the neck (effort) extend the head (resistance).

The **second-class lever** (Figure 4.11B) has the resistance in the middle. A good example is the wheelbarrow in which the handle is lifted (effort) to move the weight of the wheelbarrow (resistance) on the front wheel (the fulcrum). In this type of lever, a smaller force is able to lift a larger force. However, the handle is moved up a greater distance, with a

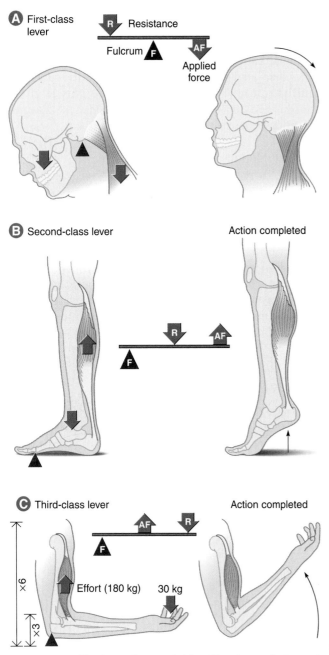

FIGURE **4.11.**   The Lever System. **A,** First-Class Lever; **B,** Second-Class Lever; **C,** Third-Class Lever

greater speed than the actual weight. Muscles attached to bones in this manner are able to lift greater weights at the expense of distance and speed. An example of such an attachment in the body is the calf muscle when standing on your toes; the calf muscle (effort) lifts the body and the bodyweight passes through the ankle (resistance) on the stationary toes (fulcrum).

Third-class levers (Figure 4.11C), the most common, have the effort applied to the center. Flex your arm: the biceps muscle is attached to the bone in the forearm, the lever; the elbow is the fulcrum. Contrac-

tion of the biceps attached to the middle of your forearm raises your hand. In this arrangement, force is compromised; however, the speed and distance moved are increased.

For a mathematical example, when the biceps contracts, it must exert about 180 kg (397 lb) tension to support a 30 kg (66 lb) weight held in the hand (the distance of the hand with the resistance is 6 times further away from the fulcrum than the attachment of the biceps). However, the hand moves 45 cm (18 in) when the site of attachment of the biceps moves only 7.5 cm (3 in). Therefore, the force exerted is six times the weight supported, but the distance the weight moves is six times the distance moved by the insertion point of the muscle. This example gives an idea of how speed and force can be altered by the site where the muscle is attached on a bone.

Type of Muscle Fiber

The proportion of fast twitch, slow twitch, and intermediate fibers also determines the characteristic of muscle contraction. This is considered in detail in the section on muscle performance, **page 194.**

Availability of Nutrients and Oxygen

The availability of nutrients and oxygen also affect the characteristics of muscle contraction. To a large extent, this is determined by the blood flow to the muscle and the capacity of the muscle to use nutrients and oxygen. The presence of myoglobin and glycogen storage in the muscle also plays a part.

MUSCLE TONE

Muscle tone is defined as the resting tension in a muscle. In any muscle, certain motor units are always active. Although this activity is too small to cause muscle shortening, it makes the muscle firm in consistency. This is one cause of muscle tone. Muscle tone is also a result of the viscoelastic property of muscle. This reflects the elastic tension of muscle fibers and the osmotic pressure of cells.

Tone in a muscle stabilizes the position of bones and joints. For example, muscle tone maintains body posture. Muscle tone also helps prevent sudden, uncontrolled changes in the position of bones and joints. If tone is reduced, the muscle feels limp and flaccid. Muscles with moderate tone feel firm and solid. If the tone is increased, the resting muscle feels rigid and resists passive movement.

MUSCLE SPINDLES

Muscle tone is maintained by stimulation of specialized tissue (**muscle spindles**) scattered within the muscle. Muscle spindles are modified muscle fibers: 3–10 fibers that are surrounded by a capsule, giving it a spindle shape (see Figure 4.12). The ends of the muscle spindle capsule are attached to endomysium and perimysium. The muscle spindles are located parallel to other muscle fibers, and their length is altered as the whole muscle stretches or contracts. On average, the length of the muscle spindle varies between 2–4 mm (0.08–0.16 in). The number of muscle spindles in each muscle is variable. Muscles of the arms and legs have the highest number, with the muscles of the hand and foot having an abundance.

The specialized muscle fibers in the muscle spindle are known as **intrafusal fibers.** The actin and myosin in the intrafusal fibers are concentrated toward the ends of the capsule. The intrafusal fibers have their own sensory and motor nerve supply. The **gamma motor neurons** supply these fibers in comparison with the other regular muscle fibers (**extrafusal fibers**) that are supplied by **alpha motor neurons.** Because the cell bodies of both motor neuron types lie in the central nervous system, the brain can control the contraction of intrafusal and extrafusal fibers. When the gamma motor neurons are stimulated, the proteins (actin and myosin) concentrated at the ends of the muscle spindle contract, stretching the middle of the muscle spindle.

In addition to the motor nerves, the center of the muscle spindle is surrounded by special sensory nerves that generate impulses every time the *length* of the muscle spindle is altered. The impulses are conveyed to the cerebral cortex, providing feedback with regard to muscle position. Impulses are conveyed to the cerebellum (see **page 348**) as well. This helps the brain coordinate muscle contraction. The sensory nerves also synapse (communicate) with motor neurons that innervate the muscle in question. Thus, reflexively (a reflex is an automatic, involuntary motor response to sensory stimulation), the muscle contracts when stretched to prevent overstretching the muscle. This reflex (**stretch reflex**) also helps alter the muscle tone according to changes in posture (see **page 334** for details). Thus, the muscle spindles function as **stretch receptors** that inform other neurons in the brain and spinal cord of muscle length and the rate at which the muscle is stretching.

Because muscle spindles have their own motor supply, the degree of stretch of the muscle spindle can

Distribution of Muscle Spindles

Muscles that must be precisely controlled, such as those of the hands and feet, have more muscle spindles per unit area as compared with others. Back muscles, which are mainly used for stabilizing the skeleton, have fewer muscle spindles.

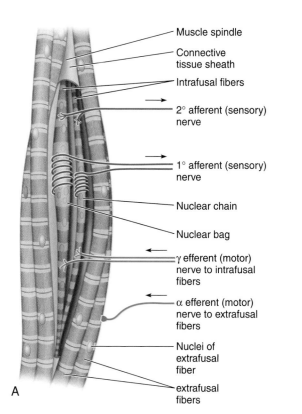

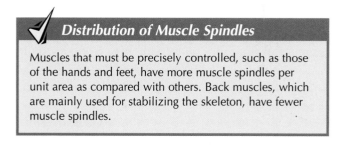

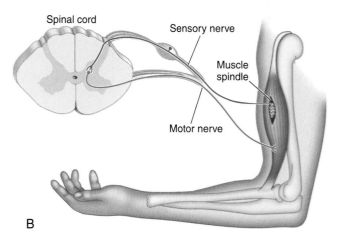

FIGURE 4.12.   Muscle Spindle. **A,** Structure of the Muscle Spindle; **B,** Schematic Representation of Stretch Reflex Regulation of Muscle Length

be altered by gamma motor neuron. For example, if the gamma motor neurons are stimulated before the muscle is lengthened, the middle of the muscle spindle is stretched even before the muscle actually lengthens. This, in turn, stimulates the sensory neurons located at the center of the spindle. By altering the degree of shortening of the contractile ends of the muscle spindle, the sensitivity of the sensory part of the muscle spindle can be regulated. Note that the muscle spindle can be stretched by two mechanisms: (1) by stretch of the whole muscle, and (2) by stimulation of the gamma motor neurons that produce contraction of the ends of the muscle spindle.

The activity and sensitivity of muscle spindles can be altered by exercise training. Thus, training can produce an increase in the resting tone of exercised muscles.

TENDON ORGANS

In addition to muscle spindles that sense change in muscle length, **Golgi tendon organs** (GTO), located in the tendons, monitor muscle tension (see Figure 4.13). GTO are sensory nerve endings that are wrapped around the collagen fibers of tendons. About 10 to 15 muscle fibers are attached to each GTO. When the muscle contracts, the stretch of the collagen

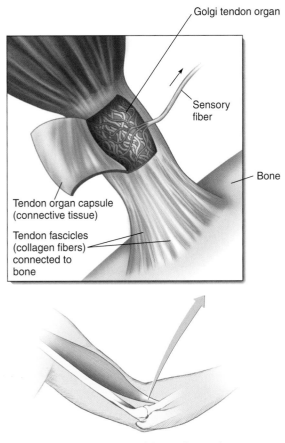

FIGURE **4.13.** Structure of the Golgi Tendon Organ

Golgi tendon organ

Sensory fiber

Bone

Tendon organ capsule (connective tissue)

Tendon fascicles (collagen fibers) connected to bone

fibers stimulates the GTO, which convey impulses to interneurons located in the central nervous system. These neurons inhibit the motor neuron innervating the muscle in question and produce reflex muscle relaxation. In this way, the Golgi tendon organs protect the muscle from contracting with excessive force and speed and becoming injured (see **page 337**).

OTHER PROPRIOCEPTORS

In addition to the muscle spindles and Golgi tendon organs, receptors present in the capsules of joints and ligaments respond to pressure and acceleration and deceleration of joint movement. They convey information regarding joint movement and position to the brain.

ISOTONIC AND ISOMETRIC CONTRACTIONS

Based on the pattern of tension production, muscle contraction can be classified as **isotonic** or **isometric.** In isotonic contraction, the tension *(tonus)* developed is constant *(iso,* meaning equal) while the length of the muscle changes. Examples of isotonic contraction are walking, running, and skipping. There are two types of isotonic contraction—**concentric** and **eccentric.** In concentric contraction, the muscle shortens. In eccentric contraction, the muscle lengthens during contraction (i.e., the muscle tension is less than the resistance and the muscle is stretched by the resistance). An example of eccentric contraction is lowering a book on a table. The resistance developed is less than that required for lifting the book, and the book (resistance) stretches the muscle. Eccentric contractions prevent rapid changes in length that may damage muscle tissue and help absorb shock when jumping or walking.

In isometric contraction, the muscle length *(metric,* measure) remains the same *(iso-,* meaning equal), and the tension varies. A good example is trying to lift a weight when you are unable to do so. Tension develops in the muscle, but the muscle does not shorten to lift the weight. Daily activity involves a combination of isotonic and isometric contractions of muscle.

Muscle Energetics

The muscle requires energy for contraction to take place and energy is derived from ATP.

$$ATP \rightarrow ADP + P + energy$$

As previously explained, ATP is required for actin-myosin interaction. It is also required for actively pumping calcium into the sarcoplasmic reticulum from the sarcoplasm after the contraction process and maintaining the ionic concentration in the muscle fiber by the action of the Na-K ATPase pump located in the cell membrane. These are only some activities that require ATP.

It is not possible for the body to have the tremendous supply of ATP demanded when a muscle contracts. Instead, the body has enough ATP and other high-energy compounds to *begin* contraction. Typically, a single muscle fiber has enough ATP to support only about 10 twitches or isometric contraction that can last for just 2 seconds; however, it can generate ATP at almost the same rate as the demand through various metabolic processes.

The ATP produced in the muscle fiber at rest is used to transfer energy to creatine and phosphate to form another high-energy compound, creatine phosphate, present in the cell.

$$ATP \rightarrow ADP + phosphate + energy$$

$$Creatine + phosphate + energy \rightarrow creatine\ phosphate + ADP$$

When needed, this compound is broken down by creatine phosphokinase to liberate energy that can be used to form ATP.

$$Creatine\ phosphate \rightarrow creatine + phosphate + energy$$

$$ADP + phosphate + energy \rightarrow ATP$$

At rest, a muscle fiber has about six times as much creatine phosphate as ATP. This store is sufficient to produce about 70 twitches or tetanic, isometric contractions that last about 15 seconds. If the fiber must sustain its contractions for longer than this, it must rely on other mechanisms for energy. This may be accomplished by breaking down glucose to lactic acid. Glucose may be made available by the breakdown of stored glycogen or glucose from the blood. All of the above can be achieved without the supply of oxygen.

AEROBIC METABOLISM

The sarcoplasm of the muscle has numerous mitochondria. The mitochondria have the enzymes necessary for breaking down glucose, amino acids, and fatty acids to produce large amounts of ATP in the presence of oxygen. The necessary substrates (e.g., glucose) and oxygen are brought to the muscle by blood. The sarcoplasm also has specialized proteins (myoglobin) that, similar to hemoglobin, combines with oxygen reversibly. In addition, the muscle has some glucose stored in the sarcoplasm in the form of glycogen.

At rest, the energy required by the muscle is provided by aerobic metabolism. The mitochondria absorb the substrate, mostly in the form of fatty acid, ADP, phosphate ions and oxygen from the sarcoplasm and, in the presence of oxygen, forms ATP from each molecule. This process of producing ATP is complex and involves numerous intermediary steps and many enzymes present inside the mitochondria. This biochemical process is known as the **Krebs cycle** or the **tricarboxylic acid cycle** or **TCA cycle,** in which the carbon atoms of the substrate molecule are converted to carbon dioxide and the hydrogen ions generated in the cycle are converted to water.

When the muscle begins to contract, pyruvic acid (derived from glucose) is used as the substrate in the TCA cycle, rather than fatty acid.

ANAEROBIC METABOLISM

Even in the absence of oxygen, the muscle is able to manufacture some ATP (see Figure 4.14). However, few ATP can be produced in this way. Also, the metabolites formed change the pH of the environment and prolonged muscle activity cannot be maintained.

In this type of metabolism, glucose is broken down to pyruvic acid in the cytoplasm of the cell to produce ATP. This process is called **glycolysis.** Because glycolysis can take place without the presence of oxygen, it is known as **anaerobic metabolism.** Production of energy through anaerobic metabolism is an inefficient way to generate ATP. When glucose is broken down to two pyruvic acid molecules, it forms only 2 ATP. However, if the two molecules were used in the TCA cycle in the presence of oxygen in the mitochondria, 34 (17 + 17) ATP could be generated. However, glycolysis is important because it can proceed without the supply of oxygen.

During peak activity, when the muscle is deprived of the ready-made ATP and creatine phosphate, it breaks down glycogen stored in the sarcoplasm to form glucose. This glucose is, in turn, broken down to pyruvic acid and ATP for immediate use. If oxygen is available and adequate, pyruvic acid enters the TCA cycle to produce more ATP.

Glycolysis:

$$Glucose \rightarrow 2\ pyruvic\ acid + 2ATP$$

If pyruvic acid production by glycolysis is faster than is used by the mitochondria in the TCA cycle, pyruvic acid is converted into lactic acid in the presence of the enzyme lactate dehydrogenase.

$$Pyruvic\ acid \rightarrow lactic\ acid$$

Accumulating lactic acid is a disadvantage because it enters the body fluids and easily dissociates into lactate ions and hydrogen ions. This tends to alter the pH of the body fluids. Although buffers in the cell and the body fluids try to prevent pH fluctua-

Myofascial Trigger Points (TrPs)

TrPs are identified as localized spots of tenderness in a nodule or a palpable taut band of muscle fibers. Patients complain of aching pain characteristic of deep tissue pain. The pain is often referred to a site some distance from the TrP that is specific to individual muscles. It is interesting to note that there is a high degree of correspondence between published locations of TrPs and classical acupuncture points for the relief of pain. Pressure on the nodule elicits the familiar pain sensation. Because of pain, there is resistance to passive stretch of muscle.

TrPs are believed to be caused by dysfunction of the motor endplate. The dysfunction results in an abnormal increase in production and release of ACh at rest. This results in depolarization of the sarcolemma with release of calcium from the sarcoplasmic reticulum and sustained shortening of sarcomeres (taut band). The shortening of muscle fiber compresses the local blood vessels, reducing the nutrient and oxygen availability. This, in turn, results in release of substances that sensitize pain receptors (pain).

TrPs are responsive to stretch therapy used in massage. By lengthening the sarcomeres and reducing the overlap between actin and myosin molecules, the energy consumption of the local tissue is reduced. Blood flow to the muscle fibers is also restored when the muscles are relaxed by stretch.

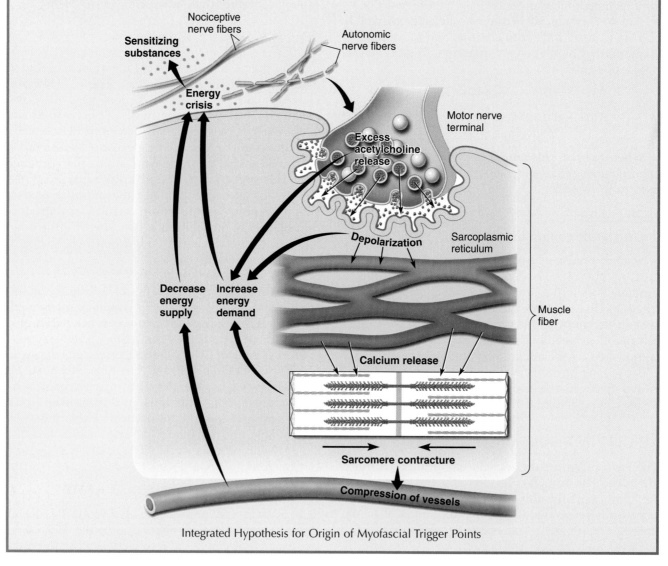

Integrated Hypothesis for Origin of Myofascial Trigger Points

tions, their defenses are limited. Eventually, the pH changes slightly and this then alters the function of various enzymes (the activity of enzymes largely depends on the pH) and the muscle fiber has difficulty contracting.

In summary, *at rest*, the demand for ATP is low, and the supply of oxygen is enough for the mito-chondria to produce surplus ATP using fatty acid. This ATP is used to build up a reserve of creatine phosphate and glycogen from glucose. Fatty acid and glucose are absorbed from the blood.

During *moderate levels of activity*, the demand for ATP increases. This demand is met by the production of ATP by the mitochondria. Because oxygen supply by the blood is sufficient at this level of activity, the mitochondria form ATP from pyruvic acid. The pyruvic acid is derived from glucose which, in turn, is derived by breaking down glycogen stores. If glycogen stores are depleted, amino acids and lipids may be broken down. Hence, the contribution of glycolysis to the production of energy is minimal.

At *high levels of activity*, the ATP demands are enormous, and the mitochondrial activity is at its maximum. At this point, even if the blood flow is good, the rate of oxygen diffusion from the blood into the cell is not fast enough. The mitochondria can only supply about one-third of the ATP required. The remaining ATP is generated by glycolysis. When the production of pyruvic acid by glycolysis is faster than can be used by the mitochondria, it is converted into lactic acid.

EFFICIENCY OF MUSCLE WORK

The amount of mechanical output from the muscle in relation to the unit of energy put into the muscular system has been calculated as 20% to 25%. This means that for a given action, the muscle is using four to five times the amount of energy to produce the action. The remaining energy is converted to heat. This is why a lot of heat is produced when muscles are exercised vigorously. The heat is dissipated by various regulatory mechanisms in the body, such as production of sweat.

> ### HYPERTHYROIDISM AND HEAT INTOLERANCE
>
> Muscles generate about 85% of the body heat required to maintain normal temperature. In individuals with hyperthyroidism, the muscles produce more heat, even when resting, as a result of increased metabolism. This is responsible for the heat intolerance experienced by those with hyperthyroidism.

MUSCLE RECOVERY

During the recovery period, the muscle returns to its normal state, and the heat that was produced during metabolism must be dissipated. The muscle reserves of glycogen and creatine phosphate and others must be rebuilt. The lactic acid that was formed must be recycled. It may take several hours for the muscle to recover after a moderate level of activity. After peak levels of activity, it may take a week for the muscle to return to its original state.

Fortunately, the lactic acid produced can be recycled; it is converted to pyruvic acid when the level of pyruvic acid is low. This happens soon after exertion. The pyruvic acid made in this way can enter the TCA cycle to produce ATP or it can be converted by special enzymes to glucose and then to glycogen. The lactic acid that enters the blood is taken up by the liver and converted to glucose. The glucose may be stored as glycogen in the liver or it may enter the blood and be used again by skeletal muscle.

During recovery, the oxygen needs of the body rise. This oxygen is used for recovering ATP that was used during muscle contraction. The amount of oxygen required to bring the muscle to its pre-exertion level is known as the **oxygen debt** or **recovery oxygen**

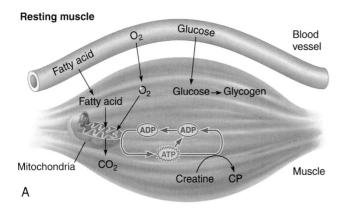

Resting muscle

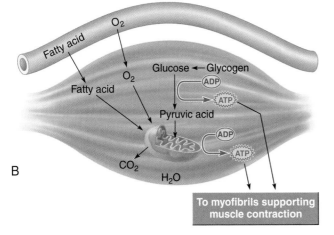

Muscle at moderate activity

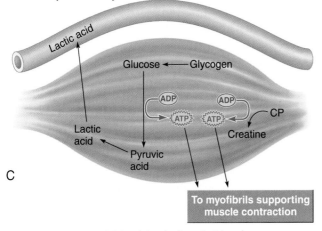

Muscle at peak activity

FIGURE **4.14.**   Metabolism in Muscle

Terms Relating to Abnormal Muscle Contractions

Contracture or **rigor** in the physiologic sense is a state of muscle contractile activity without electrical activity. Clinically, contracture is shortening of muscle caused by remodeling of connective tissue that may include joint capsules and ligaments and reduction in the number of sarcomeres. Such changes are seen when the muscle is kept in a shortened position for a long time.

Convulsions are abnormal, uncoordinated tetanic contractions of varying groups of muscles.

Cramps are painful muscle spasms.

Fasciculation is a visible, involuntary twitch of the muscles of a motor unit of short duration. There is no accompanying movement across the joint.

Fibrillation is an abnormal type of contraction in which individual fibers contract asynchronously.

Hypertonia is an increase in muscle tone (e.g., rigidity, spasticity).

Hypotonia is a decrease in muscle tone.

Myalgia is pain originating in muscle.

Myoma is tumor of muscle (e.g., leiomyoma).

Myositis is inflammation of muscle.

Repetitive strain injury is muscle pain induced by muscular activity at work that is close to or beyond the muscle's tolerance.

Rigidity denotes muscle spasm that involves both agonistic and antagonistic muscles. It is associated with certain nervous conditions such as Parkinson's disease.

Spasm is a persistent contraction of muscle that cannot be released voluntarily.

Spasticity is muscle spasm observed in conditions such as hemiplegia and brain or spinal cord injury. It is a result of the increased excitability of the stretch reflex (see **page 334**). Here, resistance to passive movement increases with increased speed of movement.

Tic is an involuntary spasmodic twitch of muscle, usually seen in the face.

Tremor is a repetitive, involuntary, oscillatory movement caused by alternate or synchronous, but irregular, contraction of opposing muscle groups.

consumption. Until the oxygen debt is repaid, the individual continues to breathe at a much faster rate and depth than normal.

The tissue involved in oxygen consumption during the recovery period are the skeletal muscles that must restore ATP, glycogen, and creatine phosphate to former levels. The liver uses ATP to convert lactic acid to glucose. ATP is also used by sweat glands to increase sweat secretion to dissipate heat by evaporation and bring the body temperature back to normal.

MUSCLE FATIGUE

Sometimes, the muscle may find it difficult to contract even when stimulated by the nerve. This state is known as **muscle fatigue.** The cause of fatigue is varied and depends on the type of activity. It may be the result of an interruption to the chain of events responsible for muscle contraction—the central nervous system (CNS), peripheral nervous system, neuromuscular junction, and muscle fiber. Following peak activity, the muscle becomes fatigued as a result of the depletion of ATP, creatine phosphate, and glycogen. The lowering of pH (acidity) as a result of lactic acid buildup may also play a part. Prolonged exercise, such as running a marathon, may result in physical damage to the sarcoplasmic reticulum, changes in T tubules, ionic imbalances, and fatigue. Exercise induced alteration in content of CNS neurotransmitters, such as dopamine, ACh, and serotonin, has been implicated as the cause of psychic or perceptual changes that reduce the ability to continue exercising. Fatigue may also be a result of failure of the action potential to cross over the neuromuscular junction. The actual cause of this failure is unknown.

Fatigue may occur more rapidly if the intracellular reserves are low, such as in malnutrition. It is also important to have adequate blood flow to the muscle. Any problems with circulation, such as cardiac problems or tight clothing, that impede blood flow to the muscle, can speed the onset of fatigue. Similarly, any condition that affects the normal blood oxygen concentration can induce fatigue quickly. Respiratory problems and low levels of oxygen carrying capacity of the blood (e.g., low red blood cell count, reduced hemoglobin) can all result in early fatigue.

MUSCLE PERFORMANCE

The performance of the muscle is measured by the tension or **power** produced and the duration that a particular activity can be maintained—the **endurance.** The power and endurance in a muscle are determined by the type of muscle and the level of physical conditioning or training.

Types of Muscle Fibers

Skeletal muscle fibers are classified into three types, according to the speed at which they respond to stimulus. The three types are **fast fibers, slow fibers,** and **intermediate fibers.**

Fibromyalgia Syndrome

Fibromyalgia syndrome is a common medical condition characterized by widespread pain and tenderness to palpation at multiple, anatomically defined soft tissue body sites. Although many of the sites are located in muscle, it is now believed that the pain is a result of alteration to the perception of pain at the central nervous system level and not specifically from muscle pathology.

Fast Fibers

The fast fibers are also known as **fast twitch, fast glycolytic,** or **type IIB fibers.** Most skeletal muscle fibers in the body are fast fibers. These fibers respond to a stimulus in 0.01 second. They are large in diameter, with huge reserves of glycogen, densely packed myofibrils, and few mitochondria. The presence of more myofibrils helps these muscles generate a lot of tension; however, because they rely largely on anaerobic metabolism, they fatigue rapidly. As a result of the lower number of capillaries per unit area, these fibers appear pale to the naked eye.

Slow Fibers

The slow fibers, however, are smaller and take about three times longer to contract after stimulus than fast fibers. Slow fibers are also known as **slow twitch** or **slow oxidative fibers.** Slow fibers have an extensive network of capillaries and numerous mitochondria. In addition, slow fibers contain a large amount of myoglobin, a red pigment. Myoglobin is similar to the oxygen carrying hemoglobin protein in the blood. Myoglobin has an affinity for oxygen and makes oxygen available when needed. Structurally, these fibers are equipped to contract for a long period without becoming fatigued (i.e., they have increased endurance). Because these fibers have more blood flowing through them and more myoglobin, these muscles appear red to the naked eye.

Intermediate Fibers

Intermediate fibers have the properties of both slow and fast fibers. They are also known as **type IIA** or **fast oxidative-glycolytic fibers.** Similar to fast fibers, they appear pale because they contain less myoglobin. They have more endurance than fast fibers because they have more capillaries per unit area.

The percentage of fast, slow, and intermediate fibers varies. For instance, muscles that must move rapidly for short intervals have a larger proportion of fast fibers—sometimes with no slow fiber at all. The eye muscles and the small muscles of the hand are typical examples. Muscles that are constantly contracting to maintain movement and posture, such as calf muscles and back muscles, have a larger propor-

WHITE AND RED CHICKEN MEAT

The chicken breast has "white" meat because the chicken uses the muscles to move the wings for only a short period, such as in getting away from a predator. The "red" meat that you see in the delicatessen contains more slow fibers. The thigh and drumstick of chicken meat is red because the chicken uses these muscles continually for walking.

tion of slow fiber. The proportion of fast and slow fibers in each muscle is determined genetically. However, it is possible for fibers to change from slow or fast to intermediate type by physical conditioning. For example, if a muscle with more fast fibers is used repeatedly for events that require endurance, the fast fibers may adapt by changing to intermediate fibers.

MUSCLES AND HORMONES

Many hormones affect the metabolism in the muscle fiber. *Growth hormone* (a hormone secreted by the pituitary gland) together with *testosterone* (the male hormone secreted primarily by the testis) stimulate the formation of contractile proteins and the enlargement of muscles. A synthetic hormone (*anabolic steroid*) that resembles testosterone is taken by some athletes to increase the size and power of their muscles.

The *thyroid hormone* can also stimulate the metabolism of both active and resting muscles.

A Summary of the Role of CNS in Muscle Function Control

The structure of the muscle, neuromuscular junction, the role of motor neuron, and motor unit has already been discussed (see Figure 4.15).

Neural control mechanisms located in the central nervous system affect the motor neuron in response to stimuli from the internal and external environment. Tracts (bundles of axons) descend from the brain to affect spinal neurons that eventually stimulate the muscle fiber. Neurons from the cerebral cortex are responsible for discrete movements. Neurons from other areas of the brain control posture and muscle tone. Neurons from the cerebellum help coordinate movement. Neurons in the spinal cord and other areas of the CNS control many muscle functions, such as spinal reflexes occurring at the subconscious level.

Physical Conditioning

EXERCISE TRAINING PRINCIPLES

The effects of training depend on the metabolic pathways used during training. Hence, the type of training should be geared to activating the metabolic pathway primarily used by the activity in which the person is involved. Figure 4.16 shows the energy pathways used for different types of exercises.

Altering training duration, frequency, and intensity in such a way to **overload** the muscle results in a training response. The response is **specific** to the type

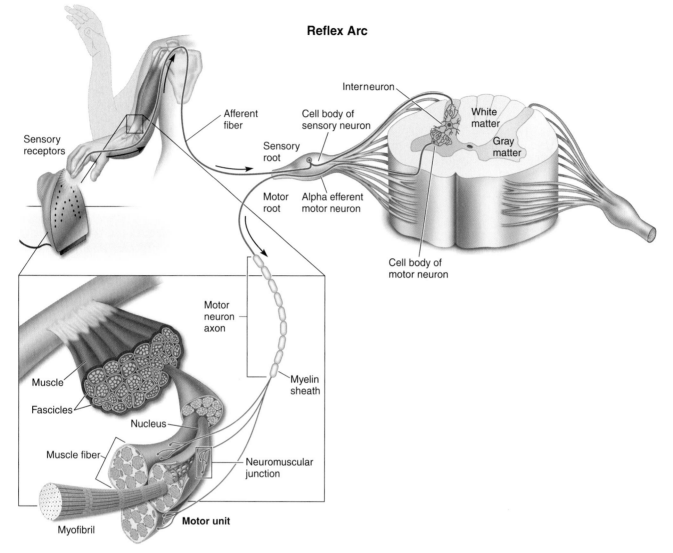

Reflex Arc

FIGURE 4.15.   An Example of the Role of Nervous System in Muscle Function

of overload imposed. For example, if swimming is the mode of training, greater response would be seen only when tested by swimming. This is because adaptations take place in the specifically trained muscles. Figure 4.16 shows the energy pathways used for different types of exercises.

 Physical Fitness

Physical fitness is the ability to carry out daily tasks with vigor and alertness, without undue fatigue, and with ample energy to enjoy leisure-time pursuits and meet unforeseen emergencies.

"Physical fitness is not only one of the most important keys to a healthy body, it is the basis of dynamic and creative intellectual activity. Intelligence and skill can only function at the peak of their capacity when the body is strong. Hardy spirits and tough minds usually inhabit sound bodies" (John F. Kennedy).

The training response varies among **individuals.** For example, the individual's genetic make-up and relative fitness at the beginning of training play an important part. Therefore, exercise programs should be designed for the specific individual.

Unfortunately, the adaptations that occur with training decrease rapidly when training stops. Within 1 to 2 weeks of **detraining,** the physiologic adaptations significantly reduce and many of the improvements are lost within 1 to 2 months.

ADAPTATION TO TRAINING

Metabolic Adaptations

As mentioned, the adaptation to training depends on the energy pathways used during training. When a person uses activities that involve stressing the anaerobic metabolism, as in sprint-power training, the levels of ATP, creatine phosphate, free creatine, and

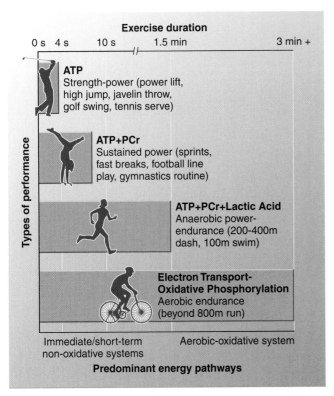

Exercise duration

0 s 4 s   10 s   1.5 min   3 min +

ATP
Strength-power (power lift, high jump, javelin throw, golf swing, tennis serve)

ATP+PCr
Sustained power (sprints, fast breaks, football line play, gymnastics routine)

ATP+PCr+Lactic Acid
Anaerobic power-endurance (200-400m dash, 100m swim)

Electron Transport-Oxidative Phosphorylation
Aerobic endurance (beyond 800m run)

Immediate/short-term non-oxidative systems   Aerobic-oxidative system

Predominant energy pathways

FIGURE **4.16.** Comparison of Activity With the Energy Pathways Used

glycogen are increased in individual muscle fibers of those muscles used in training. The levels of enzymes and myoglobin used in this metabolic pathway are also increased. There is also an increased capacity to generate lactate.

When aerobic training is used, the adaptations occur to improve transport and use of oxygen. The muscle fibers in trained muscles contain larger and more mitochondria and enzymes used in aerobic metabolism than those in untrained muscle. The capacity to use fat for energy is also increased. This is of benefit because it helps conserve glycogen stores. There is also an increase in the capacity to use carbohydrates during exercise. The changes occurring in the fiber type vary according to the overload used. The muscles used in training **hypertrophy.** Hypertrophy denotes an increase in fiber *size;* the number of muscle fibers does not increase. As a result of the presence of testosterone, hypertrophy is more prevalent in men than in women. Training for power combined with a high protein diet speeds the process of hypertrophy.

Cardiovascular Adaptations

The cardiovascular adaptations resulting in improved oxygen delivery to the muscle are summarized in Figure 4.17.

The size of the heart changes as a result of increased chamber volume and the thickness of the muscle wall. These changes vary with the type of activity. In endurance training, the volume increases more than the thickness of the walls. In power training, such as wrestling or weight lifting, the thickness of the wall showed a more significant increase.

There is a decrease in resting and exercise heart rate and an increase in stroke volume and maximal cardiac output. The drop in heart rate is attributed to increased parasympathetic activity and decreased sympathetic activity. The change in stroke volume is a result of increased left ventricular volume, greater compliance (capacity to stretch) of the heart tissue, longer time between contractions that increase diastolic filling, and a general improvement in the contractility of the heart. The change in maximal cardiac output is directly related to the changes in stroke volume.

There is a marked increase in plasma volume soon after the beginning of training. This increase contributes to the increase in stroke volume, end-diastolic volume, oxygen transport, and temperature regulation during exercise.

There is an improvement in the capacity of trained muscles to extract oxygen from the blood. The blood flow to the trained muscles and distribution of cardiac output is also altered. There is decreased blood flow to the kidney and gastrointestinal tract and increased cutaneous blood flow. The latter facilitates the dissipation of heat produced during exercise. There is an increase in total muscle blood flow as a result of increased cardiac output, increased cross-sectional areas of blood vessels and number of capillaries per gram of muscle tissue.

Postexercise Muscle Soreness

Excessive or unaccustomed eccentric (lengthening) contractions are responsible for postexercise soreness. It appears 8–24 hours after activity, peaks during the first 1–2 days, and resolves in 5–7 days. The muscle is swollen, tender, and resists stretch as a result of pain. There is pain on contracting voluntarily. Muscle soreness is caused by disruption of the structure of myofibrils resulting from mechanical overload. The injury sensitizes the pain receptors in muscle. Muscle soreness resembles a sterile inflammation and is not caused by accumulation of lactate as was once believed.

Stretching

Regular stretching is important especially during the healing of a muscle tear. Stretching promotes correct orientation of the collagen fibers and counteracts the natural tendency of maturing fibrous tissue to shorten and pucker. The aim is to have a soft, elongated, and flexible scar, with the collagen fibers parallel to the direction of the pull of muscle.

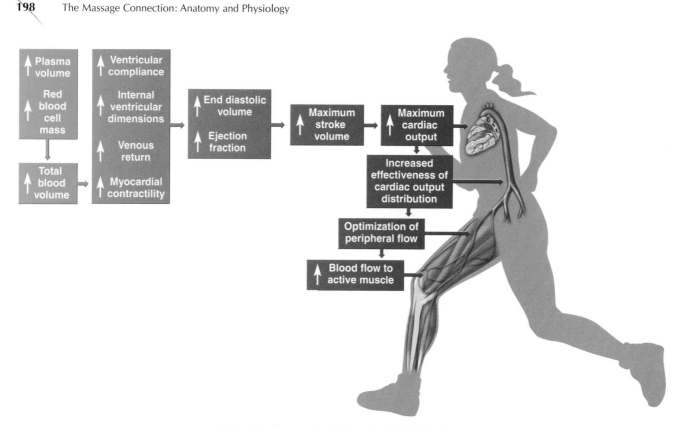

FIGURE **4.17.**   Cardiovascular Adaptations With Aerobic Training

The blood flow to the heart muscle is also modified with training. There is an increase in cross-sectional area of coronary blood vessels, recruitment of collateral vessels, and number of capillaries. This contributes to better oxygen supply to the myocardium.

Training has the capacity to reduce both systolic and diastolic blood pressure during rest and exercise.

Changes in the blood lactate concentrations have also been observed with training. There is a decrease in the rate of formation and clearance of lactate during exercise. Trained individuals also tolerate a more acidic pH than untrained counterparts. This implies that the body's capacity to regulate acid-base balance is improved with training.

Pulmonary Adaptations

One significant adaptation is the improvement in breathing efficiency. Changes in the respiratory muscles result in reduced use of oxygen for respiration. This, in turn, reduces the fatiguing effects of exercise on the respiratory muscles and frees oxygen for use by the active muscles. In trained individuals, the respiratory rate is decreased during exercise and the tidal volume (volume of air breathed in per breath) is increased. This is advantageous because it allows for a longer time for oxygen extraction from the inspired air. It must be noted that these adaptive changes are specific to the type of exercises used and type of training (i.e., observed when the specifically trained muscles are used).

Others

In addition to the adaptations described above, training reduces body fat, increases fat-free body mass, improves temperature regulation, and increases work capacity. Psychologically, it increases the sense of well-being.

FACTORS AFFECTING RESPONSE TO TRAINING

A number of factors affect the magnitude of adaptational changes described above. The *initial level of aerobic fitness* has a bearing on the improvements seen with training. As expected, those at a lower fitness level can expect greater improvements. With endurance training, the average improvement ranges from 5% to 25%.

A major factor that affects improvement is *exercise intensity.* Exercise intensity can be measured in many ways. The energy expended per unit time, the percentage of maximal oxygen capacity (VO$_2$ max), power output, lactate levels, exercise heart rate or percentage of maximum heart rate, metabolic rate, and rating of perceived exertion are some measures used (the details of these measures are beyond the scope of this book). In general, physiologic improvements are seen when the exercise intensity increases the heart rate to 55% to 70% of maximal heart rate. An approximation of maximal heart rate can be calculated by subtracting the individual's age in years from 220 ($HR_{max} = 220 -$ age [yr]).

Twenty to 30 minutes of continuous exercise at 70% HR_{max} have been shown to produce optimum training effects. Shorter duration of training—as low as 3 to 5 minutes daily—have produced effects in poorly conditioned individuals. Longer exercise duration at a lower intensity has been shown to be beneficial as well. Higher intensity training of shorter duration also shows significant improvement.

The effect of different training frequency (i.e., 2- or 5-day training) is controversial. In general, more frequency is beneficial when lower intensity is used or weight loss is desired. To produce weight loss, each exercise session should last at least 60 minutes and it should be at an intensity that uses 300 kcal or more.

In terms of exercise type, it has been found that the effects are similar as long as the exercise involves large muscle groups. Bicycling, running, walking, climbing stairs, rowing, in-line skating, and skipping rope are examples of exercises that involve large muscle groups and provide sufficient overload to improve aerobic capacity. The adaptation to exercise may be seen within a few weeks and excessive exercise does not speed improvement. It has been shown that the frequency and duration of exercise may be reduced to maintain a level of improvement. However, the intensity of exercise must be maintained.

Another factor that affects the physiologic responses is genetic endowment. Although the proportion of slow and fast muscle fibers in a specific muscle is genetically determined, fibers can change to intermediate type by activity.

METHODS OF TRAINING

The method of training should match the type of activity. For activities, such as football or weightlifting, in which the body relies on energy derived from ATP and phosphocreatine, the muscles in question must be engaged in repeated 5–10 second maximal bursts of exercise.

If the activity extends beyond 10 seconds, the body relies on energy derived by glycolysis and with resultant production of lactic acid. For such activities, the individual may have to train in bouts of about 1-minute maximum exercise with a short rest in between.

For aerobic training, the goal is to improve the capacity of the body to deliver oxygen to the muscle and to improve the capacity of the muscle to extract and utilize the oxygen. **Interval training, continuous training,** and **Fartlek training** are some methods used.

In interval training, high intensity exercise and short rest are alternated. In this way, a person is able to perform a large amount of high intensity exercise. An impossible feat if they had to do the exercise continuously. Physiologically, interval training results in less build up of lactate and muscle fatigue. The intensity, duration of exercise, and rest will depend on the improvements desired.

Continuous training involves exercise of longer duration at a lower intensity. Fartlek training is a blend of continuous training and interval training in which the person runs at fast and slow speeds over level and uphill terrain.

EFFECT OF OVERTRAINING

Many athletes experience the syndrome of overtraining. Here, the athlete fails to adapt to training, with deterioration of normal performance. The athlete has difficulty recovering completely after a workout. Muscle soreness and stiffness; increased susceptibility to infection; gastrointestinal disturbances; sleep disturbances; loss of appetite; overuse injuries; fatigue; altered reproductive function; and mood changes such as apathy, depression, and irritability are some other symptoms. These changes are attributed to biologic and psychological influences.

Overtraining syndrome is described as two clinical forms: **sympathetic** (less common) and **parasympathetic** (more common). The sympathetic form may reflect a perpetual stimulation of the sympathetic system as a result of the interaction of increased training, competition, and other stresses of day-to-day living. The parasympathetic form is characterized by overstimulation of the parasympathetic system during rest and exercise. It may result from interactions between overload of the neuromuscular, endocrine, nervous, psychological, immunologic, and metabolic (glycogen depletion, amino acid imbalances) factors. There are changes in the function and relationship between the hypothalamus, pituitary, gonads, and adrenal glands.

Overtraining may be prevented by adequate rest and recovery between training and proper nutrition and hydration during training. Athletes with overtraining syndrome may require weeks and sometimes even months of rest to recover.

TRAINING DURING PREGNANCY

A number of women exercise during pregnancy. It has been found that the physiologic changes in the

> ### ✚ Muscle Tear
>
> If a muscle is stretched suddenly or too far, some fibers will tear and bleeding will occur in the muscle. In the commonly occurring muscle pull or strain, only a small proportion of fibers are involved.
>
> Such injuries occur soon after beginning the activity, especially when the individual has not stretched and warmed-up adequately or when the weather is cold. It may occur late in a game when the athlete is tired and movements are less coordinated.
>
> Treatment of muscle tears should be performed with care. Immediately, rest, ice, compression, and elevation should be employed to reduce bleeding. Subsequently, stretching and graded active exercises should be started early. In general, total rest is detrimental to muscle injuries because wasting of muscle occurs together with formation of scar tissue. Scar tissue in muscle contracts and is not elastic. Also, it is weak and may tear easily when the muscle is stressed again. However, the treatment should be modified if a large proportion of muscle is torn.

maternal cardiovascular system follow normal response patterns. The stress on the mother offered by moderate exercise is mainly a result of the additional weight gain. There is no evidence to show that moderate exercise during pregnancy increases the risk of fetal death or low–birth-weight. Fetal hypoxia, fetal hypothermia, and low fetal glucose supply are potential risks of intensive maternal training.

MUSCLE ATROPHY

Muscles that are not used extensively reduce in size. This process is known as **atrophy.** Both tone and mass are lost if the muscle is not regularly stimulated by motor nerves. Atrophy is seen in those individuals paralyzed by spinal injuries (**denervation atrophy**). It can occur even if the nerves are intact. For example, **disuse atrophy** occurs in limbs that have been in a cast.

Cardiac, Smooth, and Skeletal Muscle

The basic contractile process is the same in cardiac, smooth, and skeletal muscle, with movement produced by the action of the myofilaments actin and myosin. However, because the requirements in terms of speed and force of contraction are different, the structure of cardiac and smooth are slightly different than skeletal muscle.

CARDIAC MUSCLE

The cardiac muscle (see Figure 4.18; also see page 482) present in the walls of the heart is used to propel blood from the chambers, requiring each chamber to contract in one accord. Relaxation should also be synchronous for blood to fill the chamber. To meet these needs, the structure is altered.

Cardiac muscle is branched and has specialized regions on the sarcolemma where it comes in contact with the adjoining cell. These specialized regions, intercalated disks, contain proteins (desmosomes) that hold adjacent cells together and transmit the force generated from muscle to muscle. Intercalated disks also contain gap junctions, which are specialized channels that allow action potentials (impulses) to travel from one cell to another. Because of the presence of intercalated disks, cardiac muscle is able to

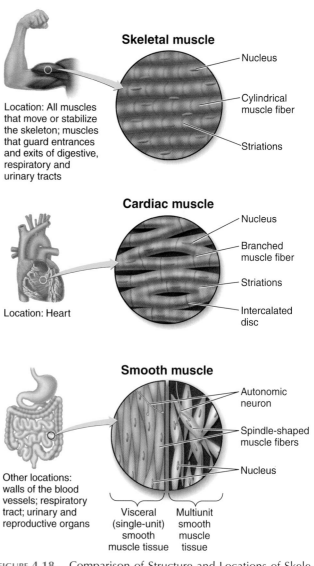

FIGURE **4.18.** Comparison of Structure and Locations of Skeletal, Cardiac, and Smooth Muscles

contract together as a functional syncytium (as if it functioned as one muscle fiber). The myosin and actin filaments are arranged in an orderly manner; and cardiac muscle, like skeletal muscle, looks striated.

Because the heart must alter its force of contraction according to regional requirements, its contraction is not only regulated by nerves, but also by hormones and ionic contents of the blood among others. For example, adrenaline in blood can speed contraction and calcium levels can alter the excitability and contractility of the heart. Unlike skeletal muscle that relies on a stimulus from a nerve fiber, the cardiac muscle can respond to action potentials produced by specialized cardiac muscle fibers belonging to the conducting system of the heart (see page 489). In response to a stimulus, the cardiac muscle fiber remains contracted for a longer period (about 10 to 15 times the duration of skeletal muscle).

Cardiac muscle does not have the capacity to regenerate.

SMOOTH MUSCLE

Smooth muscle is spindle-shaped with no striations. Because the demands made of smooth muscle for speed and force of contraction is considerably less, actin and myosin filaments are scattered in the cytoplasm; hence, the lack of striations. The sarcoplasm does not contain transverse tubules and has few sarcoplasmic reticulum for calcium storage. However, smooth muscle has specialized calcium binding regulatory proteins called **calmodulin,** which is similar to troponin in skeletal muscle. The sarcoplasm of smooth muscle contains scattered filaments (**dense bodies**) that are equivalent to the Z disks in the skeletal muscle. Dense bodies are also found attached to the sarcolemma. Other filaments interconnect adjacent dense bodies. The force generated by the sliding between the scattered actin and myosin filaments is generated to the dense bodies that, in turn, cause shortening of the muscle fiber.

Smooth muscle contractions are slower and last longer than those of skeletal or cardiac muscle. The lack of T tubules and scarce sarcoplasmic reticulum for calcium is one reason for the slower start and longer duration; therefore, it takes longer for calcium to diffuse into the cell and initiate sliding between the actin and myosin. The shortening produced in smooth muscle is also considerable, a result of the slow diffusion of calcium from the cell to the outside.

A special feature of smooth muscle is the ability to stretch and shorten to a greater extent and still maintain contractile function. Smooth muscle, like skeletal muscle, has muscle tone. This is important in the gut where the walls must maintain a steady pressure on the contents. It is also important in blood vessels that must maintain pressure.

Smooth muscle, similar to cardiac muscle, responds to changes in the local environment and factors such as hormones, ions, pH, temperature, and stretch.

There are two types of smooth muscle. The **single unit,** or **visceral smooth muscle fibers,** form large networks and are connected by gap junctions. This enables the smooth muscle to contract in waves when stimulated at one end of the organ. This is the more common type and it is found in the walls of small arteries and veins and walls of hollow organs.

The **multiunit smooth muscle** fibers act independently. Similar to skeletal muscle fiber, each muscle fiber is innervated, with few gap junctions between adjacent cells. Therefore, each fiber must be stimulated separately to produce contraction. These fibers are found in the walls of large arteries, bronchioles, arrector pili muscle attached to hair follicles, and muscles of the eye that control the size of the pupil and shape of the lens.

Smooth muscle can regenerate more than other muscle tissue, but much less than epithelial tissue.

Muscle Terminology and Major Muscles of the Body

MUSCLE TERMINOLOGY

It is important for massage therapists and other bodyworkers dealing with soft tissue to become familiar with terms relating to muscle and muscle contraction.

The most stationary point of muscle attachment, usually the proximal point, is called the **origin.** The **insertion** is the point of muscle attachment that is more mobile and moves with the bone, usually the more distal point. The changes produced to the joint by the contraction of the muscle are called the **action(s)** of the muscle. The action of a muscle can be identified by knowledge of its origin and insertion which, in turn, enables health professionals to effectively treat individuals who have difficulty executing certain move-

---

✔ **Plasticity**

Because the thick and thin filaments are not organized in smooth muscles, there is no direct relationship between tension developed and resting length in smooth muscle. A stretched smooth muscle soon adapts to its new length and retains the ability to contract on demand. This ability to function over a wide range of lengths is called plasticity.

✓ *Names of Muscles*

According to:

Organization of the fascicles (direction in which the muscle fibers run)
Obliquus—oblique direction of muscles
Rectus—parallel direction of fascicles
Transversus—transverse direction of fascicles

Location (region of the body)
Abdominis—in the abdomen
Anconeus—elbow
Anterior—in the front
Auricularis—near the ear
Brachialis—in the arm
Capitis—in the head
Carpi—in the wrist
Cervicis—in the neck
Clavius/cleido—near the clavicle
Coccygeus—near the coccyx
Costalis—near the ribs
Cutaneous—near the skin
Externus, extrinsic—toward the superficial/outer part of the body
Femoris—near the femur
Genio—near the chin
Glosso—tongue
Hallucis—big toe
Ilio—near the ilium
Inferioris—inferior
Inguinal—groin region
Internus, intrinsic—in the deeper/inner regions
Lateralis—away from the midline
Lumborus—lumbar region
Medialis/medius—toward the midline
Nasalis—nose
Nuchal—back of the neck
Oculo—near the eye
Oris—near the mouth
Palpebrae—eyelid area
Pollicis—thumb
Popliteus—behind the knee
Posterior—toward the back
Psoas—loin region
Radialis—radius
Scapularis—near the scapula
Superioris—superior
Temporalis—near the temple
Thoracic—thoracic region
Tibialis—tibia
Ulnaris—ulna

Structure (unique features of the muscle)
Alba—white
Biceps—has two heads or points of origin
Gracilis—graceful/slender
Triceps—has three heads or points of origin

Size
Brevis—small
Lata—wide
Latissimus—widest
Longus—long muscle
Magnus—big
Major—bigger
Maximus—biggest
Minimus—smallest
Minor—small

Shape
Deltoid—shaped like a triangle or delta
Orbicularis—circular
Piriformis—pear-shaped
Platys—flat
Rhomboideus—shaped like a rhomboid
Serratus—saw-toothed appearance
Splenius—bandage
Teres—long and round
Trapezius—trapezoid shape
Vastus—great

Actions
Abductor—moves away from midline
Adductor—moves towards midline
Buccinator—action of muscle when a trumpet is blown
Depressor—to lower
Extensor—increases angle between articulating bone
Flexor—reduces angle between articulating bone
Levator—to elevate
Pronator—moves forearm so that the palm faces back
Risorius—action of muscle when one laughs
Rotator—produces a rotating movement
Supinator—moves forearm so that the palm faces front
Sartorius—like a tailor (tailors used to sit cross-legged and this muscle produces this action)

ments. It must be remembered that difficulty moving specific bones is not always a result of malfunction of muscles that produce the movement. Problems in joint architecture, ligament structure, and skin over the joint, among others, may restrict movement.

Depending on the attachment site of a muscle to a bone, the joint can be moved in many directions.

These directions of movement have specific terms, and the standard terms for all movements are explained on **page 128.**

The movements produced by muscles are grouped according to their primary actions. A muscle is considered to be a **prime mover,** or **agonist,** if it is the main muscle or one of the main muscles producing a particular movement. For example, the biceps brachii is the prime mover for flexion of the forearm. **Antagonists** are prime movers that oppose the action of the agonist. In the above example, the triceps brachii located in the back of the upper arm is the antagonist.

A muscle that assists a prime mover in performing the movement is called a **synergist.** Synergists may assist by producing more pull at the insertion point or stabilizing the point of origin of the prime mover. They include muscles that often help the prime mover initiate the action when the power produced by the prime mover is not at its maximum. **Fixators** are muscles that stabilize the origin of the prime mover to increase efficiency.

NAMES OF MUSCLES

One of the most daunting tasks for any health professional is to learn the names of muscles. But this process is simplified if the meaning of certain terms is understood. Many muscles are named according to *organization of the fascicle, location, structure, size, shape, action, origin, insertion, and other striking features.* Some examples are given in **page 202.**

Origin and Insertion of Muscles

Knowledge of origin, insertion, and action of muscles is important for massage therapists to better serve their clients. This knowledge enables the therapist to

target specific groups of muscles according to their actions. Both agonists and antagonists of particular movements can be worked on effectively. Strokes can be directed in relation to the direction of the fascicles for maximum benefit. The therapist will be able to recommend innovative passive and active exercises according to the client's symptoms. Therefore, the therapist should have a thorough knowledge of muscle anatomy and physiology. The muscles in this book are described according to their actions in different regions.

THE AXIAL MUSCULATURE

Muscles Responsible for Facial Expression Changes

These muscles (see Figure 4.19 and Chapter Appendix Table 4.1) originate from the bones of the skull. The connective tissue surrounding the fascicles of these muscle fibers are woven into the connective tissue of the dermis of the skin. In this way, when the muscles contract, the skin moves and alters the expression on the face. All these muscles are innervated (receive nerve supply/stimulation) by the facial nerve (cranial nerve VII). As with all paired muscles, the right half of the face is innervated by the right nerve and the left side by the nerve on the left.

The larger muscles of facial expression are detailed in Chapter Appendix Table 4.1.

Muscles of Mastication

These muscles (see Figure 4.20 and Chapter Appendix Table 4.2) move the jaw and help chew and move food around the mouth. Most of these muscles are innervated by the trigeminal nerve (cranial nerve V).

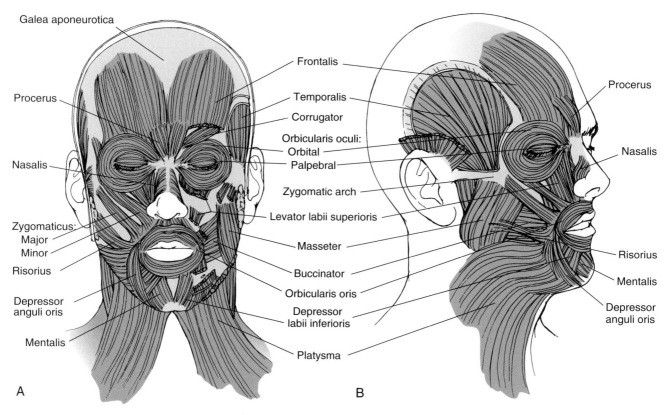

FIGURE **4.19.** Muscles of Facial Expression. **A,** Anterior View; **B,** Lateral View

Muscles of the Tongue

There are many tongue muscles, all names beginning with the region of origin and ending with the term *glossus,* meaning tongue. These muscles originate from the styloid process of the temporal bone (Figure 3.8), soft palate, hyoid bone, and medial surface of mandible around the chin; they are called **styloglossus, palatoglossus, hyoglossus,** and **genioglossus,** respectively. Together they move the tongue in all directions, enabling speech and movement of food in preparation for swallowing. Most muscles of the tongue are innervated by the hypoglossal nerve (cranial nerve XII).

Muscles of the Pharynx

These muscles are responsible for the swallowing process. Because the pharynx serves as a common passage for both food and air, all passages other than that of the food must be closed when food is swallowed (see **page 545**). Many pharyngeal muscles are present. (The individual names are not addressed by the book because they are not relevant to the audience. The student is encouraged to read an anatomy textbook for medical students for the individual names of pharyngeal muscles.)

Most muscles are innervated by the glossopharyngeal nerve (cranial nerve IX) and the vagus nerve

(cranial nerve X). Some muscles of the palate are innervated by the trigeminal nerve (cranial nerve V) and the accessory nerve (cranial nerve XI). The complexity of the swallowing process is realized when a nerve is injured; the person has difficulty swallowing and speaking. The food may enter the larynx and lead

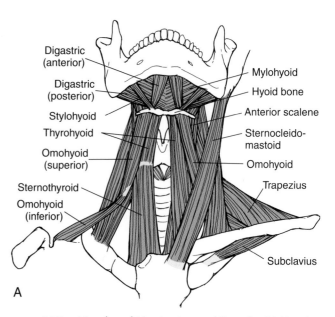

FIGURE **4.20.** Muscles of Mastication and Suprahyoid Muscles. **A,** Anterior View

(continued)

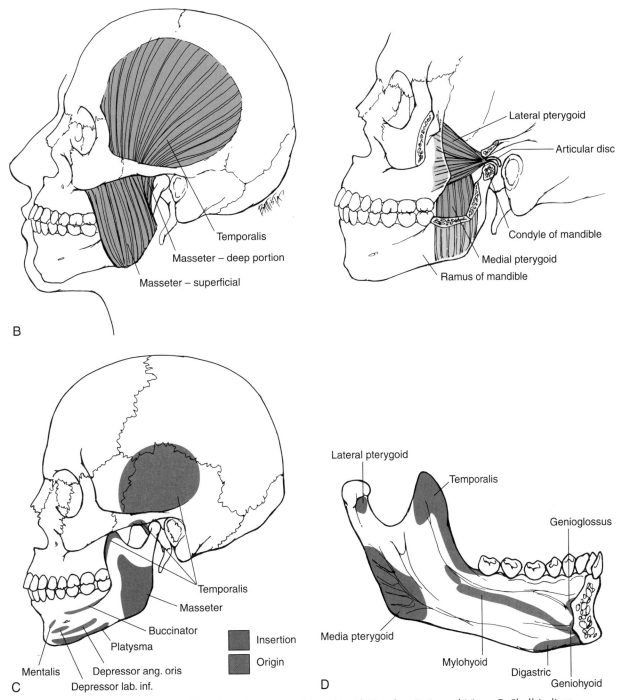

FIGURE **4.20., cont'd**   Muscles of Mastication and Suprahyoid Muscles. **B,** Lateral View; **C,** Skull Indicating Origin and Insertion of Muscles; **D,** Left Half of Mandible-Medial View

to lower respiratory tract infections and may also regurgitate into the nose.

Muscles of the Head and Neck

The muscles of the head and neck help position and move the head and assist with breathing, swallowing, and coughing.

Muscles of the Anterior Aspect of Neck

These muscles (see Figures 4.20A and 4.21) depress the mandible, tense the floor of the mouth, control the position of the larynx, and help provide a stable foundation for the muscles of the tongue and pharynx. The points of attachment of these muscles include the hyoid bone, the cartilages of larynx, the clavicle, and sternum.

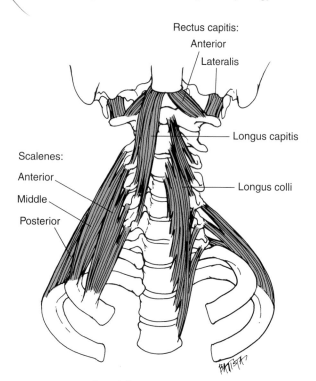

FIGURE **4.21.** Muscles of the Anterior Aspect of the Neck With Origin and Insertion

The **sternocleidomastoid** muscle becomes prominent in the front of the neck when the head is turned to one side. The sternocleidomastoid is the largest anterior muscle, acting on the head and neck. The origins and insertions of the small muscles of the neck are listed in Chapter Appendix Table 4.3. The names of many of these muscles suggest the origin and insertion (e.g., sternohyoid, stylohyoid, geniohyoid, thyrohyoid, sternothyroid, omohyoid). The sternocleidomastoid is innervated by the accessory nerve (cranial nerve XI).

Deep Muscles of the Neck, Anterior to the Cervical Spine

Deep skeletal muscles, posterior to the pharynx, just anterior to the cervical vertebrae help flex the cervical spine. The **longus capitis** extends from the transverse processes of the cervical vertebrae to the occipital bone and helps flex the head. Rotation of the head is aided by muscles (**longus cervicis**) that extend from the body of cervical and thoracic vertebrae to the transverse processes. All of these muscles are spinal muscles.

Muscles in the Posterior Aspect of Neck

Straplike muscles (see Figure 4.22 and Chapter Appendix Table 4.4) extending from the spinous and transverse processes of the thoracic and cervical vertebrae to the occipital bone help keep the head erect and extend and hyperextend the head. These muscles are covered by the origin of the trapezius.

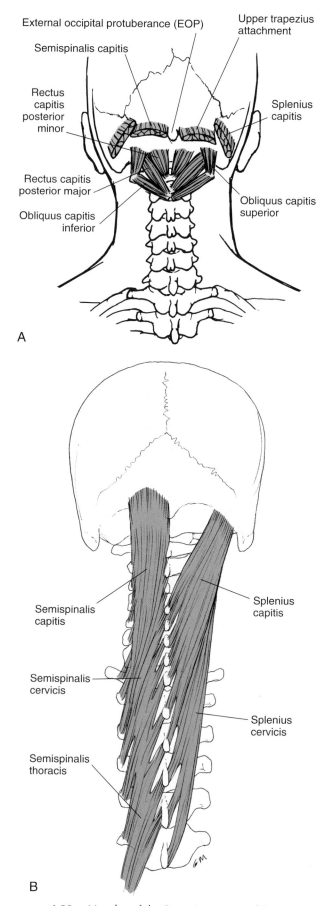

FIGURE **4.22.** Muscles of the Posterior Aspect of the Neck

The cervical muscles are those often injured in whiplash. In this condition, usually caused by car accidents, the head is thrown forward and then backward like a whip, injuring the structures in front and the back of the neck.

Muscles of the Trunk

The trunk muscles include those of the spine, thorax, abdomen, and pelvis. They help stabilize the trunk when the head and extremities move; protect the spine; and help maintain posture, breathing, coughing, straining. The abdominal muscles support and protect the viscera.

Muscles of the Spine

Some muscles of the spine (Chapter Appendix Table 4.5) have been described with the muscles of the neck. The muscles that move the spine are covered

Erector Spinae and Spinal Movement

The erector spinae is recruited completely during almost all movements of the spine. However, different groups are recruited according to the movement. The muscles closer to the spine favor extension and hyperextension and those farther away favor lateral flexion. Rotation is accomplished by those parts that have a diagonal line of pull with respect to the long axis.

posteriorly by large superficial muscles, such as the trapezius and latissimus dorsi.

The Spinal Extensors

The muscles that extend the spine are known as the **spinal extensors,** or **erector spinae,** muscles. They include the superficial and deep layers of muscles (see Figure 4.23).

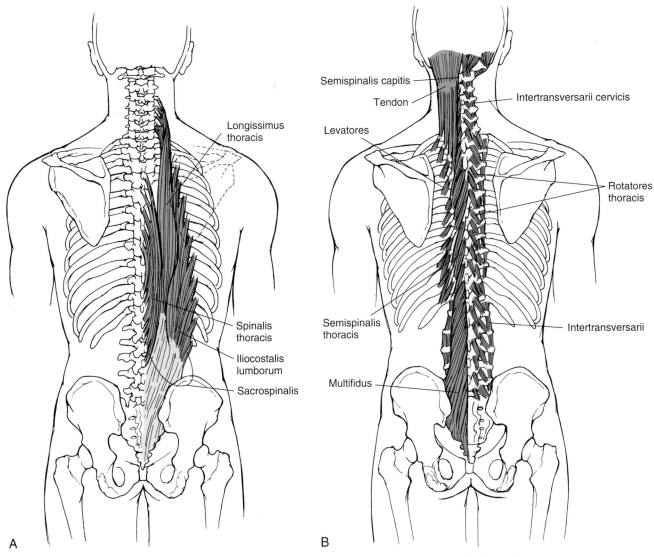

FIGURE **4.23.** Muscles of the Spine. **A,** Erector Spine; **B,** Intervertebral Muscles

The Superficial Muscles

The superficial layer of muscles can be divided (from medial to lateral) into the **spinalis, longissimus,** and **iliocostalis** divisions. The longissimus and iliocostalis are not distinct in the lower lumbar and sacral regions and are known as the **sacrospinalis** muscles. When muscles on both sides contract, the spine is extended. Contraction of one side bends the spine laterally (lateral flexion).

The spinalis group: The semispinalis muscles arise from the transverse processes of the spines and insert into the adjacent spinous processes. The spinalis muscles go from spinous process of one vertebra to spinous processes of others located above.

The longissimus group: The longissimus group extends from the transverse processes of lower vertebrae to those located above or to the ribs.

The iliocostalis group: The iliocostalis muscles extend from the ribs to the transverse processes of vertebrae and/or the ribs located above.

All spinal muscles are innervated by spinal nerves that exit from the spinal cord in the specific region of the muscle.

The Deep Muscles

The deep layer of muscles consists of smaller muscles that interconnect vertebrae and help stabilize the vertebral column. They also help extend or rotate the spine and are important for adjusting positions of individual spines. It is important for an athlete to stretch and warm these small muscles before any major activity. These muscles include the **intertransversarii, rotatores, interspinales,** and **multifidus.**

Spinal Flexors

Although all of the above muscles help with extension and rotation, there are few muscles that help with flexion. Certain large muscles of the trunk serve as major flexors of the spine; the **longus capitis** and **longus cervicis** rotate and flex the neck, and the **quadratus lumborum** muscles in the lumbar region flex the spine (Figure 4.24).

The origin, insertion, and action of individual groups of spinal muscles are listed in Table 4.5. The spinal muscles located in the neck have been previously discussed. It is not possible for the massage therapist to access individual muscles of the spine, and an idea of the general grouping of these muscles and general direction of fibers would suffice for most therapists.

Muscles of the Abdomen

The muscles of the abdomen (see Figure 4.24 and Chapter Appendix Table 4.6) are large and sheetlike,

with the fascicles running in different directions. These powerful muscles help protect the internal organs and flex and rotate the spine. The arrangement of the muscles is similar in the cervical, thoracic, and abdominal region because they all develop in the fetus from the same origin.

Located in the neck are the scalenes; in the thorax, the external intercostals, internal intercostals, and transversus thoracis; and in the abdomen, the external obliques, internal obliques, and transversus abdominis. The thoracic and the abdominal muscles are in three layers (see Chapter Appendix Tables 4.6 and 4.7). The innermost layer has fascicles running transversely. The internal intercostals and internal obliques (the middle layer) have muscle fascicles running upward and medially, similar to forward slashes (////). The outermost layer (the external intercostals and external obliques) has fibers running downward and medially, similar to backward slashes (\\\\) or the direction that hands are placed into pants pockets.

In addition to the oblique muscles described above, straplike muscles are seen in the cervical, thoracic, and abdominal regions. These muscles have fascicles running parallel and vertical. In the abdomen, the rectus abdominis runs near the midline from the xiphoid process to the pubic bone. A thick, connective tissue sheet, the **linea alba,** is seen in the midline, separating the right and the left rectus. The rectus muscle are segmented transversely by connective tissue (**transverse inscriptions**) and are respon-

---

✚ Cause of Hernia and Prolapse

The three muscle layers of the abdomen are powerful and can exert tremendous pressure on the internal organs if they contract. Because the diaphragm closes the abdominal cavity superiorly and the pelvis and the pelvic muscles close off the abdominopelvic cavity inferiorly, the abdominal contents, in effect, lie in a closed cavity. If the pressure inside the abdomen is constantly increased, such as in weight lifters and those with chronic cough, the organs are forced into weak areas of the cavity.

The weaker areas are around the umbilicus, the inguinal (groin) region, and around the opening through which the esophagus enters the abdomen, among others. When the intestines/organs are forced into these abnormal openings, they can become trapped and tissue death can occur if the blood supply to the trapped part is stopped. This condition is called **hernia.**

In individuals with weakened perineal muscles, the pelvic organs may descend and, in severe cases, protrude outside the body cavity. An example of this is **prolapse** of the uterus, in which the uterus descends into the vagina.

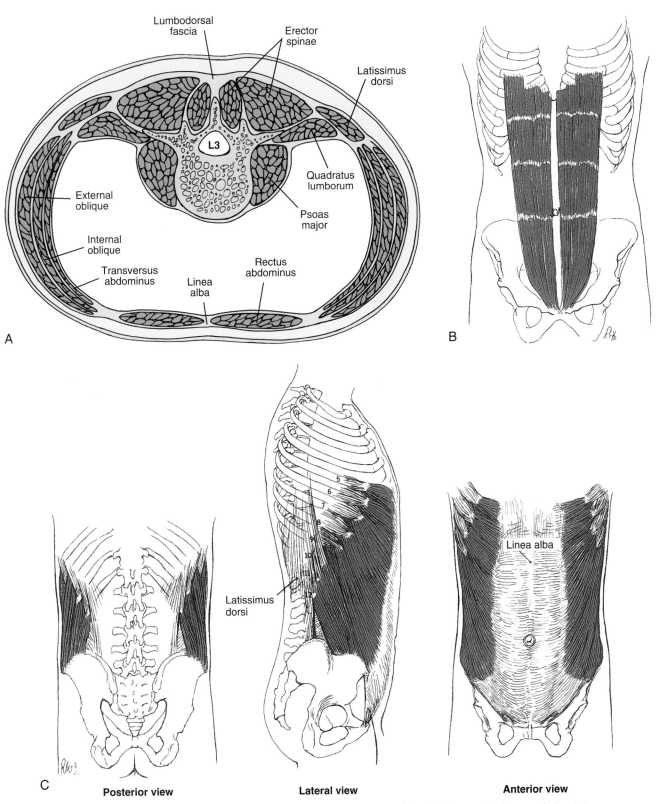

FIGURE 4.24. Muscles of the Abdomen. **A,** Transverse Section of the Abdomen; **B,** Rectus Abdominis; **C,** External Oblique

(continued)

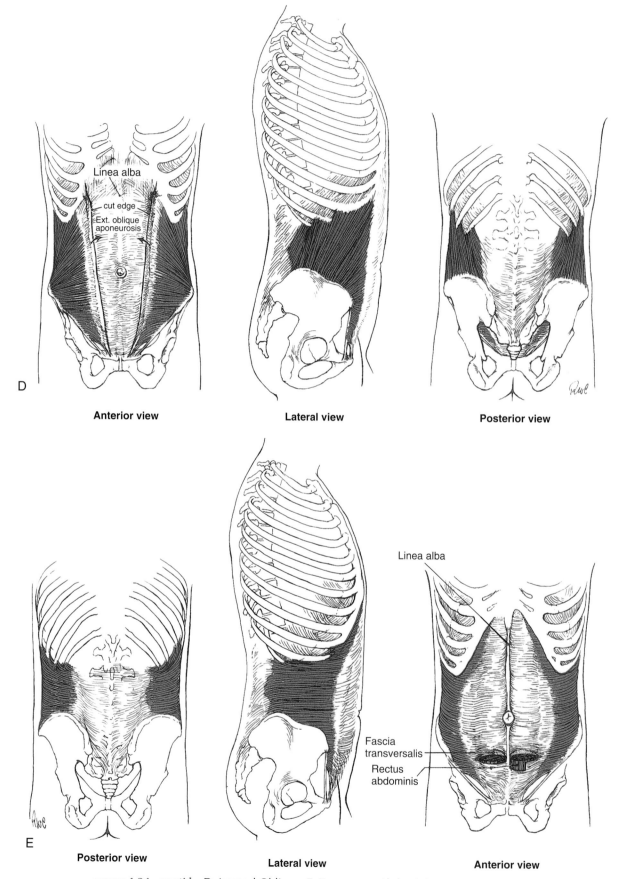

D

Linea alba
cut edge
Ext. oblique aponeurosis

Anterior view   **Lateral view**   **Posterior view**

E

Posterior view   **Lateral view**   **Anterior view**

Linea alba

Fascia transversalis

Rectus abdominis

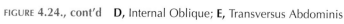

FIGURE **4.24., cont'd**   **D,** Internal Oblique; **E,** Transversus Abdominis

sible for the transverse indentations seen in front of the abdomen of a muscular individual.

Muscles of the Thorax

Many powerful muscles that support the shoulder girdle are attached to the thorax (see Figures 4.25, 4.27, and 4.28). Anteriorly, the pectoral group—the pectoral major and minor—are attached. Posteriorly, large muscles, such as the trapezius superiorly and latissimus dorsi inferiorly, cover the thorax before they reach their points of insertion. Muscles that support the scapula, such as the rhomboids, lie deep to the trapezius over the thorax. Posteriorly, closer to midline and deep to the trapezius, are the muscles of the spine (previously described). In the sides, the thoracic cage is covered by the serratus anterior, which has an origin with a saw-toothed appearance. This muscle inserts into the medial border of the scapula. Because all of the above muscles are involved with the pectoral girdle, only the deepest layers are described here. For details of the other muscles, see Muscles That Move the Shoulder.

Together with the intercostals, the diaphragm (see Figures 4.25, 4.26, and Table 4.7) is an important muscle involved in respiratory movements. It is a sheet of muscle with a central connective tissue section. The diaphragm separates the thoracic cavity from the abdominopelvic cavity, and structures passing from one cavity to the other pierce through the diaphragm. It, therefore, has a circular origin and inserts into the connective tissue sheet in the center, the **central tendinous sheet.** The diaphragm is a powerful muscle used during inspiration. It is innervated by the phrenic nerve that descends all the way from cervical regions C3–C5.

Muscles of the Pelvic Floor

There are many muscles that extend from the sacrum and coccyx to the ischium and pubis, supporting the

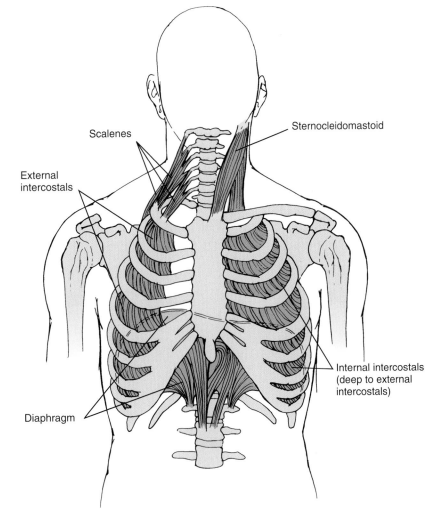

FIGURE **4.25.** Muscles of the Thorax

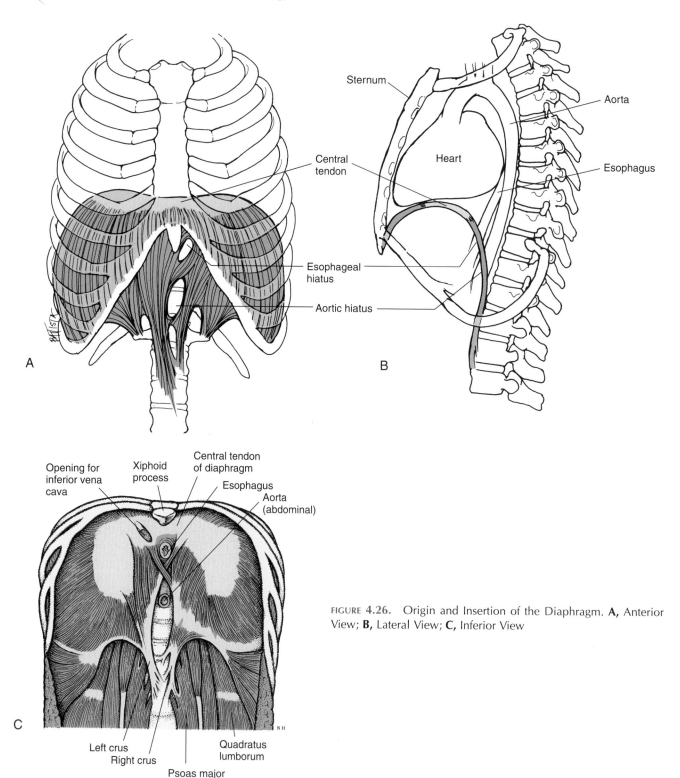

FIGURE **4.26.** Origin and Insertion of the Diaphragm. **A,** Anterior View; **B,** Lateral View; **C,** Inferior View

organs of the pelvic cavity, flexing the sacrum and coccyx, and controlling the movement of material through the urethra, vagina (females), and the anus. These muscles form the **pelvic floor,** or **perineum.** Sphincters—circular muscles—guard the openings and provide voluntary control. In males, some super-ficial muscles compress the base and stiffen the penis and help with ejaculation of semen and passage of urine. (The names of the individual muscles are be-yond the scope of this book. The student is encour-aged to refer to any standard anatomy textbook for details of these muscles.)

The Diaphragm

Because the liver is below the diaphragm, the right side of the diaphragm is higher than the left. Pregnant women tend to rely more on the movement of the intercostal muscles for breathing because the diaphragmatic movements are restricted, especially late in pregnancy.

Because the diaphragm is supplied by the phrenic nerve arising in the cervical region, irritation to the diaphragm can often reflect as pain (referred pain) in the shoulder because the skin of the shoulder is supplied by sensory nerves arising in the cervical regions C3–C5.

Winging of the Scapula

Loss of the serratus anterior seriously impairs the ability to reach forward with the arm because that action must be accompanied by abduction of the scapula to align the glenoid fossa in a forward direction. Similarly, subjects who have paralysis of the serratus anterior are typically unable to raise their arms overhead because of muscular insufficiency in upward rotation. This muscle, along with the rhomboids, holds the scapula close to the rib cage; paralysis of the serratus anterior can result in "winging of the scapula." (See figure on page 326.)

THE APPENDICULAR MUSCULATURE

The appendicular musculature includes muscles that help stabilize and position the pectoral and pelvic girdle and move the upper and lower limbs.

To make it more practical and applicable to bodyworkers, the muscles of the pectoral girdle and upper limbs are described in four groups; each group, in turn, being subdivided according to the movements they perform. The four groups are: (1) Muscles that position and move the shoulder girdle; (2) Muscles that move the arm; (3) Muscles that move the forearm and wrist; and (4) Muscles that move the palm and fingers.

Muscles That Position and Move the Shoulder Girdle

These muscles (Figure 4.27 and Chapter Appendix Table 4.8) stabilize the scapula and clavicle. As mentioned, the only joint in the pectoral girdle that articulates with the axial skeleton is at the sternoclavicular joint. The scapula and the clavicle are held in

place by the numerous muscles that originate from the axial skeleton.

Muscles That Move the Arm

The muscles that move the arm (Figure 4.28 and Chapter Appendix Table 4.9) cross the shoulder joint

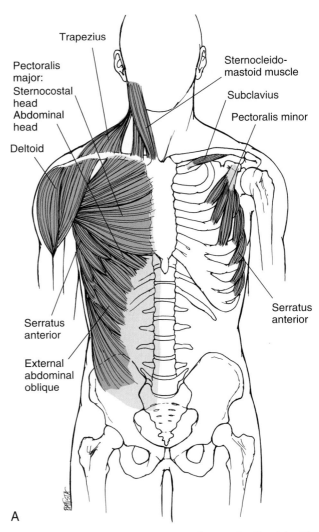

FIGURE **4.27.**   Muscles That Position and Move the Shoulder Girdle. **A,** Anterior View   *(continued)*

Rotator Cuff Muscles

The infraspinatus, supraspinatus, subscapularis, and teres minor are the **rotator cuff** muscles and they are a frequent site of injury in athletes. The rotator cuff muscles are grouped together because (1) they all have rotational functions on the humerus, and (2) their tendons are interwoven into the capsule to form a musculotendinous cuff around the joint. The rotator cuff muscles act together to hold the head of the humerus against the glenoid fossa and stabilize the joint. They contract along with the deltoid during abduction and flexion. If the deltoid contracted alone, its line of pull would cause the humerus to hit the acromion process. If the rotator cuff muscles contracted alone they would depress the head of the humerus. Acting together, the deltoid and cuff muscles produce proper abduction and flexion.

Damage to the rotator cuff is more common in those who engage in repetitive movements that include holding the arm above the head.

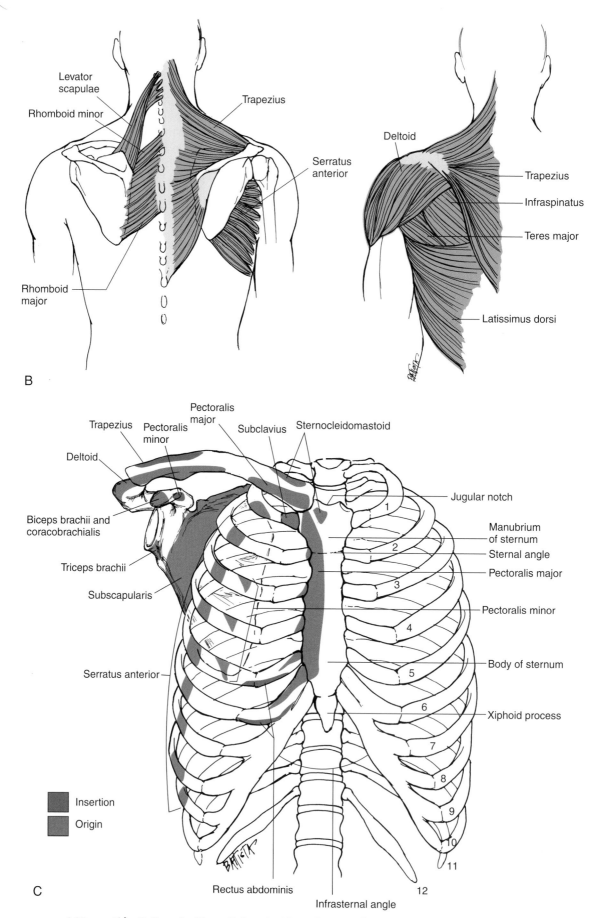

B

Levator
scapulae

Trapezius

Rhomboid minor

Serratus
anterior

Rhomboid
major

Deltoid

Trapezius

Infraspinatus

Teres major

Latissimus dorsi

Pectoralis
major

Trapezius   Pectoralis   Subclavius   Sternocleidomastoid
              minor

Deltoid

Jugular notch

Biceps brachii and
coracobrachialis

Manubrium
of sternum

Sternal angle

Pectoralis major

Triceps brachii

Subscapularis

Pectoralis minor

Serratus anterior

Body of sternum

Xiphoid process

Insertion

Origin

Rectus abdominis

Infrasternal angle

C

FIGURE 4.27., cont'd   B, Posterior View; C, Anterior View of Bones, Showing Origin and Insertion of Muscles

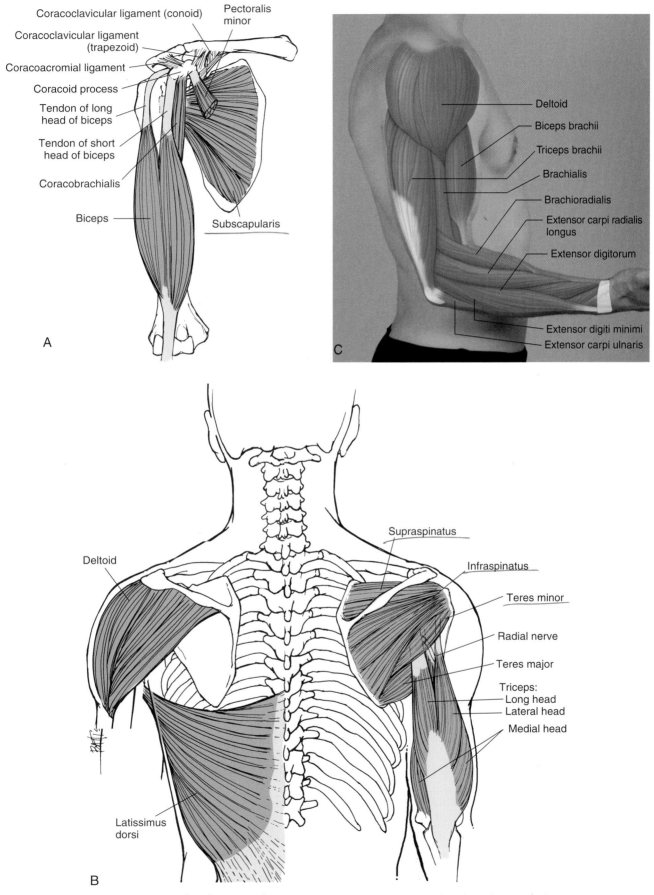

FIGURE **4.28.**   Muscles That Move the Arm. **A,** Anterior View; **B,** Posterior View; **C,** Lateral View
(continued)

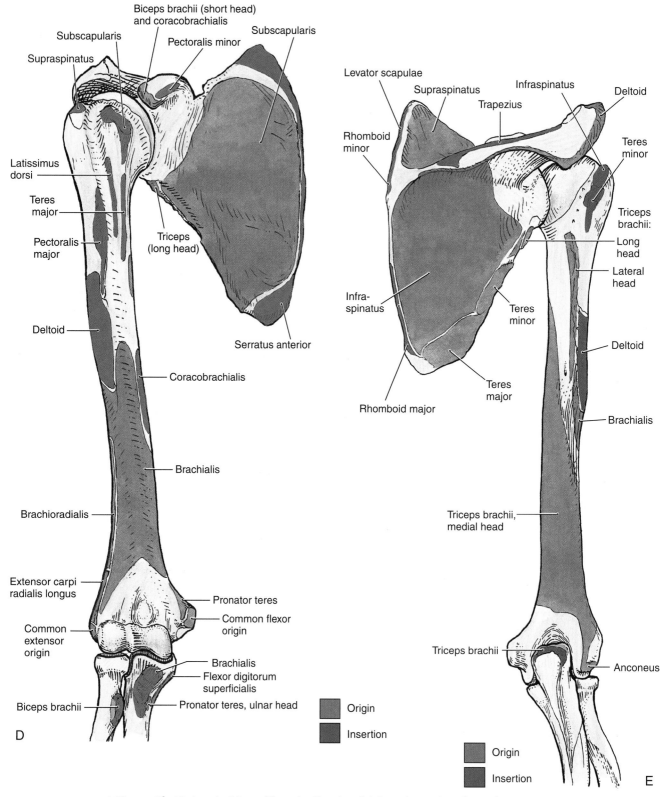

FIGURE **4.28., cont'd** **D,** Anterior View of Scapula, Showing Origin and Insertion of Muscles; **E,** Posterior View of Bones, Showing Origin and Insertion of Muscles

✓ *Muscles Moving Scapula*

Place the thumb and long finger along the scapular spine of your partner. When palpating, note the movements of the scapula as the arm is moved through the full range of flexion-extension, abduction-adduction, and internal-external rotation. Identify the groups of muscles involved in each movement.

and attach to the humerus, around or close to the humeral head. They originate posteriorly from the scapula and the vertebrae. Anteriorly, the muscles originate from the sternum, the cartilage of ribs 2–6, and the clavicle.

Muscles That Move the Forearm and Wrist

The muscles that move the forearm and wrist (see Figure 4.29 and Chapter Appendix Table 4.10) generally have their origins in the humerus (except for biceps brachii and the triceps brachii) and cross the elbow and/or wrist joint. At the elbow, the muscles

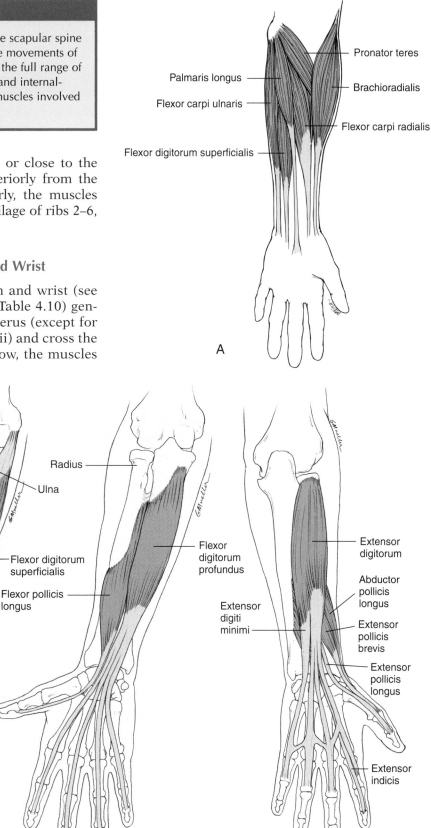

FIGURE 4.29. Muscles That Move the Forearm and Wrist. **A,** Anterior View of Right Upper Limb; **B,** Anterior View (Superficial); **C,** Anterior View (Deep); **D,** Posterior view   *(continued)*

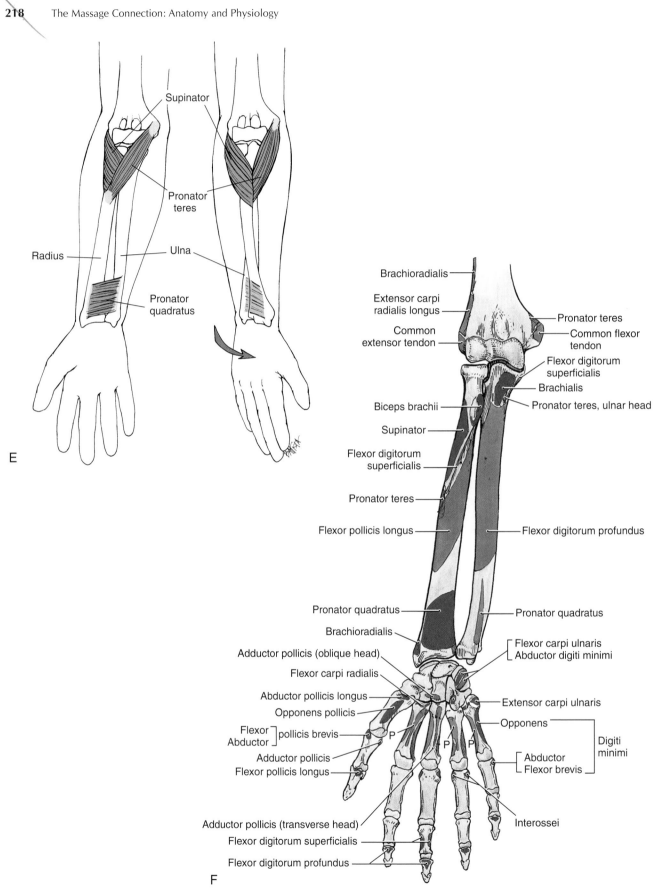

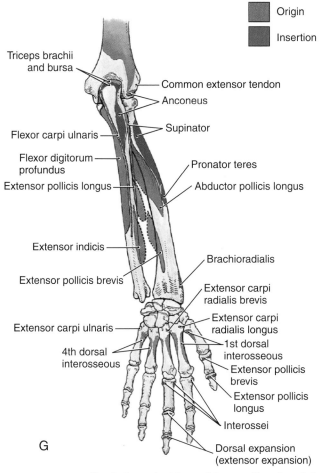

Origin

Insertion

Triceps brachii and bursa

Common extensor tendon

Anconeus

Flexor carpi ulnaris

Supinator

Flexor digitorum profundus

Pronator teres

Extensor pollicis longus

Abductor pollicis longus

Extensor indicis

Brachioradialis

Extensor pollicis brevis

Extensor carpi radialis brevis

Extensor carpi ulnaris

Extensor carpi radialis longus

4th dorsal interosseous

1st dorsal interosseous

Extensor pollicis brevis

Extensor pollicis longus

Interossei

G

Dorsal expansion (extensor expansion)

FIGURE **4.29., cont'd G,** Posterior View of Bones, Showing Origin and Insertion of Muscles

produce flexion and extension of the forearm. In addition, some muscles, by rotating the radius over the lower end of the ulna, pronate (palm faces posteriorly) and supinate (palm faces anteriorly) the forearm.

Flexion, extension, abduction, and adduction are movements that are brought about at the wrist. *Note that all the extensors arise on the lateral aspect of humerus and flexors on the medial aspect.*

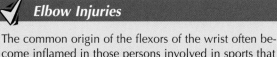

Elbow Injuries

The common origin of the flexors of the wrist often become inflamed in those persons involved in sports that require forceful flexion of wrist (e.g., baseball). This condition is known as **pitcher's arm, tennis elbow, or medial epicondylitis.**

Similarly, the common origin of the extensors can become inflamed in golfers. This condition is known as **golfer's elbow, or lateral epicondylitis.**

Muscles of Wrist and Hand

There are eight forearm muscles that originate on or just above the epicondyles of the humerus and insert distal to the wrist. What are they?

There are 25 muscles or muscle groups that are movers of the joints of the wrist and hand. The extrinsic muscles (15 muscles) are those that have their muscle bellies between the elbow and the wrist and the tendons insert in the hand. Intrinsic muscles are the remaining 10 muscles or muscle groups that originate and insert within the hand.

Muscles That Move the Palm and Fingers

Many muscles involved in moving the palm and fingers (see Figure 4.30 and Chapter Appendix Table 4.11) are located in the forearm, with just the tendons extending onto the palm. This is an efficient way of increasing finger mobility and maintaining strength. Imagine how bulky the hand would be if all the muscles controlling the fingers arose in the palm! These muscles, the **extrinsic muscles,** primarily provide strength and are responsible for crude control of the hand. For finer control, small muscles arising from the carpals and metacarpals are known as the **intrinsic muscles** of the hand.

Carpal Tunnel

The tendons of the muscles rising from the forearm are held in place against the carpals by connective tis-

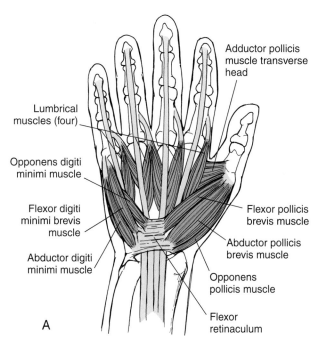

Adductor pollicis muscle transverse head

Lumbrical muscles (four)

Opponens digiti minimi muscle

Flexor digiti minimi brevis muscle

Abductor digiti minimi muscle

Flexor pollicis brevis muscle

Abductor pollicis brevis muscle

Opponens pollicis muscle

Flexor retinaculum

A

FIGURE **4.30.** Muscles That Move the Palm and Fingers. **A,** Anterior View

(continued)

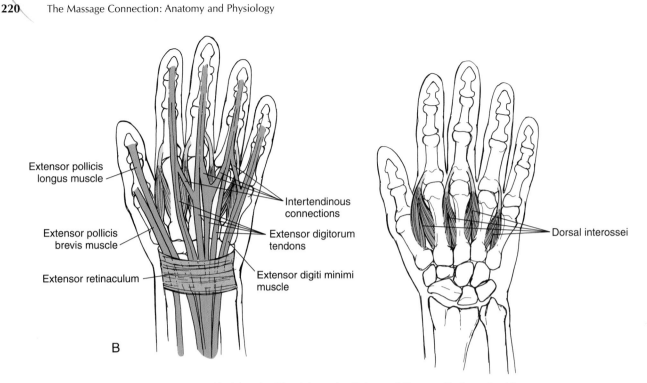

Extensor pollicis longus muscle

Extensor pollicis brevis muscle

Extensor retinaculum

Intertendinous connections

Extensor digitorum tendons

Extensor digiti minimi muscle

Dorsal interossei

B

FIGURE 4.30., cont'd   Muscles That Move the Palm and Fingers. **B,** Posterior View

sue sheets called **retinaculum.** The flexors are held in place by the **flexor retinaculum** and the extensors by the **extensor retinaculum.** The flexor retinaculum is a stamp-sized sheet of connective tissue running anteriorly across the carpals. It forms a tunnel—carpal tunnel—through which nine flexor tendons and the median nerve pass (see Figure 4.31 and **Figure 3.43**). The carpal tunnel is a narrow, rigid passage formed by the carpal bones of the wrist and the tough, inelastic **transverse carpal ligament,** or flexor retinaculum. As the tendons pass through the tunnel, they are surrounded by connective tissue sheaths (**tendon sheaths** or **synovial sheaths**) that are filled with synovial fluid. These sheaths reduce friction between the tendons as they move, lying close together in the wrist area. The median nerve in the carpal tunnel carries impulses to the muscles of the thumb and sensations from the skin over the thumb and the palmar surface of the lateral three and a half fingers.

The intrinsic muscles of the hand adduct, abduct, flex, and extend the fingers. Muscles are also present that help oppose the thumb and little finger. The bellies of the muscles that specifically move the thumb form a bulge on the lateral side of the palm called the **thenar eminence.** Those moving the little finger form a smaller bulge called the **hypothenar eminence.**

An Overview of Innervation of the Upper Limb

The muscles of the upper limb (see Figure 4.32 and Chapter Appendix Table 4.12) are innervated by nerves that arise from the cervical and upper thoracic segments of the spinal cord: C5–C8 and T1 (with contributions from C4 and T2). The nerve fibers (axons from these segments) form a network in the neck called the **brachial plexus** (see **page 325**). From this network, after dividing and subdividing, five large nerves (nerve fiber bundles) are formed that go down

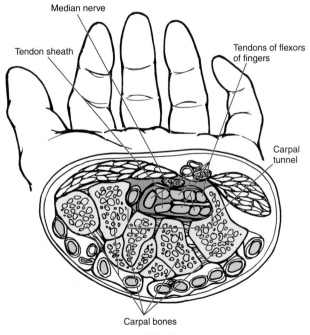

Median nerve

Tendon sheath

Tendons of flexors of fingers

Carpal tunnel

Carpal bones

FIGURE 4.31.   The Carpal Tunnel

Compartments in the Leg

The muscles of the forearm and the leg are compartmentalized by thick, connective tissue. Blood vessels and nerves enter each compartment to supply specific muscles. Occasionally, pressure can build up in these compartments if there is injury or inflammation. Because the connective tissue sheets are strong, they do not allow expansion to take place as fluid accumulates in the inflamed compartment. This results in pressure on the nerves and blood vessels and pain. This condition is known as **compartment syndrome.**

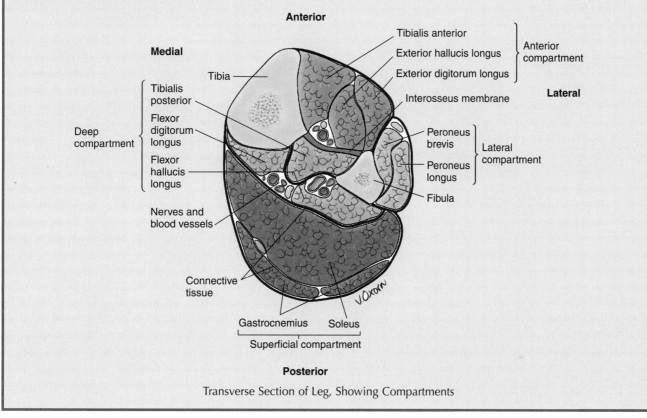

Transverse Section of Leg, Showing Compartments

the arm to innervate the muscles. The nerves are the **axillary, musculocutaneous, median, ulnar,** and **radial.**

A general description of the nerve supply of these muscles is given in Chapter Appendix Table 4.12.

MUSCLES OF THE LOWER LIMB

The muscles of the lower limb will be addressed in three functional groups: (1) muscles that move the

 Intramuscular Hematoma of Thigh

The **dead leg, charley horse,** or **cork thigh injury** is a result of a direct blow to the thigh, usually involving the vastus lateralis or intermedius. The blood vessels in the muscle may rupture, with bleeding inside the muscle. The muscle enclosed in its fascial compartment becomes bulkier as a result of the bleeding and inflammation, thereby, restricting flexion of the knee.

 HAMSTRINGS

The hamstrings are so named because these tendons can be used to suspend ham during curing.

thigh; (2) muscles that move the leg; and (3) muscles that move the foot and toes.

Muscles That Move the Thigh

The muscles that move the thigh arise from the pelvis, except for the psoas that arises from the lower thoracic and lumbar vertebrae (see Figure 4.33 and Chapter Appendix Table 4.13). Those arising posteriorly help extend the thigh, and those arising anteriorly help flex the thigh. Medially placed muscles (inner thigh) help adduction and those inserted laterally on the femur, help abduction. Muscles that are inserted medially and in the anterior aspect of the femur help rotate the leg medially. Those inserted into the lateral or posterior aspect of the femur produce

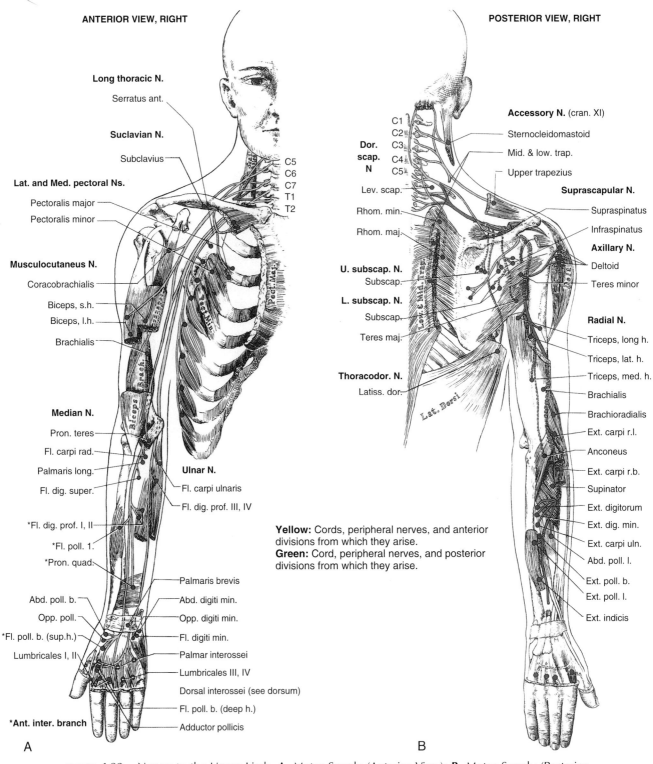

ANTERIOR VIEW, RIGHT

Long thoracic N.
Serratus ant.

Suclavian N.
Subclavius

C5
C6
C7
T1
T2

Lat. and Med. pectoral Ns.
Pectoralis major
Pectoralis minor

Musculocutaneus N.
Coracobrachialis
Biceps, s.h.
Biceps, l.h.
Brachialis

Median N.
Pron. teres
Fl. carpi rad.
Palmaris long.
Fl. dig. super.
*Fl. dig. prof. I, II
*Fl. poll. 1.
*Pron. quad.

Abd. poll. b.
Opp. poll.
*Fl. poll. b. (sup.h.)
Lumbricales I, II

Ulnar N.
Fl. carpi ulnaris
Fl. dig. prof. III, IV

Palmaris brevis
Abd. digiti min.
Opp. digiti min.
Fl. digiti min.
Palmar interossei
Lumbricales III, IV
Dorsal interossei (see dorsum)
Fl. poll. b. (deep h.)
Adductor pollicis

*Ant. inter. branch

A

POSTERIOR VIEW, RIGHT

C1
C2
C3
C4
C5

Dor.
scap.
N

Accessory N. (cran. XI)
Sternocleidomastoid
Mid. & low. trap.
Upper trapezius

Lev. scap.
Rhom. min.
Rhom. maj.

Suprascapular N.
Supraspinatus
Infraspinatus

Axillary N.
Deltoid
Teres minor

U. subscap. N.
Subscap.
L. subscap. N.
Subscap.
Teres maj.

Radial N.
Triceps, long h.
Triceps, lat. h.
Triceps, med. h.
Brachialis
Brachioradialis
Ext. carpi r.l.
Anconeus
Ext. carpi r.b.
Supinator
Ext. digitorum
Ext. dig. min.
Ext. carpi uln.
Abd. poll. l.
Ext. poll. b.
Ext. poll. l.
Ext. indicis

Thoracodor. N.
Latiss. dor.

Lat. Dorsi

B

Yellow: Cords, peripheral nerves, and anterior divisions from which they arise.
Green: Cord, peripheral nerves, and posterior divisions from which they arise.

FIGURE 4.32.   Nerves to the Upper Limb. **A,** Motor Supply (Anterior View); **B,** Motor Supply (Posterior View) *(continued)*

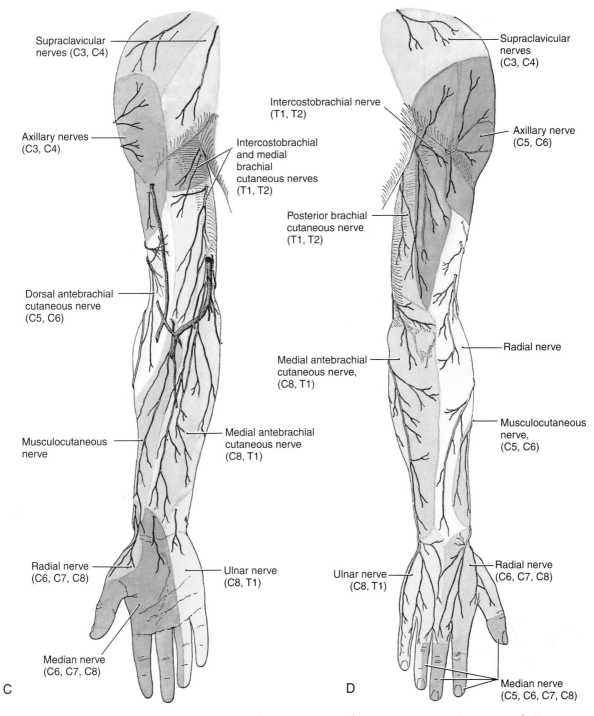

Supraclavicular
nerves (C3, C4)

Axillary nerves
(C3, C4)

Intercostobrachial
and medial
brachial
cutaneous nerves
(T1, T2)

Dorsal antebrachial
cutaneous nerve
(C5, C6)

Musculocutaneous
nerve

Medial antebrachial
cutaneous nerve
(C8, T1)

Radial nerve
(C6, C7, C8)

Ulnar nerve
(C8, T1)

Median nerve
(C6, C7, C8)

C

Intercostobrachial nerve
(T1, T2)

Supraclavicular
nerves
(C3, C4)

Axillary nerve
(C5, C6)

Posterior brachial
cutaneous nerve
(T1, T2)

Radial nerve

Medial antebrachial
cutaneous nerve,
(C8, T1)

Musculocutaneous
nerve,
(C5, C6)

Ulnar nerve
(C8, T1)

Radial nerve
(C6, C7, C8)

Median nerve
(C5, C6, C7, C8)

D

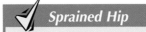

FIGURE **4.32., cont'd**   Nerves to the Upper Limb. **C,** Sensory Supply (Anterior View); **D,** Sensory supply (Posterior View)

lateral rotation. By knowing the origin and insertion of the muscles, the primary and secondary actions can be identified.

The gluteus maximus is the largest muscle located posteriorly. It inserts into a thick connective tissue sheet, the **iliotibial tract.** This tract is responsible for the indentation produced in the lateral part of the thigh when standing. The tract inserts into the upper

> ### Sprained Hip
>
> A forced extension of the hip may sprain the anterior iliofemoral ligament. This causes flexor spasm of the hip, tenderness over the front of the hip, and pain on extension. Recovery may take 3 to 4 months. Hip strengthening and mobilizing exercises are important.

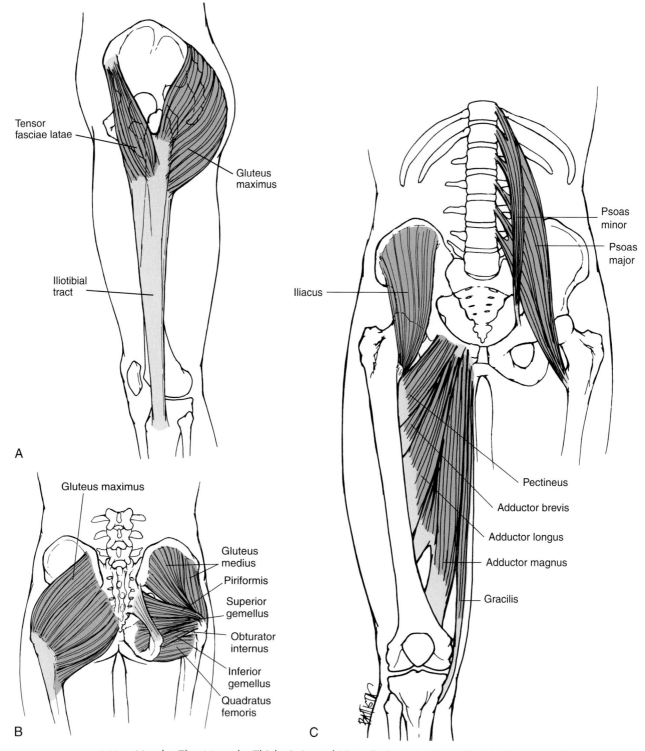

FIGURE **4.33.**   Muscles That Move the Thigh. **A,** Lateral View; **B,** Posterior View (Deep); **C,** Anterior View
(continued)

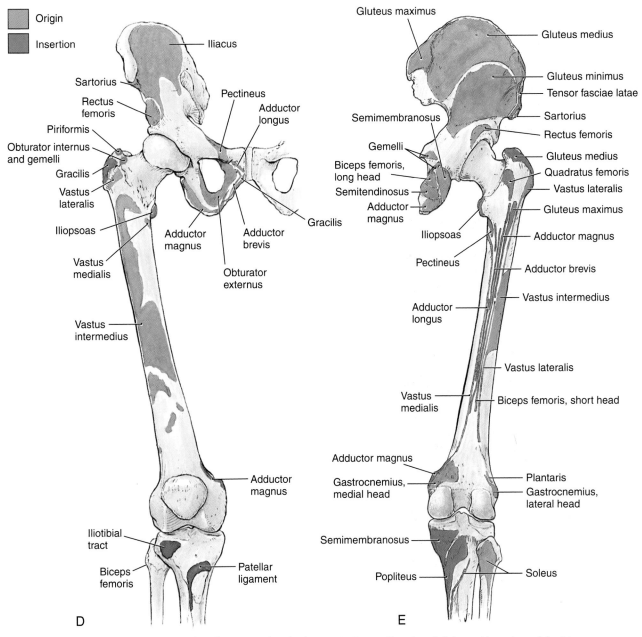

Origin

Insertion

Iliacus
Sartorius
Rectus femoris
Pectineus
Adductor longus
Piriformis
Obturator internus and gemelli
Gracilis
Vastus lateralis
Iliopsoas
Adductor magnus
Adductor brevis
Gracilis
Vastus medialis
Obturator externus
Vastus intermedius
Adductor magnus
Iliotibial tract
Biceps femoris
Patellar ligament

D

Gluteus maximus
Gluteus medius
Gluteus minimus
Tensor fasciae latae
Semimembranosus
Sartorius
Rectus femoris
Gemelli
Gluteus medius
Biceps femoris, long head
Quadratus femoris
Semitendinosus
Vastus lateralis
Adductor magnus
Gluteus maximus
Iliopsoas
Adductor magnus
Pectineus
Adductor brevis
Vastus intermedius
Adductor longus
Vastus lateralis
Vastus medialis
Biceps femoris, short head
Adductor magnus
Plantaris
Gastrocnemius, medial head
Gastrocnemius, lateral head
Semimembranosus
Popliteus
Soleus

E

FIGURE **4.33., cont'd**   Muscles That Move the Thigh. **D,** Hip Bone, Showing Origin and Insertion of the Muscles (Anterior View); **E,** Hip Bone, Showing Origin and Insertion of the Muscles (Posterior View)

end of tibia and helps brace the knee laterally. Table 4.13 shows the origin, insertion, and action of the muscles that move the thigh.

Muscles That Move the Leg

The arrangement of muscles in the lower limb is similar to that of the upper limb (see Figure 4.34 and Chapter Appendix Table 4.14). It must be remembered that flexion at the knee results in moving the lower leg posteriorly, unlike the upper limb where

Action of Rectus Femoris and Hamstrings

The rectus femoris and hamstrings serve as agonists and antagonists in many movements of the hip and knee. If the hip is flexed and the knee extended, the rectus is the agonist and the hamstrings become the antagonist. The opposite happens when the movement is reversed.

When both the hip and the knee are flexed simultaneously, both the hamstrings and rectus femoris are agonists at one joint and antagonists at the other!

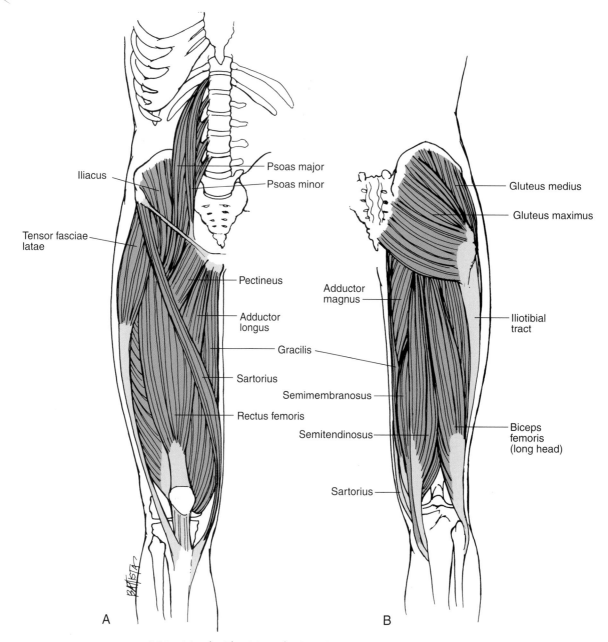

FIGURE **4.34.** Muscles That Move the Leg. **A,** Anterior View; **B,** Posterior View *(continued)*

flexion of the elbow results in anterior movement of the forearm. The extensor group of muscles is located in the anterior and lateral aspect of the thigh; the flexors are located posteriorly and medially.

Muscles That Move the Foot and Toes

As in the forearm, extrinsic muscles of the foot are located in the anterior and posterior aspect of the tibia (see Figure 4.35 and Chapter Appendix Table 4.15). Those located posteriorly help with plantar flexion, and the muscles located anteriorly help extend or dorsiflex the foot. The large muscles located in the posterior aspect of the calf form a strong, thick tendon called the **Achilles tendon,** or **tendo calcaneus** or **calcaneal tendon.** It is formed by the fusion of the soleus and gastrocnemius muscles.

Intrinsic Muscles of the Toes

Like the intrinsic muscles of the hand, numerous muscles help adduct, abduct, flex, and extend the toes (see Figure 4.36 and Chapter Appendix Table 4.16). They arise from the tarsals and insert into the phalanges.

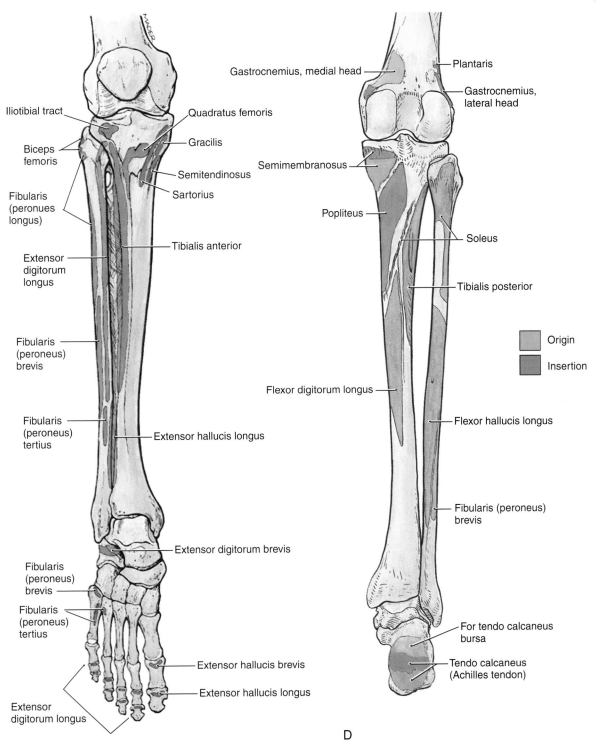

Iliotibial tract

Biceps femoris

Fibularis (peronues longus)

Extensor digitorum longus

Fibularis (peroneus) brevis

Fibularis (peroneus) tertius

Fibularis (peroneus) brevis

Fibularis (peroneus) tertius

Extensor digitorum longus

Quadratus femoris

Gracilis

Semitendinosus

Sartorius

Tibialis anterior

Extensor hallucis longus

Extensor digitorum brevis

Extensor hallucis brevis

Extensor hallucis longus

C

Gastrocnemius, medial head

Plantaris

Gastrocnemius, lateral head

Semimembranosus

Popliteus

Soleus

Tibialis posterior

Flexor digitorum longus

Flexor hallucis longus

Fibularis (peroneus) brevis

For tendo calcaneus bursa

Tendo calcaneus (Achilles tendon)

Origin

Insertion

D

FIGURE **4.34.**, cont'd   Muscles That Move the Leg. **C,** Bones, Showing Origin and Insertion of Muscle (Anterior View, Dorsal Aspect of Foot); **D,** Bones, Showing Origin and Insertion of Muscle (Posterior View)

Shinsplints

Shinsplints is a rather loose term that describes pain in the shin caused by activities such as running. The tugging of the medial border of the tibia by the fascia covering the soleus, gastrocnemius muscles, and other muscles, causes the periosteum to rise up from the bone with resultant inflammation.

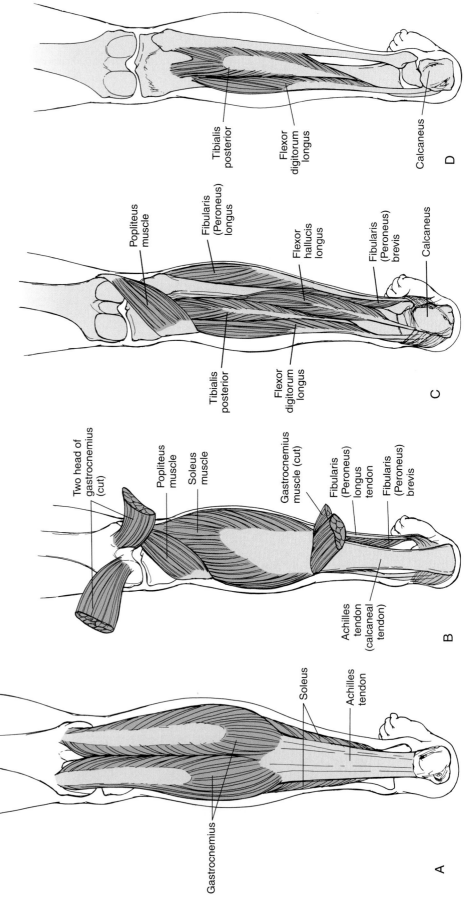

Gastrocnemius

Soleus

Achilles tendon

A

Two head of gastrocnemius (cut)

Popliteus muscle

Soleus muscle

Gastrocnemius muscle (cut)

Fibularis (Peroneus) longus tendon

Fibularis (Peroneus) brevis

Achilles tendon (calcaneal tendon)

B

Popliteus muscle

Fibularis (Peroneus) longus

Flexor hallucis longus

Fibularis (Peroneus) brevis

Calcaneus

Tibialis posterior

Flexor digitorum longus

C

Tibialis posterior

Flexor digitorum longus

Calcaneus

D

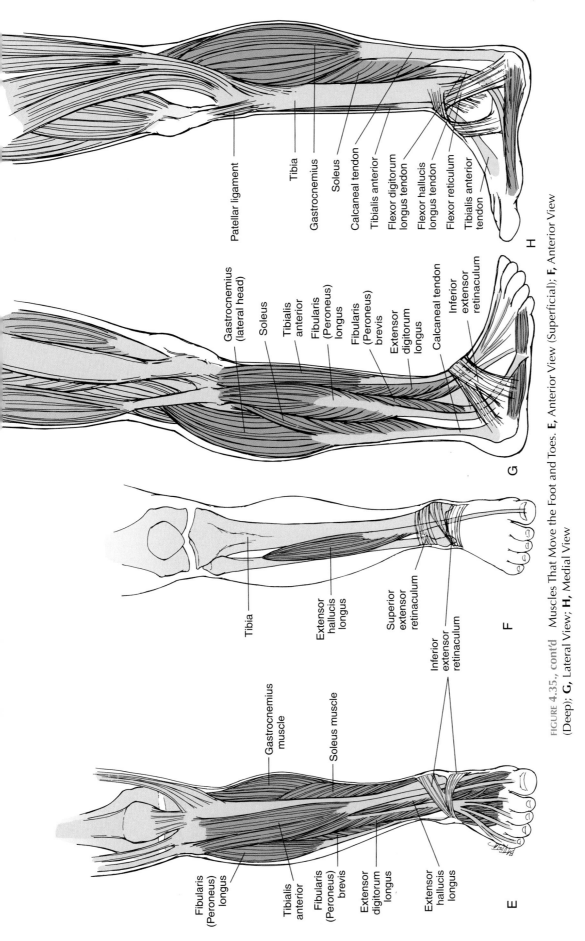

Patellar ligament

Tibia

Gastrocnemius

Soleus

Calcaneal tendon

Tibialis anterior

Flexor digitorum longus tendon

Flexor hallucis longus tendon

Flexor reticulum

Tibialis anterior tendon

H

Gastrocnemius (lateral head)

Soleus

Tibialis anterior

Fibularis (Peroneus) longus

Fibularis (Peroneus) brevis

Extensor digitorum longus

Calcaneal tendon

Inferior extensor retinaculum

G

Tibia

Extensor hallucis longus

Superior extensor retinaculum

Inferior extensor retinaculum

F

Fibularis (Peroneus) longus

Tibialis anterior

Fibularis (Peroneus) brevis

Extensor digitorum longus

Extensor hallucis longus

Gastrocnemius muscle

Soleus muscle

E

FIGURE 4.35., cont'd   Muscles That Move the Foot and Toes. **E,** Anterior View (Superficial); **F,** Anterior View (Deep); **G,** Lateral View; **H,** Medial View

Adductor and Iliopsoas Strains

These strains occur in the belly of adductor longus or adductor magnus and are a result of forced abduction or resisted adduction. It is a common injury in football.

Injury to the iliopsoas muscle is commonly referred to as a groin strain. Because the belly of psoas major extends up to its attachments into the transverse process of the lumbar vertebra, a strain here may result in abdominal pain and tenderness on deep palpation.

"Tom, Dick, and Harry" Muscles

The tendon of the tibialis posterior crosses the ankle and midtarsal joints with the tendon of the flexor digitorum longus and the flexor hallucis longus and functions with them at these joints. These three muscles are often referred to as the **Tom, Dick,** and **Harry** muscles. Tom for tibialis posterior; Dick for flexor digitorum longus; and Harry for flexor hallucis longus.

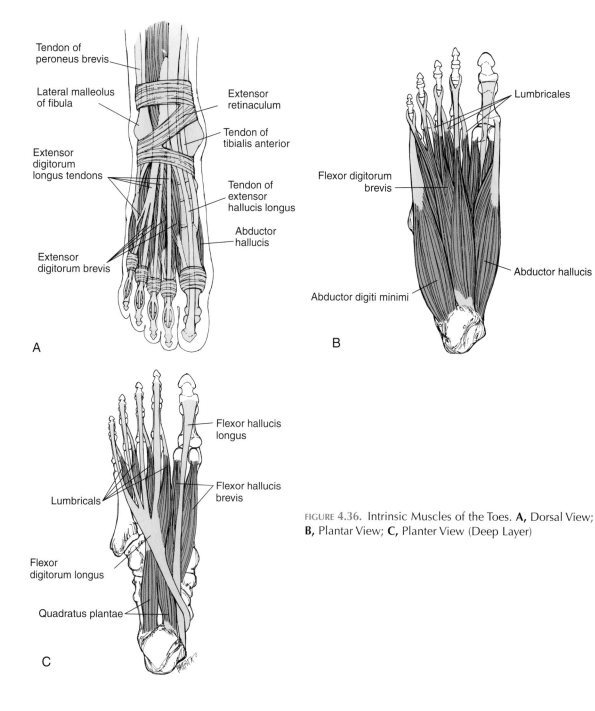

FIGURE **4.36.** Intrinsic Muscles of the Toes. **A,** Dorsal View; **B,** Plantar View; **C,** Planter View (Deep Layer)

An Overview of Lower Limb Innervation

The muscles of the lower limb are innervated by nerves that arise from the lumbar (with contribution from T12, L1–L4) and sacral (L4–L5, S1–S3) segments of the spinal cord. These nerves initially form a network known as the **lumbosacral plexus** (see **page 328**). Of the many nerves that arise from this plexus (see Figure 4.37), the **sciatic nerve** (L4–L5, S1–S3) is the largest (it is the largest nerve in the body). The sciatic nerve, with its two main divisions—**tibial** and **common fibular (peroneal) nerves**—supplies the skin of most of the leg and foot, muscles of the posterior thigh, and all the muscles of the leg and foot.

Muscular System and Aging

The slower movement, weakness, and altered physical appearance are largely a result of changes in the muscular and skeletal system.[1]

With age, the muscles decrease in size as a result of loss of muscle fibers and atrophy of individual muscle fibers. There is also a loss of motor units. There is greater loss of fast twitch fibers, partly a result of aging and partly a result of disuse. The vascularity decreases and more fat is deposited in the muscle. The atrophied muscles are replaced with fibrous tissue, reducing elasticity. Changes in muscle, as well as the nervous system, slow movement and decrease strength and endurance. The rate of loss of strength and endurance can be significantly reduced by resistance exercise. Changes in the vertebral column, stiffening of ligaments and joints, and hardening of tendons result in mild flexion of the vertebrae, hips, knees, elbows, wrists, and neck.

The changes in muscle function may be partly attributed to effects of age on the nervous system. The extrapyramidal system (see **page 361**) is impaired and this results in mild tremors at rest. There is a decline in the number of spinal cord axons and in nerve conduction velocity. Voluntary responses that involve reaction and/or movement are slower; however, the decline is less in those who maintain an active lifestyle.

Muscular System and Massage

Most of the therapist's work is likely to be related to the muscular system. There are too many muscle-related problems, however, and they cannot all be discussed in this section.

Massage is beneficial in treating many musculoskeletal problems,[2-6] such as tendinitis, sprain, tenosynovitis, and low back pain. It reduces swelling, increases blood flow, relieves pain and muscle spasm, and mobilizes fibrous tissue, and also improves muscle action and induces a state of general relaxation. Early institution of massage not only decreases pain but also accelerates the rate of functional recovery.

The gradual compression produced by strokes such as effleurage reduces muscle tone and induces a general state of relaxation that relieves muscle spasm.[7] The relaxation is produced by the localized stretch effect that lengthens sarcomeres in the immediate vicinity of the applied pressure. Strokes that involve application of firm pressure accelerate blood and lymph flow and improve tissue drainage. Kneading promotes the flow of tissue fluid and causes reflex vasodilation and marked hyperemia; this reduces swelling and helps resolve inflammation. Vigorous kneading decreases muscle spasm and can stretch tissues shortened by injury. Petrissage is particularly useful for stretching contracted or adherent fibrous tissue and will relieve muscle spasm. Acting deeper than kneading, petrissage also promotes the flow of body fluids and resolves long-standing swelling. Substances released by ischemic tissue that sensitize pain receptors are also dispersed, relieving pain. Friction massage[2] breaks down scars and prevents scar tissue from matting muscle fibers together.

Postexercise effleurage reduces subsequent muscle soreness and pain by rapidly reducing lactate concentration in the muscle cells. This has been shown to be a more effective treatment than either rest or a conventional active warm-down program.[8-11] Massage can also be used to prevent denervated muscle from losing both bulk and contractile capability, assisting subsequent rehabilitation.[12] Massage has been successfully used for prevention of delayed-onset muscle soreness[13] and as an adjuvant therapy for conditions such as carpal tunnel syndrome,[14] low back pain (not involving nervous dysfunction),[15-17] and joint sprains.[18]

Heat is often used during massage.[19] Local heat can be applied by immersion in hot water, hot towels, paraffin wax baths, electrically heated pads, infrared lamps, or infrared lasers. The latter have the capacity to penetrate deep tissue. Heat causes local vasodilation, increased cell metabolism, pain relief, relaxation of muscle spasm, increased range of motion, and decreased stiffness.[19] Some of the effects of heat on deeper structures is believed to be a result of reflex mechanisms. By stimulating other afferent fibers, heat reduces the number of impulses carried to the brain by pain fibers (gate-control theory).[19,20] Muscle relaxation may be produced by a reduction of gamma motor neuron and alpha motor neuron activity.[19] Heat also increases the extensibility of collagen. By increasing blood flow, it speeds the removal of pain-

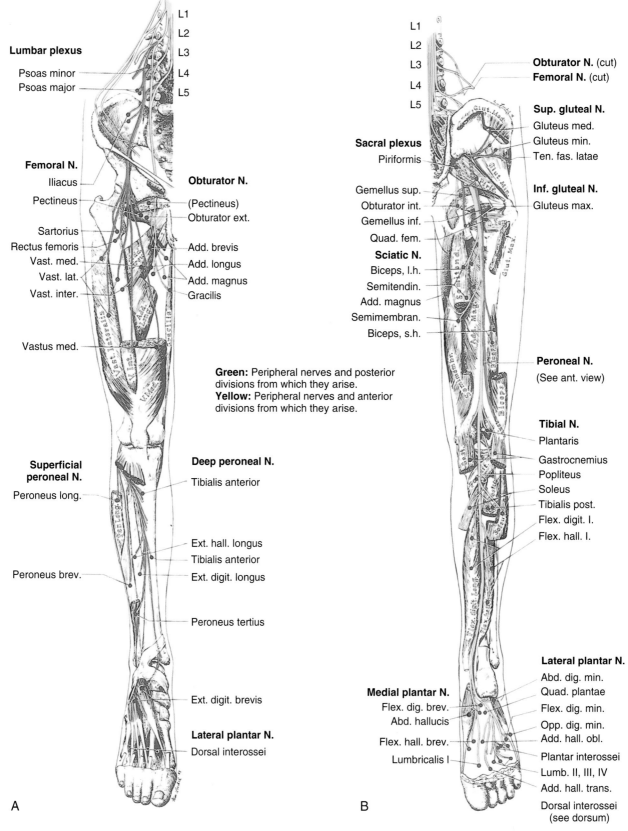

L1
L2
L3
L4
L5

Lumbar plexus
Psoas minor
Psoas major

Femoral N.
Iliacus
Pectineus

Sartorius
Rectus femoris
Vast. med.
Vast. lat.
Vast. inter.

Vastus med.

Obturator N.
(Pectineus)
Obturator ext.
Add. brevis
Add. longus
Add. magnus
Gracilis

Green: Peripheral nerves and posterior divisions from which they arise.
Yellow: Peripheral nerves and anterior divisions from which they arise.

Superficial peroneal N.
Peroneus long.

Peroneus brev.

Deep peroneal N.
Tibialis anterior

Ext. hall. longus
Tibialis anterior
Ext. digit. longus

Peroneus tertius

Ext. digit. brevis

Lateral plantar N.
Dorsal interossei

A

L1
L2
L3
L4
L5

Obturator N. (cut)
Femoral N. (cut)

Sup. gluteal N.
Gluteus med.
Gluteus min.
Ten. fas. latae

Sacral plexus
Piriformis

Gemellus sup.
Obturator int.
Gemellus inf.
Quad. fem.
Sciatic N.
Biceps, l.h.
Semitendin.
Add. magnus
Semimembran.
Biceps, s.h.

Inf. gluteal N.
Gluteus max.

Peroneal N.
(See ant. view)

Tibial N.
Plantaris
Gastrocnemius
Popliteus
Soleus
Tibialis post.
Flex. digit. I.
Flex. hall. I.

Medial plantar N.
Flex. dig. brev.
Abd. hallucis
Flex. hall. brev.
Lumbricalis I

Lateral plantar N.
Abd. dig. min.
Quad. plantae
Flex. dig. min.
Opp. dig. min.
Add. hall. obl.
Plantar interossei
Lumb. II, III, IV
Add. hall. trans.
Dorsal interossei (see dorsum)

B

FIGURE 4.37.   Nerves to the Lower Limb. **A,** Motor Supply (Anterior View); **B,** Motor Supply (Posterior View)

(continued)

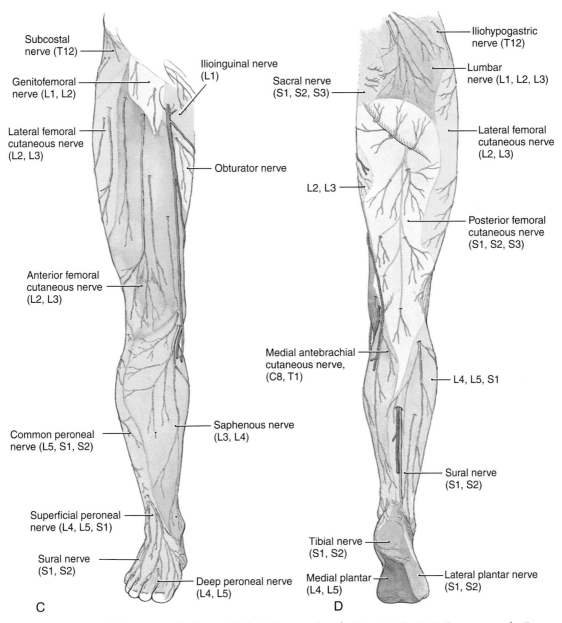

Subcostal
nerve (T12)

Genitofemoral
nerve (L1, L2)

Lateral femoral
cutaneous nerve
(L2, L3)

Anterior femoral
cutaneous nerve
(L2, L3)

Common peroneal
nerve (L5, S1, S2)

Superficial peroneal
nerve (L4, L5, S1)

Sural nerve
(S1, S2)

Ilioinguinal nerve
(L1)

Obturator nerve

Saphenous nerve
(L3, L4)

Deep peroneal nerve
(L4, L5)

C

Iliohypogastric
nerve (T12)

Sacral nerve
(S1, S2, S3)

Lumbar
nerve (L1, L2, L3)

Lateral femoral
cutaneous nerve
(L2, L3)

L2, L3

Posterior femoral
cutaneous nerve
(S1, S2, S3)

Medial antebrachial
cutaneous nerve,
(C8, T1)

L4, L5, S1

Sural nerve
(S1, S2)

Tibial nerve
(S1, S2)

Medial plantar
(L4, L5)

Lateral plantar nerve
(S1, S2)

D

FIGURE 4.37., cont'd   Nerves to the Lower Limb. **C,** Sensory Supply (Anterior View); **D,** Sensory supply (Posterior View)

causing substances. Before the application of heat, therapists must ensure that the client has normal temperature and pain perception to determine a safe level of heat. Therapists should also make sure that the local circulation is not impaired. Deep heat (e.g., infrared, ultrasound) should be avoided in areas that contain large amounts of fluid, such as the eye, joints, and acutely inflamed tissue because high thermal energy can build up. Deep heat should also be avoided over tissue containing metallic objects.

Cold may also be used therapeutically.[21] The term *cold* refers to removal of heat (i.e., one feels a sensation of cold if the temperature is lower than that of the body area to which it is applied). The temperature is described as *tepid* if it is 26.7–33.9°C (80–93°F); *cool*

if it is 18.3–26.7°C (65–80°F); *cold* if it is 12.8–18.3°C (55–65°F), and *very cold* if it is below 12.8°C (55°F). Substances may be used in solid forms (ice, carbon dioxide, snow), liquid forms (water), or gaseous forms (ethyl chloride, alcohol, ether; they extract heat during evaporation) for eliciting cold sensations.

Although it sounds unappealing, application of cold (cryotherapy) is a more effective way of producing deep vasodilation than heat. Application of cold also has a pain-relieving effect and reduces muscle spasm.[22] Cooling produces analgesia by reducing the rate of conduction through nerves. When the skin is cooled, it initially causes local vasoconstriction; however, after 5 to 10 minutes, the blood flow through superficial and deep tissue increases and then oscillates.

The increased blood flow raises the temperature and improves tissue nutrition. Ice applied for short periods causes vasoconstriction and reduces bleeding. Prolonged application will cause vasodilation by tissue injury and increase tissue hemorrhage. Melting ice is the most effective way to chill the skin.

The therapist must remember that muscle is made up of different kinds of tissue. Although the bulk of the muscle is muscle tissue, the tension produced in the muscle is transmitted to the bone via *connective tissue* in the form of fascia, tendons, and aponeurosis. The pressure, stretching, friction, and movement exerted during a therapeutic session can make this connective tissue more pliable and have a beneficial effect.

All connective tissue exhibits **thixotropy.**[23] This is the property by which connective tissue becomes more fluid and pliable when exposed to heat, friction, and/or movement and becomes more solid when exposed to cold and/or is unused. This inherent property is a result of the ground substance and collagen, elastic, and reticular fibers it is made of. The application of heat and cold in therapy capitalizes on this property of connective tissue.

As in any tissue, when injury occurs, it is followed by inflammation and healing. While healing, the connective tissue fibers/fascia of adjacent muscles may adhere (stick) to each other. These adhesions, other than restricting movement of muscle, may trap nerves and blood vessels supplying the muscle, producing further complications. Appropriate application of heat/cold and massage, passive, and active movements at the right time can prevent adhesion formation in tissue.

Another fact that should be remembered is that structures, such as tendons, fascia, aponeurosis and ligaments, that are made up of connective tissue with a high proportion of nonliving collagen fibers take a longer time to heal because of their structure as well as the reduced blood supply. Hence, treatment regimens that are too early, vigorous, or overenthusiastic should not be given when treating conditions related to these structures.

The tone of the muscle may vary from person to person. In some individuals who are paralyzed, the tone may be increased, and the muscle may be fixed in awkward positions that result from contractures. In other individuals, the limb may lie limp, with no tone at all. Both conditions are a result of dysfunction of the nervous system. It is important for the therapist to assess the client carefully and be fully equipped with all relevant information about the disorder. If in any doubt, it is better to get advice from a medical professional.

Some clients may be taking medications such as painkillers, anti-inflammatory drugs, or even muscle relaxants that depress pain sensations. It should be ensured that the client has not taken such medications. If using these medications, therapy should only begin after the effects have worn off.

Trigger points are locations in tissue that are hypersensitive and painful when compressed. Therapeutic work on trigger points of various muscles[24] seems to have a positive outcome, and it is worthwhile to master the techniques needed to identify and treat these regions.

Many problems related to muscle may be a result of the occupation of the client or a result of bad posture. An important element of therapy should be proper history taking and physical assessment. Details of occupation and work-related stresses and strains that may be the cause of the ailment should be obtained, and client education and strategies should be planned accordingly.

Lastly, but most importantly, the therapist should ensure that the techniques and posture used during a massage are ergonomically healthy in order to prevent problems to themselves such as musculotendinous and nerve impingement injuries.[25]

REFERENCES

1. Kenney RA. Physiology of Aging: A Synopsis. 2 Ed. Chicago: Year Book Medical, 1989.
2. Chamberlain GJ. Cyriax's friction massage: A review. J Orthoped Sports Physic Ther 1982;4:16–22.
3. Clews W. Effects of massage in athletes with rotator cuff tendinitis. Excel 1988;4(4):12–15.
4. Goats GC. Massage and arthritis—modern applications of an ancient art. Arthritis Today 1992;2:3–4.
5. Hammer WI. The use of transverse friction massage in the management of chronic bursitis of the hip or shoulder. J Manipulative Physiol Ther 1993;16(2):107–111.
6. Peng J. 16 cases of scalenus syndrome treated by massage and acupoint-injection. J Trad Chin Med 1999;19(3):218–220.
7. Andrade CK, Clifford P. Outcome-Based Massage. Baltimore: Lippincott Williams & Wilkins, 2001.
8. Hemmings B, Smith M, Graydon J, Dyson R. Effects of massage on physiological restoration, perceived recovery, and repeated sports performance. Br J Sports Med 2000;34(2):109–115.
9. Hemmings BJ. Massage effects on regeneration, recovery and performance in sport: recent research and implications for the management of athletes. Physiother Sport 1999;22(2):7–11.
10. Newman S. Canadian athletes and massage. Coaching Rev 1986;May/June:16–20.
11. Newman S. Canada's case for sports massage. Coaching Review 1986;May/June:20–25.
12. Mein EA, Richards DG, McMillin DL, McPartland JM. Physiological regulation through manual therapy. Phys Med Rehabil: A State of the Art Review 2000;14(1):27–42.
13. Gulick DT, Kimura IF. Delayed onset muscle soreness: What is it and how do we treat it? J Sport Rehabil 1996;5:234–243.
14. Stoll ST, Simmons SL. Inpatient rehabilitation and manual medicine. Phys Med Rehabil: A State of the Art Review 2000;14(1):85–106.
15. Kinalski R. The comparison of the results of manual therapy versus physiotherapy methods used in treatment of patients with low back pain syndromes. J Manual Med 1989;4(2):44–46.
16. Hernandez-Reif M, Field T, Krasnegor J, Theakston H, Burman I. Chronic lower back pain is reduced and range of motion improved with massage therapy. Intern J Neurosci 2000;99:1–15.

17. Ernst, E. Massage therapy for low back pain: A systematic review [In Process Citation]. J Pain Symptom Manage 1999;17:65–69.

18. Lei Z. Treating dislocation of small joints of thoracic vertebrae by manipulation with palm pressing and shaking. J Trad Chin Med 1993;13(1):52–53.

19. Duncombe A, Hopp JF. Modalities of physical treatment. Phys Med Rehabil: State of the art reviews 1991 Oct;5(3 Musculoskeletal Pain):493–519.

20. Melzack R, Vetere P, Finch L. Transcutaneous electrical nerve stimulation for low back pain. A comparison of TENS and massage for pain and range of motion. Phys Ther 1983;63(4):489–493.

21. Bierman W. Therapeutic use of cold. JAMA 1954;157(14):1189–1192.

22. Bugaj R. The cooling, analgesic and rewarming effects of ice massage on localized skin. Phys Ther 1975;55(1):11–19.

23. Juhan D. A Handbook for Bodywork—Job's Body. New York: Station Hill Press, 1987.

24. Travell JG, Simons DG. Myofascial pain and dysfunction. The Trigger Point Manual, vol 1. Baltimore: Williams & Wilkins, 1983.

25. Greene L. Save your hands! Injury prevention for massage therapists. Gilded Age Press. 1995, Coconut Creek, Florida.

SUGGESTED READINGS

Bale P, James H. Massage, warm-down and rest as recuperative measures after short-term intense exercise. Physiother Sport 1991;13:4–7.

Balke B, Anthony J, Wyatt F. The effects of massage treatment on exercise fatigue. Clin Sports Med 1989;1(4):189–196.

Boyek K, Watson R. A touching story. Elderly Care 1994; 6(3):20–21.

Branstrom MJ. Interactive Physiology—Muscular system. A.D.A.M. Software and Benjamin/Cummings Publishing, 1995, San Francisco, CA.

Cafarelli E, Flint F. The role of massage in preparation for and recovery from exercise. An overview [Review]. Sports Med 1992;14(1):1–9.

Clarkson GM. Musculoskeletal Assessment: Joint Range of Motion and Manual Muscle Strength. 2nd Ed. Philadelphia: Lippincott Williams & Wilkins, 2000.

Cochran-Fritz S. Physiological effects of therapeutic massage on the nervous system. Intern J Alternative Complementary Med 1993;11(9):21–25.

Corbett M. The use and abuse of massage and exercise. Practitioner 1972;208:136–139.

Crosman LJ, Chateauvert SR, Weisberg J. The effects of massage to the hamstring muscle group on range of motion. J Orthop Sports Phys Ther 1984;6(3):168–172.

Danneskiold-Samsoe B, Christianson E, Lund B, Anderson RB. Regional muscle tension and pain (fibrositis), effect of massage on myoglobin in plasma. Scand J Rehabil Med 1982;15:17–20.

Davies S, Eiches L. Healing touch. Nurs Times 1995;91(26):42–43.

deGroot J, Chusid JG. Correlative neuroanatomy. 20th Ed. San Matoe: Appleton & Lange, 1985.

Fraser J, Ross Kerr J. Psychophysiological effects of back massage on elderly institutionalized patients. J Adv Nurs 1993;18(2): 238–245.

Gam AN, Warming S, Larsen LH, Jensen B. Treatment of myofascial trigger points with ultrasound combined with massage and exercise—a randomized controlled trial. Pain 1998;77(1):73–79.

Goats GC. Massage—The scientific basis of an ancient art: parts 1 and 2. Br J Sports Med 1994;28(3):149–155.

Graham D. Massage, Manual Treatment, Remedial Movements, History, Mode of Application and Effects: Indications and Contraindication. Philadelphia: J.P. Lippincott, 1913.

Grant AE. Massage with ice (cryokinetics) in the treatment of painful conditions of the musculoskeletal system. Arch Phys Med 1964;45:233–238.

Guthrie RA, Martin RH. Effect of pressure applied to the upper thoracic (placebo) versus lumbar areas (osteopathic manipulative treatment) for inhibition of lumbar myalgia during labor. J Am Osteopath Assoc 1982;82:247–251.

Harmer PA. The effect of preperformance massage on stride frequency in sprinters. Athl Training J NATA 1991;26:55–59.

Jisaying W. The mechanism and the effects of Chinese traditional massage treatment on traumatic lumbar pain. J Trad Chin Med 1986;6(3):168–170.

Kendall FP, McCreary EK, Provance PG. Muscles, testing and function. 4th Ed. Baltimore: Williams & Wilkins, 1993.

Konrad K, Tatrai T, Hunka A. Controlled trial of balneotherapy in treatment of low back pain. Ann Rheum Dis 1992;51(6):820–822.

Longworth JCD. Psychopysiological effects of slow stroke back massage in normotensive females. Adv Nurs Sci 1982;4:44–61.

Lundeberg T, Nordemar R, Ottson D. Pain alleviation by vibratory stimulation. Pain 1984;20:25–44.

Lundeberg T. Long-term results of vibratory stimulation as a pain-relieving measure for chronic pain. Pain 1984;20:13–23.

McArdle WD, Katch FI, Katch VL. Exercise Physiology: Energy, Nutrition, and Human Performance. 5th Ed. Baltimore: Lippincott Williams & Wilkins, 2001.

Melzack R, Jeans ME, Stratford JG, Monks RC. Ice massage and transcutaneous electrical stimulation: comparison of treatment for low back pain. Pain 1980;9:209–917.

Melzack R. The McGill pain assessment questionnaire, major properties and scoring methods. Pain 1975;1:277–299.

Mense S, Simons DG, Russell IJ. Muscle Pain: Understanding Its Nature, Diagnosis, and Treatment. Baltimore: Lippincott Williams & Wilkins, 2001.

Morelli M, Seaborne DE, Sullivan SJ. H-reflex modulation during manual muscle massage of human triceps surae. Arch Phys Med Rehabil 1991;72(11):915–919.

Morelli M, Seaborne DE. Changes in H-reflex amplitude during massage of triceps surae in healthy subjects. J Orth Sports Phys Ther 1990;12(2):55–59.

Nawroth A. Massage—The anthroposophic approach. J Anthroposophic Med 1995;12(2):43–49.

Nordschow M, Bierman W. Influence of manual massage on muscle relaxation. Phys Ther 1962;42:653–657.

Premkumar K. Pathology A to Z. 2nd Ed. Calgary: VanPub Books, 1999.

Rinder AN, Sutherland CJ. An investigation of the effects of massage on quadriceps performance after exercise fatigue. Complementary Ther Nurs Midwifery 1995;1:99–102.

Rodenburg JB, Steenbeek D, Schienreck P, et al. Warm-up, stretching and massage diminish harmful effects of eccentric exercise. Inter J Sports Med 1994;15(7):414–419.

Scull CW. Massage—Physiological basis. Arch Phys Med 1945;26:159–167.

Smith LL, Keating MN, Holbert MN, et al. The effects of athletic massage on delayed onset muscle soreness, creatine kinase, and neutrophil count: A preliminary report. J Sports Phys Ther 1994;19:93–99.

Viitasalo J, Niemela K, Kaappola R, Korjus T, Levola M, Monomen H, et al. Warm underwater water-jet massage improves recovery from intense physical exercise. Eur J Appl Phys 1995;71: 432–438.

Wainapel SF, Thomas AD, Kahan BS. Use of alternative therapies by rehabilitation outpatients. Arch Phys Med Rehabil 1998;79(8):1003–1005.

Wakim KG. Physiologic effects of massage. In: Licht S, ed. Massage, Manipulation and Traction. Huntington, NY: Robert E. Keirger, 1976:38–42.

Westland G. Massage as a therapeutic tool, part 2. Brit J Occupational Ther 1993;56(5):177–180.

Wilkins RW, Halperin MH, Litter J. The effects of various physical procedures on circulation in human limbs. Ann Intern Med 1950;33:1232–1245.

Wood EC. Beard's massage: Principles and Techniques. Philadelphia: W.B. Saunders, 1974.

Wu L, Jin Y. Application of finger pressure to ankle sprains. J Trad Chin Med 1993;13(4):299–302.

Yackzan L, Adams C, Francis KT. The effects of ice massage on delayed muscle soreness. Am J Sports Med 1984;12:159–165.

Yang Z, Hong J. Investigation on analgesic mechanism of acupuncture finger-pressure massage on lumbago. J Trad Chin Med 1994;14(1):35–40.

Ylinen J, Cash M. Sports Massage. London: Stanley Paul, 1988.

Yu C. 55 cases of lumbar muscle strain treated by massage. Intern J Clin Acupuncture 1999;10(2):189–190.

Yurtkuran M, Kocagil T. TENS, electroacupuncture and ice massage: comparison of treatment for osteoarthritis of the knee. Am J Acupuncture 1999;27(3-4):133–140.

Zelikovski A, Kaye C, Fink G, et al. The effects of the modified intermittent sequential pneumatic device (MISPD) on exercise performance following an exhaustive exercise bout. Br J Sport Med 1993;27:255–259.

 # Review Questions

Multiple Choice
Choose the best answer to the following questions:

1. A motor unit consists of
   A. a skeletal muscle and all of its supplying neurons.
   B. a nerve and all of the skeletal muscles supplied by the nerve.
   C. a neuron and all of the skeletal muscle fibers that it stimulates.
   D. all of the skeletal muscles that accomplish a single movement.

2. Consider the list of actions below. Which would classify as isotonic contractions?
   A. Pushing against a stationary wall
   B. Chewing gum
   C. Writing a letter
   D. B and C
   E. All of the above

3. During moderate levels of exercise, the process that provides the richest supply of ATP for muscle contraction is
   A. the use of creatine phosphate.
   B. anaerobic glycolysis.
   C. aerobic respiration.
   D. the use of ATP storage in muscle.

4. The connective tissue that surrounds the most muscle tissue is
   A. endomysium.
   B. perimysium.
   C. epimysium.

5. Of the following, the smallest structure is the
   A. myofibril.
   B. muscle fascicle.
   C. myofilament.
   D. muscle fiber.

6. If the motor nerve to a muscle is injured, the muscle
   A. loses tone.
   B. atrophies.
   C. hypertrophies.
   D. A and B are correct.
   E. A and C are correct.

7. When muscle length is 75% of optimal, the force of the muscle contraction would be
   A. maximal.
   B. less than maximal.

8. The cause of staircase phenomenon can be explained by
   A. availability of calcium in the sarcoplasm.
   B. a more rapid action potential.
   C. an increased number of acetylcholine receptors.
   D. more myofibrils.

9. During aerobic metabolism, a molecule of glucose can yield _____ ATP.
   A. 2
   B. 36
   C. 30
   D. 40

10. Paralysis of which of the following would make an individual unable to flex her knee?
   A. Hamstrings
   B. Gluteal muscles
   C. Soleus
   D. Tibialis anterior
   E. Quadriceps

Fill-In
Complete the following:
a. The following table compares the characteristics of skeletal, cardiac, and smooth muscle. Fill in the empty cells.

Characteristics	Skeletal	Cardiac	Smooth
Striations (yes, no)	✓	✓	
Intercalated disks		✓	
Appearance (cylindrical, branched, fusiform)			
Innervation (motor neuron, autonomic nerves)			
Location (attached to skeleton, etc.)			
Control (voluntary, involuntary)			

Complete the following:
b. The following table compares the characteristics of fast twitch, slow twitch, and intermediate muscle fibers. Fill in the empty cells.

Characteristics	Fast Twitch	Slow Twitch	Intermediate
Diameter (e.g., large)			
Glycogen content (e.g., large)			
Number of mitochondria			
Color			
Primary type of metabolism (aerobic, anaerobic)			
Capillaries (abundant, few)			
Myoglobin content			

c.

1. One substance in muscle that stores oxygen until oxygen is needed by mitochondria is __Myoglobin__ .

2. During exercise lasting longer than 10 minutes, more than 90% of ATP is provided by the __aerobic__ (aerobic, anaerobic) breakdown of pyruvic acid.

3. In general, __red__ (red, white) fibers are more suited for endurance exercise than for short bursts of energy.

d. Arrange the following steps involved in muscle contraction in the correct sequence.

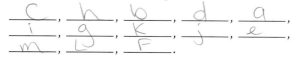

__C__ , __h__ , __b__ , __d__ , __a__ ,
__i__ , __g__ , __k__ , __j__ , __e__ ,
__m__ , __l__ , __F__ .

A Summary of the Steps Involved in Muscle Contraction

a. This potential change is communicated directly into the sarcoplasm via the T tubules

b. ACh binds to ACh receptors on the sarcolemma and this results in opening of sodium channels

c. Action potentials or impulses from the central nervous system come down the nerve axon of the motor nerve when movement must occur

d. The rush of sodium into the sarcoplasm causes the inside of the cell to become positive as compared to the outside

e. ATP provides the energy for the bound myosin head to pivot towards the M line

f. The cycle continues and the muscle fiber shortens as long as calcium is bound to troponin

g. Calcium binds to troponin

h. The impulse, on arriving at the myoneural junction, causes the ACh vesicles to fuse with the nerve cell membrane and release its contents into the synaptic cleft

i. The sarcoplasmic reticulum releases calcium into the sarcoplasm as a result of the potential change

j. Myosin binds to the uncovered active site on actin

k. Binding of calcium to troponin causes troponin to shift tropomyosin and uncover the active site for myosin on the actin

l. Attachment of another ATP to the bound myosin head causes it to release from the actin and bind to another molecule of actin

m. ADP and P are released when the myosin head pivots

e. *Name one or more muscle that is used to produce the following actions:*

1. To turn the palm so that it faces forward __supinator__

2. To bend the elbow to touch the tip of the shoulder __biceps brachii__

3. To flex the hip joint __psoas major__

4. To stand up tall (extend the vertebral column) __erector spinae__

5. To breathe in __diaphragm__

6. To plantar flex __gastrocnemius__

True–False
(Answer the following questions T, for true; or F, for false):

F a. Muscle spindles are spindle-shaped smooth muscles.

T b. The Golgi tendon organ is a sensory receptor.

T c. Smooth muscles are found in respiratory bronchi.

F d. A second-class lever is the most common muscle arrangement.

F e. The muscle fibers of the sartorius are bipennate.

T f. Oxygen debt is the amount of oxygen required to bring the muscle to its pre-exertion level.

T g. The wheelbarrow is an example of a second-class lever.

T h. The hamstrings antagonize the action of quadriceps.

T i. The peroneus longus, tibialis major, gracilis, and sartorius are all muscles located in the lower limb.

F j. The trapezius, pectoralis minor, teres minor, deltoid, and sternocleidomastoid are all attached to the scapula.

Matching
a. *Match the following muscles that move the shoulder girdle with their actions:*

1. __a__ levator scapulae   a. elevates
2. __c__ serratus anterior   b. depresses
3. __d__ rhomboideus major   c. abducts
        and minor   d. adducts
4. __b__ pectoralis minor
5. __a,b,d__ trapezius

b. *Match the following muscles that move the humerus with their actions:*

1. __b__ pectoralis major   a. abducts arm; flexes arm (anterior fascicles)
2. __a__ deltoid   b. flexes; adducts; medially rotates
3. __c__ latissimus dorsi   c. extends; adducts; medially rotates

c. *Match the following muscles that move the forearm with their actions:*

1. __b__ brachialis   a. flexes and supinates forearm
2. __a__ biceps brachii   b. flexes forearm
3. __d__ triceps brachii   c. flexes palm; abducts palm
4. __c__ flexor carpi radialis   d. extends forearm

d. *Match the following terms with their meaning:*

1. __b__ psoas   a. in the wrist
2. __f__ deltoid   b. loin region
3. __e__ serratus   c. groin region
4. __a__ carpi   d. thumb
5. __i__ rectus   e. saw-toothed appearance
6. __c__ inguinal   f. shaped like a triangle
7. __j__ latissimus   g. big toe
8. __h__ nuchal   h. back of the neck
9. __d__ pollicis   i. parallel direction of muscle fascicles
10. __g__ hallucis   j. widest

Short Answer Questions

1. What are the effects of physical training on the cardiovascular system?
2. What are the changes that occur in the skeletal muscle with aging?
3. What are the causes of muscle fatigue?
4. What are the factors that affect speed, direction, and force of contraction of muscle?

Case Studies

a. Mary is a 15-year-old swimmer, aspiring to reach the Olympics. She has been diagnosed with shoulder impingement syndrome and has been referred to a massage therapist and a local phys-

iotherapist. The massage therapist decides to assess the shoulder of the client.
  A. What muscles are involved with movements of the shoulder joint?
  B. What are their origins, insertions, and actions?

b. A therapist working at a sports clinic marvels at the differences between the bodies of athletes involved in short-distance running and those running marathons.
  A. What is the difference in the structure of the muscles of these two groups of athletes?
  B. How do muscles primarily obtain energy for each of their activities?
  C. What are the factors that affect recovery of muscle in general?
  D. What is muscle fatigue?
  E. What are the different types of muscle fibers?

c. Some clients at the sports clinic are in wheelchairs. The therapist noticed a dramatic difference between the well-developed, hypertrophied, firm muscles of the upper limb and the hardly discernible muscles of the lower limb of some of the athletes with spinal cord injury.
  A. Why is there a difference in the muscles of the upper and lower limb?
  B. How do muscles contract? What are the steps involved in muscle contraction?
  C. What is the role of nerves in the contraction of muscle?
  D. What are the factors that affect muscle contraction?
  E. What is meant by atrophy, hypertrophy, and spasticity?
  F. What is a motor unit?
  G. What is the structure of a myoneural junction?

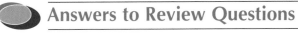

Answers to Review Questions

Multiple Choice

1. C
2. D
3. C
4. C
5. C
6. D
7. B
8. A
9. B
10. A

Fill-In

a.

Characteristics	Skeletal	Cardiac	Smooth
Striations (yes, no)	Yes	Yes	No
Intercalated disks	No	Yes	No
Appearance (cylindrical, branched, fusiform)	Cylindrical	Branched	Fusiform
Innervation (motor neuron, autonomic nerves)	Motor neuron	Autonomic	Autonomic
Location (attached to skeleton, etc.)	Attached to skeleton	Around Heart	Blood vessels; bronchi; gut, etc.
Control (voluntary, involuntary)	Voluntary	Involuntary	Involuntary

b.

Characteristics	Fast Twitch	Slow Twitch	Intermediate
Diameter (e.g., large)	Large	Small	Intermediate
Glycogen content (e.g., large)	Large	Small	Intermediate
Number of mitochondria	Few	Numerous	Some
Color	Pale	Red	Pale
Primary type of metabolism (aerobic, anaerobic)	Anaerobic	Aerobic	Both
Capillaries (abundant, few)	Few	Abundant	Intermediate
Myoglobin content	Less	Large amounts	Less

c.

1. myoglobin
2. aerobic
3. red

d. c; h; b; d; a; i; g; k; j; e; m; l; f

e.

1. supinator
2. biceps brachii
3. psoas major
4. erector spinae
5. diaphragm
6. gastrocnemius

True–False

a. false, they have skeletal muscle fibers.
b. true
c. true
d. false, third class is most common.
e. false
f. true
g. true
h. true
i. true
j. false (sternocleidomastoid is not)

Matching

a. 1. a; 2. c; 3. d; 4. b; 5. a, b or d (depending on position)
b. 1. b; 2. a; 3. c
c. 1. b; 2. a; 3. d ; 4. c
d. 1. b; 2. f; 3. e; 4. a; 5. i; 6. c; 7. j; 8. h; 9. d; 10. g

Short-Answer Questions

1. see **page 197**
2. see **page 231**
3. see **page 194**
4. see **page 184**

Case Studies

a. see Chapter Appendix Table 4.8
b. see pages:
 A. 195 (fast fibers/slow fibers)
 B. See figure 4.16
 C. 193 (muscle recovery)
 D. 194 (muscle fatigue)
 E. 195
c. see pages:
 A. 197 (hypertrophy), upper limb
   200 (atrophy), lower limb
 B. 181 (box: a summary of the steps involved in muscle contraction)
 C. 181 (excitation contraction-coupling)
 D. 184 (sentence: some factors that affect . . .)
 E. 200 (atrophy); 197 (hypertrophy);
   194 (spasticity)
 F. a motor neuron and all the muscle fiber it innerates
 G. See figure 4.5

Coloring Exercise

Label the structures in the given diagrams, and color the structures, using the color code.
a. In the diagram of a muscle fiber, label the marked structures. Using the color code, color the sarcoplasmic reticulum blue; t tubule pink; sarcoplasm yellow; myofibrils brown; mitochondria red and nucleus black.

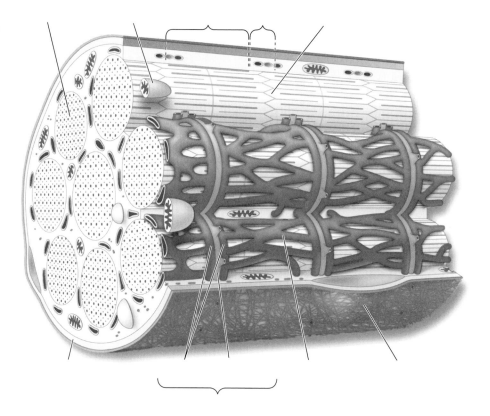

b. In the myoneural junction diagram, label the structures indicated. Color the nerve ending *yellow* and the muscle fiber *brown,* the synaptic cleft *orange,* and the acetylcholine vesicles *purple.* Outline the sarcolemma of the motor endplate in *black.*

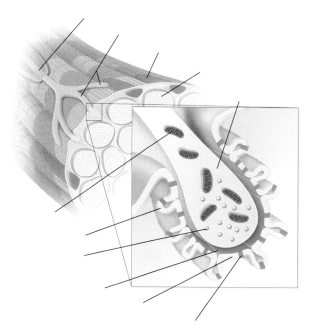

c. The following is a diagram of the scapula and humerus (anterior and posterior view). Shade the scapula *yellow* and the humerus *orange.* For the following muscles:

Label the **origins** on the **scapula:** supraspinatus; infraspinatus; teres minor, teres major, deltoid; subscapularis, coracobrachialis; biceps brachii; triceps brachii (long head); deltoid

Label the **insertions** on the **scapula:** trapezius, levator scapulae, rhomboideus minor, rhomboideus major, serratus anterior, pectoralis minor

Label the **insertions** on the **humerus:** supraspinatus, infraspinatus, teres minor; deltoid. Shade all origins red and all insertions blue.

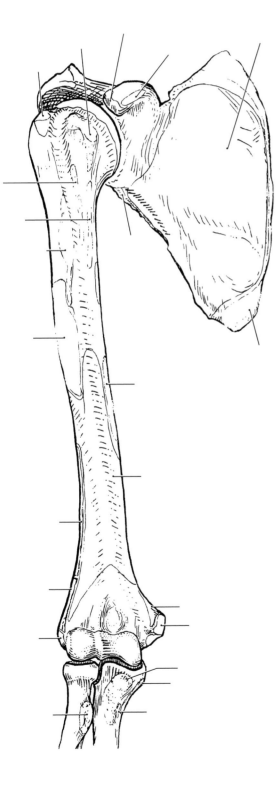
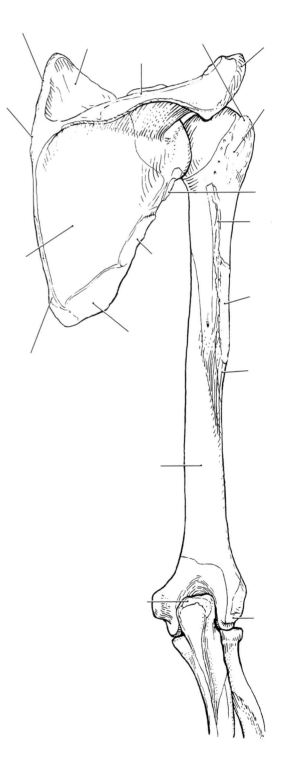

d. The following is a diagram of the arm (anterior and posterior views). Shade the humerus *yellow;* the ulna *orange;* and radius *green.*

Label the **origins:**

On the **humerus:** brachialis; brachioradialis; pronator teres

On the **radius:** pronator teres

On the **ulna:** pronator quadratus

Label the **insertions:**

On the **humerus:** coracobrachialis; teres major; pectoralis major; deltoid; latissimus dorsi; subscapularis; supraspinatus

On the **radius:** biceps brachii; pronator teres; pronator quadratus; brachioradialis

On the **ulna:** brachialis

Shade the origins in red and the insertions in blue.

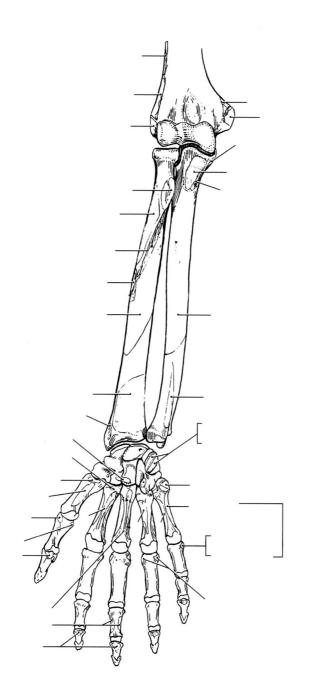
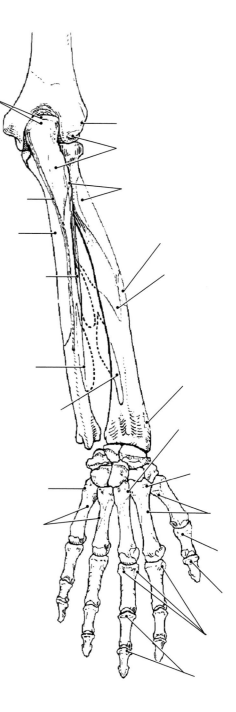

e. The following is a diagram of the femur; and leg (anterior and posterior views). Shade the femur *green;* the tibia *purple;* and the fibula *pink*

Label the **origins:**

On the **tibia:** tibialis anterior

On the **fibula:** extensor digitorum longus; extensor hallucis longus

Label the **insertion:**

On the **tibia:** semimembranosus; sartorius; patellar tendon; gracilis; semitendinosus

On the **fibula:** biceps femoris. Shade the origins in red and the insertions in blue.

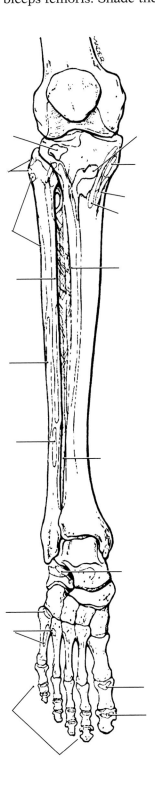
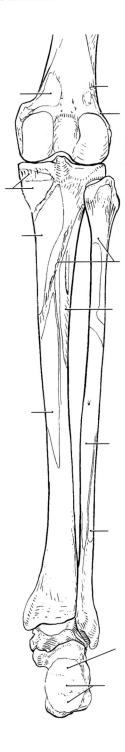

Table 4.1

Muscles Responsible for Facial Expressions

Name	Origin	Insertion	Action	Nerve Supply
Muscles in the cheek and lip region				
Orbicularis oris	Alveolar border of maxillae and mandible; muscle fibers of other muscles surrounding the mouth	Lips; most fibers into the deep surface of the skin and mucous membrane; becomes continuous with muscles that insert into the lips	Constricts the opening of the mouth; protrusion of the lips	VII
Buccinator	Alveolar processes of maxillae and mandible	Skin and mucosa of the lips; blends with orbicularis oris	Compresses cheek against teeth	VII
Depressor labii	Mandible	Skin of lower lip; blends with muscle fibers of lip	Depresses lip	VII
Levator labii	Maxillae	Skin and muscle of upper lip	Raises upper lip	VII
Mentalis	Mandible	Skin of chin	Protrudes and raises lower lip	VII
Depressor anguli oris	Anterolateral surface of mandible	Angle of mouth	Depresses the angle of the mouth	VII
Risorius	Connective tissue around angle of mandible	Angle of mouth	Draws corner of mouth to the side	VII
Zygomaticus (major and minor)	Zygomatic bone	Angle of mouth; blends with muscle fibers of lip	Draws the corner of the mouth back and up	VII
Depressor septi	Maxilla superior to the central incisor tooth	Nasal septum	Widens the nasal opening	VII
Muscle in the eye region				
Orbicularis oculi	Medial margin of orbit	Skin around eyelid	Closes eye	VII
(6 other muscles move the eyeball, which originate from the bones of the orbit and insert on the eyeball)				
Muscle in the nose region				
Nasalis (transverse and alar)	Maxilla	Bridge of nose; corners of nose	Compresses the bridge and narrows the nasal opening (transverse); elevates corners and widens the nasal opening (alar)	VII
Muscles in the scalp region				
Occipitofrontalis (has two bellies; frontal and occipital)	Epicranial aponeurosis (sheet of connective tissue running over the scalp)—frontal belly; Superior nuchal line of occipital bone and mastoid process of temporal bone—occipital belly	Skin of eyebrow and bridge of nose—frontal belly; Epicranial aponeurosis—occipital belly	Raises eyebrows; wrinkles forehead transversely—frontal belly; Pulls scalp posteriorly—occipital belly	VII
Corrugator supercilii	Medial end of the superciliary arch of frontal bone	Skin above the supraorbital margin (eyebrow)	Draws the eyebrows together, resulting in vertical wrinkles in forehead	VII
Procerus	Fascia covering the inferior part of the nasal bone and the superior portion of the lateral nasal cartilage	Skin over the inferior aspect of the forehead, between the eyebrows	Draws medial angle of the eyebrow inferiorly to wrinkle skin transversely over the bridge of nose	VII
Muscle in the neck region				
Platysma	Acromion of scapula and fascia covering the superior part of pectoralis major and deltoid muscles (i.e., upper part of chest)	Inferior border of mandible; skin and muscles of cheek; corner of mouth and lateral half of lower lip	Tenses skin of neck; depresses mandible; depresses corner of mouth and lower lip	VII

Table 4.2

Muscles of Mastication

Name	Origin	Insertion	Action	Nerve Supply
Masseter	Maxilla and zygomatic arch	Lateral surface of mandibular ramus; coronoid process of the mandible	Elevates mandible (clenches teeth); protraction (superficial fibers) and retraction of mandible; minimal side-to-side movement	V
Temporalis	Along the temple (frontal, parietal, and temporal bones)	Coronoid process and ramus of mandible	Elevates and retracts mandible	V
Medial Pterygoid	Medial surface of lateral pterygoid plate of the sphenoid bone; maxilla	Medial surface of mandibular ramus and angle	Elevates, protracts, and moves mandible from side to side	V
Lateral Pterygoid	Lateral surface of greater wing of sphenoid bone	Condyle of mandible and temporomandibular joint	Depresses jaw; protracts; moves mandible from side to side	V
Suprahyoid muscles				
Digastric	*Posterior belly:* mastoid process of the temporal bone *Anterior belly:* base of the mandible, near midline	Hyoid bone (The muscle passes through a fibrous loop attached to the hyoid bone that changes the course of the muscle.)	Depresses mandible; elevates hyoid bone	V, VII
Stylohyoid	Styloid process of the temporal bone	Body of the hyoid bone	Elevates and retracts hyoid bone	VII
Mylohyoid	Mandible	Body of hyoid bone; connective tissue (median fibrous raphe) from the middle of the mandible to the hyoid bone	Depresses mandible; elevates the floor of mouth and hyoid bone	V
Geniohyoid	Posterior aspect of the middle of mandible	Anterior aspect of body of the hyoid bone	Elevates and protracts hyoid bone; depresses the mandible	XII

Table 4.3

Muscles in the Anterior Aspect of Neck

Name	Origin	Insertion	Action	Nerve Supply
Sternocleidomastoid	Superior margin of sternum (sternal head) and medial aspect of clavicle (clavicular head)	Mastoid process of temporal bone	*If acting bilaterally:* Flexes the neck; draws head anteriorly and elevates chin; *Bilaterally with insertion fixed:* Draws sternum superiorly during deep inspiration; *Unilaterally:* Rotates head to opposite side; laterally flexes neck	XI (spinal); C2–C3
Scalenes (anterior, medius, and posterior)	Transverse process of cervical vertebrae	Superior surface of first two ribs	Flexes neck; ipsilateral neck lateral flexion; contralateral neck rotation; elevates the ribs	anterior: C4–C6 medius: C3–C8 posterior: C6–C8
Longus colli (inferior oblique, superior oblique, and vertical)	*Inferior oblique:* Anterior aspect of the bodies of T1–T3; *Superior oblique:* Transverse processes of C3–C6; *Vertical:* Bodies of T1–T3 and C5–C7	*Inferior oblique:* Anterior aspect of transverse processes of C5–C6; *Superior oblique:* Anterior arch of the atlas *Vertical:* Bodies of T1–T3 and C5–C7	Flexes neck; contralateral neck rotation	C2–C7
Longus capitis	Transverse processes of C3–C6	Inferior surface of the occipital bone anterior to the foramen magnum	Flexes head	C1–C3
Rectus capitis (anterior and lateralis)	Anterior and superior aspect of the atlas	Inferior surface of the basilar aspect of the occipital bone (anterior to the occipital condyle)	Flexes head; ipsilateral lateral flexion of the head (lateralis)	C2–C3

The scalenes and sternocleidomastoid are brought into action in people with breathing difficulties (e.g., asthmatics).

Table 4.4

Muscles in the Posterior Aspect of Neck

Name	Origin	Insertion	Action	Nerve Supply
Semispinalis capitis	Transverse processes of lower and upper thoracic vertebra	Occipital bone (between inferior and superior nuchal line)	*Bilaterally:* Extends head; *Unilaterally:* Extends and tilts head to one side	C2–T1
Semispinalis cervicis	Transverse processes of upper thoracic spine	Spinous processes of C2–C5	Extends vertebral column; rotates to opposite side	C2–T5
Splenius capitis	Spinous processes of 7th cervical, upper three or four thoracic vertebrae, and lower part of ligamentum nuchae	Mastoid process of temporal bone and lateral part of superior nuchal line of occipital bone	*Bilaterally:* Extends head; *Unilaterally:* Tilts and rotates head to same side	Capitis: C3–C6
Splenius cervicis	Spinous process of T3–T6	Transverse processes of C1–C3	*Bilaterally:* Extends or hyperextends head and neck; *Unilaterally:* Laterally flexes and rotates head and neck	C4–C8
Longissimus capitis (*considered part of erector spinae*)	Articular processes of C5–C7 and transverse processes of T1–T5	Mastoid process of temporal bone	*Bilaterally:* Extends neck; *Unilaterally:* Rotates head to side	C3–C8
Longissimus cervicis (*considered part of erector spinae*)	Transverse processes of T1–T5	Transverse processes C2–C6	*Bilaterally:* Extends neck, *Unilaterally:* Rotates head to side	C3–T6
Levator scapulae	Transverse processes of C1–C4	Superior part of medial border of scapula	*Unilaterally:* Elevates and adducts scapula; rotates scapula (glenoid faces down); Laterally flexes neck to same side and rotates neck to same side; *Bilaterally:* Extends neck	C3–C5
Rectus capitis posterior (major and minor)	Spinous process of axis (major); posterior arch of the atlas (minor)	On and close to inferior nuchal line	Extends head; rotates head ipsilaterally	C1
Obliquus capitis (superior and inferior)	*Superior:* Transverse process of atlas *Inferior:* Spine and lamina of axis	*Superior:* Occipital bone between superior and inferior nuchal line; *Inferior:* Posterior aspect of transverse process of atlas	Rotates head ipsilaterally; extends head; lateral flexion	C1

Table 4.5

Muscles of the Spine

Name	Origin	Insertion	Action	Nerve Supply
Superficial muscles (extensors of spine): made up of the spinalis, longissimus, and iliocostalis groups.				
Spinalis Group				
Semispinalis thoracis	Transverse processes of T6–T10	Spinous processes of C5–T4	Extends and rotates vertebral column	Thoracic spinal nerves
Spinalis thoracis	Spinous processes of T11–L2	Spinous processes of T1–T8	Extends and rotates vertebral column	Lower cervical and thoracic spinal nerves
Longissimus Group				
Longissimus thoracis *(includes longissimus capitis and cervicis, described in Table 4.4)*	Broad sheet of connective tissue and transverse process of lower thoracic and upper lumbar vertebrae; with iliocostalis, forms sacrospinalis	Inferior surface of ribs and transverse process of upper thoracic vertebrae	Extends spine; bends spine to same side; depresses ribs	Lower cervical thoracic and lumbar spinal nerves
Iliocostalis Group				
Iliocostalis thoracis	Medial aspect of the superior border of lower 7 ribs	Angles of upper ribs and transverse process of last cervical vertebra	Stabilizes thoracic vertebrae during extension; extends and laterally flexes vertebrae	T7–L2
Iliocostalis lumborum	Medial part of iliac crest and sacrospinal aponeurosis	Inferior surface of angles of lower 7 ribs	Extends spine; laterally flexes vertebral column, rotates ribs	T7–L2
Deep muscles (extensors of spine)				
Multifidus	Sacrum and transverse process of each vertebra	Spinous process of vertebra, located about five vertebrae above origin	Extends and rotates vertebrae	Dorsal rami of the spinal nerves
Rotatores	Transverse process of each vertebra	Spinous process of vertebra above origin	Extends and rotates vertebrae	Dorsal rami of the spinal nerves
Interspinales	Spinous processes of each vertebra	Spinous process of vertebra above origin	Extends vertebral column	Dorsal rami of the spinal nerves
Intertransversarii	Transverse process of each vertebra	Transverse process of vertebra above origin	Bends vertebral column laterally	Dorsal and ventral rami of the spinal nerves
Muscles of spine (flexor of spine)				
Quadratus lumborum	Iliac crest	12th rib and transverse process of L1–L4	Flexes spine; depresses ribs; assists in extension; *Bilaterally:* With the diaphragm fixes the last two ribs during expiration; *With insertion fixed:* Elevates pelvis	T2, L1–L4

Table 4.6

Muscles of the Abdomen

Name	Origin	Insertion	Action	Nerve Supply
External oblique	Lower 8 ribs	Linea alba and anterior part of iliac crest	*Bilaterally:* Flexes vertebral column; tilts pelvis posteriorly; supports and compresses the abdominal viscera; depresses thorax and assists with respiration; *Unilaterally:* Depresses ribs; Laterally flexes the vertebral column approximating the thorax and iliac crest; (along with lateral fibers of internal oblique of same side), rotates the vertebral column (with the internal oblique on the opposite side); when the pelvis is fixed, the right external oblique rotates thorax counterclockwise, and the left rotates the thorax clockwise	T6–T12
Internal oblique	Thoracolumbar fascia; iliac crest; lateral half of inguinal ligament	Cartilage of lower 3–4 ribs; xiphoid process; linea alba	*Bilaterally:* Flexes vertebral column; depresses thorax and assists in respiration; compresses and supports the lower abdominal viscera in conjunction with the transversus abdominis; *Unilaterally:* Rotates thorax backward (in conjunction with the anterior fibers of the external oblique on the opposite side); the right internal oblique rotates the thorax clockwise, and the left rotates the thorax counterclockwise on a fixed pelvis; lateral fibers (along with the lateral fibers of the external oblique on the same side) laterally flexes the vertebral column approximating the thorax and pelvis	T6–T12, L1
Transversus abdominis	Cartilage of lower 6 ribs; thoracolumbar fascia; lateral part of inguinal ligament	Linea alba and pubis; iliac crest	Compresses abdomen	T6–T12, L1
Rectus abdominis	Superior surface of pubis	Xiphoid process; inferior surface of cartilage of ribs 5–7	Flexes vertebral column by approximating the thorax and pelvis; with the pelvis fixed, moves thorax toward the pelvis; with the thorax fixed, moves pelvis towards the thorax; depresses ribs	T5–T12

Table 4.7

Muscles of the Thorax

Name	Origin	Insertion	Action	Nerve Supply
External intercostals	Inferior border of each rib	Superior border of lower rib	Elevates ribs, increasing the volume of the thoracic cavity—inspiratory muscle	T1–T12
Internal intercostals	Superior border of each rib	Inferior border of rib above origin	Depresses ribs, reducing thoracic volume—expiratory muscle	T1–T12
Transversus thoracis	Inner surface of inferior part of sternum and adjacent costal cartilages	Cartilage of ribs 2–6	Depresses ribs, reducing thoracic volume for forceful expiration	T7–T12
Diaphragm	Xiphoid process (sternal); cartilages of ribs 4–10 (costal); body of upper 2–3 lumbar vertebrae (lumbar)	Fibers converge to central tendinous sheet	Increases volume of thoracic cavity; decreases volume of abdomino-pelvic cavity—inspiratory muscle	phrenic, C3–C5

Table 4.8

Muscles That Position and Move the Shoulder Girdle

Name	Origin	Insertion	Action	Nerve Supply	Muscle Diagram
Posteriorly located muscles					
Trapezius	Long origin from the occipital bone, ligamentum nuchae; spinal processes of C7 and all thoracic vertebrae	V-shaped insertion from the lateral one-third of clavicle, acromion, and spine of scapula	(Depends on the fibers contracting) elevates, depresses, adducts, rotates scapula; elevates clavicle; extends head and neck; acts as accessory muscle of respiration	XI (accessory nerve)	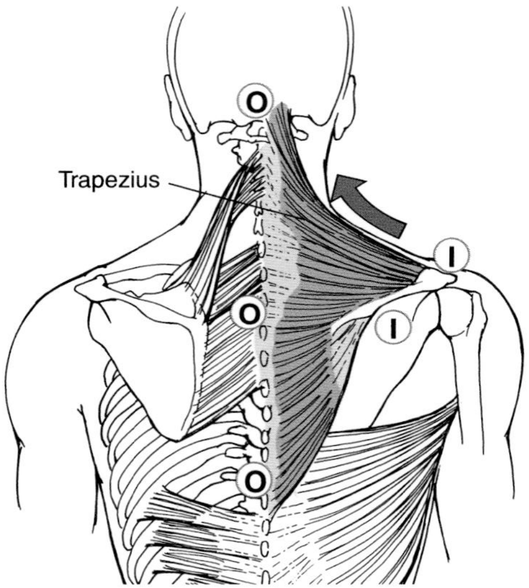 Trapezius
Rhomboideus major	Spinous processes of T2–T5 vertebrae	Medial border of scapula from spine to inferior angle	Adducts, elevates, and rotates the scapula (glenoid cavity faces caudally); helps stabilize scapula	C4–C5 (dorsal scapular)	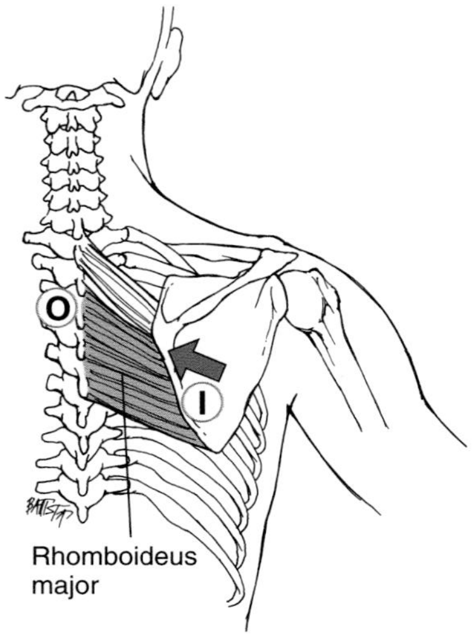 Rhomboideus major

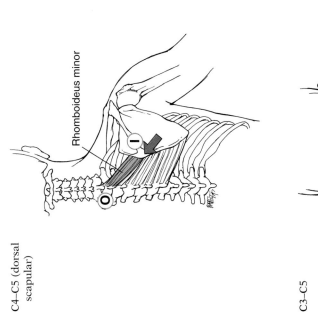

Continued

Muscle	Origin	Insertion	Action	Innervation
Rhomboideus minor	Spinous processes of C7 and T1; inferior part of ligamentum nuchae	Medial border of scapula near spine	Adducts, elevates, and rotates the scapula (glenoid cavity faces caudally); stabilizes scapula	C4–C5 (dorsal scapular)

Superiorly located muscle

Muscle	Origin	Insertion	Action	Innervation
Levator scapulae	Transverse processes of C1–C4	Superior part of medial border of scapula	Unilaterally: Elevates and adducts scapula; rotates scapula (glenoid faces down); lateally flexes neck to same side; rotates neck to same side; Bilaterally: extends neck	C3–C5

Table 4.8

Muscles That Position and Move the Shoulder Girdle (Continued)

Name	Origin	Insertion	Action	Nerve Supply	Muscle Diagram
Laterally located muscle					
Serratus anterior	Anterior and superior aspect of ribs 1–9	Anterior aspect of the medial border of scapula	Protracts, abducts, rotates the inferior angle laterally and glenoid cavity of scapula cranially; stabilizes scapula by holding medial border firmly against the rib cage; lower fibers may depress scapula, upper fibers may elevate it slightly; starting from a position with the humerus fixed in flexion and the hands against a wall or floor, acts to displace the thorax posteriorly (e.g., push-up); with insertion fixed, may act in forced inspiration	C5–7 (long thoracic nerve)	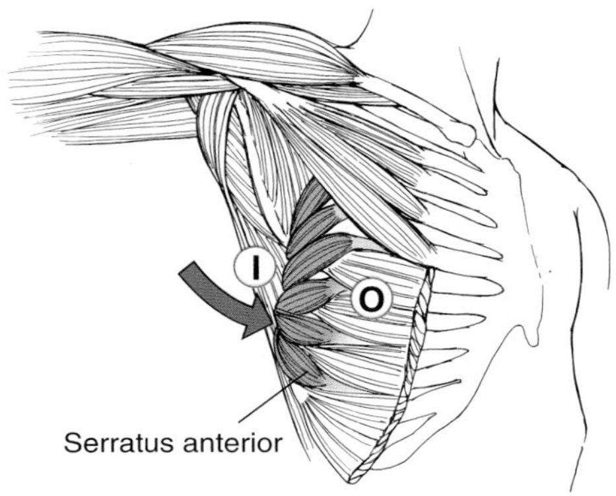 **Anteriolateral view** Serratus anterior

Anteriorly located muscles

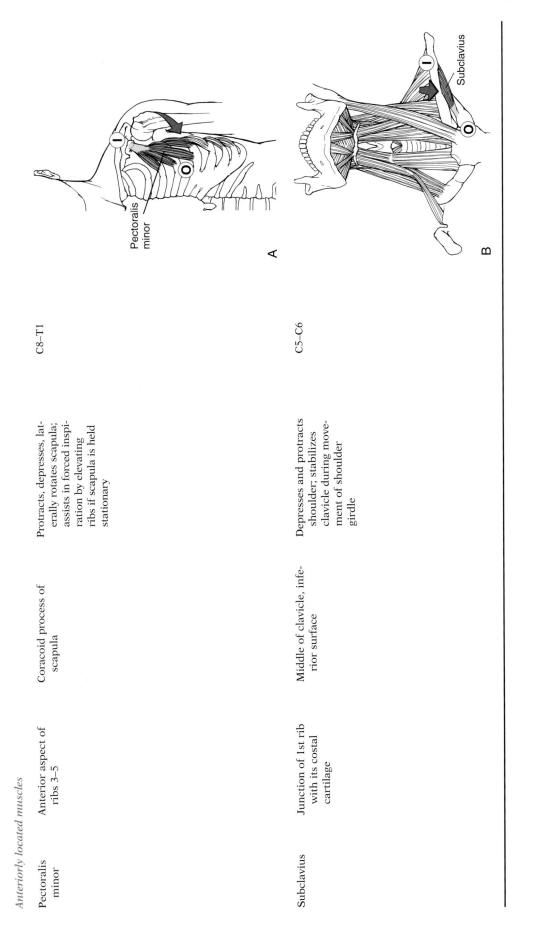

| Pectoralis minor | Anterior aspect of ribs 3–5 | Coracoid process of scapula | Protracts, depresses, laterally rotates scapula; assists in forced inspiration by elevating ribs if scapula is held stationary | C8–T1 |
| Subclavius | Junction of 1st rib with its costal cartilage | Middle of clavicle, inferior surface | Depresses and protracts shoulder; stabilizes clavicle during movement of shoulder girdle | C5–C6 |

Table 4.9 Muscles That Move the Arm

Name	Origin	Insertion	Action	Nerve Supply	Muscle Diagram
Anteriorly located muscles					
Pectoralis major	Body of sternum, cartilage of 2–6 ribs, aponeurosis of external oblique (sternocostal); medial half of clavicle (clavicular)	Greater tubercle of humerus and lateral lip of the bicipital groove of humerus	Flexes; adducts; medially rotates humerus; with insertion fixed, may assist in elevating the thorax as in forced inspiration	C5–C8, T1	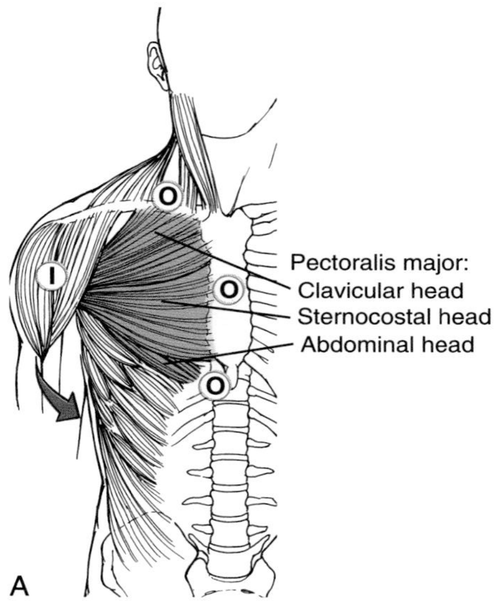

(*Pectoralis minor lies beneath the pectoralis major, but manipulates the scapula.*)

Name	Origin	Insertion	Action	Nerve Supply	Muscle Diagram
Deltoid (*deltoid or triangular muscle covering anterior and posterior part of shoulder*)	Lateral third of clavicle (anterior); acromion process (middle) and spine of the scapula (posterior)	Deltoid tuberosity of humerus	Flexes arm and medially rotates shoulder joint (anterior fibers); abducts arm (middle fibers); extends arm and laterally rotates shoulder joint (posterior fibers)	C5–C6 (axillary nerve)	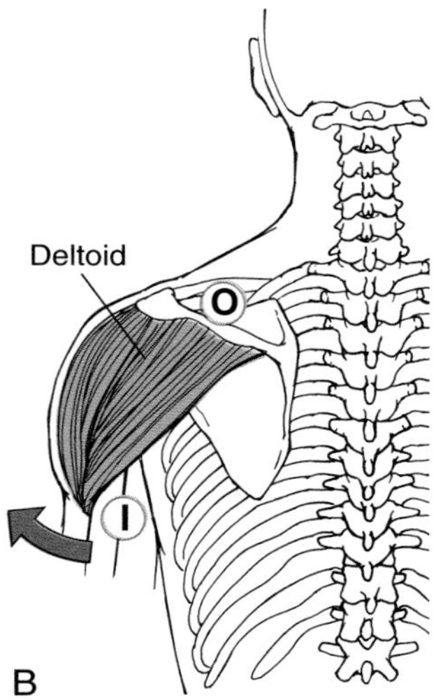

Continued

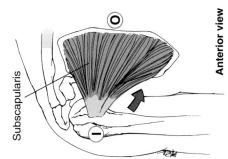

Anterior view

Coracobrachialis

Subscapularis

Anterior view

Coraco-brachialis

Coracoid process of scapula

Middle third of medial margin of humerus

Adducts and flexes arm; stabilizes humerus

C5–C7 (musculo-cutaneous)

Posteriorly located muscles

Subscapularis *(rotator cuff muscle)*

Subscapular fossa of scapula

Lesser tubercle of humerus

Medially rotates humerus; stabilizes shoulder joint

C5–C6

Table 4.9
Muscles That Move the Arm (Continued)

Name	Origin	Insertion	Action	Nerve Supply	Muscle Diagram
Anteriorly located muscles					
Supraspinatus *(rotator cuff muscle)*	Supraspinous fossa of scapula	Greater tubercle of humerus	Abducts arm (assists at start of movements); stabilizes shoulder joint	C5–C6	
Infraspinatus *(rotator cuff muscle)*	Infraspinous fossa of scapula	Greater tubercle of humerus	Laterally rotates humerus; stabilizes shoulder joint	C5–C6	

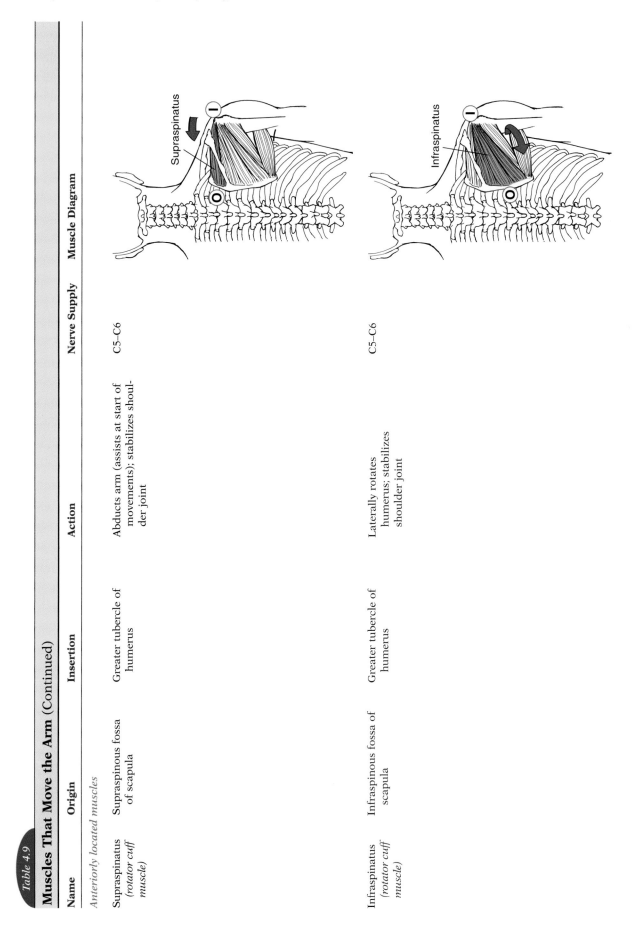

Continued

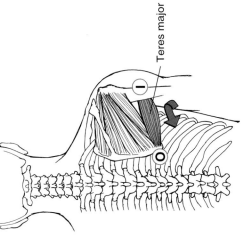

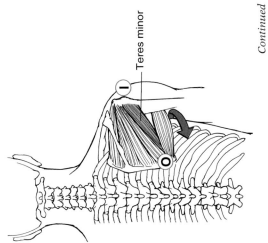

Teres major

Lower third of lateral border and inferior angle of scapula

Medial lip of intertubercular groove of humerus

Medially rotates humerus; adducts arm; extends shoulder

C5–C7

Teres minor
(rotator cuff muscle)

Upper two-thirds of lateral border of scapula

Greater tubercle of humerus

Laterally rotates humerus; adducts arm (weakly); stabilizes shoulder joint

C5–C6
(axillary)

Table 4.9

Muscles That Move the Arm (Continued)

Name	Origin	Insertion	Action	Nerve Supply	Muscle Diagram
Posteriorly located muscles					
Latissimus dorsi	Spinous processes of lower six thoracic vertebrae and lumbar vertebrae; thoracolumbar fascia; 8–12 ribs; inferior angle of scapula	Floor or bicipital groove	*Unilaterally:* Extends; adducts; medially rotates arm; depresses the shoulder girdle; *Bilaterally:* Assists in hyperextending spine and anteriorly tilting the pelvis, or in flexing the spine, depending on its relation to the axes of motion; *With insertion fixed:* Assists in lateral flexion of the trunk, assists in tilting the pelvis anteriorly and laterally; may act as an accessory muscle of respiration	C6–C8	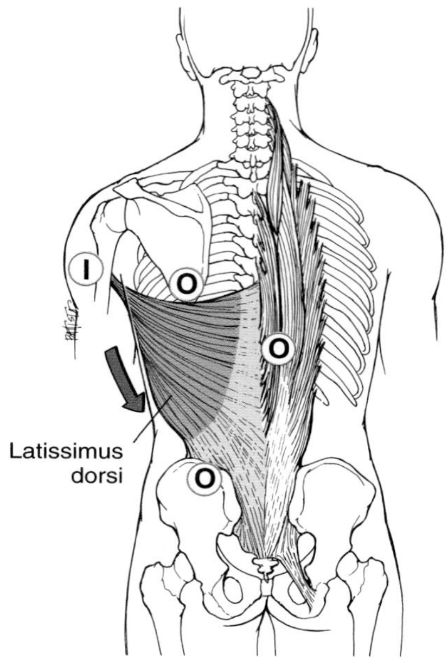 Latissimus dorsi
Triceps brachii (long head)	Infraglenoid tuberosity of scapula	Olecranon process of ulna	Extends arm; assists in adduction and extension of the shoulder joint	C6–C8 (radial)	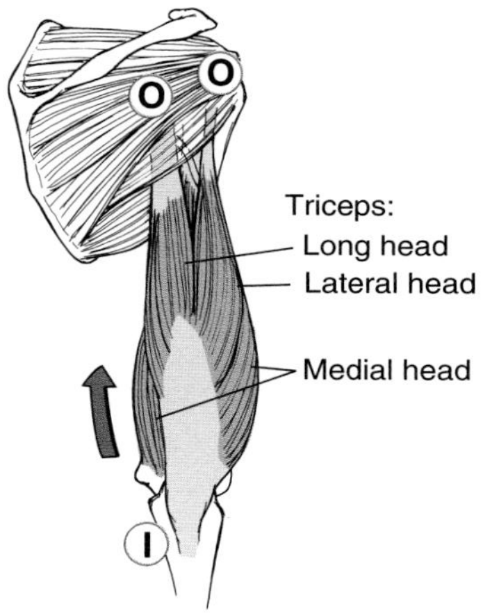 Triceps: Long head, Lateral head, Medial head

Continued

Table 4.10

Muscles That Move the Forearm and Wrist

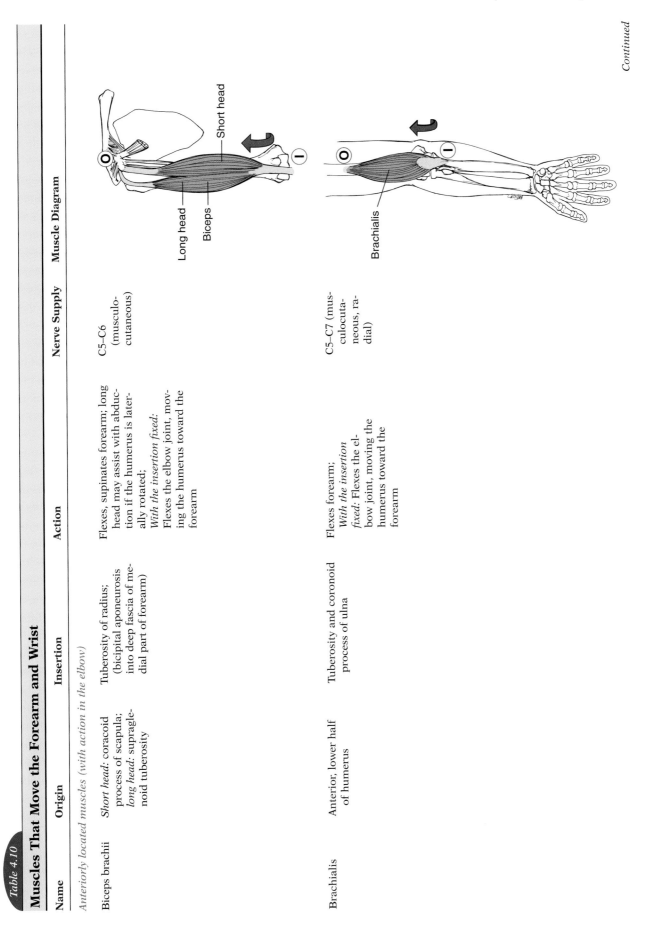

Anteriorly located muscles (with action in the elbow)

Name	Origin	Insertion	Action	Nerve Supply	Muscle Diagram
Biceps brachii	*Short head:* coracoid process of scapula; *long head:* supraglenoid tuberosity	Tuberosity of radius; (bicipital aponeurosis into deep fascia of medial part of forearm)	Flexes, supinates forearm; long head may assist with abduction if the humerus is laterally rotated; *With the insertion fixed:* Flexes the elbow joint, moving the humerus toward the forearm	C5–C6 (musculocutaneous)	
Brachialis	Anterior, lower half of humerus	Tuberosity and coronoid process of ulna	Flexes forearm; *With the insertion fixed:* Flexes the elbow joint, moving the humerus toward the forearm	C5–C7 (musculocutaneous, radial)	

Table 4.10

Muscles That Move the Forearm and Wrist (Continued)

Name	Origin	Insertion	Action	Nerve Supply	Muscle Diagram
Brachio-radialis	Upper two-thirds of lateral supra-condylar ridge of humerus	Lateral aspect of styloid process of radius	Flexes forearm and assists in pronating and supinating the forearm	C5–C6 (radial)	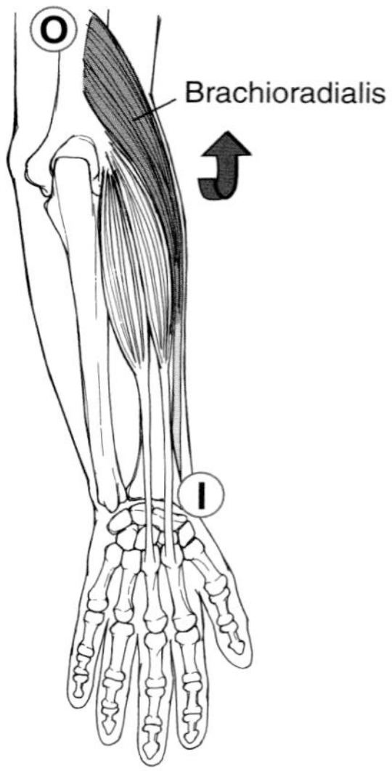
Supinator	Lateral epicondyle of humerus and ulna	Anterolateral surface of upper third of radius	Supinates forearm	C6–C7 (radial)	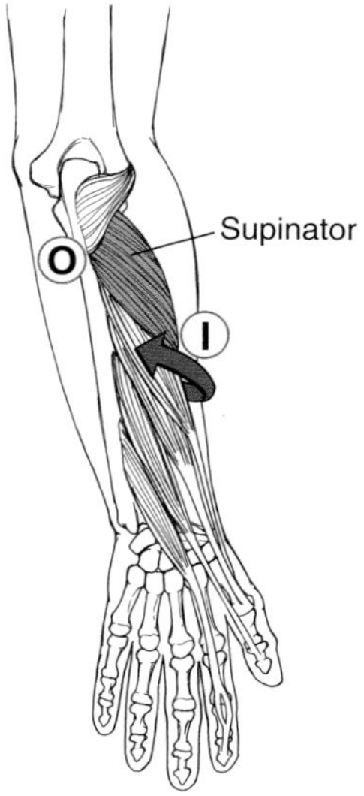

Brachioradialis

Anterior view

Supinator

Posterior view

Continued

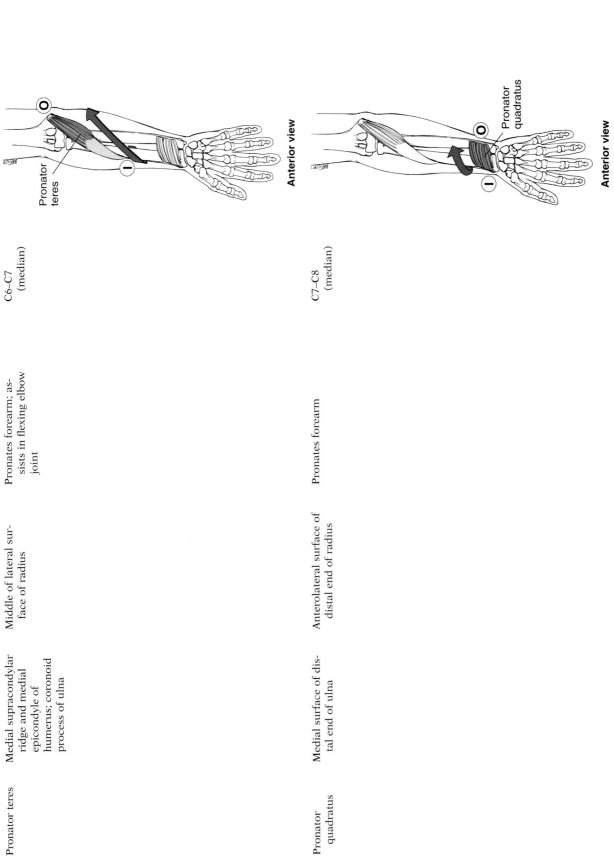

C6–C7
(median)

C7–C8
(median)

Pronates forearm; assists in flexing elbow joint

Pronates forearm

Middle of lateral surface of radius

Anterolateral surface of distal end of radius

Medial supracondylar ridge and medial epicondyle of humerus; coronoid process of ulna

Medial surface of distal end of ulna

Pronator teres

Pronator quadratus

Table 4.10

Muscles That Move the Forearm and Wrist (Continued)

Posteriorly located muscles (with action at the forearm)

Name	Origin	Insertion	Action	Nerve Supply	Muscle Diagram
Anconeus	Lateral epicondyle of humerus, posterior surface	Olecranon process of ulna	Extends arm	C7–C8 (radial)	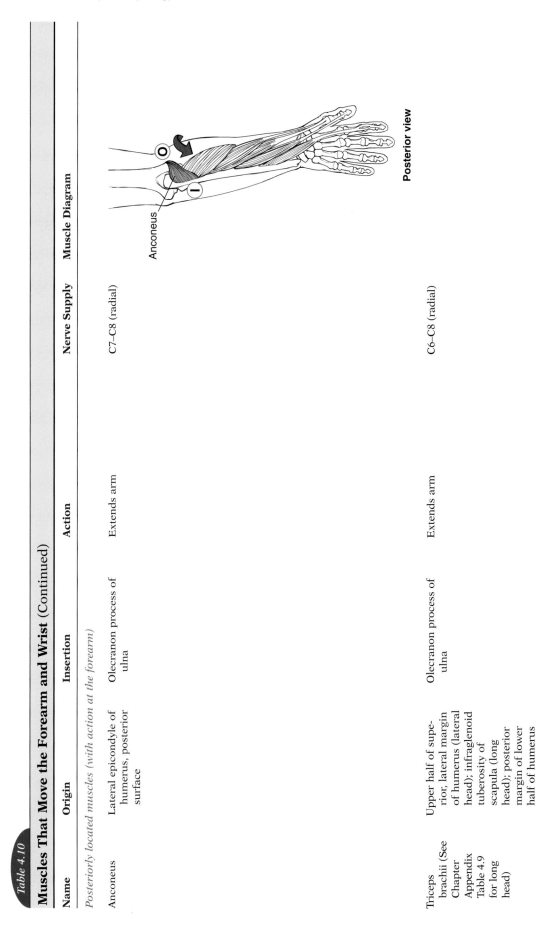
Triceps brachii (See Chapter Appendix Table 4.9 for long head)	Upper half of superior, lateral margin of humerus (lateral head); infraglenoid tuberosity of scapula (long head); posterior margin of lower half of humerus (short head)	Olecranon process of ulna	Extends arm	C6–C8 (radial)	

Anconeus

Posterior view

Continued

Anteriorly placed muscles (with action at the wrist)

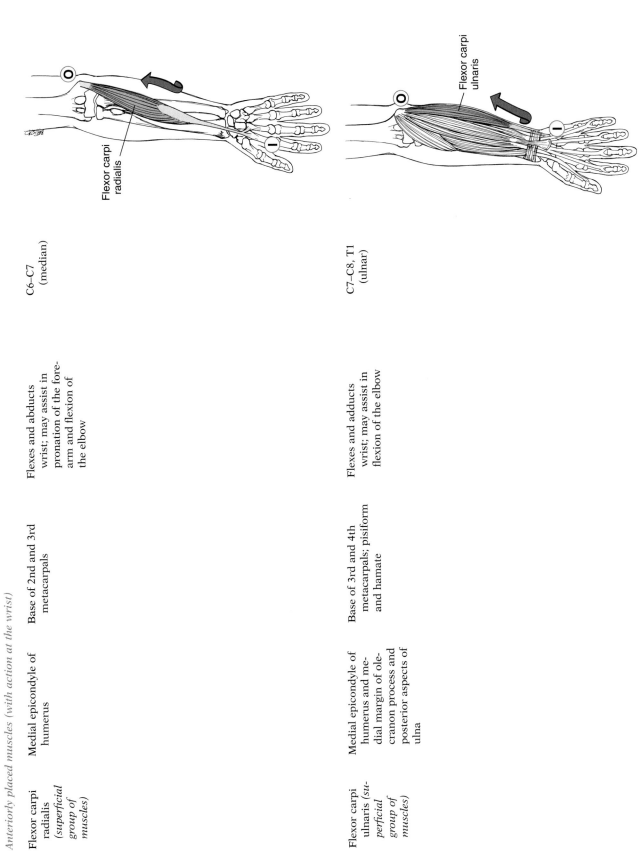

C6–C7
(median)

C7–C8, T1
(ulnar)

Flexes and abducts
wrist; may assist in
pronation of the fore-
arm and flexion of
the elbow

Flexes and adducts
wrist; may assist in
flexion of the elbow

Base of 2nd and 3rd
metacarpals

Base of 3rd and 4th
metacarpals; pisiform
and hamate

Medial epicondyle of
humerus

Medial epicondyle of
humerus and me-
dial margin of ole-
cranon process and
posterior aspects of
ulna

Flexor carpi
radialis *(su-
perficial
group of
muscles)*

Flexor carpi
ulnaris *(su-
perficial
group of
muscles)*

Table 4.10

Muscles That Move the Forearm and Wrist (Continued)

Name	Origin	Insertion	Action	Nerve Supply	Muscle Diagram
Anteriorly located muscles (with action at the forearm)					
Palmaris longus (*superficial group of muscles*)	Medial epicondyle of humerus	Palmar aponeurosis	Tense palmar fascia, flexes the wrist and may assist in flexion of elbow	C6–C7 (median)	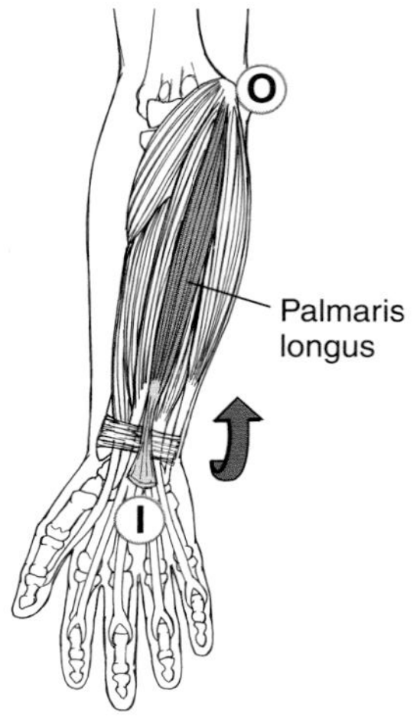 Palmaris longus Anterior view
(Note that all the flexors of palm arise from the medial epicondyle.)					
Posteriorly placed muscles (with action at the wrist)					
Extensor carpi radialis longus	Lower third of lateral supracondylar ridge of humerus	Base of 2nd metacarpal	Extends and abducts wrist; assists in flexion of the elbow	C6–C7 (radial)	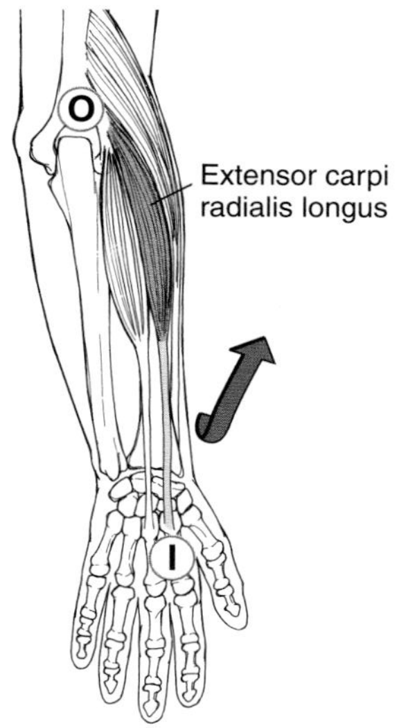 Extensor carpi radialis longus Posterior view

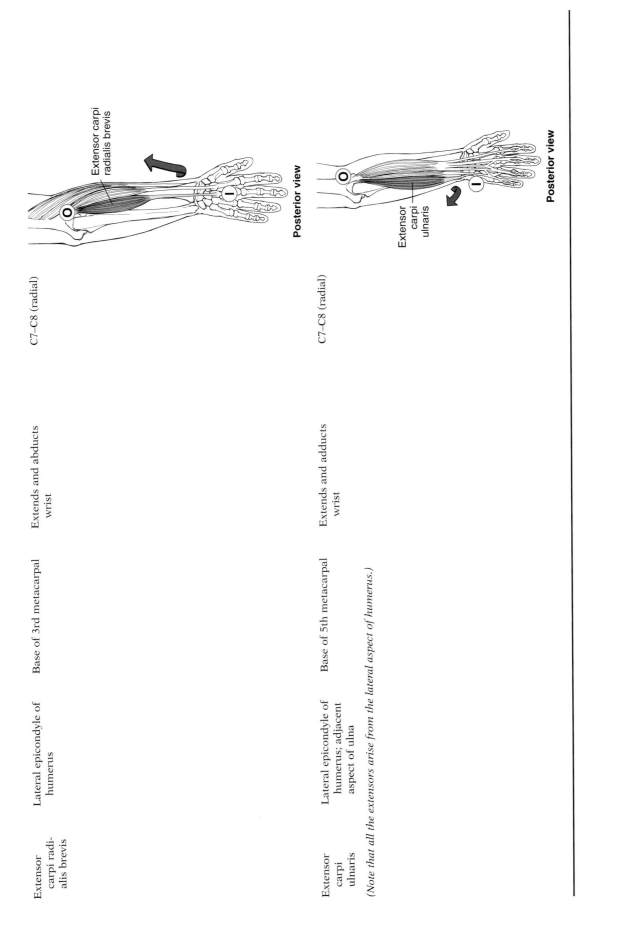

Extensor carpi radialis brevis

C7–C8 (radial)

Extends and abducts wrist

Base of 3rd metacarpal

Lateral epicondyle of humerus

Extensor carpi radialis brevis

Posterior view

Extensor carpi ulnaris

C7–C8 (radial)

Extends and adducts wrist

Base of 5th metacarpal

Lateral epicondyle of humerus; adjacent aspect of ulna

(Note that all the extensors arise from the lateral aspect of humerus.)

Posterior view

Table 4.11

Muscles That Move the Palm and Fingers (Continued)

Anteriorly located muscles (deep to the muscles moving the wrist)

Name	Origin	Insertion	Action	Nerve Supply	Muscle Diagram
Flexor digitorum superficialis	Medial epicondyle of humerus; proximal anterior surface of ulna and radius	Four tendons split into two slips and attached into 2nd phalanx of fingers (except thumb);	Flexes wrist; flexes fingers, especially 2nd phalanx; assists in flexion of the metacarpophalangeal joints	C8, T1 (median)	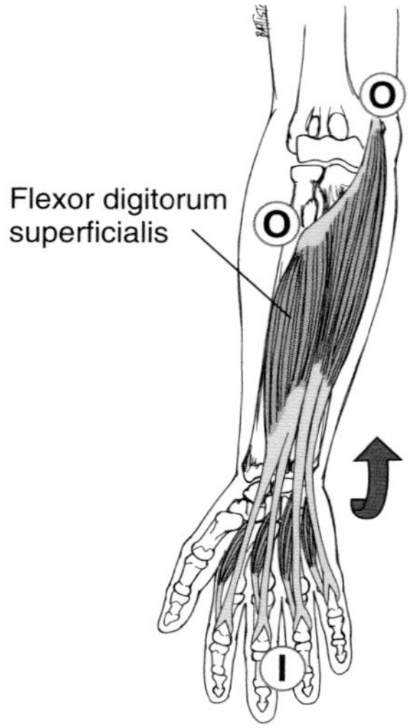 Flexor digitorum superficialis — Anterior view
Flexor digitorum profundus	Proximal three-fourths of antero-medial aspect of ulna; coronoid process and interosseous membrane	Base of distal phalanges of fingers	Flexes wrist; flexes fingers; flexes distal interphalangeal joints of index, middle, ring, and little fingers, and assists in flexion of proximal interphalangeal and metacarpophalangeal joint	C8, T1 (lateral portion: median; medial portion: ulnar)	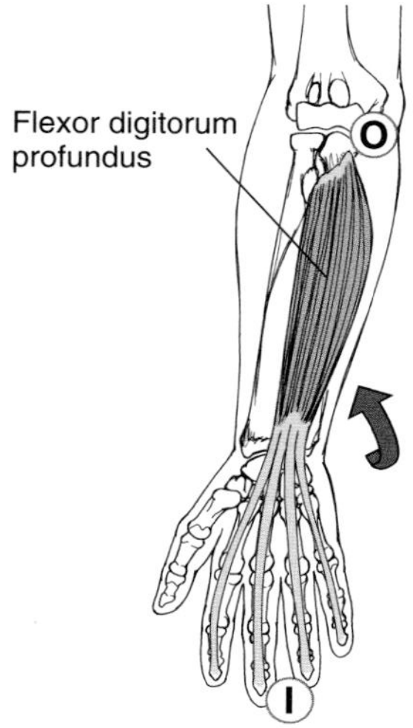 Flexor digitorum profundus — Anterior view

Continued

Flexor pollicis longus

Medial epicondyle of humerus, middle of anterior shaft of radius; interosseous membrane

Distal phalanx of thumb

Flexes the interphalangeal joint of thumb, assists in flexion of the metacarpophalangeal and carpometacarpal joints, and may assist in flexion of the wrist

C7–C8 (median)

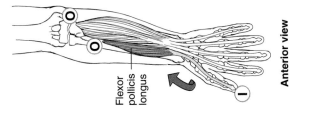
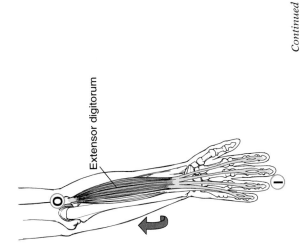

Flexor pollicis longus

Anterior view

Posteriorly located muscles

Extensor digitorum

Lateral epicondyle of humerus

Dorsal surface of phalanges of all fingers

Extends fingers; extends the metacarpophalangeal joints and, in conjunction with the lumbricals and interossei, extends the interphalangeal joints of the 2nd through 5th digits; assists in abduction of the index, ring, and little fingers; assists in extension and abduction of the wrist

C7–C8 (radial)

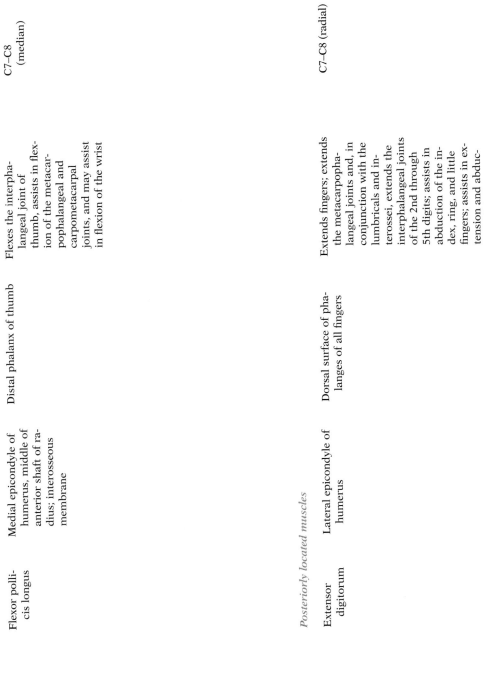

Extensor digitorum

Table 4.11

Muscles That Move the Palm and Fingers (Continued)

Name	Origin	Insertion	Action	Nerve Supply	Muscle Diagram
Anteriorly located muscles (deep to the muscles moving the wrist)					
Abductor pollicis longus	Proximal, posterior surface of ulna and radius	Lateral margin of 1st metacarpal	Abducts and extends the carpometacarpal joint of the thumb; abducts (radial deviation) and assists in flexion of the wrist	C7–C8 (radial)	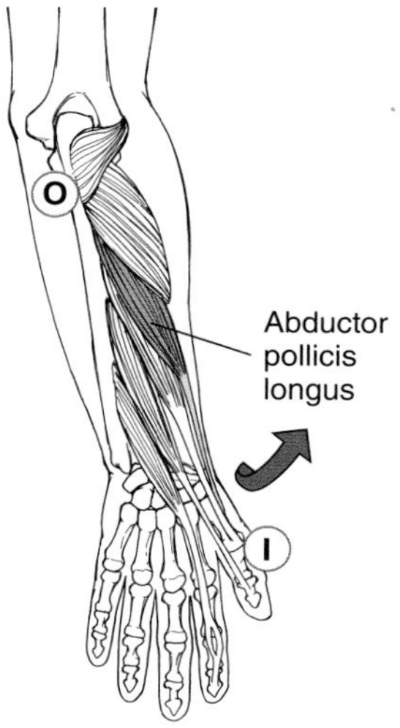 Abductor pollicis longus **Posterior view**
Extensor digiti minimi	Common extensor origin on the lateral epicondyle of the humerus	Dorsal surface of proximal phalanx of fifth digit	Extends the metacarpophalangeal joint and, in conjunction with the lumbricalis and interosseus, extends the interphalangeal joints of the little finger; assists in abduction of the little finger	Nerve root: C7–C8 (radial)	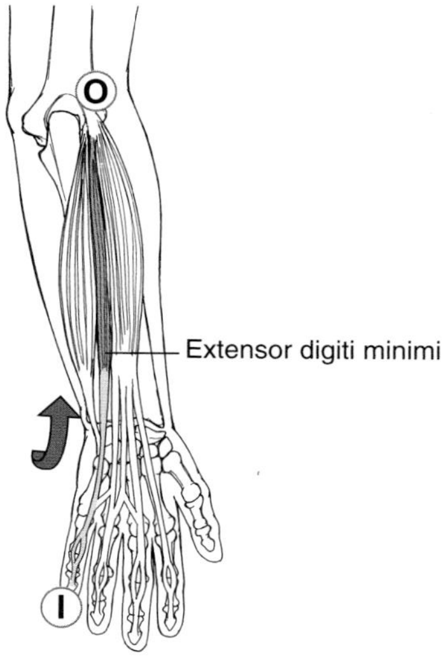 Extensor digiti minimi **Posterior view**

Intrinsic muscles of the hand (muscles that originate and insert in the hand)

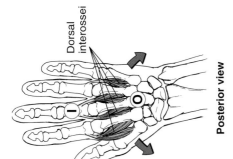

Posterior view

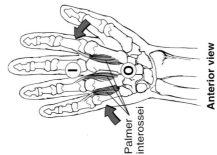

Anterior view

Muscle	Origin	Insertion	Action	Innervation
Dorsal interossei *(first–fourth)*	Adjacent sides of metacarpal bones	All insert into the dorsal digital expansions (in the base of the proximal phalanx) of either the index, middle, or ring fingers	Abducts 2nd to 4th fingers from the axial line through the 3rd digit; assists in flexion of metacarpophalangeal joints and extension of interphalangeal joints of the same fingers; the first assists in adduction of the thumb	C8, T1 (ulnar)
Palmar interossei *(first–fourth)*	Side of the shaft of all metacarpal bones (ulnar side, 1st and 2nd; radial side, 3rd and 4th) except middle metacarpal	All insert into the dorsal digital expansions at the sides of bases of proximal phalanges of all digits (except the middle)	Adducts the thumb, index, ring, and little finger toward the axial line through the 3rd digit; assists in flexion of metacarpophalangeal joints	C8, T1 (ulnar)

Continued

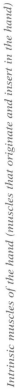

Table 4.11

Muscles That Move the Palm and Fingers (Continued)

Anteriorly located muscles (deep to the muscles moving the wrist)

Name	Origin	Insertion	Action	Nerve Supply	Muscle Diagram
Lumbricalis	Tendons of flexor digitorum profundus of each finger	Radial aspects of the dorsal expansion of the corresponding index, middle, ring, and little fingers	Extends the interphalangeal joints and simultaneously flexes the metacarpophalangeal joints of the 2nd through 5th digits; extends the interphalangeal joints when the metacarpophalangeal joints are extended	Medial two lumbricalis—C8, T1 (ulnar), lateral two lumbricalis—C8, T1 (median)	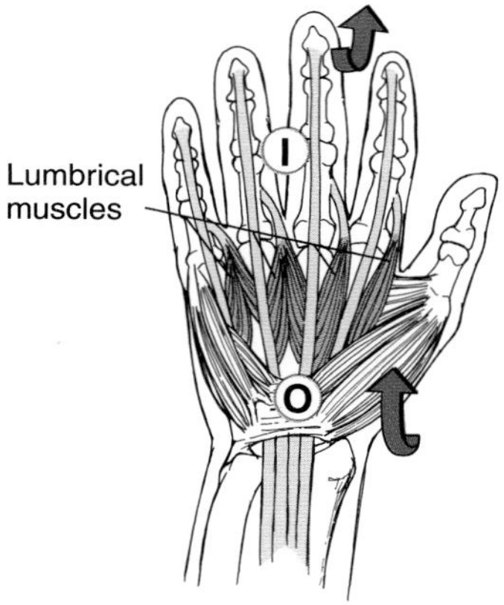 Lumbrical muscles **Anterior view**
Abductor digiti minimi	Pisiform bone; tendon of flexor carpi ulnaris	Ulnar aspect of the base of the proximal phalanx of the little finger; dorsal digital expansion of the little finger	Abducts, assists in opposition, and may assist in flexion of the metacarpophalangeal joint of the little finger; may assist in extension of interphalangeal joints	C8, T1 (ulnar)	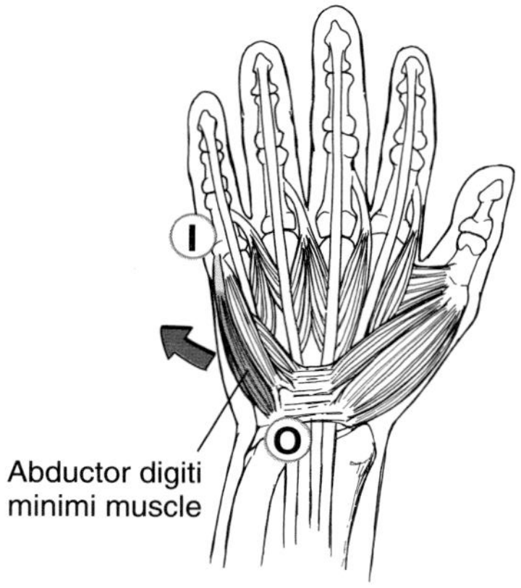 Abductor digiti minimi muscle **Anterior view**

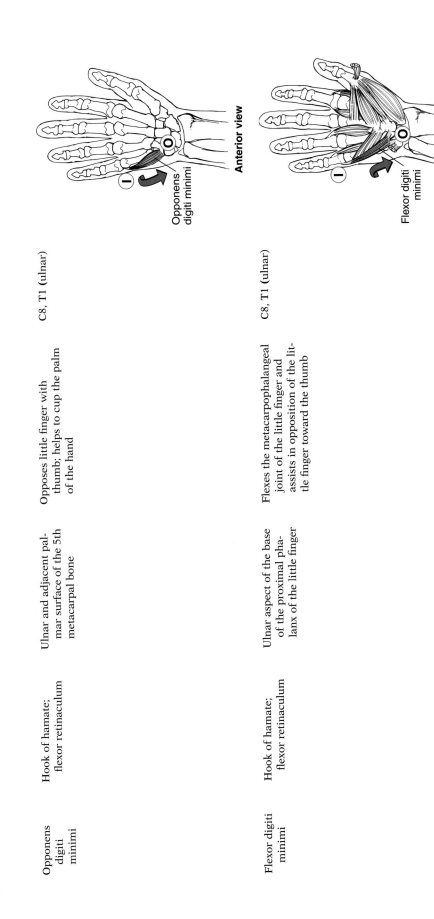

Continued

Opponens
digiti
minimi

Hook of hamate;
flexor retinaculum

Ulnar and adjacent pal-
mar surface of the 5th
metacarpal bone

Opposes little finger with
thumb; helps to cup the palm
of the hand

C8, T1 (ulnar)

Flexor digiti
minimi

Hook of hamate;
flexor retinaculum

Ulnar aspect of the base
of the proximal pha-
lanx of the little finger

Flexes the metacarpophalangeal
joint of the little finger and
assists in opposition of the little finger toward the thumb

C8, T1 (ulnar)

Table 4.11

Muscles That Move the Palm and Fingers (Continued)

Anteriorly located muscles (deep to the muscles moving the wrist)

Name	Origin	Insertion	Action	Nerve Supply	Muscle Diagram
Flexor pollicis brevis	*Superficial head:* Flexor retinaculum and the tubercle of the trapezium bone *Deep head:* Capitate and trapezoid bones and the palmar ligaments of the distal row of carpal bones	Radial side of the base of the proximal phalanx of the thumb	Flexes the metacarpophalangeal and carpometacarpal joints of the thumb; assists in opposition of the thumb toward the little finger; may extend the interphalangeal joint	*Superficial head:* C8, T1 (median) *Deep head:* C8, T1 (ulnar)	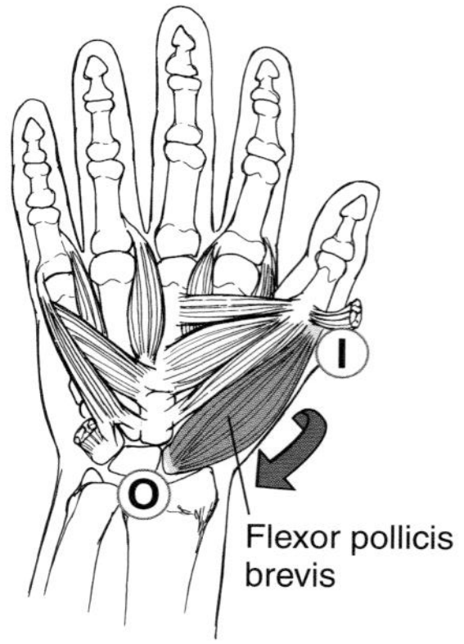 Flexor pollicis brevis **Anterior view**
Extensor pollicis brevis	Posterior aspect of the radius below the abductor pollicis longus; posterior surface of the interosseous membrane	Dorsal aspect of the base of the proximal phalanx of the thumb	Extends the metacarpophalangeal joint of the thumb, extends and abducts the carpometacarpal joint, and assists in abduction of the wrist	C7–C8 (radial)	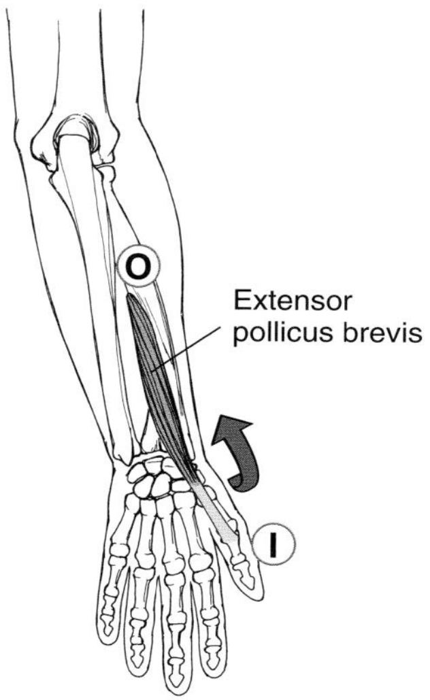 Extensor pollicus brevis **Posterior view**

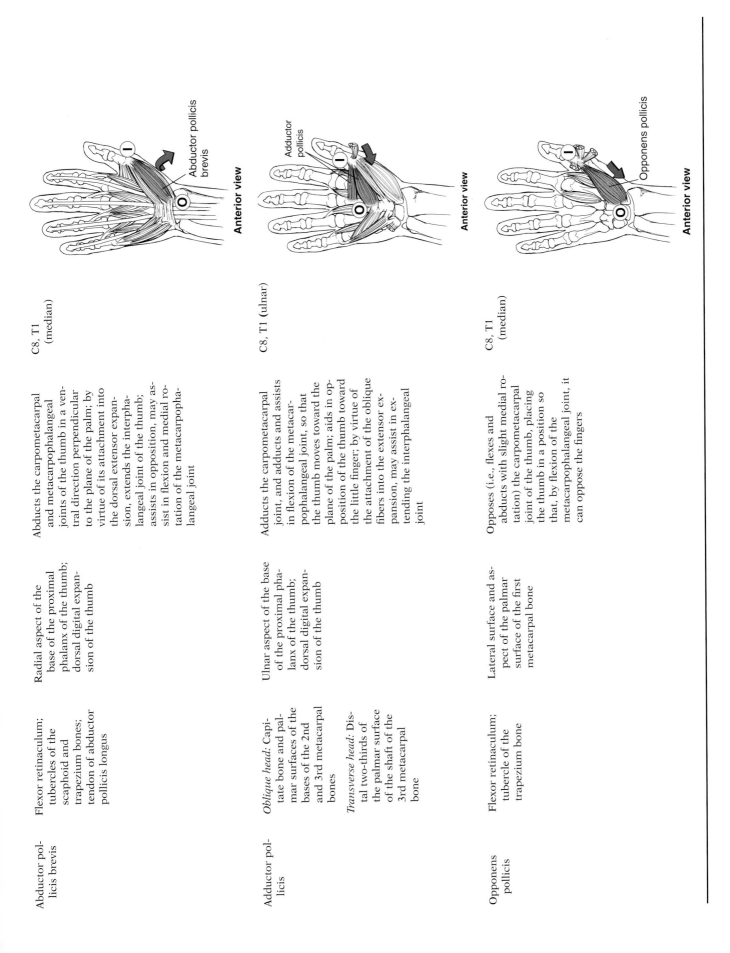

Muscle	Origin	Insertion	Action	Innervation	Illustration
Abductor pollicis brevis	Flexor retinaculum; tubercles of the scaphoid and trapezium bones; tendon of abductor pollicis longus	Radial aspect of the base of the proximal phalanx of the thumb; dorsal digital expansion of the thumb	Abducts the carpometacarpal and metacarpophalangeal joints of the thumb in a ventral direction perpendicular to the plane of the palm; by virtue of its attachment into the dorsal extensor expansion, extends the interphalangeal joint of the thumb; assists in opposition, may assist in flexion and medial rotation of the metacarpophalangeal joint	C8, T1 (median)	*Abductor pollicis brevis — Anterior view*
Adductor pollicis	*Oblique head:* Capitate bone and palmar surfaces of the bases of the 2nd and 3rd metacarpal bones; *Transverse head:* Distal two-thirds of the palmar surface of the shaft of the 3rd metacarpal bone	Ulnar aspect of the base of the proximal phalanx of the thumb; dorsal digital expansion of the thumb	Adducts the carpometacarpal joint, and adducts and assists in flexion of the metacarpophalangeal joint, so that the thumb moves toward the plane of the palm; aids in opposition of the thumb toward the little finger; by virtue of the attachment of the oblique fibers into the extensor expansion, may assist in extending the interphalangeal joint	C8, T1 (ulnar)	*Adductor pollicis — Anterior view*
Opponens pollicis	Flexor retinaculum; tubercle of the trapezium bone	Lateral surface and aspect of the palmar surface of the first metacarpal bone	Opposes (i.e., flexes and abducts with slight medial rotation) the carpometacarpal joint of the thumb, placing the thumb in a position so that, by flexion of the metacarpophalangeal joint, it can oppose the fingers	C8, T1 (median)	*Opponens pollicis — Anterior view*

Table 4.12

An Overview of Innervation of the Upper Limb (also see page 325)

Name	Muscle Innervated	Disability Caused by Damage
Axillary	Main abductor of shoulder (deltoid)	Weakness in abduction of shoulder
Musculocutaneous	Flexors of elbow (except brachioradialis)	Weakness in flexing elbow
Median	Flexors of wrist and fingers; pronators of forearm; thenar muscles	Difficulty in opposing thumb; (if nerve affected in carpal tunnel); weakness in flexion of wrist and fingers and pronation seen as well, if the nerve is affected more proximally
Ulnar nerve	Intrinsic muscles of hand	Difficulty adducting and abducting fingers; hands appear like claws (claw hands) due to the unopposed action of unaffected muscles
Radial nerve	Triceps; extensors of elbow, wrist	"Wrist drop." Wrist flexed; cannot extend fingers and abduct thumb, as in hitchhiking; can be caused by compression of the nerve against bone when using crutches or draping arm over a chair

Continued

Table 4.13

Muscles That Move the Thigh

Name	Origin	Insertion	Action	Nerve Supply	Muscle Diagram
Posteriorly located muscles					
Gluteus maximus	Iliac crest of ilium; sacrum; coccyx and thoracolumbar fascia; sacrotuberous ligament	Iliotibial tract and gluteal tuberosity of femur	Extends and laterally rotates thigh; lower fibers assist in adduction of the hip joint; upper fibers assist in abduction; by its insertion into the iliotibial tract, helps to stabilize the knee in extension	L5, S1–S2	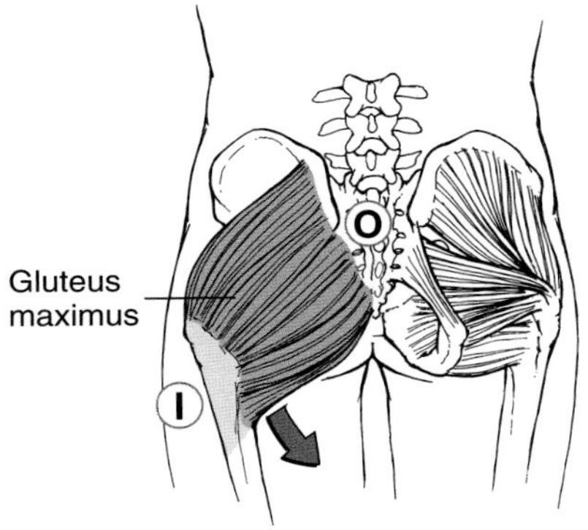 Gluteus maximus
Gluteus medius	Anterior iliac crest; lateral surface between superior and inferior gluteal lines	Greater trochanter of femur	Abducts and medially rotates thigh; the anterior fibers medially rotate and may assist in flexion of the hip joint; the posterior fibers laterally rotate and may assist in extension	L4–L5, S1	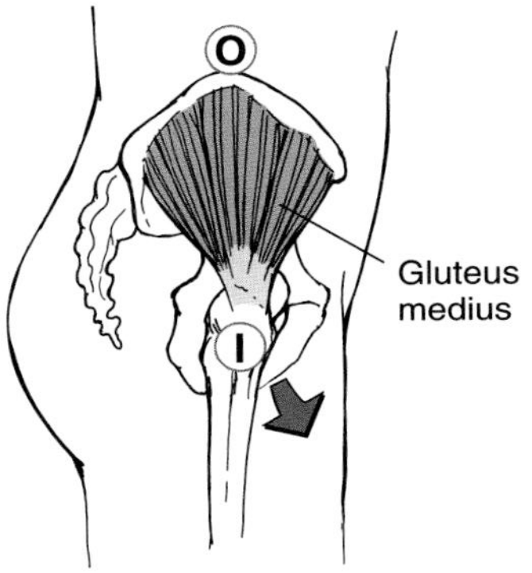 Gluteus medius
Gluteus minimus	Lateral surface of ilium between inferior and anterior gluteal lines	Greater trochanter of femur	Abducts and medially rotates thigh; may assist in flexion of the hip joint	L4–L5, S1	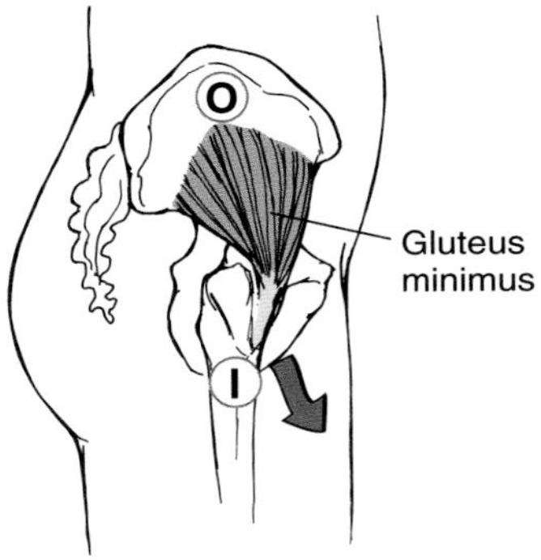 Gluteus minimus

Table 4.13

Muscles That Move the Thigh (Continued)

Name	Origin	Insertion	Action	Nerve Supply	Muscle Diagram
Laterally located muscles					
Tensor fasciae latae	Iliac crest and area between anterior iliac spines	Iliotibial tract	Flexes; abducts; medially rotates thigh; tenses the fascia lata; and may assist in knee extension	L4–L5, S1	
Obturators (externus and internus)	Margins of obturator foramen	Trochanteric fossa of femur	Laterally rotates thigh	Externus: L3–L4 Internus: L5, S1	

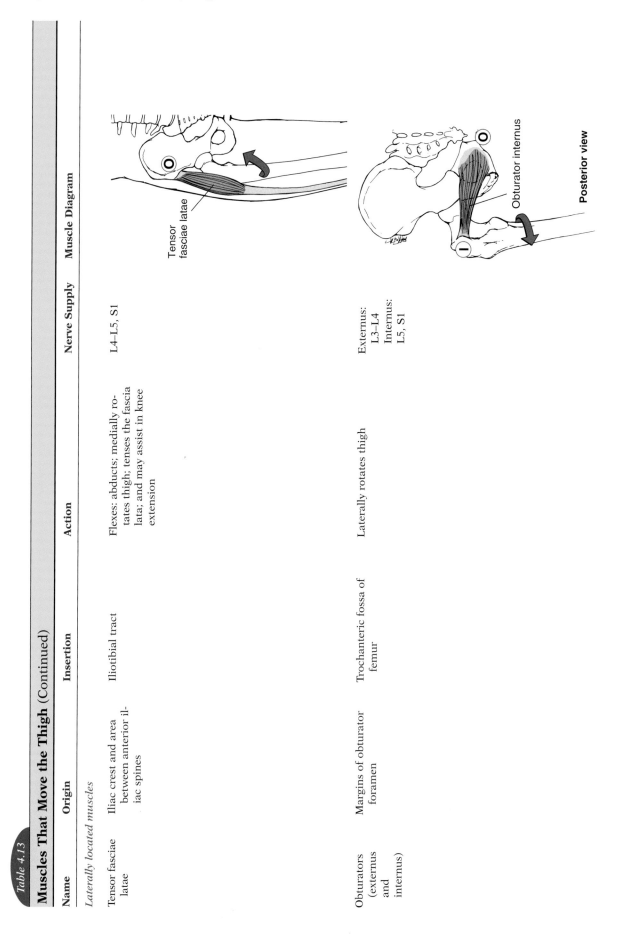

Tensor fasciae latae

Obturator internus

Posterior view

Continued

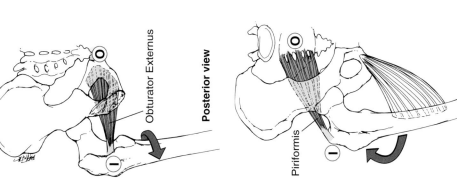

Obturator Externus

Posterior view

Piriformis

Anterior view

Piriformis

Anterolateral surface of sacrum; sacrotuberous ligament

Greater trochanter of femur

L5, S1–S2

Laterally rotates and abducts thigh

Table 4.13

Muscles That Move the Thigh (Continued)

Name	Origin	Insertion	Action	Nerve Supply	Muscle Diagram
Medially located muscles					
Adductor brevis	Inferior ramus of pubis	Linea aspera of femur	Adducts; flexes and medially rotates thigh	L2–L3	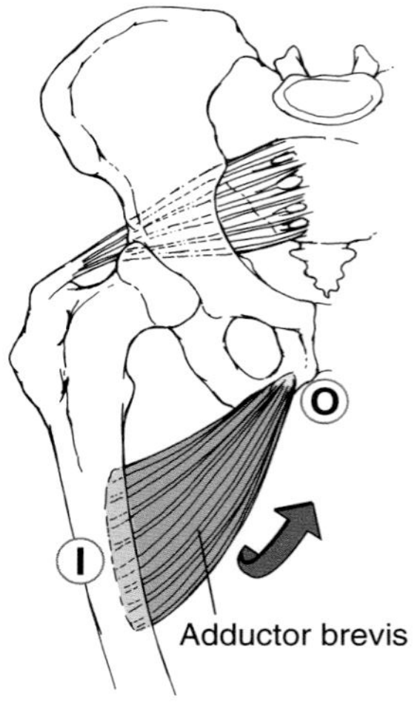 Adductor brevis Anterior view
Adductor longus	Inferior ramus of pubis	Linea aspera of femur	Adducts; flexes and medially rotates thigh	L2–L4 (obturator nerve)	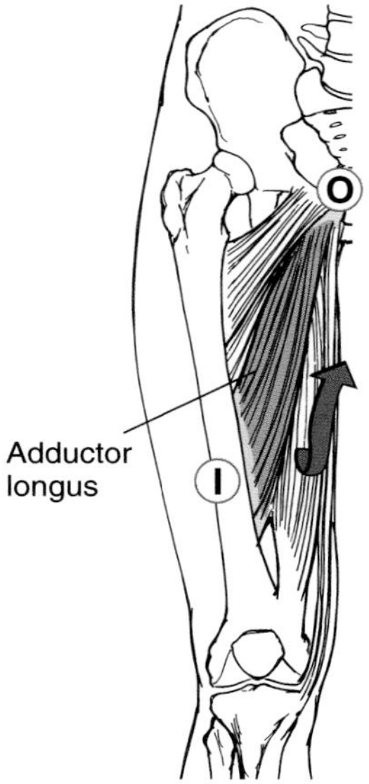 Adductor longus Anterior view

Continued

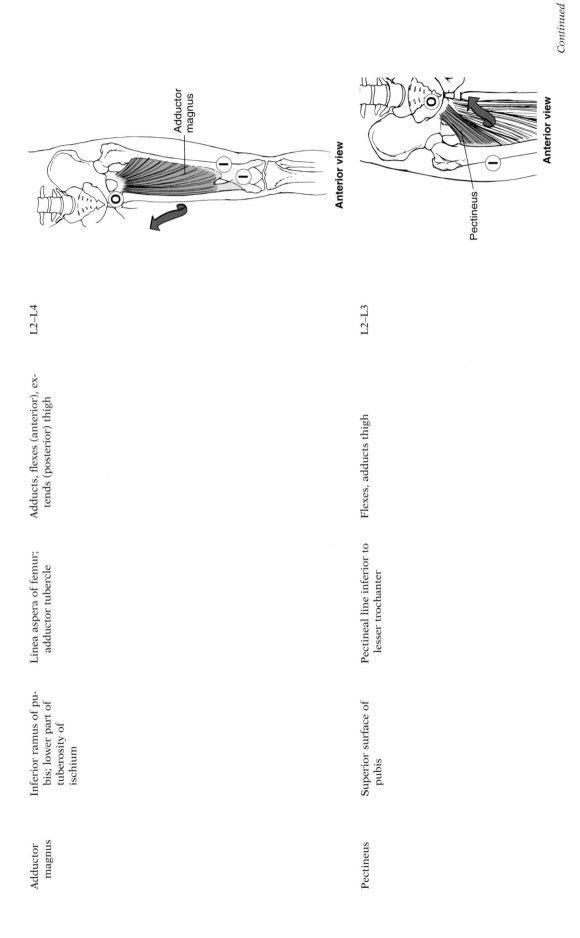

| Adductor magnus | Inferior ramus of pubis; lower part of tuberosity of ischium | Linea aspera of femur; adductor tubercle | Adducts, flexes (anterior), extends (posterior) thigh | L2–L4 |
| Pectineus | Superior surface of pubis | Pectineal line inferior to lesser trochanter | Flexes, adducts thigh | L2–L3 |

Table 4.13

Muscles That Move the Thigh (Continued)

Name	Origin	Insertion	Action	Nerve Supply	Muscle Diagram
Gracilis	Inferior ramus of pubis and ischium	Anterior surface of tibia, inferior to medial condyle	Adducts thigh; flexes leg; assists in medial rotation of thigh when legs flexed	L2–L3	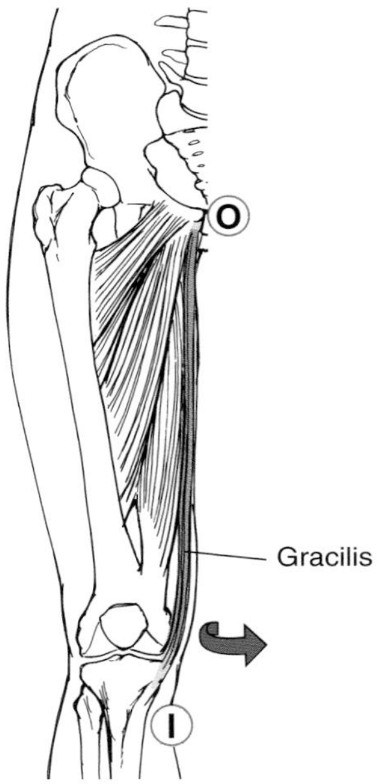 Gracilis / **Anterior view**
Anteriorly located muscles					
Iliacus (*part of iliopsoas*)	Iliac fossa of ilium; ala of sacrum and adjacent ligaments	Distal to lesser trochanter tendon fused with that of psoas	Flexes thigh; *With insertion fixed:* Flexes lumber spine	L2–L3 (femoral nerve)	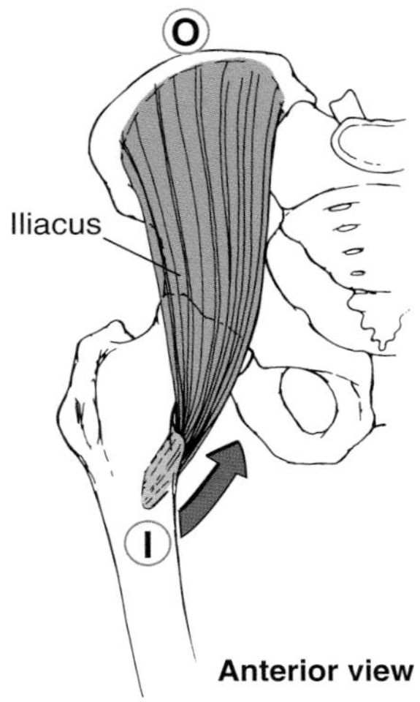 Iliacus / **Anterior view**

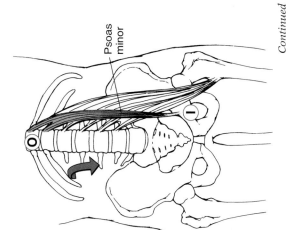

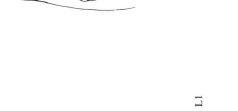

Psoas major

Psoas minor

Anterior view

Continued

Muscle	Origin	Insertion	Action	Innervation
Psoas major *(part of iliopsoas)*	Body and transverse process of T12–L5	Tendon fuses with iliacus and inserts distal to lesser trochanter	Flexes thigh; *With insertion fixed:* Flexes lumbar spine	L1–L3
Psoas minor	T12–L1 vertebral bodies and intervertebral disks	Ilium inner surface (iliopectineal eminence and line)	Flexion of trunk and lumbar spine	L1

(Iliacus and psoas are together known as the iliopsoas.)

Table 4.13

Muscles That Move the Thigh (Continued)

Name	Origin	Insertion	Action	Nerve Supply	Muscle Diagram
Rotators					
Gemellus superior	Dorsal aspect of the spine of the ischium	Medial aspect of the greater trochanter	Lateral rotation of thigh	L5, S1	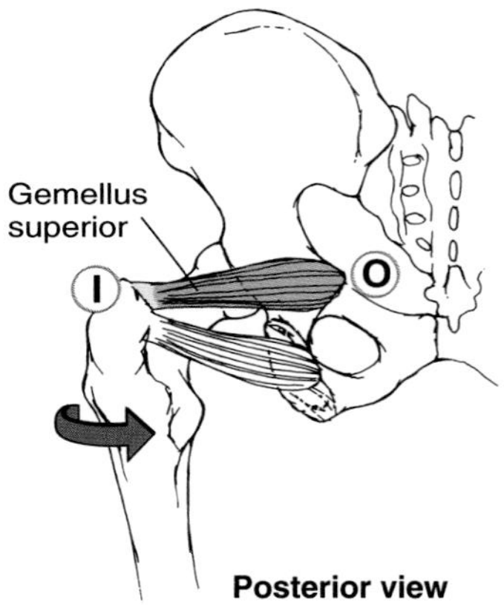 Gemellus superior — Posterior view
Gemellus inferior	Superior aspect of the tuberosity of the ischium	Medial aspect of the greater trochanter	Lateral rotation of thigh	L5, S1	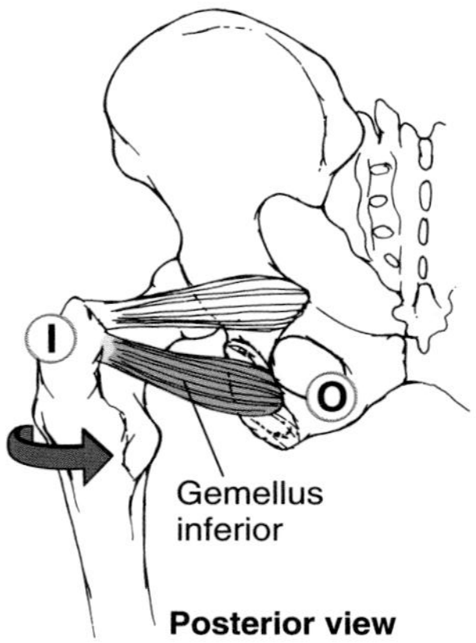 Gemellus inferior — Posterior view
Obturator externus	(see laterally located muscles)				
Obturator internus	(see laterally located muscles)				

Continued

Muscles That Move the Leg

Table 4.14

Anteriorly located muscles

Name	Origin	Insertion	Action	Nerve Supply	Muscle Diagram
Rectus femoris (one of quadriceps femoris)	Anterior inferior iliac spine; superior acetabular rim	First into patella then via patellar ligament to tibial tuberosity	Extends leg; flexes thigh	L2–L4	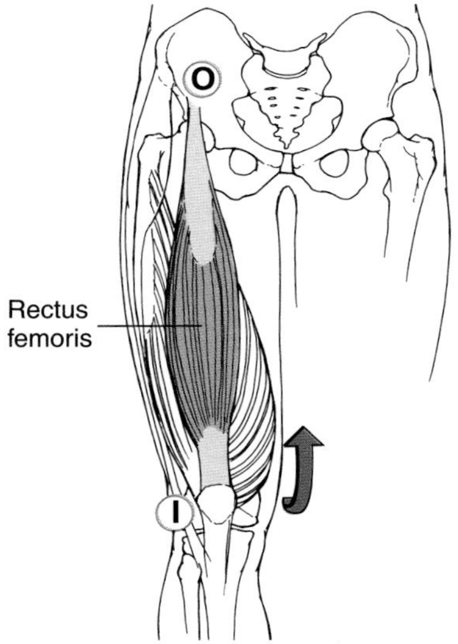 Rectus femoris
Vastus intermedius (one of quadriceps femoris)	Anterolateral surface of femur along linea aspera (distal half)	First into patella then via patellar ligament to tibial tuberosity	Extends leg	L2–L4	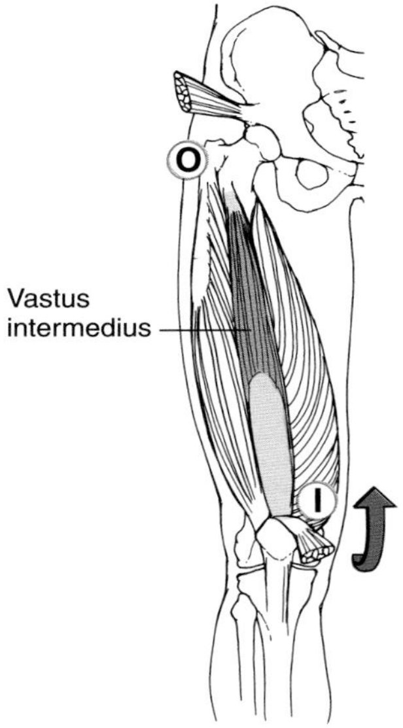 Vastus intermedius

Table 4.14

Muscles That Move the Thigh (Continued)

Name	Origin	Insertion	Action	Nerve Supply	Muscle Diagram
Rotators					
Vastus lateralis (*one of quadriceps femoris*)	Anterior and inferior to greater trochanter, along linea aspera (distal half)	First into patella then via patellar ligament to tibial tuberosity	Extends leg	L2–L4	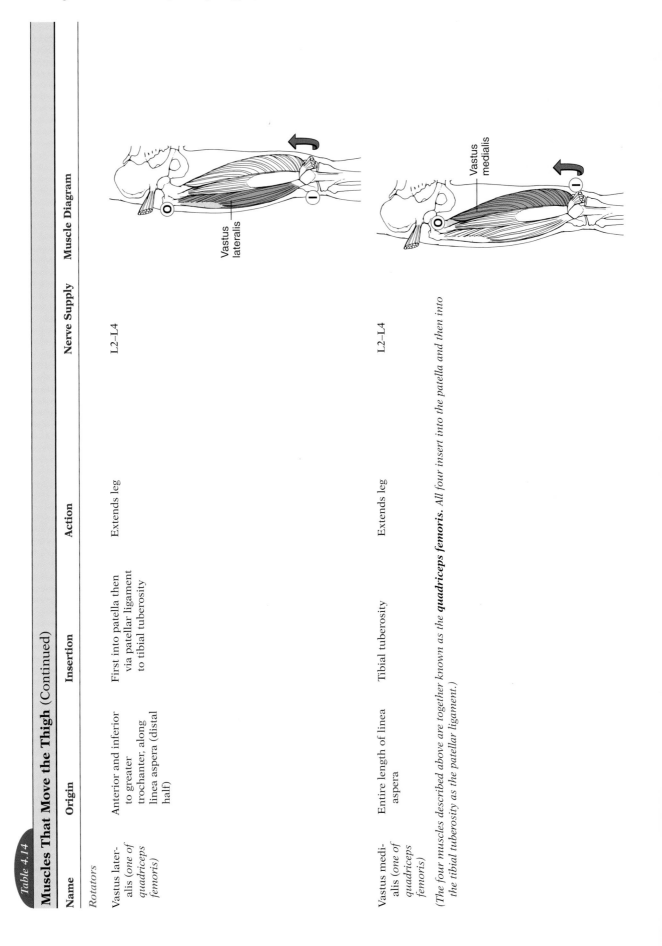
Vastus medialis (*one of quadriceps femoris*)	Entire length of linea aspera	Tibial tuberosity	Extends leg	L2–L4	

(*The four muscles described above are together known as the* **quadriceps femoris**. *All four insert into the patella and then into the tibial tuberosity as the patellar ligament.*)

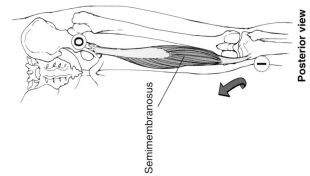

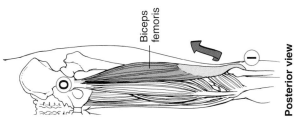

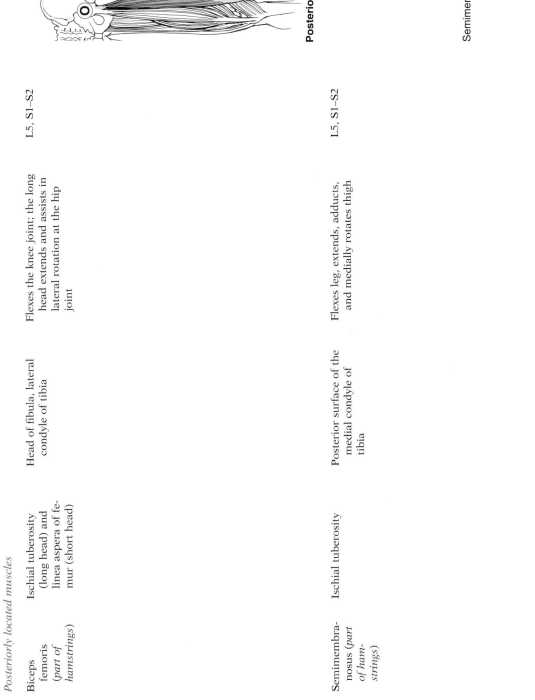

Continued

Posteriorly located muscles

Biceps femoris *(part of hamstrings)*	Ischial tuberosity (long head) and linea aspera of femur (short head)	Head of fibula, lateral condyle of tibia	Flexes the knee joint; the long head extends and assists in lateral rotation at the hip joint	L5, S1–S2
Semimembranosus *(part of hamstrings)*	Ischial tuberosity	Posterior surface of the medial condyle of tibia	Flexes leg, extends, adducts, and medially rotates thigh	L5, S1–S2

Table 4.14

Muscles That Move the Thigh (Continued)

Name	Origin	Insertion	Action	Nerve Supply	Muscle Diagram
Semitendinosus (*part of hamstrings*)	Ischial tuberosity	Posteromedial surface of tibia	Flexes and medially rotates leg, extends, adducts, and medially rotates thigh	L5, S1–S2	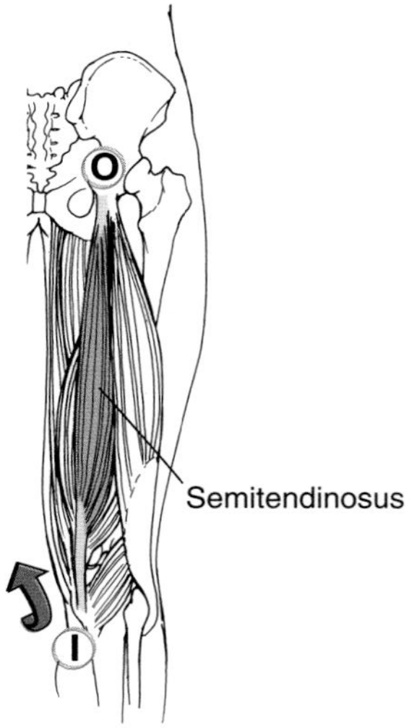

(*The three muscles—biceps femoris, semimembranosus, and semitendinosus—are called* **hamstrings.**)

Semitendinosus

Posterior view

Sartorius	Anterior superior iliac spine	Medial surface of tibia, near tibial tuberosity	Flexes and assists in medial rotation of leg; flexes and laterally rotates thigh	L2–L3	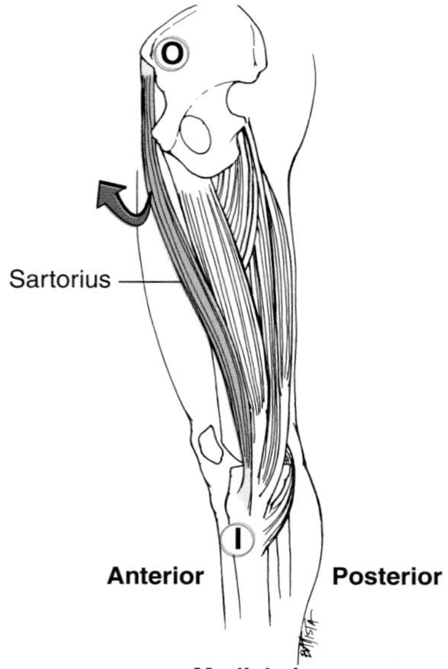

Sartorius

Posterior

Anterior

Medial view

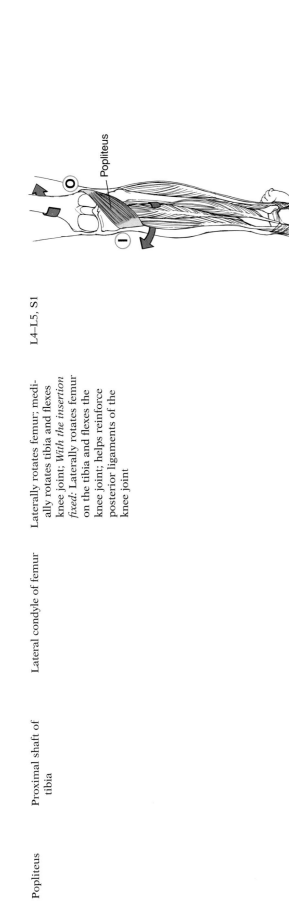

| Popliteus | Proximal shaft of tibia | Lateral condyle of femur | Laterally rotates femur; medially rotates tibia and flexes knee joint; *With the insertion fixed:* Laterally rotates femur on the tibia and flexes the knee joint; helps reinforce posterior ligaments of the knee joint | L4–L5, S1 |

Table 4.15

Muscles That Move the Foot and Toes

Name	Origin	Insertion	Action	Nerve Supply	Muscle Diagram
Posteriorly located muscles					
Gastrocnemius	Femoral condyles and posterior surface of femur	Posterior surface of calcaneus	Plantar flexion; flexion of leg at knee joint	S1–S2	
Soleus	Head and proximal shaft of fibula; posteromedial shaft of tibia	Posterior surface of calcaneus	Plantar flexion	S1–S2	

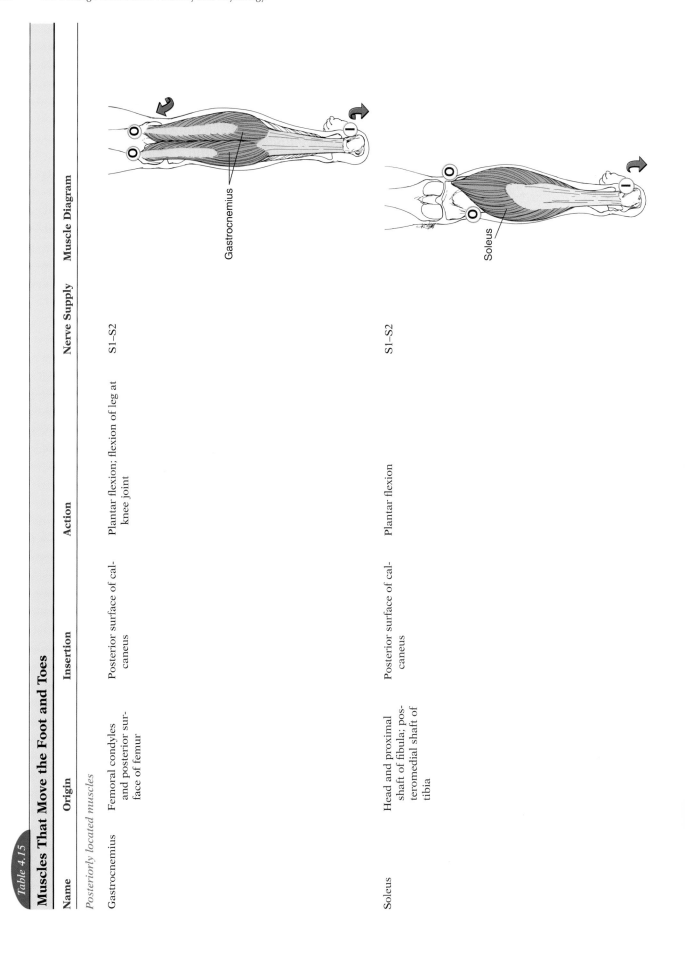

Gastrocnemius

Soleus

Continued

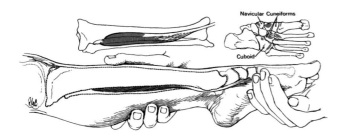

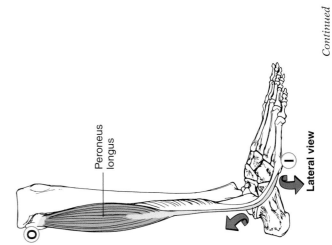

Peroneus longus

Lateral view

Muscle	Origin	Insertion	Action	Nerve
Tibialis posterior	Most of the interosseous membrane, lateral part of posterior surface of tibia; proximal two thirds of medial surface of fibula; adjacent intermuscular septa	Tuberosity of navicular bone and by fibrous expansions to cuneiforms; cuboid; bases of second, third and fourth metatarsal bones	Inverts foot; assists in plantar flexion	L(4), 5, S1
Peroneus longus	Lateral condyle of tibia; head of fibula	Base of 1st metatarsal	Everts foot; plantar flexion at ankle; supports longitudinal arch of foot	L5, S1

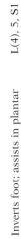

Table 4.15

Muscles That Move the Foot and Toes (Continued)

Name	Origin	Insertion	Action	Nerve Supply	Muscle Diagram
Peroneus brevis	Lateral margin of fibula (middle)	Base of 5th metatarsal	Everts foot; assists in plantar flexion of ankle	L5, S1	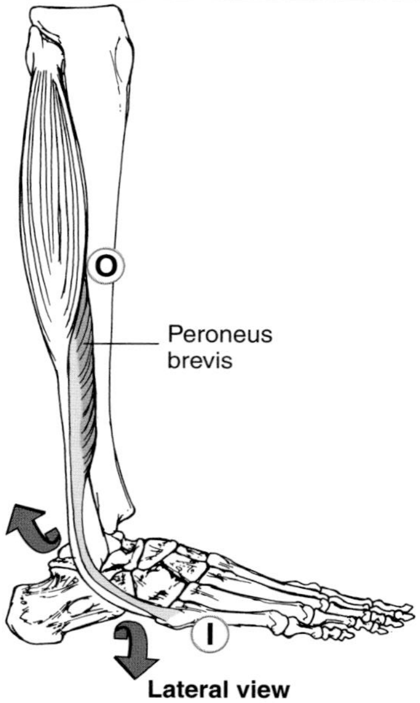
Flexor digitorum longus	Posteromedial surface of tibia	Inferior surface of phalanges of toes 2–5	Plantar flexion of toes 2–5; assists in plantar flexion of ankle joint and inversion of foot	L5, S1–S2	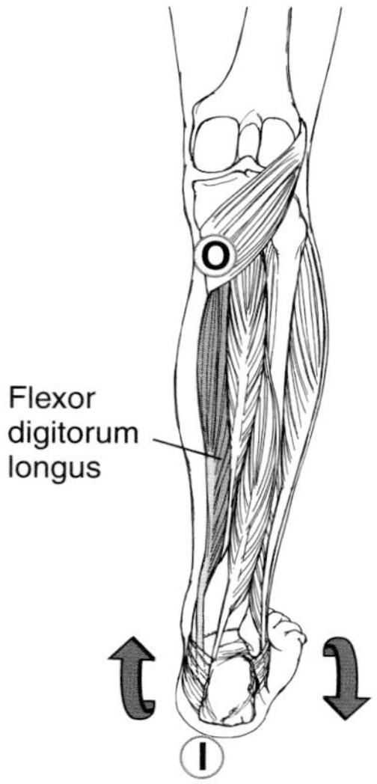

Peroneus brevis

Lateral view

Flexor digitorum longus

Continued

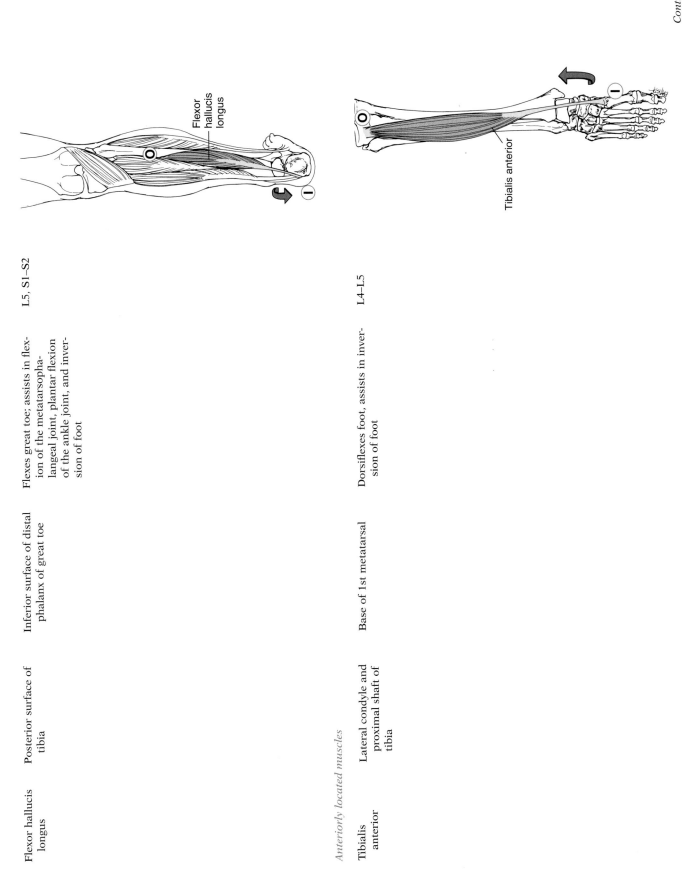

Flexor hallucis longus

Posterior surface of tibia

Inferior surface of distal phalanx of great toe

Flexes great toe; assists in flexion of the metatarsophalangeal joint, plantar flexion of the ankle joint, and inversion of foot

L5, S1–S2

Anteriorly located muscles

Tibialis anterior

Lateral condyle and proximal shaft of tibia

Base of 1st metatarsal

Dorsiflexes foot, assists in inversion of foot

L4–L5

Table 4.15

Muscles That Move the Foot and Toes (Continued)

Name	Origin	Insertion	Action	Nerve Supply	Muscle Diagram
Extensor digitorum longus	Lateral condyle of tibia; anterior surface of fibula	Superior surfaces of phalanges of toes 2–5	Extends toes 2–5; assists in dorsiflexion of ankle joint and eversion of foot.	L5, S1	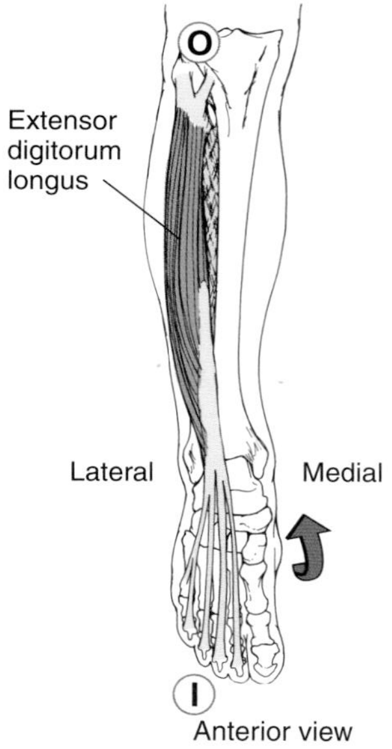 Medial / Lateral / Anterior view / Extensor digitorum longus
Extensor hallucis longus	Anterior surface of tibia	Superior surface of distal phalanx of great toe	Extends great toe; assists in inversion of foot and dorsiflexion at ankle joint	L5	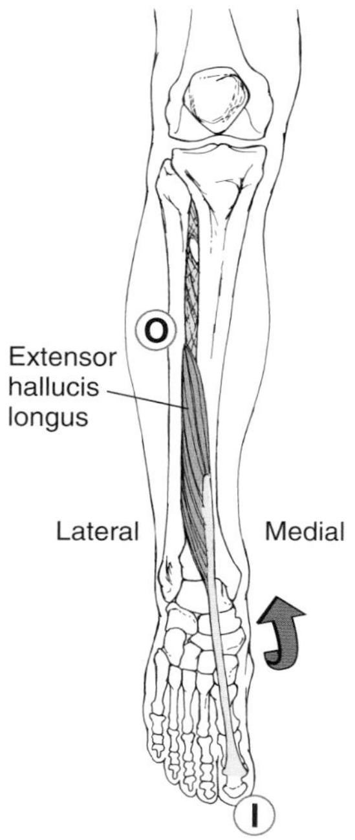 Medial / Lateral / Extensor hallucis longus

Table 4.16

Intrinsic Muscles of the Toes

Name	Origin	Insertion	Action	Nerve Supply	Muscle Diagram
Extensor digitorum brevis	Anterior superolateral surface of the calcaneum	Medial part of the muscle (extensor hallucis brevis): dorsal aspect of the base of the proximal phalanx of the great toe tendons to the 2nd, 3rd, and 4th toes: into the lateral aspect of the corresponding extensor digitorum longus tendons	Extends the metatarsophalangeal joints of digits 1–4 and assists in extending the interphalangeal joints of digits 2–4	L5, S1	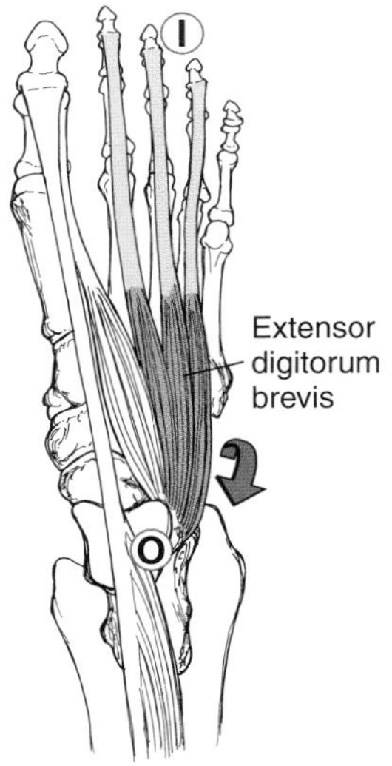 Extensor digitorum brevis — Dorsal surface of the foot
Extensor hallucis brevis	Distal part of superior and lateral surfaces of calcaneus, lateral talocalcaneal ligament, and apex of inferior extensor retinaculum	Dorsal surface of base of proximal phalanx of great toe	Extends metatarsophalangeal joint of great toe	L4–L5, S1	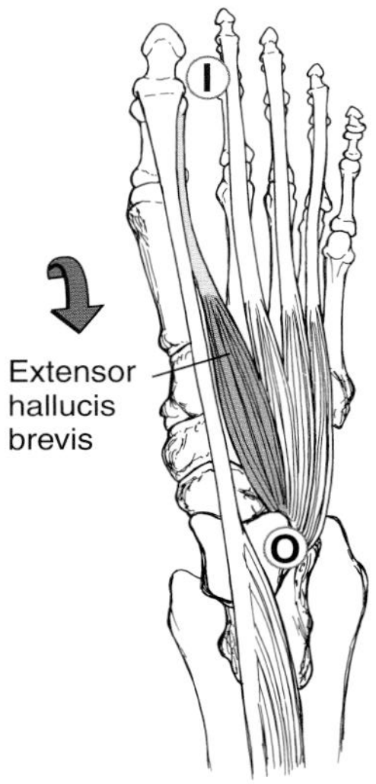 Extensor hallucis brevis — Dorsal surface of foot

Continued

Table 4.16

Intrinsic Muscles of the Toes (Continued)

Name	Origin	Insertion	Action	Nerve Supply	Muscle Diagram
Abductor hallucis	Medial process of the calcaneal tuberosity; flexor retinaculum and plantar aponeurosis	Medial aspect of the base of the proximal phalanx of the great toe	Abducts and assists in flexion of metatarsophalangeal joint of the great toe, assists with adduction of foot	S1–S2	
Flexor hallucis brevis	Medial part of the plantar surface of the cuboid bone and adjacent part of the lateral cuneiform bone	Medial and lateral aspects of the base of the proximal phalanx of the great toe	Flexes the metatarsophalangeal joint of the great toe	S1–S2	

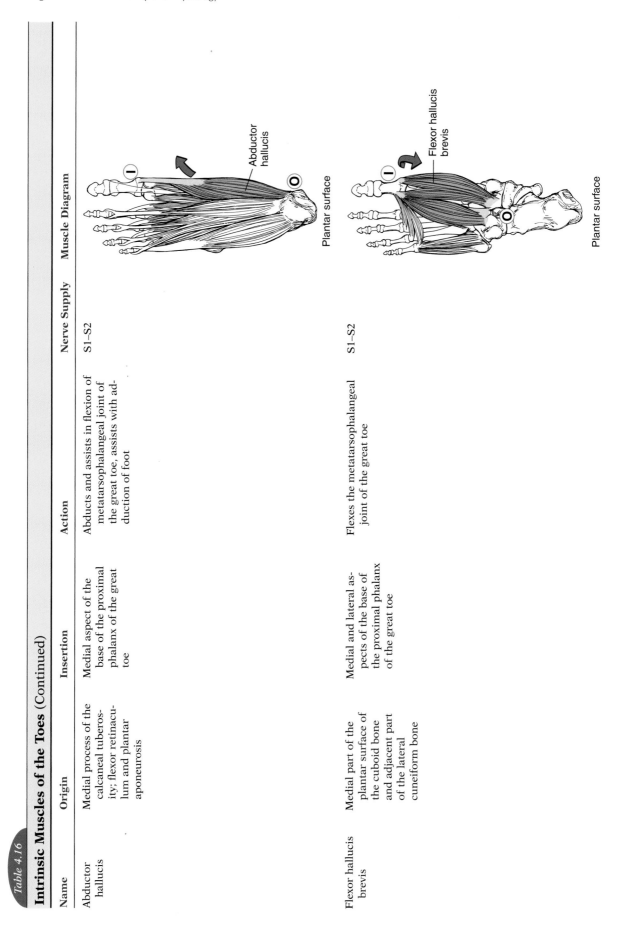

Abductor hallucis

Plantar surface

Flexor hallucis brevis

Plantar surface

Continued

Flexor digitorum brevis

Plantar surface

Flexor digiti minimi

Plantar surface

Muscle	Origin	Insertion	Action	Nerve
Flexor digitorum brevis	Medial process of the calcaneal tuberosity; plantar fascia	Medial and lateral aspects of the middle phalanges of the lateral four toes	Flexes proximal interphalangeal joints, and assists in flexion of metatarsophalangeal joints of 2nd–5th digits.	S1–S2 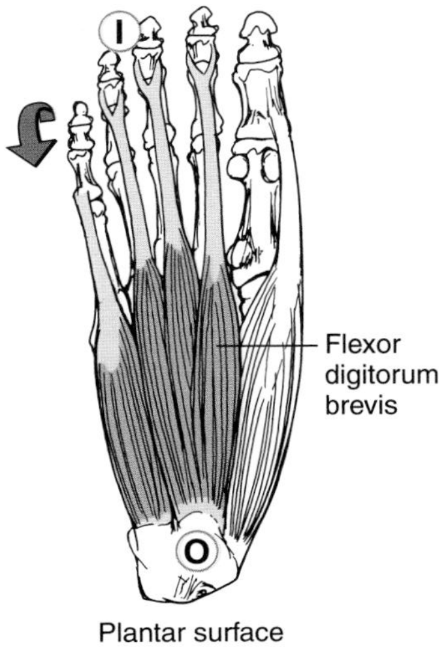
Flexor digiti minimi brevis	Medial plantar aspect of the base of 5th metatarsal; sheath of peroneus longus	Lateral side of the base of proximal phalanx of 5th toe	Flexion of the metatarsophalangeal joint of the 5th toe	S2–S3 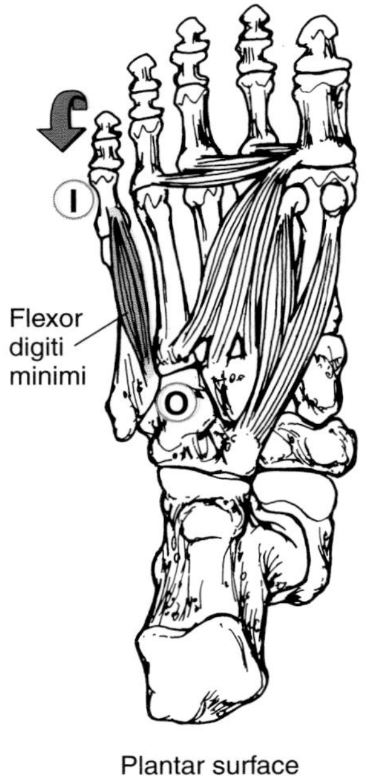

Table 4.16

Intrinsic Muscles of the Toes (Continued)

Name	Origin	Insertion	Action	Nerve Supply	Muscle Diagram
Lumbricalis	First lumbricalis: medial aspect of flexor digitorum longus tendon; 2nd to 4th lumbricalis: adjacent sides of the flexor digitorum longus tendons	Medial aspects of dorsal digital expansions on the proximal phalanges of the lateral four toes	Flexes metatarsophalangeal joints and assists in extending interphalangeal joints of 2nd–5th digits	S2–S3	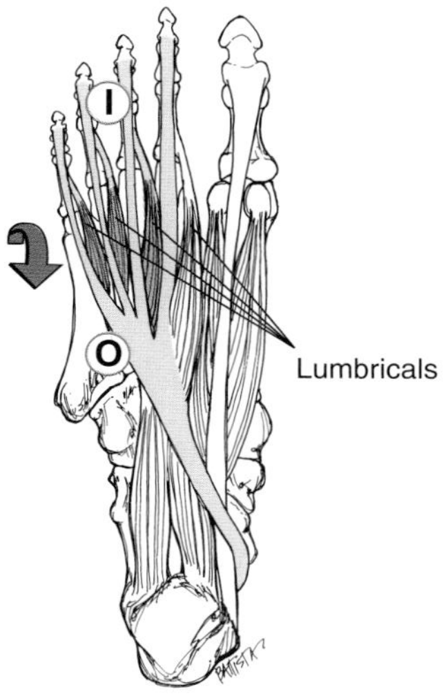
Adductor hallucis	Base of second, third and fourth metatarsals (oblique head) and metatarsophalangeal plantar ligaments (transverse head)	Lateral aspect of proximal phalanx of big toe	Adduction of the proximal phalanx of the big toe towards the second toe; assists in flexing the metatarsophalangeal joint of big toe	S1, 2	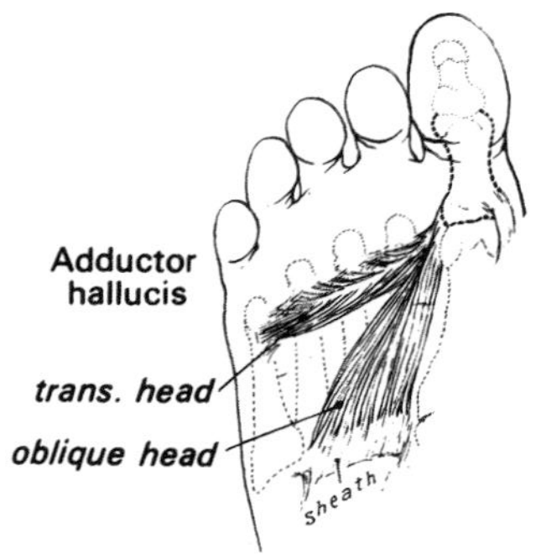

Lumbricals

Plantar surface

Adductor hallucis

trans. head

oblique head

Continued

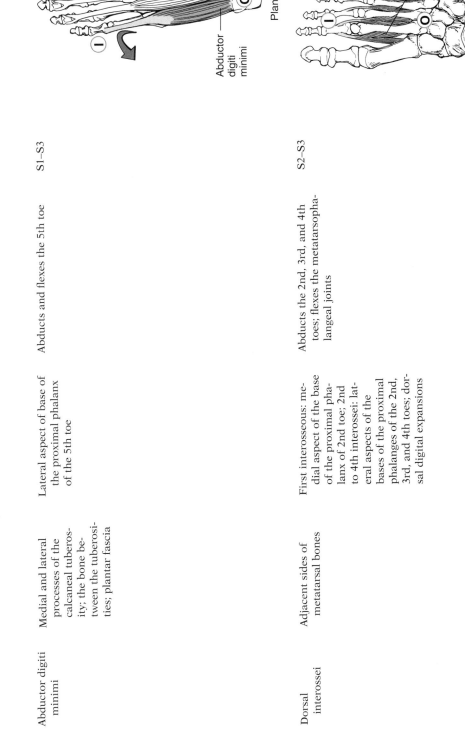

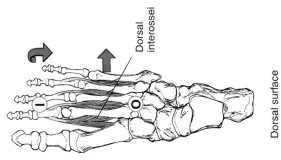

Plantar surface

Abductor digiti minimi

Dorsal interossei

Dorsal surface

Abductor digiti minimi	Medial and lateral processes of the calcaneal tuberosity; the bone between the tuberosities; plantar fascia	Lateral aspect of base of the proximal phalanx of the 5th toe	S1–S3	Abducts and flexes the 5th toe
Dorsal interossei	Adjacent sides of metatarsal bones	First interosseous: medial aspect of the base of the proximal phalanx of 2nd toe; 2nd to 4th interossei: lateral aspects of the bases of the proximal phalanges of the 2nd, 3rd, and 4th toes; dorsal digital expansions	S2–S3	Abducts the 2nd, 3rd, and 4th toes; flexes the metatarsophalangeal joints

Table 4.16

Intrinsic Muscles of the Toes (Continued)

Name	Origin	Insertion	Action	Nerve Supply	Muscle Diagram
Plantar interossei	Bases and medial aspects of the 3rd, 4th, and 5th metatarsal bones	Medial aspects of the bases of the proximal phalanges of the 3rd–5th toes; dorsal digital expansions	Adducts 3rd–5th toe; flexes the metatarsophalangeal joints	S2–S3	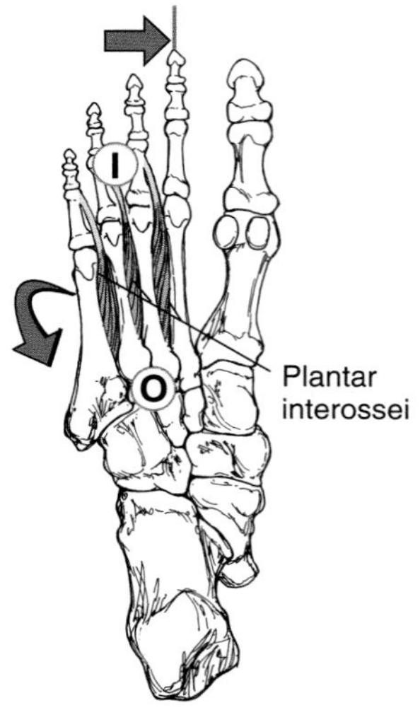

Plantar interossei

Plantar surface

Nervous System

Objectives   **On completion of this chapter, the reader should be able to:**

- Identify the parts of a typical neuron and the functions of the different components.
- Classify the neurons according to structure and function.
- Explain how myelin sheaths are formed in the peripheral nervous system (PNS) and central nervous system (CNS).
- List the different types and functions of neuroglia.
- Explain how a resting membrane potential is created in an excitable cell.
- Describe how an action potential is generated and propagated.
- Name the factors that can affect the speed of transmission in a neuron.
- Describe the structure of a synapse.
- Describe how transmission occurs across synapses.
- Give examples of neurotransmitters and their role in synaptic transmission.
- Describe the process of neuron regeneration.
- List the factors that affect regeneration.
- Classify sense organs.
- Describe how various sensations are perceived.
- Define pain.
- Compare acute and chronic pain.
- Describe, in brief, some theories used to describe pain.
- Explain the mechanism of pain and pain responses.
- Define visceral pain.
- Describe referred pain.
- Explain the possible process of referred pain.
- Identify the body areas where various visceral organs tend to produce referred pain.
- List the various strategies available for managing acute pain.
- List the various strategies available for managing chronic pain.
- Identify, given a diagram, the various structures on a transverse section of the spinal cord.
- Explain the role of white mater and gray mater of the spinal cord.
- Describe the different types of information carried by a typical spinal nerve.
- List the structures innervated by a typical spinal nerve.
- Define a dermatome.
- Explain the basis of the dermatomal pattern.
- List the various nerve plexus found in the body.
- Describe the course of major nerves arising in the brachial and lumbosacral plexus.
- Describe a reflex arc.
- List the components of a reflex arc.
- List the different reflexes and the situations in which each type comes into play.

- Explain how higher centers modify the response produced by a reflex.
- Describe the structure of a muscle spindle and explain its role in stretch reflexes.
- Trace the path taken by various sensations from the point of stimulus to the brain.
- Identify, given diagrams, the major regions of the brain and describe their functions.
- Identify, given a diagram, the motor, sensory, and association areas of the brain.
- Name the location and functions of the limbic system, thalamus, hypothalamus, basal ganglia, cerebellum, vestibular apparatus, reticular formation, pons, and medulla.
- Name the different cranial nerves and the primary destinations and functions of each, with special reference to the olfactory, trigeminal, facial, and vagus nerves.
- Trace the major motor pathways from the brain to the skeletal muscle.
- Describe the process of voluntary muscle control and the structures involved.
- Describe the process of posture control and the structures involved.
- Identify the protective covering of the brain.
- Explain the formation, circulation, and function of the cerebrospinal fluid.
- Describe, in brief, the blood supply to the nervous system.
- Compare the structure and functions of the sympathetic and parasympathetic system.
- Name the neurotransmitters involved in these systems and the effects they have on various target organs.
- Explain the importance of dual innervation of organs in the body.
- Explain the importance of autonomic tone.
- Describe the interacting levels of control in the autonomic nervous system.
- Describe age-related changes in the nervous system.
- Describe the possible effects of massage on the nervous system.
- Explain the role of massage on pain management.

The nervous system and the endocrine system help maintain homeostasis by coordinating the various activities of the body that have been altered by changing environment and situations. The nervous system helps initiate changes quickly, with responses lasting for a short duration; the endocrine system brings slower changes of longer duration. However, both the nervous and endocrine systems work in an integrated and complementary manner.

The nervous system is also responsible for the complex processes of intelligence, learning, memory, communication, emotion, and other higher functions.

This chapter describes the structure of the nervous system and the physiologic mechanisms involved in carrying out its functions.

Organization of the Nervous System

The nervous system includes all neural tissue present in the body and accounts for just 3% of total body weight. The functional unit of the nervous system is the **neuron.** The neurons are supported and protected by specialized cells known as **neuroglia.** The organs of the nervous system are formed by the neurons, neuroglia, connective tissue, and blood vessels.

The nervous system consists of the **brain** and **spinal cord,** enclosed in the skull and vertebrae, respectively. The **sensors** sense the changes in the in-

ternal and external environment, and the **nerves** connect the sensors to the brain and spinal cord and take commands to tissue from the spinal cord to produce a response.

Classically, the brain and spinal cord are known as the **central nervous system** (CNS); the rest of the nervous system is the **peripheral nervous system** (PNS). The CNS (see Figure 5.1) helps integrate, process, and coordinate the sensory input and motor commands. For example, when you see a car hurtling directly toward you, you jump out of its path. The CNS processes the input (the sight of a car) and, based on past experiences and learning (processing and integration), decides that you need to jump out of the way. It commands the relevant muscles to contract and move the body and, perhaps, yell at the same time (coordination). Of course, more than this happens inside your body—your heart beats faster, your palms sweat, and your blood pressure increases.

The parts of the nervous system are referred to according to function. The sensors that sense changes in the internal and external environment are the **receptors.** The nerves that carry impulses from the receptors to the CNS are the **sensory nerves,** or **afferents.** The nerves that carry impulses from the CNS to the muscles or glands are the **motor nerves,** or **efferents.** The nerves that carry impulses to and from the brain are the **cranial nerves;** those that carry impulses to and from the spinal cord are the **spinal nerves.**

The organs that respond to impulses from the CNS are the **effectors.** The nerves that go to skeletal mus-

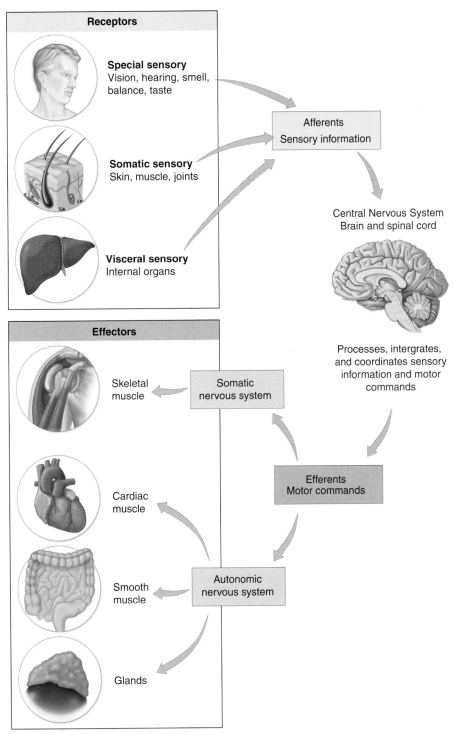

FIGURE **5.1.** Schematic Representation of the Nervous System

cle comprise the **somatic nervous system.** Reaction may take place before the stimuli reach the conscious level; this response is known as a **reflex.**

The part of the nervous system responsible for automatic, involuntary regulation of smooth muscle, cardiac muscle, and glands is the **autonomic nervous system.** This system, described later, has two divisions: the **sympathetic** and **parasympathetic divisions** (**see page 369** for details).

STRUCTURE OF THE NEURON

The structure of the neuron (see Figure 5.2), the functional unit of the nervous system, varies from site to site. Typically, a neuron has a **cell body/soma,** or **perikaryon,** with a nucleus and cytoplasm, along with the organelles normally found in a cell. The prominent rough endoplasmic reticulum is known as **Nissl bodies.** However, most neurons do not have a centriole and lose the ability to multiply. **Nuclei** are clusters of cell bodies of neurons in the CNS (naming exception, basal ganglia). These clusters in the PNS are known as **ganglia.**

Many processes lead off from the soma. The **axon** is long and helps conduct impulses *away* from the cell body. The axon may have many branches, known as **collaterals.** The collaterals help the cell communicate with more than one neuron. The **dendrites** are highly branched processes from the cell body that take impulses *to* the soma. The presence of numerous dendrites enables many neurons to have an effect on one cell.

Flow From Axon to Cell Body

Many viruses enter the CNS at the synaptic level. They are absorbed into the synaptic knob and transported to the cell body that invariably lies in the spinal cord or brain. A good example of such transport is the chicken-pox virus, which causes **shingles,** or **herpes zoster.** In this condition, the virus in the nerve cell body becomes activated, and the condition presents as a rash along the distribution of the nerve to the skin.

THE SYNAPSE

A **synapse** (see Figure 5.3) is the region where neurons communicate with each other. The axon of the neuron, which brings impulses to the synapse, belongs to the **presynaptic neuron.** The neuron which receives the

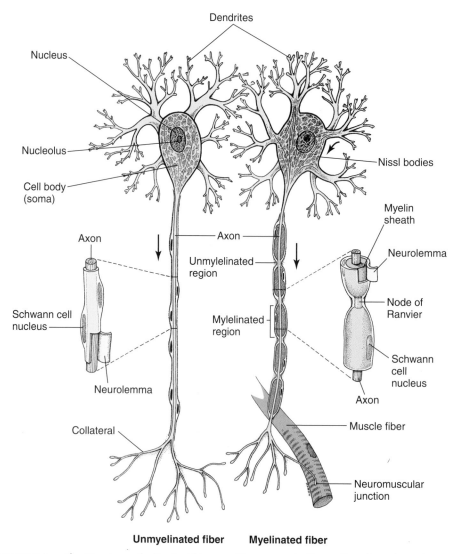

Unmyelinated fiber   Myelinated fiber

FIGURE 5.2.   The Structure of a Typical Neuron. The arrows indicate direction of conduction.

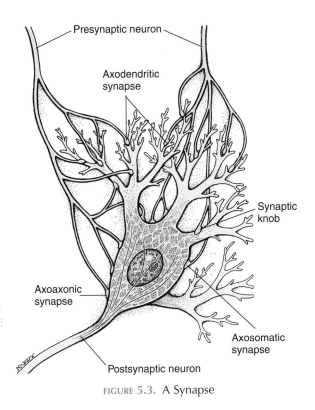

- Presynaptic neuron
- Axodendritic synapse
- Synaptic knob
- Axoaxonic synapse
- Axosomatic synapse
- Postsynaptic neuron

FIGURE 5.3. A Synapse

impulse is the **postsynaptic neuron.** The end of the axon of the presynaptic neuron is enlarged into a bulb, the **synaptic knob,** or **terminal.** The synaptic knob usually has neurotransmitters packaged in small structures called **synaptic vesicles** (Figure 5.9A; **page 312**). When the presynaptic neuron is stimulated, it releases neurotransmitters into the gap between the two neurons. These then become attached to receptors on the cell membrane of the postsynaptic neuron, producing electrical changes.

A synapse may be at a dendrite (**axodendritic),** on the soma (**axosomatic**), or along the length of the axon (**axoaxonic**). Rarely, a synapse may exist between two dendrites (**dendrodendritic**). The neurotransmitters are actually manufactured in the soma and transported down the axon. Transport of substances can also occur in the opposite direction, from the end of axon to the soma.

Neurons, in addition to communicating with each other, can communicate with another cell type. This communication is known as the **neuroeffector junction.** Such communications are seen between the neuron and muscle—**neuromuscular junction** (described in **page 181**)—and between neuron and glands—**neuroglandular junction.** Neurons also innervate fat cells.

CLASSIFICATION OF NEURONS

Neurons are classified in many ways, according to their anatomical structure and function.

Anatomical Classification

Bipolar Neurons

These neurons have two processes extending from either end of the cell body, the dendrite and the axon (see Figure 5.4). This type of neuron is rare and is found in the retina of the eye.

Unipolar Neurons

The cell body in this type lies to one side, with a single process leading off from one side of the body. This process divides at once into two processes: the axon and the dendrite. Sensory neurons are of this type.

Multipolar Neurons

This is the most common type of neuron, with the cell body having several dendrites and one axon. All the motor neurons to the skeletal muscles are of this type.

Functional Classification

The neurons may be also classified according to function. These are the **sensory, motor,** and **interneurons,** or **association neurons.** Those that take impulses *to* the CNS are known as the sensory neurons or afferent fibers. Of the sensory neurons, the **visceral afferents** innervate the organs, and the **somatic afferents** carry impulses from the surface of the body. Sensory neurons may be named according to the type of information they sense. Those afferents that sense information in the external environment are called **exteroceptors.** Afferents sensing changes in the inside of the body are called **interoceptors.**

 Drugs Acting at the Synaptic Level

A familiar example is nicotine, the ingredient in cigarettes. It binds to receptor sites and stimulates the postsynaptic membrane, producing responses similar to that resulting from stimulation of nicotinic receptors. Another example is pesticide use. Because animals also use acetylcholine as a neurotransmitter the pesticide, (by preventing the action of acetylcholinesterase, the enzyme that destroys acetylcholine in the synaptic cleft), prolongs the action of acetylcholine at the neuromuscular junction. As a result, muscles go into prolonged contraction, jeopardizing respiratory movements.

Many drugs produce an effect by altering synaptic transmission. They may (1) reduce or increase synthesis of neurotransmitters, (2) alter the rate of release of neurotransmitters, (3) alter the rate at which neurotransmitters are removed from the synaptic cleft, and (4) prevent binding of neurotransmitters to the receptors on the postsynaptic membrane.

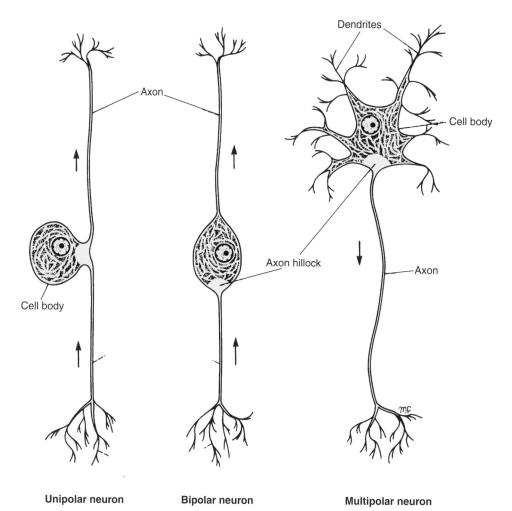

Unipolar neuron   **Bipolar neuron**   **Multipolar neuron**

FIGURE **5.4.** Anatomic Classification of Neurons. Unipolar Neuron (e.g., sensory neurons); Bipolar Neuron (e.g., neurons in the retina of the eye); and Multipolar Neuron (e.g., motor neurons to skeletal muscle). The arrows indicate the direction of transmission of nerve impulses.

Those that monitor position and movement of skeletal muscles and joints are the **proprioceptors.**

The neurons that take impulses away from the CNS are the motor neurons or efferents. **Somatic motor neurons** innervate skeletal muscles. **Visceral motor neurons** are part of the autonomic nervous system that innervates various organs of the digestive, cardiovascular, respiratory, reproductive, and renal systems.

Interneurons are neurons situated between a sensory and motor neuron or between any two neurons. Most in number, they are responsible for distribution of sensory information to different areas of the CNS and play an important role in the coordination of motor activity.

Other

Neurons are also classified on the basis of myelination (i.e., according to the presence or absence of myelin sheaths as **myelinated** or **unmyelinated** neurons).

NEUROGLIA

Neuroglia are the supporting cells. They are five times more abundant than neurons. There are four types of glial cells in the CNS: the **ependymal cells, astrocytes, microglia,** and **oligodendrocytes** and two types in the PNS: **Schwann cells,** or **neurolemmocytes,** and **satellite cells,** or **ganglionic gliocytes.**

The ependymal cells line the cavities in the brain and spinal cord and are responsible for producing, circulating, and monitoring the cerebrospinal fluid—

Multiple Sclerosis and Demyelination

In certain conditions, such as multiple sclerosis (MS), the myelin sheaths in both the CNS and PNS are slowly destroyed, with resultant reduction in rate of conduction and destruction of axons of both sensory and motor neurons. The axons are said to be demyelinated.

the fluid inside and around the CNS that cushions and protects the brain.

The astrocytes, as the name suggests, are star-shaped. They are present between the blood capillaries and the brain and spinal cord, monitoring the substances that enter and leave the brain and preventing sudden changes in the environment around the CNS. This is the **blood-brain barrier,** and the astrocytes are responsible for its creation. The astrocytes also help at the time of tissue injury. In addition, they take up neurotransmitters from the synapses, break them down and release the products, and make them available to neurons to produce more neurotransmitters. The network of astrocytes, located over the entire brain and spinal cord, form a supporting framework for the CNS. The astrocytes are the most abundant of the neuroglial cells.

Microglia are small cells similar to the monocytes and macrophages in the blood. They engulf dead cells and cellular remnants in the CNS.

Oligodendrocytes are neuroglia with long, slender processes that come in contact with cell bodies and axons in the CNS. The processes form thin sheaths in the region where they contact an axon (See Figure 5.5). This sheath is wound around the axon, serving as insulation. Because the sheath around the axon is made of many layers of the cell membrane, it is composed of 80% lipids and 20% protein.

To visualize the sheath, place a pencil on one end of a thin strip of paper and roll the paper around the pencil. The pencil represents the axon, and the paper represents the process of an oligodendrocyte. This

multilayered membranous wrapping around the axon is known as **myelin.** Each oligodendrocyte puts out many processes and each process wraps around an axon. Thus, each oligodendrocyte forms myelin around many axons (or many oligodendrocytes help myelinate one axon). Not all neurons have this wrapping; those that do are said to be **myelinated** and the others are **unmyelinated.**

Now imagine many thin strips of paper (processes of different oligodendrocytes) wrapped around the pencil (axon), separated by small gaps between the strips. This is how an axon is typically myelinated. The gaps between the myelin, known as **nodes of Ranvier** or **internodes,** help speed the impulses that travel down it, and the myelin helps insulate the axon from the surrounding interstitial fluid. The myelinated neurons conduct impulses much faster than those that are unmyelinated. The myelinated axons appear white, and the regions dominated by this type of axon tend to be white (**white matter**). The areas with cell bodies and/or unmyelinated neurons appear gray (**gray matter**). It is believed that the gray coloration is a result of the presence of Nissl bodies.

Neuroglial cells also exist in the PNS. One type, the **Schwann cells** or **neurilemmal cells,** surround axons and protect them from the surrounding interstitial fluid. They are similar in function to the oligodendrocytes of the CNS—formation of myelin (see Figure 5.5). Such protection is important as impulses are produced and propagated by ions flowing in and out of the neurons (see below). While all axons are protected by Schwann cells, some axons have the cell

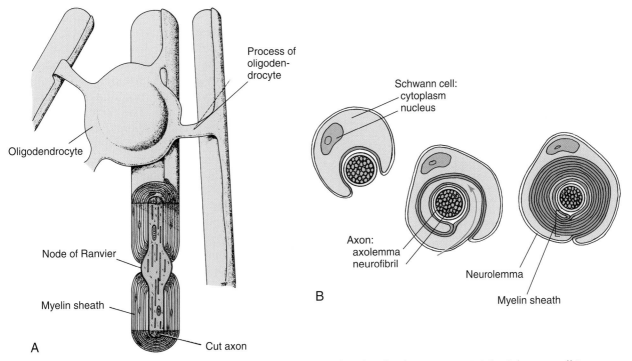

FIGURE 5.5. The Formation of Myelin Sheaths. **A,** CNS (by oligodendrocytes); **B,** PNS (by Schwann cells)

membrane of many Schwann cells wrapped around them in segments, with small gaps between the wrappings of any two Schwann cells. These are the **myelinated axons.**

One other type, **satellite cells** or **ganglionic glio-cytes,** surround the collections of cell bodies of neu-rons (ganglions) lying outside the CNS.

PRODUCTION AND PROPAGATION OF IMPULSES

Impulse formation is a complex process and is re-lated to the properties of the cell membrane (review the section on cell membrane, **page 27,** if necessary). The neurons communicate with each other by chang-ing the electrical potential inside the cell. This is achieved by movement of ions in and out of the cell and is determined by the permeability of the nerve cell membrane. The changes in the neuron (at rest and when stimulated) have been studied using minute electrodes that penetrate inside the neuron.

Resting Membrane Potential

If two electrodes are placed on the surface of the cell membrane of a neuron and connected to a measuring device (see Figure 5.6), no electrical changes are de-tected. However, if one of the electrodes is pushed into the cell and the other placed on the surface, the recording device will show that the inside of the cell is negative to that of the outside. This is known as the **resting membrane potential,** or **transmembrane potential.**

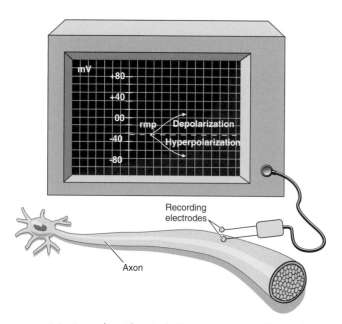

FIGURE 5.6. Recording Electrical Changes Across Cell Membrane
rmp = resting membrane potential

The resting membrane potential is caused by the distribution of ions inside and outside the neurons. The inside of the cell contains large, negatively charged organic particles, and the movement of smaller positively and negatively charged inorganic molecules occurs only through special channels. The cell membrane also has active pumps that use energy to pump ions in and out; thus, at rest, the inside is maintained more negative than the outside.

At rest, the inside of the neuron (intracellular fluid) has more potassium ions (K^+) and proteins (Pr^-), and the outside has more sodium (Na^+) and chloride ions (Cl^-). This is mainly because the cell membrane is not freely permeable to the ions. If it was, the ions would diffuse in and out to equalize the composition in and out of the cell. In this case, because of semiperme-ability, the ions only move in and out of the cell through channels on the cell membrane specific for each ion.

Membrane Channels

Membrane channels (see Figure 5.7), which are actu-ally proteins, (see **page 28**) remain closed, partly closed, or fully opened and are affected by many fac-tors. Some channels are operated by changes in volt-age (**voltage-gated channels**). At a particular voltage specific to the channel, the channel may be open, al-lowing its particular ions to move freely along the concentration gradient. At other voltages, the chan-nel may be closed, shutting off entry or exit of that ion. Some channels open fully at a positive voltage, others at a negative voltage.

Other than voltage-gated channels, certain chan-nels are operated by hormones and other chemicals (**ligand-gated channels**). These channels open when the chemical binds to receptor sites on the cell mem-brane. Other channels are regulated mechanically (**mechanically-regulated channels**).

The resting membrane potential in a neuron is about -70 millivolts (mV). The concentration differ-ence of ions (chemical gradient), as well as the dif-ference in electrical charges (electrical gradient), serve as a force to reinforce or oppose movement of ions when the channels open.

For example, when the sodium channels open, sodium tends to move into the cell (along the con-centration gradient). The electrical gradient also helps as sodium is positively charged and the inside is negative (remember that opposite charges attract). Movement of sodium will occur into the cell as long as the channels are open and the gradient exists.

When the potassium channels are open, potassium tends to move from inside the cell to the outside along the chemical gradient. Because the inside is negative, the electrical gradient will tend to oppose it.

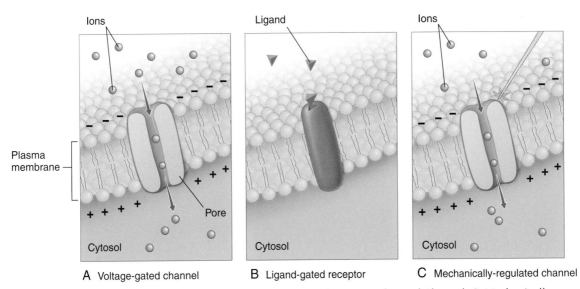

A Voltage-gated channel   B Ligand-gated receptor   C Mechanically-regulated channel

FIGURE 5.7. Membrane Channels. **A,** Voltage-Gated Channels; **B,** Ligand-Gated Channel; **C,** Mechanically-Gated Channel

At rest, there is a leak of sodium into the cell and potassium out of the cell. More potassium leaves the cell than sodium enters cell. This is one of the reasons why the inside is negative at -70 mV. To combat the leak, a pump on the cell membrane, the **sodium-potassium (Na-K) pump** or **sodium-potassium ATPase,** constantly pushes sodium out of the cell and brings potassium into the cell, using energy (see **page 30**).

Action Potential

When a cell is stimulated, sodium channels open and sodium diffuses into the cell along its electrochemical gradient. The inside becomes less negative and this is known as **depolarization.** In some cells, if potassium channels open instead, potassium moves out of the cell and the inside becomes more negative, known as **hyperpolarization.** Soon after the stimuli are removed, the cell returns to its original state and this is known as **repolarization** (see Figure 5.8).

When a neuron is sufficiently stimulated to depolarize it to a threshold value of about -60 to -55 mV, many voltage-gated sodium channels are opened and sodium rushes in, further depolarizing the cell. This depolarization is rapid and propagated throughout the cell along the axon. An **action potential** or **nerve impulse** is a rapid change in potential that is propagated along the cell. The direction of propagation of action potentials is from the dendrite or cell body down an axon.

As a result of opening and closing of other voltage-gated channels, the depolarization does not last long and the cell is repolarized to reach its original resting potential. The voltage-gated sodium channels close when the potential becomes more and more positive.

At the same time, voltage-gated potassium channels open and potassium rushes out. The resultant reduction in movement of the positively charged sodium into the cell and movement of positively charged potassium out of the cell is responsible for repolarization. The sodium-potassium pump is important in the generation of action potentials as it helps bring the ionic concentrations across the cell back to its original state.

If the stimulus is given again, another action potential results. In some neurons, many action potentials are produced continuously as long as the stimu-

> ### Action Potential and Neuronal Changes (Summary)
>
> In Summary:
> * the resting membrane potential is about -70 mV
> * when the stimulus is given to the neuron, some depolarization occurs in the area of the stimulus
> * if the depolarization reaches threshold level (i.e., about -60 mV), voltage-gated sodium channels open
> * positively charged sodium rushes in, rapidly depolarizing the neuron
> * this depolarization is propagated to the rest of the cell
> * during the rapid depolarization, voltage-gated sodium channels close and voltage-gated potassium channels open
> * sodium does not move into the cell as rapidly as before; however, positively charged potassium moves out, making the inside negative until it reaches the resting potential
> * Na-K pump actively pumps sodium out and brings potassium in, using ATP for energy and bringing the ionic concentrations back to normal.

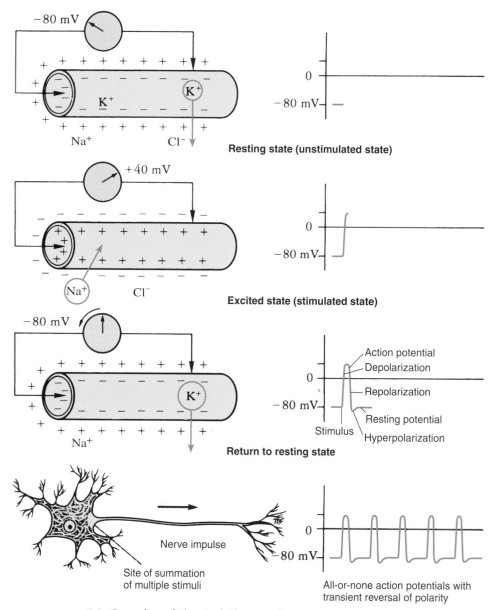

FIGURE 5.8. Recording of Electrical Changes That Occur at Rest and on Stimulation

lus remains (i.e., the stimulus does not have to be given over and over again) and the generation of action potentials stops after the stimulus is removed.

In the body, the strength of the stimulus is translated as more frequent action potentials generated per second and not as increase in amplitude of the action potential (i.e., the higher the strength, the greater the frequency).

The threshold level at which an action potential can be produced varies from neuron to neuron. For example, when a weak stimulus is used, only those neurons that have a low threshold will be stimulated. For example, if a neuron has a threshold of -55 mV, a stimulus that changes the membrane potential to -55 mV from the neuron's resting potential of -70 mV will

cause it to fire an action potential. However, no action potential will be produced in those neurons with a threshold of more than -55 mV (e.g., -50 mV).

DIFFERENCES IN PROPAGATION OF ACTION POTENTIAL IN MYELINATED AND UNMYELINATED AXONS

The action potential in an unmyelinated neuron travels slowly along the axon because every region of the axon has sodium and potassium channels. In a myelinated cell, the myelin sheath serves as insulators, preventing movement of ions through the membrane. Ions move only through the numerous channels located in the nodes and the action potential is propagated from one node of Ranvier to another, literally jumping from node to node across the myelin. Hence, propagation is rapid. This is known as **saltatory conduction.** It should be noted that jumping is only a metaphor. Actually, the action potential in one node depolarizes the membrane at the next node to threshold and a new action potential is produced there. Action potential is also faster in thicker axons. The rate of conduction ranges from 1.0 m/sec (2.25 miles per hour) in thin, unmyelinated fibers to 100 m/sec (225 miles per hour) in thick, myelinated fibers.

When the action potential reaches a synapse, it causes the release of neurotransmitters into the synaptic cleft. The neurotransmitters, in turn, produce electrical changes in the postsynaptic neuron.

SYNAPTIC TRANSMISSION

For the neurotransmitters to have an effect on the postsynaptic neuron, sufficient amounts of neurotransmitters must be released. The number of synaptic vesicles that fuse with the cell membrane of the axon terminal, to release neurotransmitters into the synaptic cleft by exocytosis, depends on the frequency of action potentials. With greater frequency, more vesicles release the neurotransmitters contained within them. The neurotransmitters become attached to receptors on the postsynaptic membrane that open chemical-gated *sodium* channels (see Figure 5.9A). If sufficient channels open, they depolarize the neuron to reach threshold potential and produce an action potential. This is an example of a **stimulatory neurotransmitter.** The potential changes that occur at the nerve junction are known as **excitatory postsynaptic potential** (EPSP).

Certain neurotransmitters become attached to receptors that open chemical-gated *potassium* channels or *chloride* channels in the postsynaptic neuron. In this case, instead of depolarization, the neuron becomes hyperpolarized (the inside becomes more negative as positively charged potassium ions move out or negatively charged chloride ions move in). As a result, it becomes more difficult for action potentials to be produced. Such neurotransmitters are known as **inhibitory neurotransmitters.** The potential changes that occur at the nerve junction are known as **inhibitory postsynaptic potential** (IPSP). From

RECEPTORS

You may recall that the term *receptor* was used to denote proteins located on the cell membrane that bind to specific hormones and chemicals. Although these endings of the sensory neurons are known as sensory "receptors," their structure is different.

the description of stimulatory and inhibitory effects, it can be seen that the synapse is the region where there is possibility of modifying the message.

Whether a neurotransmitter is inhibitory or stimulatory is dependent on the type of receptors they bind to in the postsynaptic membrane. For example, the neurotransmitter acetylcholine released by nerves in the neuromuscular junction causes skeletal muscle to contract. The same acetylcholine released by the nerves to cardiac muscle has an inhibitory effect.

Soon after neurotransmitters are released into the synaptic cleft, they are removed quickly from the area by enzymes, which break them up, or by reuptake back into the presynaptic neuron. Or, the neurotransmitter diffuses into the intercellular fluid. For example, acetylcholine is broken down by the enzyme acetylcholinesterase to acetic acid and choline. Choline enters the presynaptic neuron and is recycled. The neurotransmitters epinephrine and norepinephrine are removed in an unchanged form from the synapse by reuptake. Quick removal of neurotransmitters is important to enable the postsynaptic neuron to respond to another stimulus again.

EXAMPLES OF NEUROTRANSMITTERS

There are many neurotransmitters in the nervous system. Some examples of common neurotransmitters are norepinephrine, dopamine, serotonin, γ-aminobutyric acid (GABA), glutamate, glycine, enkephalins, endorphins, substance P, nitric oxide (yes, a gas!), among many others. Some neurotransmitters are predominant in certain areas of the nervous system. If production of these neurotransmitters is affected, the functioning of this region of the nervous system is affected.

Many drugs affect the nervous system at the synapse level. For example, symptoms of strychnine poisoning (spasm of skeletal muscles) is a result of the blocking of glycine receptors. Glycine is the neurotransmitter in neurons that inhibits motor neurons to muscle. If these neurons don't function, the motor neurons fire continuously, causing muscles to spasm. Similarly, cocaine causes euphoria by blocking dopamine removal from certain areas of the brain. Increased levels of dopamine in these synapses result in change in feeling. Valium (diazepam), an antianxiety drug, enhances the effects of GABA (an inhibitory neurotransmitter). Viagra (sildenafil) produces its action by facilitating the action of nitric oxide, and Prozac (fluoxetine), the drug prescribed for attention deficit disorder (ADD) and depression, acts by slowing down the removal of serotonin in synapses.

ELECTRICAL SYNAPSES

Most synapses are chemical synapses; however, more recently, electrical synapses (Figure 5.9B) have been

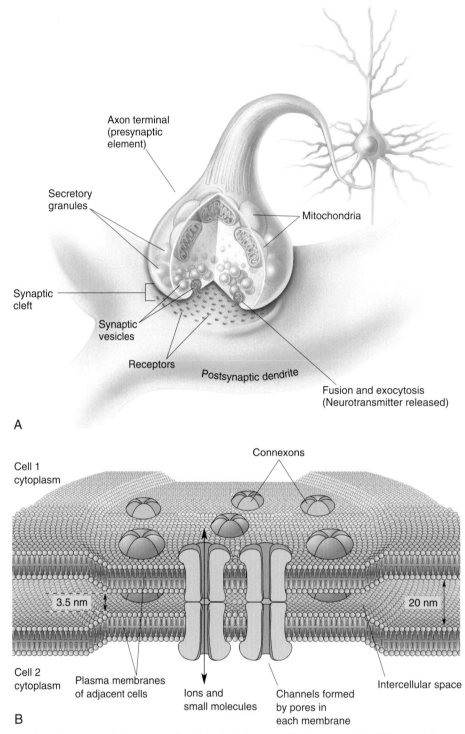

Axon terminal
(presynaptic
element)

Secretory
granules

Mitochondria

Synaptic
cleft

Synaptic
vesicles

Receptors

Postsynaptic dendrite

Fusion and exocytosis
(Neurotransmitter released)

A

Connexons

Cell 1
cytoplasm

3.5 nm

20 nm

Cell 2
cytoplasm

Plasma membranes
of adjacent cells

Ions and
small molecules

Channels formed
by pores in
each membrane

Intercellular space

B

FIGURE 5.9. Synapses. **A,** Structure of a Chemical Synapse; **B,** Structure of an Electrical Synapse

discovered in the brain. Such synapses also exist between smooth muscle cells, between cardiac cells, and between glial cells. In the region of such a synapse, there are gap junctions or connexons (**see page 32**) present between adjacent cells. These junctions allow ions to move in both directions and are a route of communication of impulses from one cell to another.

As a result of the presence of gap junctions, transmission of impulses is faster than in chemical synapses.

SUMMATION

As already mentioned, each neuron can have many synapses. Therefore, the potential changes that occur in it depend on the net effect of all synapses. Certain synapses may produce inhibitory effects and others may produce stimulatory effects. What happens in the postsynaptic neuron depends on which effect is predominant.

For example, if action potentials arrive rapidly in a synapse that has a stimulatory effect, the potential in the postsynaptic neuron may reach threshold quickly and produce an action potential. At the same time, if action potentials arrive in a synapse that produces an inhibitory effect, the postsynaptic membrane will become hyperpolarized, making it difficult for action potential to be generated. This mechanism of integrating the effects of two or more neurons by the postsynaptic neuron is known as **summation.**

FACTORS THAT AFFECT NEURAL FUNCTION

Other factors that affect neuronal functioning are the changes in the extracellular environment and the metabolic demands of the neuron. Neurons are very sensitive to pH. If the pH becomes too high (more alkaline), they start discharging action potentials spontaneously. If the pH becomes too low, the opposite happens and the nervous system shuts down.

As can be expected, fluctuating levels of ions, especially sodium, potassium, and calcium, have a marked effect on impulse production. Similarly, an increase in body temperature makes neurons more excitable.

Neurons require energy for manufacturing neurotransmitters and for maintaining ionic composition. They can be easily injured if metabolic demands are not met.

FUNCTIONAL ORGANIZATION OF NEURONS

The body has about 10 million sensory neurons, 20 billion interneurons, and one-half million motor neurons. These neurons are arranged in so many ways that impulses generated can converge on one neuron or diverge to many neurons or even have a feedback on the neuron that originally generated the impulse. All these possibilities help the body better coordinate its activities. For some different ways that impulses can be modified, see Figure 5.10.

A **diverging arrangement** allows for a wide distribution of a specific input. For example, sensory input is distributed to other neurons in the spinal cord and the brain. **Parallel processing** allows the information to be processed by different neurons at the same time and produce a response in different regions of the body. For example, if you encounter a grizzly bear face-to-face on a hike, I do not know what you would do, but I would scream and run at the same time (but, please don't do that if it actually happens). Parallel processing would help me do that.

A **converging arrangement** helps more than one neuron have an effect on a postsynaptic neuron. For example, if you are carrying a hot plate, your initial response may be to drop the plate. But if the plate contained something you did not want to loose, you could force yourself to carry it to the nearest table without it dropping. It is convergence that makes this possible. The motor neurons to your muscles have synapses with sensory neurons conveying temperature sensation, as well as neurons, from your brain. The activity of the motor neuron depends on the integrated effect of all the neurons synapsing with it. In this way, the motor neuron can be inhibited or stimulated, according to situations and altering the activity of the presynaptic neurons.

Serial processing affects only one neuron. This arrangement is seen in the way sensations are conveyed to the brain. This helps the brain discern the exact region from which the sensation originated. For example, all sensations initiated in the left big toe reach the "toe area" in the brain on the right side (Figure 5.35, **page 348**).

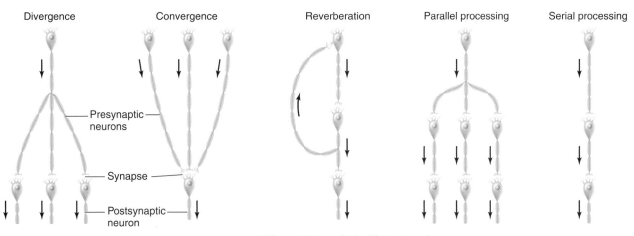

FIGURE **5.10.** Different Ways of Modifying Impulses

NEUROTROPHINS

Chemicals that promote neuron growth—neurotrophins—have been discovered during our quest to help those persons with nerve injuries. Nerve growth factor is one of them. Neurotrophins have important functions in the fetal, as well as the adult, brain. They help promote nerve growth in the fetus. In adults, they are needed for regeneration after injury and for maintenance of neurons.

By providing the appropriate environment with the help of neurotrophins, limited regeneration has been achieved in experiments done on animals with spinal cord injury.

Reverberation helps neurons down the circuit to initiate an impulse in the presynaptic neuron. Although the Figure shows a simplified version, more complicated circuits, with many neurons involved, are seen in the CNS. These circuits continue on and on until the neurons are inhibited or fatigued. An example of such circuits is the respiratory center, which helps with repetitive activities such as breathing.

STANDARD TERMS AND GROUPING

Anatomically, the neurons are arranged in a systematic and logical manner in the brain and spinal cord, with neurons having the same or similar functions invariably grouped together. Many standard terms describe these areas and groupings:

Ganglia. A collection of cell bodies of neurons (e.g., Preganglionic nerves of the sympathetic and parasympathetic nerves synapse with postganglionic neurons in a region located outside the spinal cord and brain). The collection of cell bodies of the postganglionic neurons of one region is known as a ganglion. Another example is the **dorsal root ganglion,** a collection of the cell bodies of the unipolar sensory neurons that lies just outside the spinal cord.

Centers, located in the CNS, are collections of cell bodies of neurons having the same function. For example, the vasomotor center in the brain has cell bodies of neurons involved in regulating the activities of the smooth muscles in the walls of blood vessels. If the boundary of a center can be distinctly made out in anatomic sections of the brain, it is referred to as the **nucleus.** The hypothalamus, for example, has many nuclei, some controlling sleep, some appetite.

Nerve. A nerve is a collection of axons of motor neurons, dendrites of sensory neurons, and axons/dendrites of autonomic fibers bundled together by connective tissue in the PNS. A specific nerve may or may not contain all three types of nerve fibers (i.e., motor, sensory, and autonomic). Nerves leading to or from the brain and brain stem are the **cranial nerves,** and those leading from and to the spinal cord are the **spinal nerves.**

Tracts are bundles of the axons of neurons having the same function and destination. For example, the spinothalamic tract carries pain impulses from the body to the thalamus. Many tracts, if present in the same region of the CNS, are referred to as **columns.** For example, the sensations of touch and pressure are carried by neurons whose axons lie in the posterior aspect of the spinal cord, the dorsal column.

REGENERATION AND DEGENERATION OF NEURONS

Effect of Pressure on Neurons

Neurons generally have a limited capacity to regenerate. For most neurons, cell division stops at birth. Although the whole neuron cannot be replaced if damaged, it is possible for the dendrites and axons to regenerate if the cell body is intact.

If pressure is applied to the axon of a neuron, the lack of oxygen and blood supply reduces its ability to conduct. If the pressure is released after a few hours, the neurons recover in a few weeks.

Cut Injury

More severe pressure will present with the same symptoms as a cut to the nerve. If the axon of a neuron is cut, the part of the axon distal to the cut degenerates and is phagocytized by the Schwann cells that surround it. This process is known as **Wallerian degeneration.** Macrophages come to the area and remove the debris. The Schwann cells, however, do not degenerate. Instead, they multiply along the path of the original axon. The axon stump connected to the cell body grows with multiple small branches into the injury site, guided by the cellular cord of multiplying Schwann cells. It is believed the Schwann cells secrete chemicals that attract the growing axon. If the axon grows in the right direction, it may reach its original synaptic contacts and recover. If it grows into the

Thoracic Outlet Syndrome

Thoracic outlet syndrome includes conditions that produce symptoms of pressure on structures such as nerves (in the brachial plexus) and blood vessels that exit from the thorax (posterior to the clavicle) to enter the limbs. Cervical ribs, malaligned ribs, spasm of neck muscles (scalenes), or other muscles such as the pectoralis minor lying close to the structures passing through the outlet can cause this syndrome. It is characterized by edema, numbness, tingling sensations, or weakness of the upper limbs.

wrong direction, normal function does not return. Chances of recovery are high if the cut ends of the axon are in close contact. The rate of growth of axons is about 1 mm to 2 mm per day and recovery depends on the distance the axon has to regrow to reach the structure it originally innervated (see Figure 5.11).

Many factors affect the chance of recovery. If the axon is cut close to the cell body, the cell body may die, with no chance of recovery. If a crushing type injury has occurred, partial or, often, full recovery en-

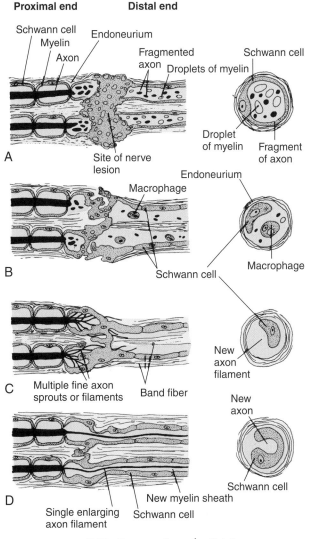

FIGURE **5.11.** Regeneration of a Cut Axon

sues. In a cutting-type injury, if the cut ends are in close contact, chance of recovery is high. However, the alignment of the cut ends also matters. It is important for the axon to grow back into the same area occupied by the original axon. If many adjacent axons are cut, the nerve must be aligned so that the right axon grows into the right area. For example, if an axon innervating skeletal muscle grows into the area occupied by a sensory nerve, the neuron eventually dies.

Injury in the CNS

Damaged neurons in the CNS have greater difficulty recovering. This is because, invariably, many neurons are involved. Also, the astrocytes (neuroglia) form scar tissue, which makes it difficult for axons to grow back. In addition, chemicals that inhibit neuron growth may be liberated in the area. After a spinal cord injury, many cells not directly injured die by **apoptosis** (cell suicide). The reason for this is not clear. Although it was believed that nerves do not multiply, it was recently discovered that new neurons are formed in certain areas of the brain (such as the area for learning). This discovery is encouraging, especially for those with injury to the CNS.

Ischemic Injury

Although the brain accounts for only 2% of the body weight, it accounts for 18% of the energy consumption at rest. Neurons rely solely on aerobic metabolism for their survival. Because they do not have stored glycogen, oxygen and glucose must be continuously supplied by the blood. Therefore, injury to neurons occurs if their blood supply is cut off for even a few seconds. The injury is in proportion to the duration of interruption of the blood supply. Stroke is a result of impairment of blood supply to areas of the brain.

Having considered the functional unit of the nervous system: the neuron and its structure and classification; how impulses are generated, propagated, and communicated to other neurons; and how the neurons recover from injury, the structures involved in sensations are addressed.

Sensory Nervous System

SENSE ORGANS AND INITIATION OF IMPULSES

The neurons that convey information about the internal and external environment—the sensory or afferent neurons—detect the actual changes in the environment by means of **sensory receptors,** which are located at that end of unipolar neurons. Sensory receptors are transducers that convert different forms of energy into action potentials. The endings of sensory nerves alone may have transducer function or they may be surrounded by other non-neural cells that produce action potentials in the neuron. In the latter case, it is known as a **sense organ.**

Some different forms of energy that receptors convert into action potentials are mechanical (touch, pressure), thermal (degrees of warmth and cold), electromagnetic (light), and chemical energy (taste, smell, oxygen content in blood, and carbon dioxide content). Each receptor responds maximally and is sensitive to one type of energy. The particular form of energy to which the receptor responds is its **adequate stimulus.** For example, the adequate stimulus for receptors in

Leprosy or Hansen's Disease

In this disorder, a bacteria—*Mycobacterium leprae*—invades the Schwann cells in cutaneous nerves and produces inflammation. It results in reduction or loss of sensation in patchy areas of the skin.

the eye is light. Sound will have no effect on them, although, if pressure is applied over the eye, flashes of light may be seen. As the sensory receptors are specialized to respond to one type of energy, it follows that there are many different kinds of receptors.

Although one learns in school that there are five senses, the body is able to sense many different senses. Table 5.1 lists some of the senses the body

CLASSIFICATION OF SENSORY NEURONS

Sensory neurons can be classified by the:
* origin of stimulus (e.g., near or far away)
* type of adequate stimulus (e.g., touch, sound)
* threshold of stimulus required for perception (e.g., low threshold; high threshold)
* rate of adaptation (e.g., rapid, slow)
* anatomic structure (e.g., free nerve ending, hair cells)
* type of sensory information they deliver to the brain (e.g., proprioceptors [sense of body position], nociceptors [sense of pain]).

Terms to describe sense organs:
Chemoreceptors are receptors stimulated by a change in the chemical composition of the environment.
Cutaneous senses are senses with receptors are located on the skin.
Exteroceptors are concerned with events near at hand.
Interoceptors are concerned with the internal environment.
Nociceptors are pain receptors often referred to as nociceptors because they are often stimulated by noxious or damaging stimuli.
Proprioceptors give information about the body in space at any given instant.
Special senses: smell, taste, vision, hearing, and rotational and linear acceleration.
Teleceptors are receptors concerned with events at a distance.
Visceral senses are senses that perceive changes in the internal environment.

Table 5.1

Receptors/Sense Organs and Sensations

Sensation	Receptor	Sense Organ
Vision	Rods and cones in retina	Eye
Hearing	Hair cells	Ear
Smell	Olfactory neurons	Nose
Taste	Taste receptors	Tongue
Acceleration	Hair cells	Ear (vestibular apparatus)
Touch-pressure	Nerve endings	Various
Warmth	Nerve endings	Various
Cold	Nerve endings	Various
Pain	Free nerve endings	
Joint position and movement	Nerve endings	Various
Muscle length	Nerve endings	Muscle spindle
Muscle tension	Nerve endings	Golgi tendon organ
Arterial blood pressure	Nerve endings	Stretch receptors in aortic arch and carotid sinus
Venous pressure	Nerve endings	Stretch receptors in walls of great veins
Inflation of lung	Nerve endings	Stretch receptors in lung
Temperature of blood in head	Neurons in hypothalamus	
Oxygen content in blood	Nerve endings?	Aortic and carotid bodies
Osmotic pressure in plasma	Cells in different parts of brain (e.g., thirst center)	
Glucose level in blood	Cells in hypothalamus (hunger center)	

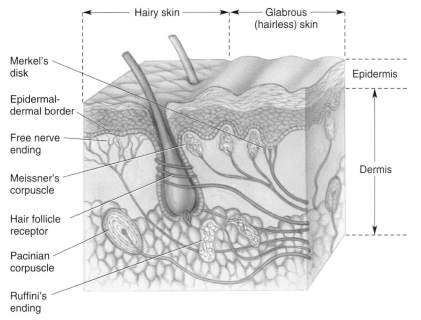

Merkel's disk

Epidermal-dermal border

Free nerve ending

Meissner's corpuscle

Hair follicle receptor

Pacinian corpuscle

Ruffini's ending

Hairy skin

Glabrous (hairless) skin

Epidermis

Dermis

FIGURE 5.12. Anatomical Structure of Certain Cutaneous Receptors

possesses. Some senses listed are complex; for example, a number of different receptors can sense different taste sensations: bitter, sweet, salt, and sour.

CUTANEOUS RECEPTORS

There are many different types of nerve endings on the skin. Some are free nerve endings, some have a capsule around them, and others have expanded tips of nerve endings. Some nerve endings are found wound around hair follicles (see Figure 5.12). Any given receptor signals or responds to only one kind of cutaneous sensation. There are four different cutaneous senses: touch-pressure, pain, cold, and warmth.

Touch Receptors

Touch receptors are present over the entire body, but are more numerous in the skin of the fingers and lips, with relatively fewer receptors in the skin of the trunk. Many are located around hair follicles. The hair acts as a lever and slight movements of the hair magnify the effect on the receptors.

Proprioceptors

Awareness of the body in space is a result of impulses from receptors located in and around joints (joint receptors), within skeletal muscle, and between tendons and muscles (see Figures 4.12 and 4.13). A conscious picture of the position of the body is a result of integration of impulses generated by these receptors and those from the eyes, muscle spindles, skin, and other tissue.

Temperature Receptors

There are two types of temperature receptors; one that responds maximally to temperatures slightly above body temperature (warmth) and one that responds to temperatures slightly below body temperature (cold). These are actually two degrees of warmth because cold is not a form of energy.

There are 4 to 10 times more cold receptors than warm receptors. Cold receptors respond to temperatures from 10–40°C (50–104°F), and warm receptors respond from 30–45°C (86–113°F). Between the temperatures 20 and 40°C (68 and 104°F), with time, the receptors adapt and conscious perception of the temperature diminishes. At temperatures above and below this, the receptors do not adapt. At temperatures above 45°C (113°F), the tissue becomes damaged and the sensation is that of pain.

Itch and Tickle

Mild stimulation, especially if produced by something that moves across the skin, causes itch and tickle sen-

---

HAVE YOU BEEN CONFUSED BY TEMPERATURE CHANGES?

We are often unable to identify the water temperature when we run our bath water. This is probably because both cold and warm receptors are stimulated between the temperatures 30–40°C (86–104°F), and the degree to which they are stimulated determines if the water is perceived as cold or hot.

sations. Free nerve endings of slow conducting, un-myelinated fibers seem to carry these sensations and repetitive, mechanical, local stimuli and/or chemicals such as histamine stimulate these receptors. Itch could possibly be a fifth cutaneous sense.

Complex sensations, such as the ability to sense **vibration;** discriminate two stimuli applied close to each other (**2-point discrimination**); and identify objects based on size, shape, consistency, and texture by handling the object without looking at it (**stereognosis**), are a result of the integration of the various cutaneous senses and require an intact cerebral cortex. A pattern of rhythmic pressure stimuli is interpreted as vibration.

Pain Receptors or Nociceptors

The stimuli for pain, pathways, and perception of pain is complex. Refer to **page 341** for a detailed discussion of pain.

AN OVERVIEW OF ELECTRICAL AND IONIC EVENTS IN RECEPTORS

The receptors convert the adequate stimuli into action potentials, similar to the electrical changes (EPSP and IPSP) that occur at the synapse. However, the electrical changes here are known as **generator potentials** and **receptor potentials.** For example, if pressure is applied over a receptor that responds to these stimuli and the electrical changes are recorded using microelectrodes inside and outside the nerve, the inside of the nerve ending which is originally negative depolarizes. This is caused, in most cases, by opening of sodium channels on the cell membrane of the nerve endings and sodium rushing in (generator potential). This seems to trigger an action potential down the nerve. Some receptors secrete neurotrans-

mitters which then stimulate the adjacent neuron and produce action potentials (receptor potential). It has been shown that if the stimuli are more intense, many action potentials at greater frequency are generated. In this way, by differences in the frequency of the action potentials, the brain is able to discern the intensity of the stimulus applied.

If a stimulus is applied for a prolonged period, the frequency of the action potentials generated declines. This phenomenon is **adaptation.** The degree to which receptors adapt varies with sense organs. In receptors that do not adapt quickly, the action potentials continue for as long as stimuli are applied. These are the **slow adaptors** or **tonic receptors.** Certain receptors trigger action potentials at the beginning and end of the application of stimulus, the **rapidly adapting receptors** or **phasic receptors.** Both types are valuable for survival. Pain and cold receptors are slow adapting and help warn the body regarding injury. Similarly, the stretch receptors that regulate blood pressure are slow adaptors. This is because the blood to the brain must be constantly monitored.

PERCEPTION OF SENSATIONS

Doctrine of Specific Nerve Energies

According to the explanation above, all stimuli seem to be converted to action potentials. If so, how does the body know what the original stimulus was? This doctrine, stated by Muller, explains how this happens. The sensation perceived depends on which part of the brain they activate. The pathway taken by action potentials generated by a sense organ is specific from sense organ to the brain. The sensation that is perceived is that for which the receptor is specialized, no matter where along the pathway the activity is initiated. For example, the sense of pressure is perceived as coming from the hand irrespective of where the sensory nerve is stimulated: pressure receptors in the hand, nerve at the elbow, the axilla, in the posterior aspect of the spinal cord where it travels, or even in the brain where it finally arrives.

Law of Projection

This law explains that wherever the nerve is stimulated in a sensory pathway, the sensation is projected (perceived) in the area of the body where the sensation normally originates. For example, if, during brain surgery on a conscious patient, the brain receiving area for impulses from the right hand is stimulated, the patient reports sensation in the right hand and not in the brain where the actual stimulation was.

💡 HOW WE SENSE

- Each sense organ or sensory receptor is specialized to convert (transduce) one form of energy into action potentials in the sensory nerves.
- Different forms (modalities) of sensation are identified by the fact that they are transmitted to the brain by different nerve pathways and synaptic connections (although all of them are in the form of nerve impulses).
- The intensity of the stimulus is identified by (1) the change in the frequency of the action potential produced, and (2) the number of receptors stimulated.
- The area/region of the body stimulated is identified by impulses from these areas reaching a specific region in the brain (stimuli to right leg reaches area representing the right leg in the cerebral cortex).

Intensity Discrimination

Again, if all stimuli are converted to action potentials, how does the body perceive variations in intensity? There are two ways by which intensity is transmitted to the brain. One is by altering the frequency of stimulation. The other is by the number of receptors that have been stimulated.

Lateral Inhibition

Another mechanism the CNS uses to better perceive sensations is lateral inhibition, in which the neuron that is most stimulated inhibits surrounding neurons via interneurons. For example, when the sound produced by striking middle C reaches the ear, the neurons that respond to this particular pitch are most stimulated. When responding by production of action potentials, they inhibit surrounding neurons that respond to the next closest pitch. This way, the sound of middle C is heard sharply.

Sensory Unit

This term is applied to a single sensory neuron and all its peripheral branches. The number of branches varies, and branches are numerous, especially in the skin. The **receptive field** of a sensory unit is the area from which a stimulus produces a response in that unit. The sensory units tend to overlap the areas supplied by other sensory units.

As the stimulus is increased, more and more sensory units are stimulated because the stimuli affect a large area. As a result, more pathways are affected, and the brain perceives more stimuli intensity.

Why Are Some Areas More Sensitive Than Others?

Some areas, such as the face, fingertips, and toes, are more sensitive than others because there are more sensory neurons innervating a unit area of skin, each with a smaller receptive area. In areas such as the back, the receptive field of each sensory neuron is large and the number of innervating nerves is less (see Figure 5.13). That is why a light touch on the face feels good. But the touch has to be more intense, covering a larger area, in regions such as the back. This is one reason why fingertips are used on the face and the entire palm is used to massage the back.

See **pages 356–358** for details of some special sensory organs (smell, taste, vestibular apparatus).

THE SPINAL CORD, SPINAL NERVES, AND DERMATOMES

From the area of supply, the peripheral branch of the sensory neuron continues toward the CNS. As a result of the way the body is developed in the embryo, there is a specific pattern in the way nerves from different regions of the skin converge to the

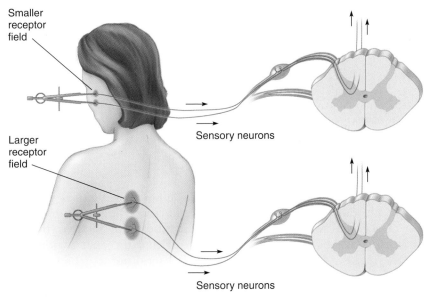

Smaller receptor field

Larger receptor field

Sensory neurons

Sensory neurons

FIGURE **5.13.** Receptive Fields

TEST YOUR SKIN SENSITIVITY

You can crudely test the sensitivity of different areas of the body by using a paper clip. Bend the clip so that the two ends are level and about a few millimeters apart. Now, ask your colleague to close her or his eyes and then touch a region of the body so that both points of the paper clip touch the body at the same time. Ask her or him to say if the touch was felt as one or two stimuli. If it was felt as one stimulus, spread the paper clip apart a little more and repeat until it is perceived as two separate stimuli. This gives you an idea of the size of the receptive field of a sensory neuron in that area. If both points of the paper clip stimulate the same receptive field, the sensation is felt as one stimulus. If each point stimulates a different receptive field, the person feels it as two. Repeat this in different regions of the body, and determine which areas can sense stimuli as two, even when the tips are close together. These areas are more sensitive because they have more sensory units per unit area of skin, with each receptive field being smaller.

Care should be taken that the test is done on bare skin as the stimuli spreads to other areas if it is performed over clothing. Also, if both tips do not touch the body at exactly the same time, it may be felt as two stimuli.

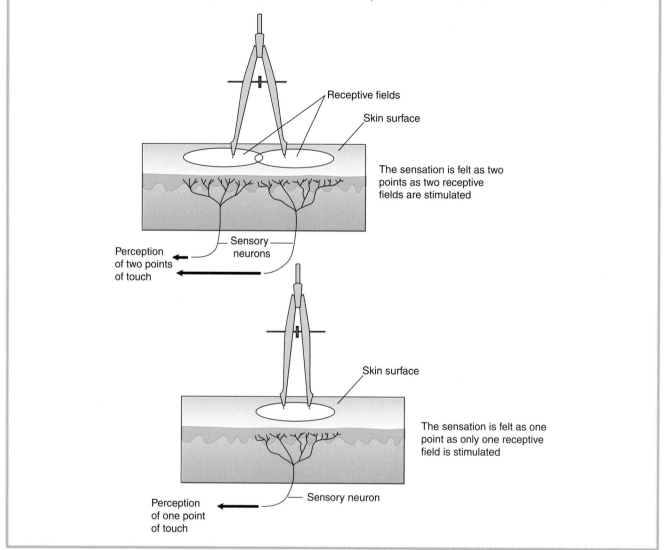

CNS. Thirty-one spinal nerves and certain cranial nerves are responsible for all body sensations. Figure 2.6 shows the area of the skin and the spinal cord segment to which sensory nerves go from specific areas of the body. The region of the body wall supplied by the cutaneous branches of a single pair of spinal nerves (right and left) is known as a **dermatome.** Although the dermatomes appear to have distinct borders, there is some overlap between adjacent areas. The sensations from the face reach the brain via cranial nerve V (trigeminal nerve). It is of interest that the anal region lies in the dermatome of the sacral nerves; the most distal segment of the spinal cord. In the embryo, this is the tail region, and the lower limb develops from the lumbar and upper sacral region.

The cell bodies of the sensory nerves are located close to the spinal cord at the location where they enter. This collection of cell bodies in each segment is known as the **dorsal root ganglion** and is seen as a slight enlargement just outside the spinal cord (see Figure 5.15). A similar ganglion is present in the route of cranial nerves that contain branches of sensory neurons.

Sensory neurons, as already mentioned, are unipolar, and the other branch leading off the cell body (axon) enters the spinal cord where it immediately synapses or travels up (and/or down) before synapsing. The pathway of the sensory impulses in the CNS is described on **page 339.**

ANATOMICAL STRUCTURE OF THE SPINAL CORD

The spinal cord in an adult is about 45 cm (18 in) long and 14 mm (0.55 in) wide. It lies in the spinal canal of the vertebral column, extending inferiorly as far as vertebra L1 and L2 (see Figure 5.14). It is

DERMATOMAL PATTERNS

An easy way to remember the dermatomal pattern is to imagine the body with the arm and legs stretched out to the sides at 180°. The dermatomes seem to stretch across as transverse strips.

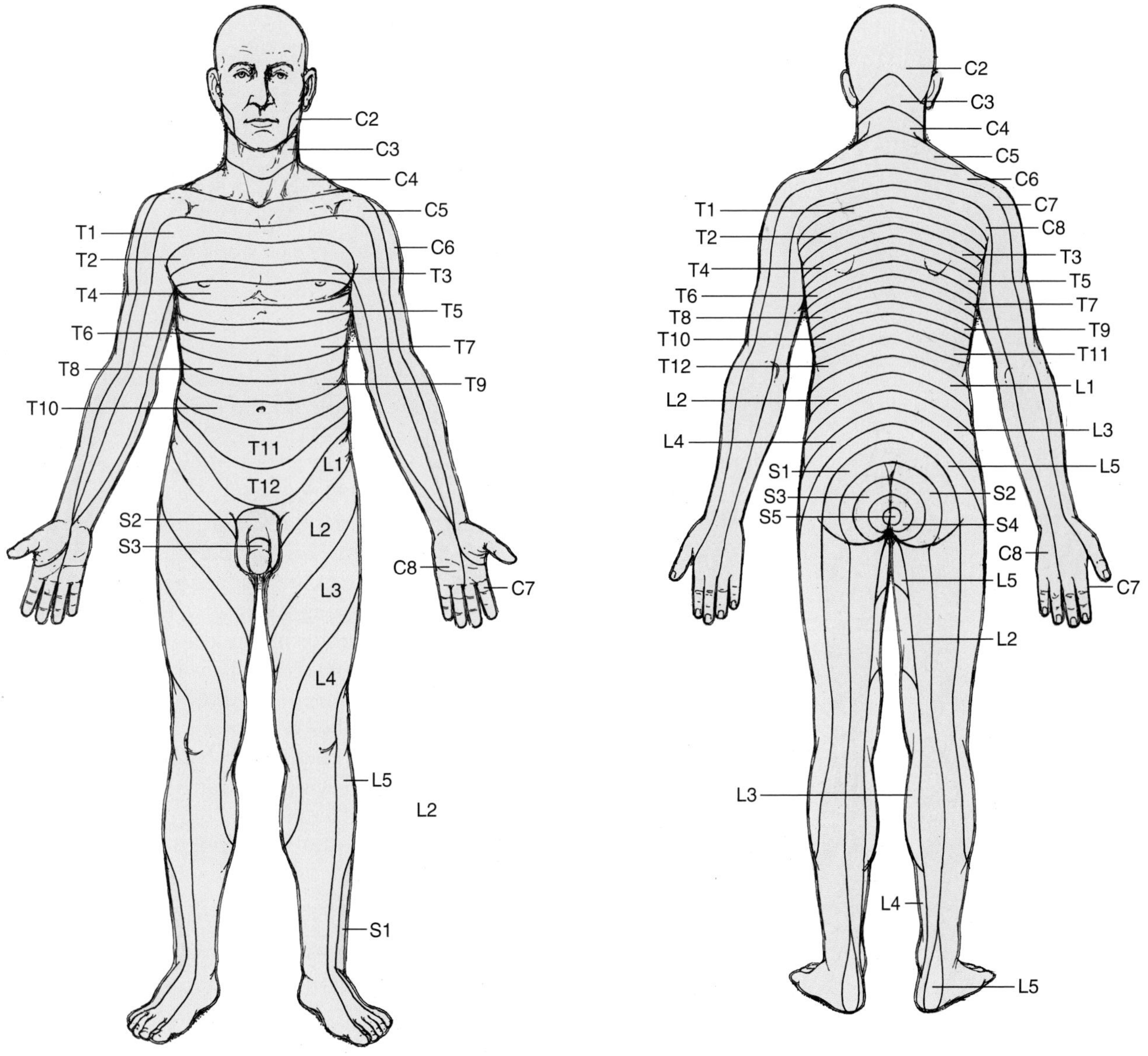

Dermatomal Patterns

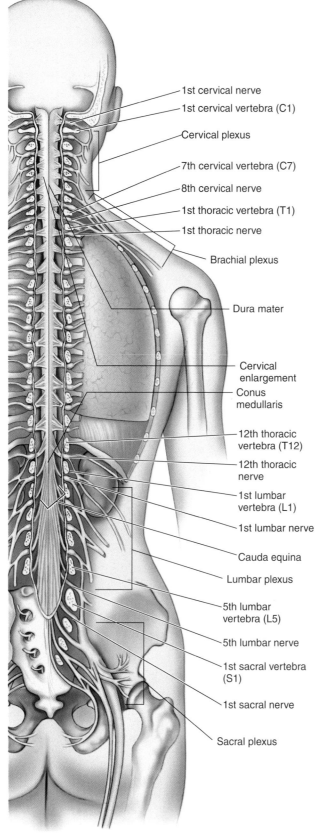

FIGURE **5.14.** Structure of the Spinal Cord—Coronal Section

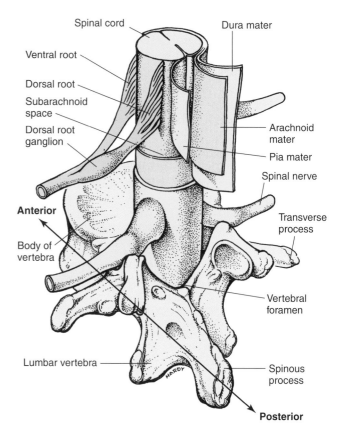

FIGURE **5.15.** Meninges and Other Structures Protecting the Spinal Cord

shorter than the vertebral column because its growth does not match that of the vertebral column during growth of the fetus and young child.

The spinal cord has 31 pairs of spinal nerves leaving through the intervertebral foramina located between the vertebrae. Some nerves are large because they supply a larger area of the body. Large nerves are seen in the lower neck region, supplying the arms, forearms, and hands. Such nerves are also seen in the lumbar and sacral regions, supplying the thighs, legs, and feet. The cord is enlarged slightly in the cervical (**cervical enlargement**) and lumbosacral (**lumbosacral enlargement**) regions, as it has to accommodate the cell bodies of a greater number of neurons. The lower end of the spinal cord becomes conical and tapers into the **conus medullaris** region. A thin, fibrous tissue extends from its tip to the sacral region, the **filum terminale.** This fibrous tissue gives longitudinal support to the spinal cord.

BELL-MAGENDIE LAW

All sensory neurons enter the spinal cord in the dorsal region, and all motor neurons leave ventrally. This principle is known as the Bell-Magendie law.

A **segment** is the part of the spinal cord that corresponds to a single pair of spinal nerves. Therefore, there are 31 segments in the spinal cord: 8 **cervical,** 12 **thoracic,** 5 **lumbar,** 5 **sacral,** and 1 **coccygeal.** Specific spinal nerves are denoted with the first letter of the spinal segment and the number. For example, the spinal nerve that is the eighth nerve arising in the cervical region is referred to as C8. Although the spinal cord is much shorter than the vertebral column, ending close to the second lumbar vertebrae, the lower lumbar and sacral segments of the spinal cord exist, although at a more superior location. Because the spinal cord is shorter than the vertebral column, the spinal nerves from the lower lumbar and sacral regions course downward to exit through the correct intervertebral foramina. These nerves combined make the lower end of the spinal cord look like a horse's tail and are referred to as the **cauda equina.**

The spinal nerves are easily indicated in relation to the vertebra. Generally, each nerve caudal to the vertebra takes its name in relation to the vertebra preceding it (i.e., the nerve between thoracic vertebrae 1 and 2 is T1). Because the first spinal nerve exits between the skull and the first cervical vertebrae, cervical spinal nerves are indicated in relation to the vertebrae following it (i.e., the nerve lying between the skull and the first vertebra is C1).

Each spinal nerve is attached to the cord by two roots—the dorsal root (sensory root) and the ventral root (motor root) (see Figure 5.15). The dorsal root is enlarged to form the dorsal root ganglion, which contains the unipolar sensory neurons with their single axon and two branches; the peripheral branch and the central branch. Two-thirds of the central branches terminate at the dorsal horn (see below) they entered. The remaining one-third ascends up the spinal cord to synapse with neurons located in the lower part of the medulla. The peripheral branch passes via the spinal nerves to sensory receptors in the body. Distal to the dorsal root ganglia, the sensory and motor roots are bound together to form a spinal nerve. Thus, spinal nerves contain both motor and sensory nerves and are considered mixed nerves. The distribution of the spinal nerves to different parts of the body is considered later.

Protection of the Spinal Cord

The vertebral column and its surrounding ligaments, tendons, and muscles separate the spinal cord from the external environment. The spinal cord must also be protected from damaging contact with the bony wall of the vertebral canal. The spinal **meninges** (Figure 5.15) provide physical stability and, along with the cerebrospinal fluid, help absorb shock. Blood vessels that supply the spinal cord pierce through the meninges.

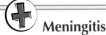

Meningitis

Meningitis is inflammation of the meninges. Usually caused by infection, it affects blood and cerebrospinal fluid circulation and destroys nerve tissue, leading to severe headache and motor and sensory complications.

Like the meninges around the brain, the spinal meninges have three layers: the **pia, arachnoid,** and **dura mater.** The spinal meninges are continuous with the cranial meninges at the foramen magnum.

The **dura mater** is a tough fibrous sheath that is the outer covering of the spinal cord. Its collagen fibers are oriented longitudinally. At the foramen magnum, it fuses with the periosteum of the occipital bone. Distally, it forms a cord that surrounds the filum terminale to form the **coccygeal ligament.** This way, it provides longitudinal stability to the spinal cord. Laterally, the dura fuses with the connective tissue surrounding the spinal nerves as they exit through the intervertebral foramen. The space between the dura and the vertebral canal is the **epidural space,** containing loose connective tissue, adipose tissue, and blood vessels.

The **arachnoid mater** is the membrane lying deep to the dura. A potential space—the **subdural space**—separates it from the dura. The arachnoid is lined by squamous epithelium. From its inner surface, delicate, loose collagen and elastic fibers extend between the epithelium and the inner layer pia. This space, the **subarachnoid space,** is filled with **cerebrospinal fluid** (CSF). The CSF, discussed on **page 367,** serves as a shock absorber and a medium that transports dissolved gases, nutrients, chemical messengers, and waste products.

The **pia mater** is firmly bound to the spinal cord. Collagen and elastic tissue from this layer extend laterally from either side of the spinal cord as the **denticulate ligament.** This ligament, after piercing the arachnoid, becomes attached to the dura, giving the spinal cord lateral stability.

Sectional Anatomy of the Spinal Cord

If a transverse section is made of the spinal cord (see Figure 5.16) and viewed, two areas are noted. Around

Epidural Block

Anesthetics are injected into the epidural space at specific points to control pain in regions supplied by spinal nerves that exit from there. This procedure is known as an epidural block.

the center, there is a gray area—the **gray matter.** Surrounding it is a white area known as the **white matter.** The cell bodies of neurons and short nerve fibers are located in the gray matter. The white matter contains neuroglia and fiber tracts. The gray matter appears as if it has many horns. Depending on the location, the horns are called the **posterior or dorsal gray horns, anterior or ventral gray horns,** and **lateral gray horns.** The cell bodies of nerves supplying skeletal muscles (motor neurons) are located in the ventral horn. The lateral horn contains cell bodies of the autonomic nerves, and the dorsal horn has cell bodies of nerves that receive impulses from the spinal nerves. At the center of the gray matter is the **central canal** through which cerebrospinal fluid flows.

Functions of the Gray Mater of the Spinal Cord

The gray matter of the spinal cord has two functions. First, synapses relay signals between the periphery and the brain in both directions. It is in the dorsal horns that sensory signals are relayed from the sensory roots of the spinal nerves to other parts of the CNS. It is mainly in the ventral and lateral horns that motor signals are relayed from the neurons descending from the brain to the motor nerves and autonomic nerves.

Second, the gray matter of the cord integrates some motor activities. For example, if you touch a hot object with your hand, the hand is withdrawn

within a few seconds. This reflex occurs even without the signals reaching the brain. Other similar reflexes that occur at the level of the cord are contraction of the extensors when standing, stretch reflexes that cause the muscle to contract when stretched and, in lower animals, the scratch reflex.

Function of the White Matter

The white matter surrounding the gray matter is white because of the myelinated fibers. It contains bundles of axons that carry impulses across spinal segments, as well as to and from the brain. The horns of the gray matter divide the white matter into three distinct columns. The two **dorsal,** or **posterior white columns,** lie between the dorsal gray horns. The two **lateral white columns** lie on each side of the cord lateral to the gray matter. Two **ventral,** or **anterior white columns,** lie anterior to the ventral gray horns. Axons from neurons having the same function, conduction speed, diameter, and myelination are bundled together as tracts in these columns. Tracts carrying sensory information *to* the brain are the **ascending tracts,** and those *from* the brain are the **descending tracts,** conveying commands from the brain to the spinal cord.

The spinal cord has two central depressions anteriorly and posteriorly. The anterior is deep and narrow and is known as the **anterior median fissure.** The posterior depression is the **posterior median sulcus.**

DISTRIBUTION OF SPINAL NERVES

To review, each of 31 spinal nerves are attached to the spinal cord via the dorsal and ventral roots. The dorsal root is enlarged to form the dorsal root ganglion. Close to the intervertebral foramen, the dorsal and ventral roots are bound together to form the spinal nerve.

As the spinal nerve continues to the periphery, it is surrounded by layers of connective tissue. The outermost layer, or **epineurium,** consists of a dense network of collagen fibers. The nerve is divided into many bundles of axons by the **perineurium,** which consists of collagen fibers that extend inward from the epineurium. Individual axons are surrounded by delicate connective tissue fibers, the **endoneurium.** The blood vessels travel along the connective tissue layers, delivering nutrients and oxygen to individual axons, Schwann cells, and connective tissue and removing waste products.

Figure 5.17 shows the distribution of a typical spinal nerve. The first branch of the spinal nerve in the thoracic and upper lumbar regions (T1–L2) carries preganglionic axons of the sympathetic nervous system (see **page 369**). These myelinated fibers appear white, and the branch is known as the **white**

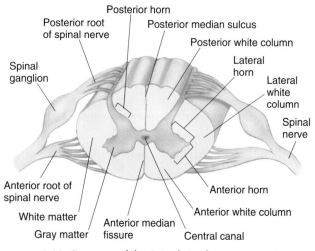

FIGURE 5.16. Structure of the Spinal Cord—Transverse Section

Posterior horn
Posterior root of spinal nerve
Posterior median sulcus
Posterior white column
Lateral horn
Lateral white column
Spinal ganglion
Spinal nerve
Anterior root of spinal nerve
White matter
Gray matter
Anterior median fissure
Anterior horn
Anterior white column
Central canal

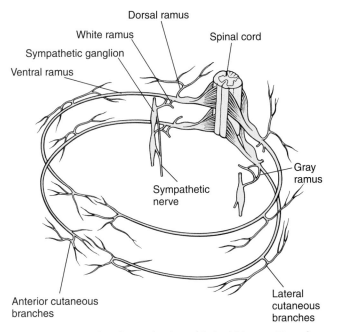

Dorsal ramus
White ramus
Spinal cord
Sympathetic ganglion
Ventral ramus
Gray ramus
Sympathetic nerve
Anterior cutaneous branches
Lateral cutaneous branches

FIGURE 5.17. Peripheral Distribution of Spinal Nerves. Dorsal ramus (**to** skeletal muscles, smooth muscles, and glands, etc., of back; **from** receptors of back); ventral ramus (**to** skeletal muscles, smooth muscles, and glands, etc., of body wall, limbs; **from** receptors of body wall, limbs); and sympathetic nerve (**to** smooth muscles, glands, and visceral organs in the thoracic and abdominopelvic cavity; **from** receptors of organs).

ramus. The axons synapse with postganglionic neurons located in the **sympathetic ganglion** that runs along the side of the vertebral column. From the sympathetic ganglion, axons of postganglionic fibers that innervate glands and smooth muscles in the body wall and limbs join the spinal nerve again as the **gray ramus.** Other postganglionic fibers of the sympathetic system that innervate the organs in the thoracic and abdominal cavity form networks and nerves in the thorax and abdomen.

The spinal nerve then branches into the **dorsal ramus** and **ventral ramus,** distal to the white and gray rami. The dorsal ramus of each spinal nerve carries sensory and motor innervation to the skin and the muscles of the back. The larger ventral ramus supplies the structures on the body wall, the limbs, and the ventrolateral areas of the body.

NERVE PLEXUS

The arrangement of spinal nerves in the segments controlling the muscles of the neck and limbs is a little complicated because, in the embryo, small muscles supplied by nerves in the ventral rami fuse to form larger muscles. These larger muscles (now identified as single muscles) have compound nerve supply (i.e., they are supplied by nerves originating from

more than one spinal segment). The ventral rami also blend their fibers with that of adjacent ones and a complex interwoven network of nerves is found. These networks are termed **nerve plexus,** and there are three major ones: the **cervical plexus, brachial plexus,** and **lumbosacral plexus** (Figure 5.14).

The Cervical Plexus

The cervical plexus consists of the ventral rami of spinal nerves C1–C5 (Figure 5.14). Nerves from here innervate muscles of the neck, shoulder, and the diaphragm (phrenic nerves C3–5). The sensory component of this plexus can be visualized on **page 321,** showing the dermatomal pattern. It supplies the skin of the ear, neck, and upper chest.

The plexus lies in relation to the first four cervical vertebrae, venterolateral to the levator scapulae muscle and scalenus medius and deep to the sternocleidomastoid muscle. Impingement of the plexus results in headaches, neck pain, and breathing difficulties and is most often a result of pressure on the nerves by the suboccipital and sternocleidomastoid muscles or by shortening of the connective tissue located in the base of the skull.

The Brachial Plexus

This plexus (Figures 5.14 and 5.18) is formed by the ventral rami of spinal nerves C5–T1. It innervates the shoulder girdle and upper limb. The ventral rami combine and divide in a specific manner as they pass from the vertebral column and neck region into the upper limbs.

Initially, the ventral rami (**roots**) combine to form three large **trunks—superior, middle,** and **inferior.** These trunks divide into **anterior** and **posterior divisions.** All the divisions pass under the clavicle and over the first rib into the axilla (armpit), where they fuse to form the three **cords—lateral, medial,** and **posterior cords.** The cords align around the axillary artery in the axilla and give rise to the major **nerves** of the upper limb. Branches from these nerves supply the skin and muscles of the upper limb.

Roots (C5–T1) → Trunks (superior, middle, inferior) → Divisions (anterior, posterior) → Cords (lateral, medial, posterior) → Nerves.

✚ Cervical Plexus and Injuries

Injury to the spinal cord above the origin of the phrenic nerve (nerve to the diaphragm, C3, 4, 5) will result in respiratory arrest because impulses cannot be sent to the diaphragm.

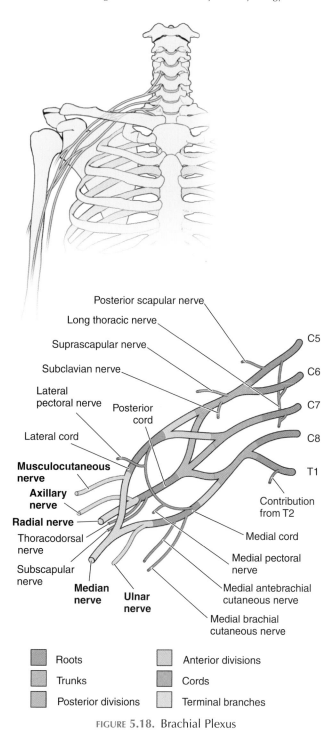

Posterior scapular nerve

Long thoracic nerve

Suprascapular nerve

Subclavian nerve

Lateral
pectoral nerve

Posterior
cord

Lateral cord

**Musculocutaneous
nerve**

**Axillary
nerve**

Radial nerve

Thoracodorsal
nerve

Subscapular
nerve

**Median
nerve**

**Ulnar
nerve**

C5

C6

C7

C8

T1

Contribution
from T2

Medial cord

Medial pectoral
nerve

Medial antebrachial
cutaneous nerve

Medial brachial
cutaneous nerve

	Roots		Anterior divisions
	Trunks		Cords
	Posterior divisions		Terminal branches

FIGURE 5.18. Brachial Plexus

The brachial plexus, being more accessible than the others, is prone for injury in the neck and axilla. Some nerves are also prone for damage, especially those branches that lie superficially. It is important for therapists to understand the relationship of the brachial plexus in the neck and axilla. In the neck, the brachial plexus lies in the posterior triangle and is covered by skin, platysma, and deep fascia. The roots lie between the scaleni anterior and medius. The plexus then becomes dorsal to the clavicle and subclavius and super-

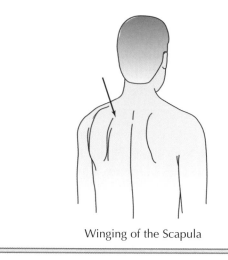

Injury to Superior Roots (C5, C6) of the Brachial Plexus

If the head is pulled forcefully from the shoulder (or vice versa), there is potential for injury to the superior roots. Such trauma may occur when a person falls on the shoulder or during delivery when unusual force is used to extract the head after the shoulder has been delivered. In a person with such an injury, the limb on the affected side is characteristically positioned. There is adduction and medial rotation of the shoulder, extension of the elbow, pronation of the forearm, and flexion of the wrist. Sensation may be lost on the lateral side of the arm. This condition is known as **Erb-Duchene palsy** or **Waiter's tip/Porter's tip position.**

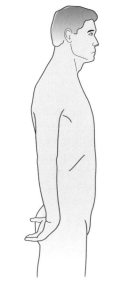

Waiter's Tip/Porter's Tip Position

Sometimes, the long thoracic nerve (C5–C7) that supplies the serratus anterior muscle may be injured, resulting in winging of the scapula where the medial border and inferior angle of the scapula move away from the thoracic cage. In this condition, it is difficult to abduct the shoulder beyond 90°.

Winging of the Scapula

ficial to the first digitation of the serratus anterior and the subscapularis to enter the axillary region. Impingement of the brachial plexus is most often a result of the scalenes, pectoralis minor, and subclavius.

The major nerves of the lateral cord are the **musculocutaneous nerve** (supplies the flexors of the arm) and the **median nerve** (supplies most muscles of the anterior forearm and certain muscles of the hand). The major nerve of the medial cord is the **ulna nerve** (supplies the anteromedial muscles of the forearm and most muscles of the hand). The **axillary** (supplies the deltoid and teres minor) and **radial nerves** (supplies the muscles on the posterior aspect of the arm and forearm) are the major nerves of the posterior cord. The muscles supplied and the area of skin innervated by each of these five nerves is given in Table 5.2.

Courses of the Major Nerves

The **axillary nerve** (C5–C6) curves around the upper and anterior aspect of the humerus to supply the deltoid and teres minor muscles and the skin of the shoulder and the shoulder joint (see Figure 5.19).

The **musculocutaneous nerve** (C5–C7) curves laterally through the deep portions of the anterior arm and then continues superficially down the lateral surface of the forearm to provide sensory innervation (see Figure 5.20). The biceps brachii, coracobrachialis, and brachialis are some major muscles innervated.

The **radial nerve** (C5–C8, T1) curves posteriorly and laterally behind the humerus and enters the forearm over the lateral epicondyle of the humerus (see Figure 5.21). Thereafter, it follows the lateral

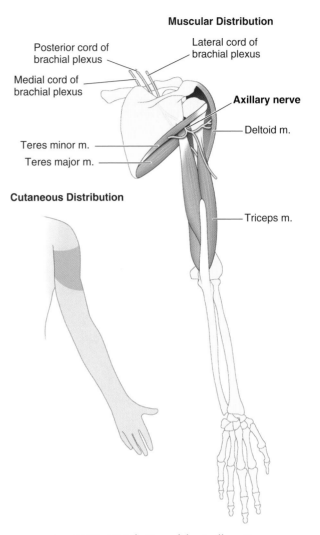

FIGURE 5.19. Distribution of the Axillary Nerve

Table 5.2

Major Nerves of Brachial Plexus and Their Distribution

Spinal Segment	Nerve	Distribution	
		Motor	*Sensory*
C5–C6	Axillary (Figure 5.19)	Deltoid; teres minor	Skin of shoulder; shoulder joint
C5–C7	Musculocutaneous (Figure 5.20)	Flexor muscles of the arm (biceps, brachialis, coracobrachialis)	Skin over lateral surface of forearm
C5–T1	Radial (Figure 5.21)	Extensor muscles of the arm and forearm (triceps; supinator; anconeus; brachioradialis, extensor carpi radialis brevis; extensor carpi radialis longus; extensor carpi ulnaris; digital extensors), abductor pollicis longus	Skin of posterolateral aspect of arm, forearm, and hand
C6–T1	Median (Figure 5.22)	Flexor muscles of the forearm (flexor carpi radialis and palmaris longus); pronators; flexors of the digits; abductor pollicis brevis	Skin over anterolateral surface of the hand
C8–T1	Ulnar (Figure 5.23)	Flexor muscles of the forearm (flexor carpi ulnaris; flexor digitorum); adductor pollicis and small digital muscles (profundus; third, and fourth lumbricals)	Skin over medial surface (two-thirds) of the hand

border of the radius and finally continues into the posterior portions of the thumb and first three fingers. The principal movements controlled by the radius are (1) extension of the elbow, (2) supination of the forearm and hand, (3) extension of the wrist, fingers, and thumb, and (4) abduction of the thumb.

The **median nerve** (C6–C8, T1) passes down the anteromedial portion of the arm, then distally in the anterolateral portions of the forearm, into the lateral palm of the hand, and into the anterior compartment of the thumb and first two fingers and lateral half of the third finger (see Figure 5.22). The median nerve

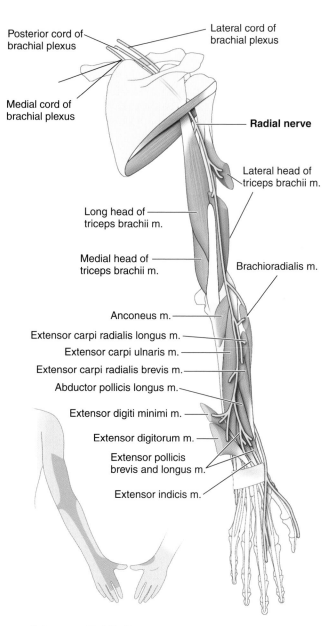

Muscular Distribution

Posterior cord of brachial plexus

Lateral cord of brachial plexus

Medial cord of brachial plexus

Radial nerve

Lateral head of triceps brachii m.

Long head of triceps brachii m.

Medial head of triceps brachii m.

Brachioradialis m.

Anconeus m.

Extensor carpi radialis longus m.

Extensor carpi ulnaris m.

Extensor carpi radialis brevis m.

Abductor pollicis longus m.

Extensor digiti minimi m.

Extensor digitorum m.

Extensor pollicis brevis and longus m.

Extensor indicis m.

Cutaneous Distribution

FIGURE 5.21. Distribution of Radial Nerve

innervates approximately the lateral two-thirds of the muscles in the anterior compartment of the forearm and the lateral third of the anterior muscles of the hand. The major movements controlled by this nerve are (1) pronation of the forearm and hand, (2) flexion of the wrist, fingers and thumb, (3) abduction of the wrist, (4) abduction of the thumb, (5) opponens motion of the thumb.

The **ulna nerve** (C8–T1) passes down the posteromedial portion of the arm, then behind the medial epicondyle of the humerus at the elbow joint and, fi-

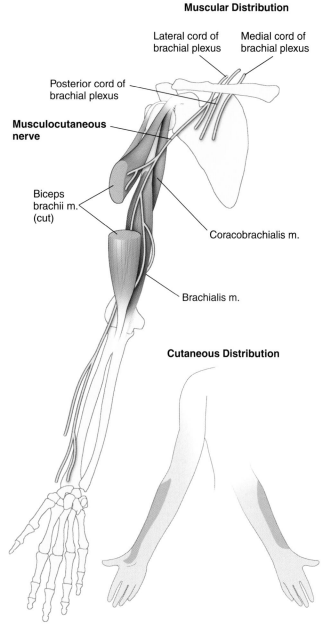

Muscular Distribution

Lateral cord of brachial plexus

Medial cord of brachial plexus

Posterior cord of brachial plexus

Musculocutaneous nerve

Biceps brachii m. (cut)

Coracobrachialis m.

Brachialis m.

Cutaneous Distribution

FIGURE 5.20. Distribution of Musculocutaneous Nerve

✚ Injuries to the Radial Nerve

The radial nerve may be injured in many ways. In people using crutches, excessive pressure may be applied on the radial nerve as it gets compressed between the crutch and the humerus. Often, when the shoulder is dislocated, this nerve is affected. It may become injured in children if their arm is yanked. It may also become injured in fracture of the shaft of the humerus or if a cast to the upper arm is applied too tightly. Improper administration of injections to the upper arm may result in radial nerve (and axillary nerve) injury.

The condition resulting from radial nerve injury is referred to as **wrist drop,** in which the person has difficulty extending the wrist and fingers and the joints of the fingers, wrist, and elbow are constantly flexed.

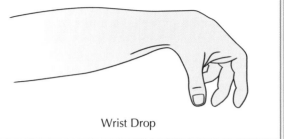

Wrist Drop

nally, alongside the ulna to enter the medial border of the hand, supplying both the anterior and posterior surfaces of the little finger and the medial half of the third finger (see Figure 5.23). The ulnar nerve innervates approximately the medial third of the muscles

✓ *Surface Anatomy of the Radial Nerve*

Try to roll the radial nerve where it runs vertically in its spiral groove on the back of the humerus, behind and below the insertion of the deltoid.

✚ Injury to the Median Nerve

The median nerve is usually injured in the forearm or wrist (carpal tunnel syndrome). If injured, the muscles of the thumb are paralyzed, with inability to oppose the thumb. There is tingling and pain or loss of sensation in the palm and fingers. Pronation and flexion of the proximal interphalangeal joints of all the fingers, the distal interphalangeal joints of the second and third fingers, and the wrist is lost or weak. In this condition, the hand has the characteristic position shown.

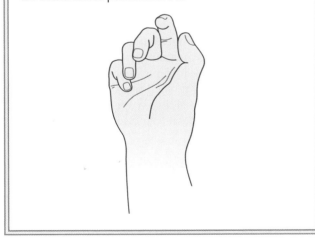

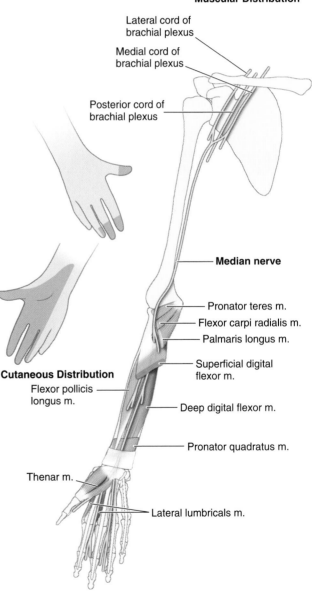

Muscular Distribution

Lateral cord of brachial plexus

Medial cord of brachial plexus

Posterior cord of brachial plexus

Median nerve

Pronator teres m.

Flexor carpi radialis m.

Palmaris longus m.

Superficial digital flexor m.

Deep digital flexor m.

Pronator quadratus m.

Lateral lumbricals m.

Cutaneous Distribution

Flexor pollicis longus m.

Thenar m.

FIGURE 5.22. Distribution of Median Nerve

in the anterior forearm and the medial two-thirds of the muscles in the anterior hand. These muscles primarily cause (1) flexion of the wrist and fingers (along with median nerve), (2) abduction of the fingers, (3) adduction of the fingers and thumb, and (4) opponens motion of the little finger.

The Lumbosacral Plexus

The lumbosacral plexus (see Table 5.3) is formed from the ventral rami of segments T12 to S4 and nerves arising from this plexus supply the pelvic girdle and the lower limbs. This plexus can be divided into the **lumbar plexus** and the **sacral plexus.**

The lumbar plexus is formed from the ventral rami of L1 to L4, with some fibers from T12. The plexus is located anterior to the transverse processes of the lumbar vertebrae on the posterior abdominal wall, ei-

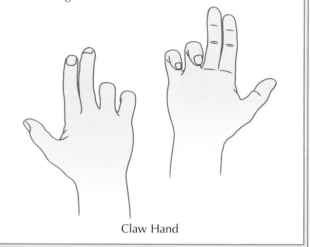

Injury to the Ulnar Nerve

The ulnar nerve is prone for injury because it passes superficially on the medial (ulnar) side of the elbow. This area is commonly referred to as the funny bone. Typically, a tingling sensation is felt along the ulna side of the forearm, hand, and the medial two digits on banging this region against an object. Severe injury to the ulnar nerve results in a condition known as **claw hand** in which there is difficulty abducting and adducting the fingers along with atrophy of the interosseus muscles, hyperextension of the metacarpophalangeal joints, flexion of the interphalangeal joints, and loss of sensation over the little finger.

Claw Hand

ther posterior to the psoas major or among its fasciculi. Nerves arising from this plexus supply the structures of the lower abdomen and anterior and medial aspect of the lower limb. The lumbar plexus is not as complex as the brachial plexus and has only roots and divisions (anterior and posterior). The major nerves are shown in Figure 5.24. The distribution of the femoral nerve and obturator nerve is shown in Figures 5.25 and 5.26.

Nerve impingement in the lumbar plexus results in pain in the lower back, abdomen, genitalia, thigh, and lower legs. Impingement is often a result of spasm of quadratus lumborum and psoas muscles and shortening of the lumbar dorsal fascia.

The sacral plexus is formed from the ventral rami of L4, L5, and S1–S4. It is located against the lateral and posterior walls of the pelvis between the piriformis and

Injury to the Obturator Nerve

This nerve may be injured during childbirth, resulting in weakness of the adductor muscles and loss of sensation in the medial aspect of thigh.

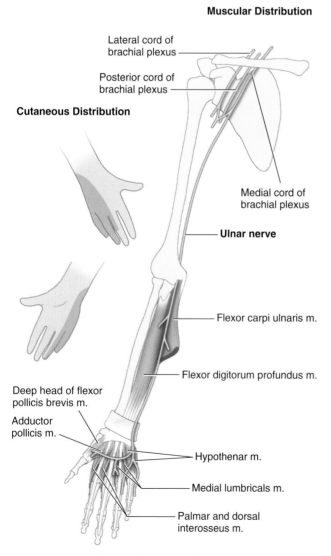

Muscular Distribution

Lateral cord of brachial plexus

Posterior cord of brachial plexus

Cutaneous Distribution

Medial cord of brachial plexus

Ulnar nerve

Flexor carpi ulnaris m.

Flexor digitorum profundus m.

Deep head of flexor pollicis brevis m.

Adductor pollicis m.

Hypothenar m.

Medial lumbricals m.

Palmar and dorsal interosseus m.

FIGURE **5.23.** Distribution of Ulna Nerve

Table 5.3		
Major Nerves of the Lumbosacral Plexus and Their Distribution		
Spinal Segment	**Nerve**	**Distribution (only certain muscles are cited)**
L2–L4	Femoral	Anterior muscles of thigh (sartorius and quadriceps)
L2–L4	Obturator	Adductors of the thigh (adductor magnus, brevis, longus; gracilis)
L4–S3	Sciatic	Two hamstrings: semimembranosus and semitendinosus; adductor magnus
	Tibial	Flexors of leg and plantar flexors of foot; flexors of toes; skin over posterior surface of leg, plantar surface of foot
	Common Fibular	Biceps femoris (short head); peroneus (brevis and longus); tibialis anterior; extensors of toes; anterior surface of leg and dorsal surface of foot; skin over anterior surface of leg and dorsal surface of foot
S2–S4	Pudendal	Muscles of the perineum, including external anal and urethral sphincters, skin over external genitalia, and related muscles

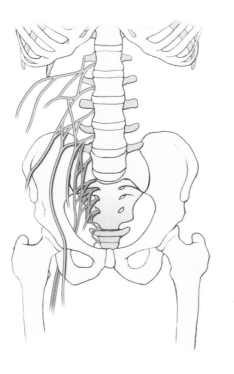

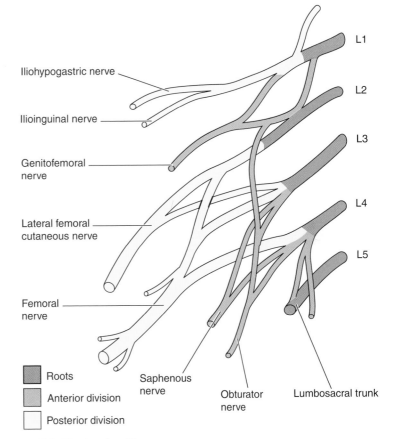

FIGURE **5.24.** The Lumbar Plexus

the internal iliac blood vessels. Nerve impingement is most often a result of the piriformis or shortening of the ligaments that stabilize the sacroiliac joint. The nerves arising from this plexus supply the lower back, pelvis, perineum, posterior surface of the lower limb, and the plantar and dorsal surface of the foot (see Figure 5.27). The sciatic nerve is the largest nerve that arises here.

Sciatic Nerve

The sciatic nerve (see Figure 5.28) is the largest nerve of the body. It is made up of two nerves, the tibial and common fibular (common peroneal), that are held together by a connective tissue sheath. It originates mainly from L5–S2 and leaves the posterior pelvis midway between the greater trochanter and ischial tuberosity. It passes posterior to the femur and deep

Muscular Distribution

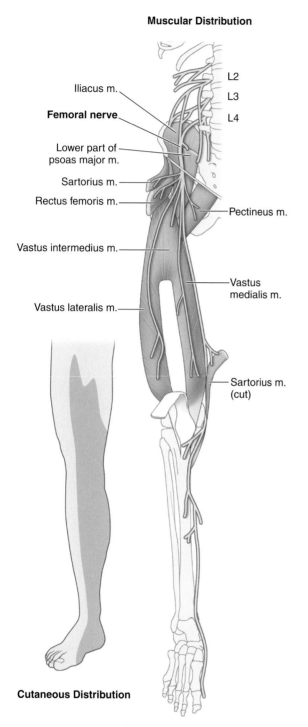

Iliacus m.

Femoral nerve

Lower part of
psoas major m.

Sartorius m.

Rectus femoris m.

Vastus intermedius m.

Vastus lateralis m.

L2

L3

L4

Pectineus m.

Vastus
medialis m.

Sartorius m.
(cut)

Cutaneous Distribution

FIGURE 5.25. Distribution of the Femoral Nerve

gastrocnemius, tibialis posterior, and the flexors of
the toes.

The common fibular nerve wraps around the lateral side of the fibula where it divides into a superficial and deep fibular branch. The superficial fibular nerve descends in the lateral leg to provide motor innervation to the peroneus muscles and cutaneous innervation to the dorsum of the foot. These muscles

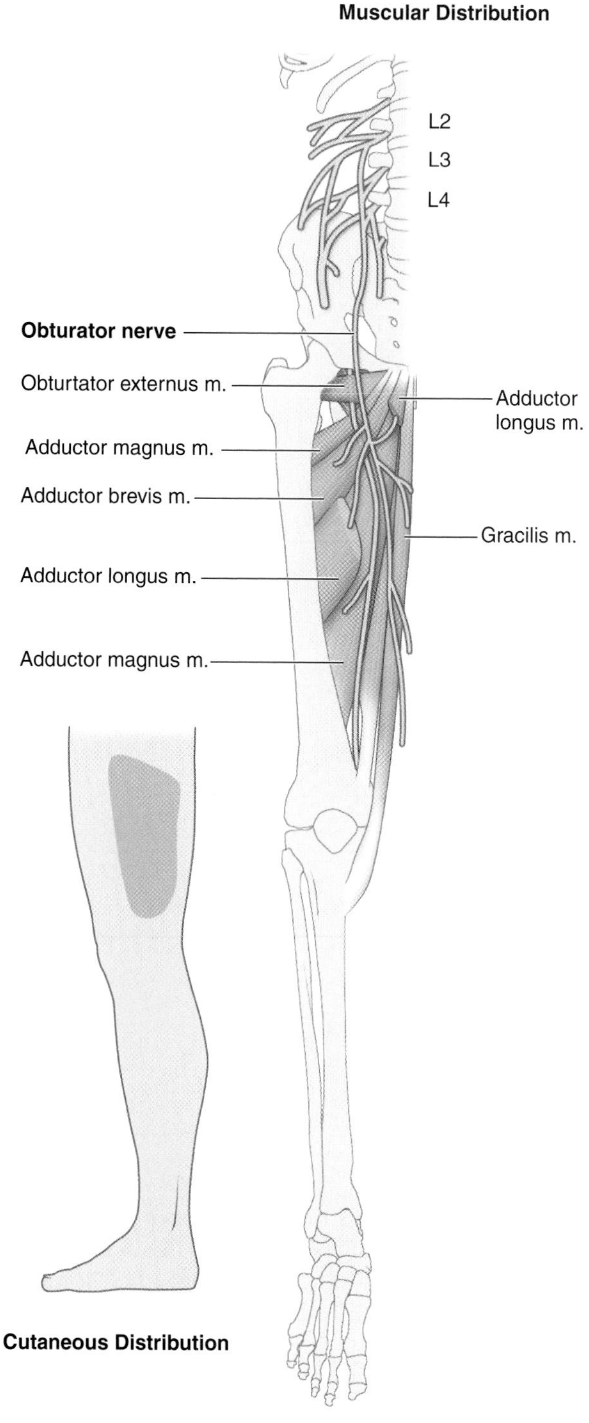

Muscular Distribution

L2

L3

L4

Obturator nerve

Obturtator externus m.

Adductor magnus m.

Adductor brevis m.

Adductor longus m.

Adductor magnus m.

Adductor
longus m.

Gracilis m.

Cutaneous Distribution

FIGURE 5.26. Distribution of the Obturator Nerve

to the long head of the biceps femoris muscle. At the popliteal fossa, the sciatic nerve divides into the common fibular and tibial nerves. The tibial nerve continues distally in the posterior compartment of the leg, lying in the gap between the tibia and the fibula and finally enters the medial side of the foot behind the medial malleolus. In its course, it supplies sensory branches to the skin as well as branches to all muscles of the back of the leg, especially the soleus,

✚ Injury to the Sciatic Nerve

The sciatic nerve is located midway between the greater trochanter and the ischial tuberosity, deep to the gluteus maximus and the piriformis. Then it travels vertically down the thigh to the apex of the popliteal fossa, deep to the hamstring muscles. The lower border of the piriformis muscle can be mapped as follows: Draw an imaginary line from the posterior superior iliac spine to the tip of the coccyx; the lower border runs along a line that joins the midpoint of the imaginary line to the top of the greater trochanter.

The sciatic nerve is often injured when there is a posterior dislocation of the hip. The nerve roots may be compressed by a herniated disk or by the enlarging uterus during pregnancy. If injections are administered improperly to the gluteal region, this nerve may become damaged. The condition of sciatic nerve injury is referred to as **sciatica.** Typically, there is a sharp pain felt in the buttock and on the posterior and lateral aspect of the thigh, leg, and foot.

Most often, the common fibular (peroneal) nerve on the lateral aspect of the leg is affected, resulting in a typical position of the foot referred to as footdrop. Here, the foot is plantar flexed and inverted, with loss of sensation on the lateral aspect of leg and dorsum of foot.

If the tibial nerve is affected, the foot takes on a typical position of dorsiflexion of the foot and eversion, with loss of sensation in the sole of the foot.

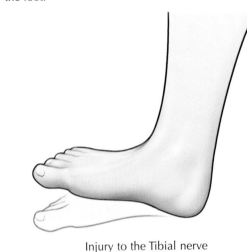

Injury to the Tibial nerve

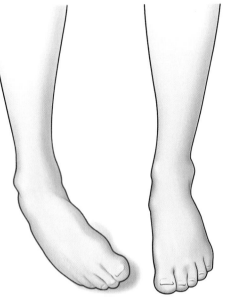

Injury to the Common Fibular (Peroneal) nerve

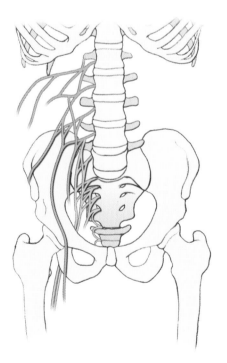

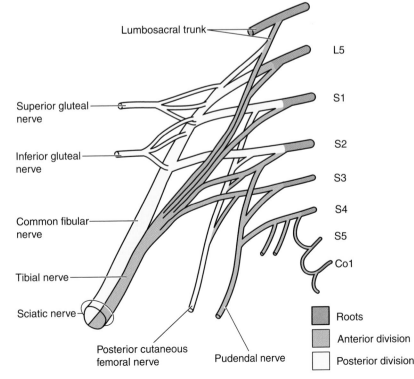

FIGURE 5.27. The Sacral Plexus

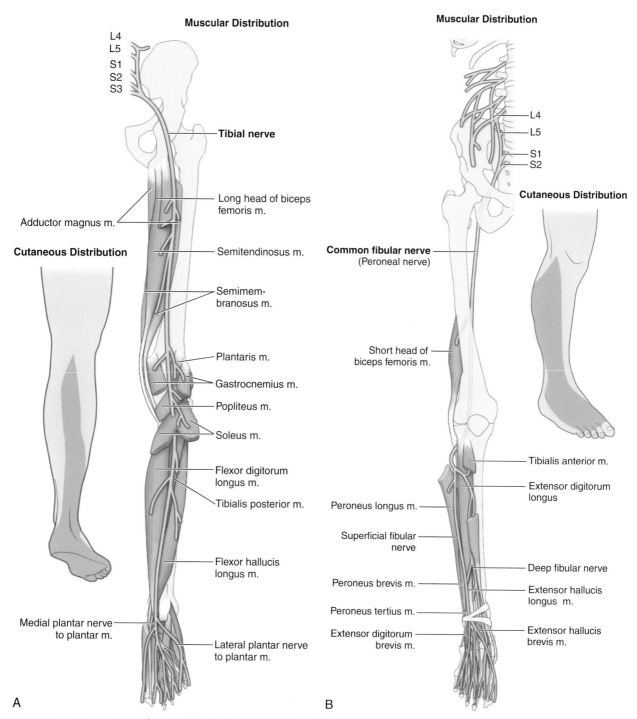

Muscular Distribution

L4
L5
S1
S2
S3

Tibial nerve

Long head of biceps femoris m.

Adductor magnus m.

Cutaneous Distribution

Semitendinosus m.

Semimem-branosus m.

Plantaris m.

Gastrocnemius m.

Popliteus m.

Soleus m.

Flexor digitorum longus m.

Tibialis posterior m.

Flexor hallucis longus m.

Medial plantar nerve to plantar m.

Lateral plantar nerve to plantar m.

A

Muscular Distribution

L4
L5
S1
S2

Cutaneous Distribution

Common fibular nerve (Peroneal nerve)

Short head of biceps femoris m.

Tibialis anterior m.

Extensor digitorum longus

Peroneus longus m.

Superficial fibular nerve

Peroneus brevis m.

Deep fibular nerve

Peroneus tertius m.

Extensor hallucis longus m.

Extensor digitorum brevis m.

Extensor hallucis brevis m.

B

FIGURE 5.28. Distribution of the Sciatic Nerve. **A,** Tibial Nerve; **B,** Common Fibular Nerve (peroneal nerve)

help evert the foot. The deep branch descends in the anterior compartment of the leg and controls the tibialis anterior and the extensor muscles of the toes. The principal action of these muscles is dorsiflexion of the toes.

Knowledge of the route taken by the major nerves and muscles and area of skin they innervate would help bodyworkers avoid regions where these nerves

lie against bone (e.g., ulnar nerve posterior to the medial epicondyle) or are superficial. Occasionally, spasm of muscles overlying the nerves (e.g., piriformis superficial to the sciatic nerve in the gluteal region) may cause pain along the region supplied by the nerve. Therapists, by relaxing these muscles or releasing trigger points, may be able to facilitate pain reduction.

REFLEXES

A **reflex** is a rapid, automatic response to a specific sensory signal. One characteristic of reflexes is that it is specific and stereotyped in terms of stimulus and response. Such reactions are important for making rapid adjustments in the body.

For a reflex to occur, certain components must be intact. A **sense organ** or **receptor** is required to detect the stimulus and convert it into action potentials. An **afferent** or **sensory neuron** is needed to transmit the action potentials generated to the spinal cord and brain. The central branch of the sensory neuron has to **synapse** with one or more interneurons or directly with the **efferent** or **motor neuron.** The efferent neuron carries the impulse to the muscle or gland (the **effector**) it innervates to produce a suitable response. The path taken by the impulse is known as the **reflex arc** and it requires all five components (see Figure 5.29).

The simplest reflex arc is one with a single synapse between the afferent and efferent neuron, known as **monosynaptic reflex.** Reflex arcs in which one or more interneurons are interspersed are known as **polysynaptic reflexes.**

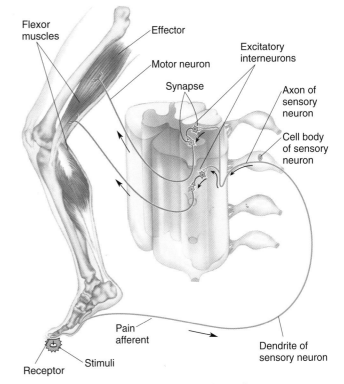

FIGURE 5.29. Components of a Reflex Arc

MONOSYNAPTIC REFLEX: THE STRETCH REFLEX

When a muscle with an intact nerve supply is stretched, it contracts. This is the **stretch reflex.** The sense organ is the muscle spindle (receptors in the muscle that respond to increase in length). The action potential generated is conducted rapidly by sensory nerves directly to the motor nerve that supplies the same muscle. For example, if the patella tendon is tapped, a stretch reflex of the quadriceps femoris causes the leg to extend. This is known as the **knee jerk** (Figure 5.30). Other such reflexes can be elicited by tapping the biceps tendon (**biceps jerk**), triceps tendon (**triceps jerk**), and Achilles tendon (**ankle jerk**).

MUSCLE SPINDLE

Knowledge of the structure and function of the muscle spindle is key to the understanding of **muscle tone.** Muscle tone is the normal resistance of the

muscle to stretch. The absence or marked increase or decrease in muscle tone in the various conditions a bodyworker encounters is a result of variations in the activity of the muscle spindle.

Structure of Muscle Spindle

The muscle spindle is described in more detail on **page 188.** In brief, each muscle spindle consists of 2–10 muscle fibers enclosed in a connective tissue capsule. The muscle fibers in the spindle are known as **intrafusal fibers,** to distinguish them from the regular muscle fibers that produce contraction, the **extrafusal fibers.** The intrafusal fibers are rather immature, with fewer striations. The striations or contractile units are located more toward the two ends of the spindle, with the nuclei located near the middle. The intrafusal fibers are positioned in parallel with

TESTING THE STRETCH REFLEXES

Physicians often check the stretch reflexes to see if they are present or absent. If any of the components of the reflex arc is damaged, a reflex cannot be elicited.

SENSITIZATION AND HABITUATION OF REFLEX RESPONSES

There is a possibility of reflex responses being altered by experience. For example, based on past experience and history of discharge in a synapse, changes can be made at the molecular level to strengthen or weaken a response. These changes are particularly important in the process of learning and memory.

the rest of the muscle fibers, and the ends of the capsule are attached to the tendon of the muscle on either side.

Sensory Nerves From the Muscle Spindle

There are two different sensory nerve endings. Some nerve endings wind around the center of the spindle, while others branch delicately on either end. These sensory neurons synapse directly with the motor neuron to the same muscle.

Motor Nerves to the Muscle Spindle

In addition to the sensory nerves that leave it, muscle spindles have motor nerves that innervate the intrafusal muscle fibers. These motor nerves are important and actually constitute 30% of the fibers in the ventral root. These motor nerves are the **gamma efferents** or **gamma motor neurons,** and the motor nerves to the extrafusal fibers are known as **alpha efferents** or **alpha motor neurons.**

Function of the Muscle Spindle

When the muscle spindle is stretched, the mechanical stimulus is converted to action potentials that travel, via the sensory nerve, directly to the motor neuron supplying the muscle, causing it to contract (Figure 5.30). If a muscle is stretched, the muscle spindle is also stretched as it lies parallel to the muscle fibers and a stretch reflex is elicited. If the muscle contracts, nothing happens because the spindle is also shortened. In this way, the spindle and its reflex connections help maintain muscle length. The muscle spindle is also able to detect changes in the rate of stretch and alter the frequency of action potentials to the extrafusal muscle fibers accordingly, to cause a smooth contraction. If muscle spindles were not present, contraction of the muscle would be jerky and tremors will be seen.

Function of the Gamma Motor Nerve

It was mentioned that the gamma motor neurons innervate the intrafusal fibers and that the contractile units of the intrafusal fibers are located toward the ends of the spindle (see Figure 5.31). If the gamma motor neuron is stimulated, it causes the intrafusal fibers to contract. Contraction of these fibers at both ends of the spindle results in stretching of the middle region of the spindle where the sensory nerves are located. The stretch is detected by the sensory nerve endings, and they produce action potentials that cause the extrafusal fibers to fire. How is this important? The nervous system, by stimulating gamma motor neurons, can make the muscle more or less sensitive to stretch. The gamma motor neurons are responsible for muscle tone.

Control of Gamma Motor Neuron Discharge

The gamma motor neurons are regulated by descending tracts from certain areas of the brain. Via these neurons, the sensitivity of the muscle spindles and, hence, the stretch reflexes and muscle tone can be altered according to change in posture. Many factors affect the gamma motor neuron discharge; for example, anxiety and stress increase its discharge, resulting in tensing of muscles and hyperactive tendon reflexes. If

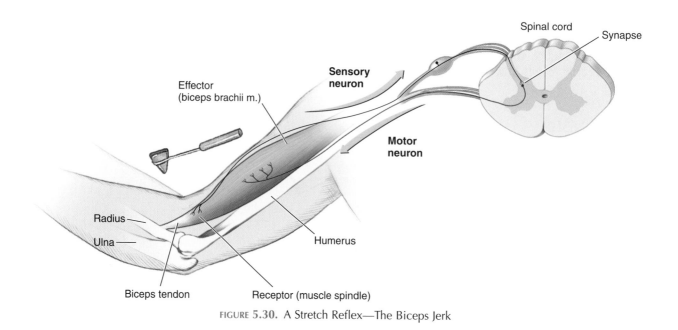

FIGURE **5.30.** A Stretch Reflex—The Biceps Jerk

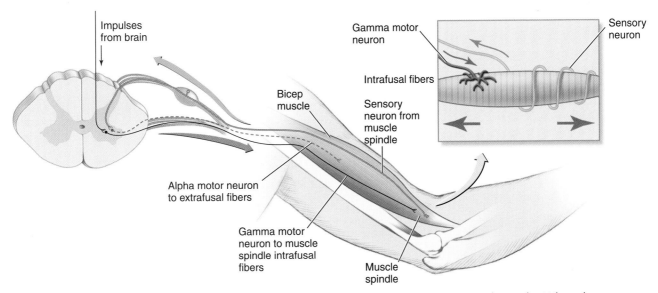

FIGURE **5.31.** Muscle Spindle, Gamma Motor Neuron, Alpha Motor Neuron, and Muscle. When the gamma motor neuron is stimulated, the intrafusal fibers of the muscle spindle contract, stretching the muscle spindle and stimulating the sensory neuron. The sensory neuron, in turn, stimulates the motor neuron to the extrafusal fiber and muscle tone is increased.

the skin of the hand on one side is stimulated by a painful stimulus, it results in increased discharge to the flexors and decreased discharge to the extensors of the same side, facilitating flexion and quick removal. At the same time, the opposite happens in the other side, adjusting posture and weight distribution.

RECIPROCAL INNERVATION

When a stretch reflex occurs, the muscles that antagonize the action of the muscle must relax. This is initiated by a simultaneous inhibition of the nerve to the antagonistic muscle. A branch of the sensory nerve synapses with an interneuron that secretes an inhibitory neurotransmitter. This way, every time an impulse travels up the sensory nerve, the motor nerve to the antagonistic muscle is inhibited (see Figure 5.32). This is known as **reciprocal innervation.**

INVERSE STRETCH REFLEX

The more a muscle is stretched, the stronger is its contraction up to a certain point when it suddenly relaxes. This is a result of stimulation of the Golgi tendon organs (see **page 190**), which are networks of nerve endings, located in series, in the tendon of a muscle. Stimulation of the sensory nerve from them inhibits the motor neuron of that muscle and stimulates that of the antagonistic muscle. This is the **inverse stretch reflex** or **tendon reflex** or **autogenic inhibition** (see Figure 5.33), a protective reflex preventing injury to the muscle and tearing of tendons from the bone.

Direct stimulation of the alpha motor neuron (innervation to the skeletal muscle) and gamma motor neuron and interplay of various reflexes help contract muscle smoothly and control the force and speed of various groups of muscle in a precise manner.

POLYSYNAPTIC REFLEXES: WITHDRAWAL REFLEX

In this type of reflex, one or more (or even hundreds) of neurons are involved. One example is the withdrawal reflex, in which a painful stimulus causes the stimulated part to withdraw. This reaction even happens in individuals who have had a spinal cord injury above the level of the segments supplying the limb tested. This is an important protective reflex and supersedes other activities.

THE FINAL COMMON PATH

Having looked at a reflex and excitation-contraction coupling in a muscle, you may have realized that all neuronal activity in the CNS that affects the muscle contraction can do so only through the motor neurons supplying the extrafusal muscles. Hence, these neurons are referred to as the **final common path.**

INPUT TO MOTOR NEURONS

The surface of a motor neuron accommodates about 10,000 synapses! At the same spinal segment, at least five inputs arrive. In addition, there are excitatory and inhibitory inputs relayed via interneurons from

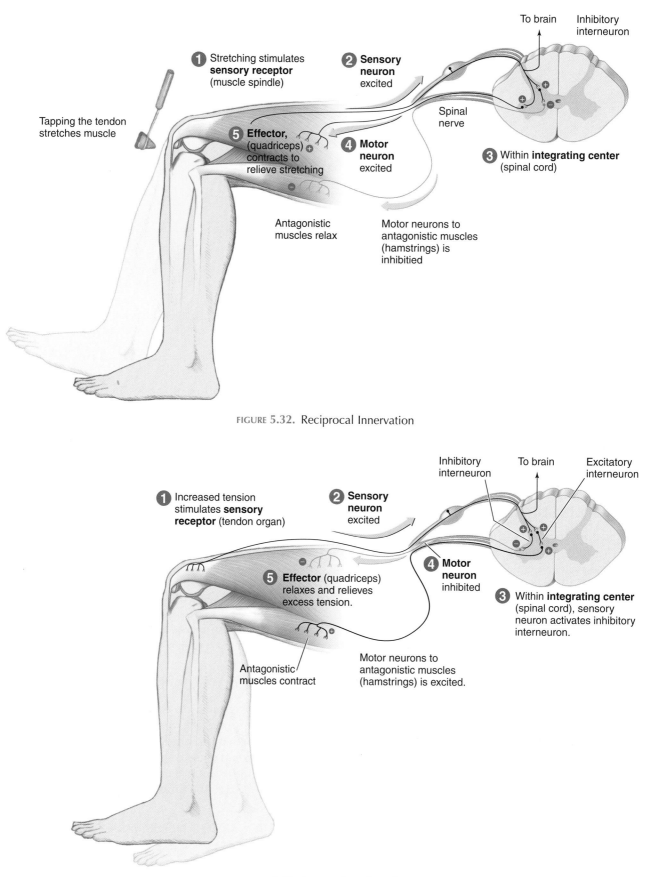

1 Stretching stimulates **sensory receptor** (muscle spindle)

Tapping the tendon stretches muscle

5 **Effector,** (quadriceps) contracts to relieve stretching

Antagonistic muscles relax

2 **Sensory neuron** excited

4 **Motor neuron** excited

Spinal nerve

Motor neurons to antagonistic muscles (hamstrings) is inhibitied

To brain   Inhibitory interneuron

3 Within **integrating center** (spinal cord)

FIGURE 5.32. Reciprocal Innervation

1 Increased tension stimulates **sensory receptor** (tendon organ)

5 **Effector** (quadriceps) relaxes and relieves excess tension.

Antagonistic muscles contract

2 **Sensory neuron** excited

4 **Motor neuron** inhibited

Motor neurons to antagonistic muscles (hamstrings) is excited.

Inhibitory interneuron   To brain   Excitatory interneuron

3 Within **integrating center** (spinal cord), sensory neuron activates inhibitory interneuron.

FIGURE 5.33. Inverse Stretch Reflex

and inhibitory inputs relayed via interneurons from other levels of the spinal cord and descending tracts from the brain. It is no wonder that we are able to accomplish such an unbelievable array of maneuvers.

PATHWAYS OF CUTANEOUS AND VISCERAL SENSATIONS

We have considered what sensory receptors are and how they convert different stimuli to action potentials and how the impulses generated make their way to the spinal cord and brain on **pages 316-319.** Now, the specific pathway taken by the various sensory impulses is considered.

As mentioned, the cell bodies of the sensory neurons are located in the dorsal root ganglia (or equivalent for cranial nerves), and the central branches enter the spinal cord (or brain). On entering, these nerves make several connections with motor neurons at the same spinal segment and those above and below. They also connect with neurons that convey the impulses to the brain.

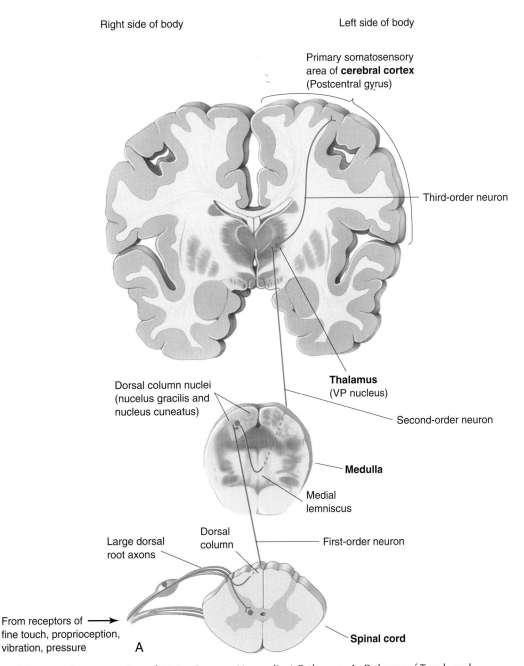

Right side of body

Left side of body

Primary somatosensory area of **cerebral cortex** (Postcentral gyrus)

Third-order neuron

Thalamus (VP nucleus)

Dorsal column nuclei (nucelus gracilis and nucleus cuneatus)

Second-order neuron

Medulla

Medial lemniscus

Dorsal column

First-order neuron

Large dorsal root axons

From receptors of fine touch, proprioception, vibration, pressure

A

Spinal cord

FIGURE 5.34. Schematic Representation of Major Sensory (Ascending) Pathways. **A,** Pathway of Touch and Pressure Sensations

(continued)

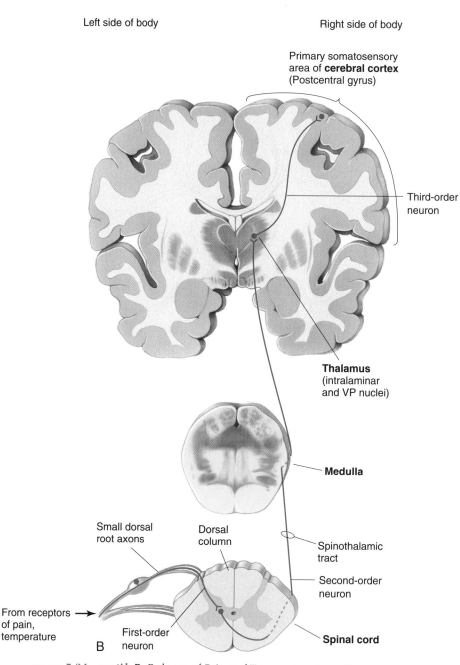

Left side of body   Right side of body

Primary somatosensory
area of **cerebral cortex**
(Postcentral gyrus)

Third-order
neuron

Thalamus
(intralaminar
and VP nuclei)

Medulla

Small dorsal
root axons

Dorsal
column

Spinothalamic
tract

Second-order
neuron

From receptors
of pain,
temperature

First-order
neuron

Spinal cord

B

FIGURE 5.34., cont'd **B,** Pathway of Pain and Temperature Sensations

DIRECT PATHWAY OF FINE TOUCH AND PROPRIOCEPTION SENSES

All fibers carrying fine touch sensations and proprioceptive sensations move to the dorsal column of the spinal cord and ascend to the medulla oblongata (see Figure 5.34A). These are **first-order neurons,** as they are the first neurons to carry impulses produced by these sensations. At the medulla, they synapse with a **second-order neuron.** The location where they synapse is known as the **nucleus gracilis** and **nucleus cuneatus,** and the tract carrying these sensations from the spinal cord/brain stem is the **fasciculus gracilis** and **fasciculus cuneatus** or the **dorsal (posterior) column.** The second order neurons cross the midline to the other side of the medulla and ascend to the thalamus (a region deep in the brain; **see page 353**) where they synapse with **third-order neurons.** The tract that carries these impulses from the medulla to the thalamus is known the **medial lemniscus.** Fibers from the thalamus carry the impulses to the sensory area of the cerebral cortex. Fibers carrying these sensations from the head join the other fibers from the rest of the body in the brainstem region and take the same path to the cerebral cortex.

The impulses carried by this tract enable a person to identify the shape, size, and texture of an object and point of stimulation; the direction of movement and position of body parts; vibratory sensations; and to identify an object by feel (**stereognosis**).

The dorsal horn can be considered as a gate that translates impulses that come into the CNS into ascending tracts. The impulses that come in via the dorsal root can be modified to some extent in the dorsal horn. Branches of fibers in the dorsal column synapse with other sensory fibers in the dorsal horn. In this way, they are able to affect the impulses generated by other sensory systems, such as pain.

DIRECT PATHWAY OF PAIN AND TEMPERATURE (AND REMAINING FIBERS OF TOUCH) SENSES

The central branches of neurons carrying impulses from pain and temperature (and some touch—crude touch) sense organs (first-order neurons) synapse with neurons located in the dorsal horn. The axons of the latter (second-order neurons) cross the midline and ascend in the anterolateral part of the spinal cord as the **ventral (anterior)** and **lateral spinothalamic tracts** (Figure 5.34B). Some fibers end in a specific region in the thalamus where they synapse with third-order neurons that convey the impulses to the cerebral cortex. Other fibers synapse with the reticular formation (see **page 366**) to maintain alertness. The anterior spinothalamic tract primarily carries impulses for itch, tickle, pressure, and crude touch sensations, and the lateral spinothalamic tract carries impulses for pain and temperature.

Although a specific pathway has been described for pain sensations, the perception of pain can be modified in various ways; hence, the major differences seen in pain perception between individuals. Definition, pain theory, pain mechanism and response, type of pain, and management of pain are described in greater detail in the box below and on the next few pages.

REPRESENTATION OF THE BODY IN THE CEREBRAL CORTEX

From the thalamus, the third-order neurons project to the cerebral cortex in a highly specific way. The region of the cerebral cortex just posterior to the **cen-**

Text continued on p. 348

✔ *Pain*

Pain is a complex and personal sensation that not only involves anatomic structures and functions, but also impacts the psychological, social, cultural, and all other aspects of the person's life.[1] It plays an important role in warning the individual and motivating him or her to seek help. Apart from its protective function, the purpose of persistent, chronic pain, even after the original injury has been treated, is still not understood and continues to bewilder both the sufferer and the treating health professionals.

The pain experience is affected by various factors. For example, the culture of the individual plays an important role in pain tolerance, although the pain threshold seems to be the same in all individuals. Physiologically, pain sensation is affected with aging. Psychologically, minimal trauma can produce excruciating pain based on past experiences. Also, the meaning of the situation plays an important part in the intensity of pain perceived. Socially, for example, the way parents react to injuries in children can alter the pain experience in children.

Definition
Because of its complexity, many definitions of pain exist. The International Association for the Study of Pain[2] describes pain as "an unpleasant sensory and emotional experience associated with actual or potential tissue damage or described in terms of such damage." Unfortunately, it is hard to objectively quantify pain or identify its nature. Therefore, one has to accept that pain is whatever the person experiencing the pain says it is and as being present whenever the person says that it is.

Pain Theories
Many theories have been suggested to explain the phenomenon. The **specificity theory** regards pain as a separate sensory modality, such as touch and warmth, that is produced when specific pain receptors are stimulated and transmitted to pain centers located in the brain. Indeed, pain pathways have been identified and traced to the brain. The pathway has been described above. Although this theory explains the way pain sensation is perceived and localized by the brain to different locations, it cannot explain the mechanism of chronic pain; pain in the amputated, nonexistent part of the limb; or pain that cannot be associated with any cause.

The **pattern theory** proposes that pain receptors share endings or pathways with other sensory modalities, and the pattern of impulses in the same neuron determines if the sensation is perceived as pain or some other sensation. For example, if the skin is lightly touched, it is perceived as touch as a result of the lower frequencies of impulses generated. If deep pressure is applied, the same receptor fires at a higher frequency, producing pain sensations.

To some extent, both specific and pattern theories are applicable because specific pain receptors have been identified and an excess of other stimuli can be perceived as pain. However, both theories fail to explain how factors such as culture, society, and psychology can alter the pain experience.

Continued

In 1965, Melzach and Wall[3] proposed a theory which is known as the **gate-control theory.** This theory proposes that there is a gating mechanism at the spinal segment where all sensory neurons enter the cord. These mechanisms modify pain sensations, with possibilities of interaction between pain and other sensations. According to this theory, there are interneurons located in the spinal segment activated by sensory fibers carrying touch sensations. These interneurons block or reduce the transmission of impulses in the adjacent pain fibers. For example, touching over or around the area of pain reduces the pain for sometime.

More recently, Melzach[4] proposed a new theory, the **neuromatrix theory.** This proposes that there is a large neural network in the brain that includes many areas, such as the limbic system, thalamus, and cerebral cortex, that are responsible for pain sensation. The genetic makeup and other sensory influences, such as input from the skin, situations that affect the interpretation of pain, culture, personality, and stress factors, determine an individual's pattern of synapses in this network and is responsible for the differences in the individual pain experience.

It is now known that the perception of pain sensations is a complex process and can be modified at many levels of the spinal cord and brain. Also, many factors cause the release of endogenous opioids (described below), which have a direct effect on nerve fibers carrying pain sensation.

Pain Mechanisms and Responses
Stimuli and Receptors

Pain stimulates receptors (free nerve endings) located over the entire body. These receptors are also known as nociceptors. The pain receptors can be stimulated by a number of strong stimuli; however, all these stimuli result in liberation of a chemical agent near the nerve ending. This agent may be from injured cells or otherwise. Some pain-producing substances are histamine, bradykinin, potassium, serotonin, acetylcholine, adenosine triphosphate, substance P, and leukotrienes.

Pain Fibers and Pathways

From the receptors, the afferent nerves travel to the spinal cord. Certain sensations are carried by small, myelinated fibers called A-delta fibers. Others are carried by unmyelinated C fibers. (A-delta and C are classifications of nerves according to the size and myelination of axons). The sharp pain that one feels soon after an injury is a result of the impulses carried by the A-delta fibers. Myelinated and larger, they carry impulses at the rate of about 5–30 m (16–98 ft) per second. The dull ache felt sometime after the injury is a result of the impulses carried by C fibers. Being small and unmyelinated, they carry impulses at a much slower rate, about 0.5–2 m (1.6–6.6 ft) per second.

At the spinal cord, these fibers communicate with other neurons in different ways: (1) They synapse with motor neurons at the same segment or that higher or lower than the segment. This communication is responsible for the withdrawal reflex that draws the body away from the damaging stimulus. (2) Certain branches ascend and communicate with the reticular activating system and hypothalamus, which is related to arousal and other accompanying autonomic changes. (3) Some reach the thalamus after crossing to the opposite side soon after they enter the segment. From the thalamus, the impulses are projected to the cerebral cortex. This helps the body localize the stimulus and also links it to past experiences. (4) Communication also occurs with the limbic system relating pain to emotions.

Mechanisms in the Body That Reduce Pain Sensation

Some neurons that originate in the brainstem and brain descend to the dorsal horn region and synapse with the ascending pain pathways, inhibiting them (see figure on page 343). One such pathway is that arising from the periaqueductal gray (PAG) region in the midbrain. Neurons from PAG synapse with the nucleus raphe magnus of the medulla that, in turn, synapse with the pain fibers in the dorsal horn. These synapses, by inhibiting the ascending pain pathways, result in fewer pain impulses reaching the cortex and less pain is perceived. PAG region is influenced by input from many regions, such as the cerebral cortex, hypothalamus, reticular formation, and spinothalamic tracts. This explains the influence of culture, society, and past experience on pain perception.

In addition to such descending tracts, the body has chemicals with the same function as synthetic painkillers. The most important of these are the endogenous opioids—**endorphins, enkephalins,** and **dynorphin.** These morphinelike substances are found in many parts of the brain and spinal cord. Many others, like serotonin and norepinephrine, have similar pain-killing functions in the CNS.

Types of Pain
Pain can be classified in many ways and treatment options vary accordingly. One way to classify pain is to identify if the source is (1) cutaneous, (2) deep somatic, (3) visceral, or (4) functional/psychogenic.

Cutaneous Pain

This type of pain arises from the skin or subcutaneous tissues (e.g., cut in finger). The source of the pain is well localized, and the pain is usually sharp, with a burning quality. Two types of sensations usually ensue. For example, if someone pinches you hard, you feel two types of pain sensations. One that is sharp, well localized, and lasting for a short time, which disappears soon after the stimulus is removed. This pain stimulates the A-delta fibers. Following the pinch, a throbbing, aching sensation is felt as a result of stimulation of the slow C fibers.

Deep Somatic Pain

This pain originates in muscles, tendons, joints, blood vessels, or bone, e.g., sprained ankle. The pain is more diffuse and may radiate to surrounding areas.

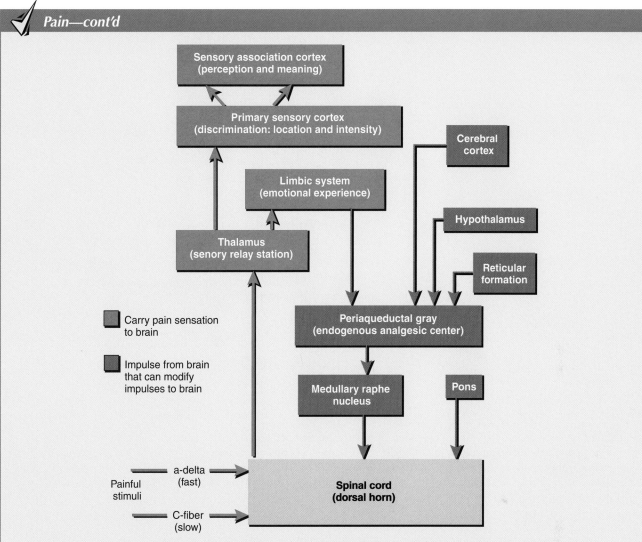

Schematic Representation of Primary Pain Pathways and Connections

Visceral or Splanchnic Pain

Visceral pain is produced by internal organs (e.g., pain produced by stomach ulcers, appendicitis, and kidney stones) It is often associated with nausea, sweating, and other autonomic symptoms. Although burning and cutting of viscera do not produce pain, stretching and reduction of blood flow to the organ can cause severe pain. This type of pain is poorly localized. One reason is because the viscera are not well represented in the cerebral cortex. Also, there are fewer pain receptors in the organs. The pain sensations from here travel via the sympathetic and parasympathetic nerves to the CNS.

Visceral pain, like deep somatic pain, produces reflex contraction of nearby skeletal muscles, usually the abdominal wall. This symptom is referred to as **muscle guarding.** Pain originating from the internal organs often produces pain, not in the organ, but in structures away from it. This is known as **referred pain.**

Referred Pain

The location of referred pain is usually to a structure that developed originally from the same dermatome as the source of pain. For example, the diaphragm originally develops from the neck area and migrates to the regions between the thorax and abdomen. That is why it is supplied by the phrenic nerve (C3–C5). C3–C5 is the location where sensory nerves from the tip of the shoulder enter (see figure on next page). Therefore, irritation of the diaphragm refers pain to the shoulder region. Similarly, the heart and the arm have the same segmental origin, and cardiac pain is often referred to the inner aspect of the left arm. In men, the testis originates in the same region as the kidney and ureter and later descends into the scrotum, dragging its nerve supply. Often, kidney stones produce pain that is felt in the scrotal region. The figure on page 344 shows other sites of referred pain.

Another reason for sites of reference is the convergence of sensory nerves from both the viscera and the superficial areas onto the same neurons (see figure on page 344). In other words, there are fewer neurons that ascend up the spinal cord than the number of neurons that bring pain sensation to it in each segment. Therefore, both sensations from the skin and viscera synapse with the same neuron that takes the impulses up to the brain. Because sensations arise more often from the skin than the viscera, the brain "learns" that activity in a given ascending pathway is from a pain stimulus in a particular somatic area. Hence, pain arising from the viscera is perceived as the somatic pain that the brain is more used to receiving.

Continued

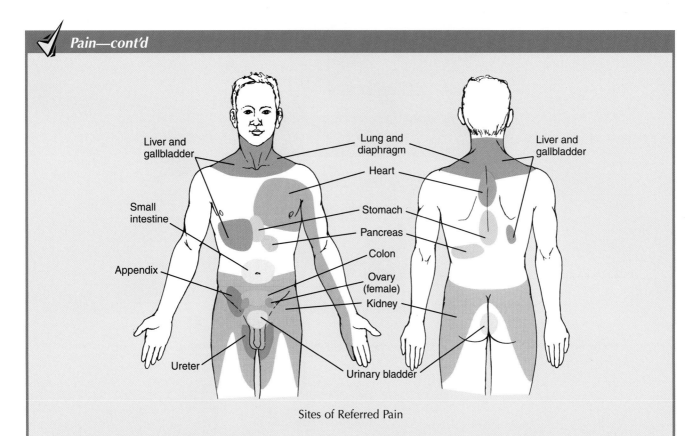

Sites of Referred Pain

It must be remembered that sites of reference are not stereotyped and, occasionally, unusual reference sites occur. Also, experience plays an important role in referred pain. For example, in patients who have had previous abdominal surgery, pain originating from abdominal organs may be referred to the site of the surgical scar. In people who have had dental work previously performed, pain originating from the maxillary sinus may be referred to the teeth where dental work was done, even if it is located far away from the sinus.

Psychogenic Pain

This is the type of pain where no physical cause can be found. However, because pain is an experience with both physical and mental components, classification of pain as psychogenic only causes confusion and more pain to the individual experiencing it. A typical example is that of people with chronic conditions, such as fibromyalgia or chronic fatigue syndrome, in which months or years may elapse before a diagnosis. Meanwhile, the pain experienced is classified as psychogenic with referrals to psychiatrists.

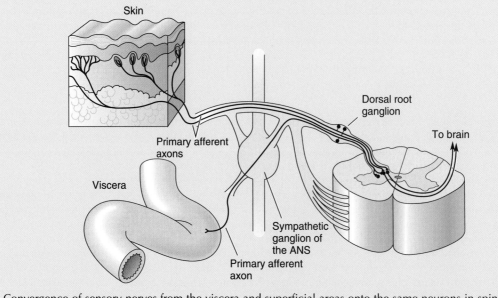

Convergence of sensory nerves from the viscera and superficial areas onto the same neurons in spinal cord.

Phantom Limb Pain

Often, people who have had part of a limb amputated complain of pain and other sensations in the region of the missing limb. This pain is partly a result of pressure on the stump of the amputated limb. The pressure initiates impulses in nerve fibers that previously came from sense organs in the amputated limb and the sensations are "projected" to where the receptors were originally located. Phantom limb pain may also be a result of changes that may have occurred along the pain pathway. (Please note that these are only two of the numerous explanations given for the origin of phantom limb pain.)

Acute and Chronic Pain

Pain is often classified according to its duration as acute and chronic. It is important to distinguish pain as acute or chronic because the cause, pathophysiology, diagnosis, and therapy vary greatly.

Acute Pain

Acute pain is often defined as pain of less than 6 months' duration. It is caused by tissue-damaging stimuli, and it is unusal for acute pain to be a result of pain of unknown origin or psychological factors. It is accompanied by anxiety, prompting the person to get professional help. Autonomic responses, such as increased heart rate, blood pressure, and muscle tension, accompany this type of pain, with all the accompanying symptoms disappearing when the pain is relieved.

Chronic Pain

This pain is classically defined as pain that has lasted for 6 months or longer. However, this definition is controversial and the International Association for the Study of Pain defines it more simplistically as pain that persists beyond the expected normal time of healing.[2] Although acute pain warns individuals of tissue injury or impending damage, chronic pain seems to have no useful function and may be associated with depression and frustration.

Management of Pain—an Overview

The management of acute pain is based on the identification of the source and treatment. However, chronic pain must be managed differently because the source is often difficult to locate. A multidisciplinary, consistent, caring, and holistic approach to pain, with involvement of the client and the client's support network, is key to chronic pain management. Because the pain experience is complex and many regions of the central nervous system can alter the sensitivity and perception of pain, many forms of therapy are available, including placebos, which can have a positive outcome.

Acute Pain

Here, the cause of the pain, its severity, and type of pain must be identified. It is difficult to assess the severity and degree of pain because pain cannot be measured objectively such as blood pressure or heart rate. Hence, a thorough history must be obtained and a systematic physical assessment performed. Some questions that need to be answered are: Is the pain *acute* or *chronic*? What is the *location* of the pain? What is the *quality* of pain? How *intense* is it? When does it occur (i.e., *timing*)? In what *setting* does the pain intensify? What are the *factors affecting* the intensity of the pain? What are the *associated manifestations*?

Abnormal Pain

In many situations in which there is abnormal and prolonged pain, the cause is not fully known. In some individuals, it is precipitated by damage to the peripheral nerves by injury or disease. Some abnormalities are defined below:

Allodynia—in this condition, intense pain is produced by a stimulus that normally does not provoke pain. For example, intense pain may be produced by even a gentle touch, such as that of clothes or wind.

Analgesia—this is the absence of pain when stimuli that normally produce pain are present or the relief of pain without loss of consciousness.

Anesthesia—a complete lack of sensation to stimuli, including pinprick. Locally, anesthesia can be produced by stopping the activity of the receptors.

Causalgia—spontaneous, intense, burning pain after a trivial injury. It may be accompanied by changes in vasomotor function.

Hyperalgesia—prolonged, severe pain produced by stimuli that would normally cause only slight pain.

Hyperesthesia—increased sensitivity to stimulation.

Hyperpathia—the threshold for pain is increased but, once it is reached, the pain is intense and burning.

Hypoalgesia—diminished pain in response to a normally painful stimulus.

Hypoesthesia—decreased sensitivity to stimulation.

Myofascial trigger points—foci of exquisite tenderness found in many muscles.

Neuralgia—pain in the distribution of a nerve or nerves.

Neuritis—inflammation of a nerve or nerves.

Neurogenic pain—pain initiated or caused by a dysfunction in the CNS.

Neuropathy—disturbance of function or pathologic change in a nerve.

Paresthesia—spontaneous, unpleasant sensations.

Thalamic syndrome—in this condition, certain parts of the thalamus are damaged, resulting in attacks of unpleasant, prolonged pain.

Continued

Most often, acute pain is a result of tissue injury. Inflammation is often present. Measures that play an important part in management include RICE: Rest (speeds healing); Ice (numbs pain receptors, constricts blood vessels, and reduces edema); Compresses (reduces bleeding, if any, and edema); and Elevation (allows gravity to help with lymphatic drainage and reduce edema).

Chronic Pain

In chronic pain, history and physical examination is important. However, it must be remembered that lack of physical findings does not mean that the pain is psychogenic. Often, there is no correlation between the intensity of pain and the amount of pathology that can be detected by examination. Each client with chronic pain must be treated individually in as caring and holistic manner as possible.

Some treatment options available, including massage, together with the physiologic basis of the approach are described. These management strategies are addressed alphabetically; they are not in order of effectiveness or all-inclusive. It must be noted that some options that work for certain individuals do not work in others, and these strategies can be used alone or in combination to maximize effectiveness.

Acupressure

Acupressure is the means of stimulating acupressure points without using needles. Pressure is applied with the thumb, finger, or any blunt instrument. The physiologic explanations are the same as that for acupuncture.

Acupuncture

Acupuncture is performed by inserting a thin needle into the skin along acupuncture meridians or paths of energy flow in the body. One way that acupuncture works is by releasing endogenous opioids. The physiologic mechanism(s) by which acupuncture works is not fully understood.

Aromatherapy

This is the use of essential oils to obtain physical and emotional well-being. As described on **page 356,** the olfactory nerve has many important connections that link it to the limbic system (emotions) and hypothalamus (endocrine function). Hence, aromas can have a profound effect on the mind and emotions and counteract stress. The oils are extracts from different parts of plants and can penetrate the skin quickly, being lipid soluble. The administration of the oils can be done in several ways; compresses, inhalation, baths, and combined with massage oil.

Biofeedback

This is a technique in which the person is made aware of the status of some body function to be able to control it at the conscious level. For example, the electrical activity in a muscle is shown on a screen, and the person is able to see the effects of imagery on the activity. This treatment is especially useful in treating migraines, tension headaches, or other forms of pain in which muscle tension is involved. Because there are nerve fibers from the cerebral cortex that can inhibit the impulses ascending in the pain pathways, this form of treatment can produce pain relief.

Cold

Cold application relieves pain by decreasing swelling from vasoconstriction and decreasing stimulation of pain nerve endings. It is believed that cold also causes release of endogenous opioids.

Distraction and Imagery

Distraction is focusing the attention on stimuli other than that of the pain. Here "sensory shielding" occurs where the attention from pain is diverted. Everyone has the experience of pain intensifying when lying quietly in bed. Often, the pain is forgotten during the day when the attention is focussed on something else.

Imagery consists of using the imagination to develop a mental picture that is relaxing and pain relieving.

Heat

Heat has been used as a form of pain relief since ancient days. Immersion in hot water, hot packs, electrically heated pads, and infrared rays are some methods used for heat application. Heat dilates local blood vessels and increases the blood flow. The increase in blood flow can reduce pain by washing away the pain-producing chemicals that have accumulated in the region. It can reduce swelling and, thereby, reduce the pressure on nerve endings. Temperature receptors are stimulated by heat and the impulses are carried by large myelinated nerve fibers that may inhibit the pain fibers in accordance to the gate-control theory. Endogenous opioids may also play a part. Heat softens collagen fibers, making them more extensible. This allows joints, tendons, and ligaments to be stretched further before stimulating the pain receptors. Therefore, heat is often used before therapy in which stretching of joint structures are involved.

Hypnosis

Hypnotic techniques alter the focus of attention and enhance imagery by using suggestions. Individuals vary widely in their ability to be hypnotized. The cause of the variation is not known. It has been hypothesized that hypnosis blocks pain from entering the conscious level by the inhibition of transmission of impulses produced by pain sensations from the thalamus to the cortex by the limbic system.

Massage

Massage certainly has an analgesic effect. The various strokes used help lymphatic drainage, reduce edema, and speed the drainage of pain-producing substances from the area. Release of histamine, as well as direct stimulation, cause local blood vessels to dilate, wash away toxins, remove edema, and bring oxygen to the area. Massage can reduce muscle spasm and improve blood flow and remove pressure on pain receptors. The touch and pressure sensations, carried by large myelinated fibers can inhibit pain fibers (gate-control theory). Massage also employs distraction and imagery techniques. The relaxation music that is often used also helps. Application of heat and/or cold has their own effects as explained above. Special techniques that help reduce adhesions can free nerves that may be producing the pain.

Music Therapy

Music has been used to reduce pain, especially postoperatively. Its positive effects have been explained in many ways. The pain relief may be a result of reduction in anxiety, inhibition of pain pathways by neurons from the cerebral cortex that may be activated by music, distraction, and/or increase in endorphins produced by music. The effect of music is also dependent on the type of person treated. It has been shown that, if used inappropriately, music can aggravate pain sensation. Therefore, it is important to check with the patient or client regarding their preferences before using relaxation tapes. Preferences with regard to familiar or unfamiliar music, volume, instrumental or otherwise, voice quality, duration, and electronic or acoustic are important and have been shown to have an effect on the outcome.

Placebo Response

This is the use of any treatment strategy that produces a positive response. The positive reaction is because of the person's belief that the treatment will be effective rather than the pain-killing properties of the strategy. The effectiveness of placebos does not indicate that the pain is psychogenic because 20% to 40% of people on whom pain has been induced by stimuli have reported pain relief with the use of placebos.

Transcutaneous Electrical Nerve Stimulation (TENS)

This is a procedure in which electrodes attached to a small portable unit are used to stimulate the skin surface over the area of pain. TENS stimulates large A-delta fibers of the skin. These fibers, according to the gate-control theory, inhibit pain-conducting fibers in the spinal cord. Research has shown that low voltage doses of electricity as applied here increase the levels of endogenous opioids in the body. About 20% to 70% of individuals with chronic pain get relief using TENS.

A TENS unit is about the size of a cigarette package and can be obtained from a local medical supply store (cost, about $100 to $650). They can also be rented for about $70 to $110 a month.

Other Forms of Therapy

Art, prayer, meditation, and laughter are other forms of therapy being used effectively.

Drugs

The use of drugs is only one aspect of controlling pain. Painkillers are termed **analgesics,** medications that act on the nervous system to decrease or eliminate pain without inducing loss of consciousness. Oral analgesics, such as aspirin, reduce inflammation and inhibit transmission of pain impulses. They are nonaddictive. Narcotic analgesics, drugs that have an effect similar to morphine, are effective, but can be addictive. Also, tolerance may develop (i.e., there is a decrease in response with continued use). Narcotics are used in individuals in whom relief cannot be obtained by other agents, in those suffering from cancer pain, or those whose life expectancy is limited.

Surgical Techniques

Surgical techniques are used to remove the cause or block the transmission of pain. Because damage to nerve cell bodies produces irreversible changes, it is used as a final option. Peripherally, nerves can be sectioned (**neurotomy**) or the dorsal root ganglion may be destroyed (**rhizotomy**). At the spinal cord level, the anterolateral region of the spinal cord, the location of pain pathways may be destroyed (**cordotomy**). Sometimes, the sympathetic nerve may be destroyed to relieve pain produced by the viscera (**sympathectomy**). In rare cases, areas of the thalamus may be destroyed (**thalamotomy**) or the prefrontal area of the cerebral cortex removed (**prefrontal lobotomy**).

In summary, pain is an individual experience and a multidisciplinary, holistic approach must be used to produce relief to the individual. Acute pain is often treated more easily than chronic pain, which is far more complex. When treating pain, it is not enough to address the physical component alone, but the emotional and spiritual aspects should also be considered. Undoubtedly, the alleviation of pain is both an art and a science.

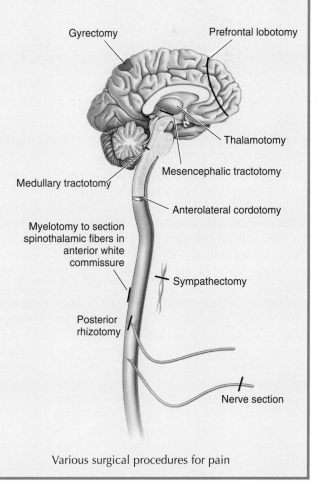

Gyrectomy
Prefrontal lobotomy
Thalamotomy
Mesencephalic tractotomy
Medullary tractotomy
Anterolateral cordotomy
Myelotomy to section spinothalamic fibers in anterior white commissure
Sympathectomy
Posterior rhizotomy
Nerve section

Various surgical procedures for pain

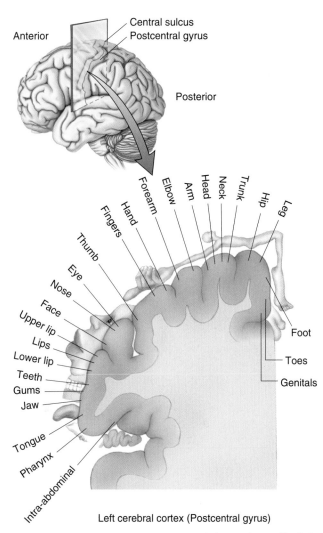

FIGURE 5.35. Sensory Representation of the Right Half of the Body in the Left Cerebral Cortex (coronal section). Note that there is a similar representation of the left half of the body in the right cerebral cortex.

tral sulcus is the sensory cortex. Central sulcus is a depression on the brain surface that runs coronally (Figure 5.35). The different parts of the body are represented in a specific order in the postcentral gyrus, with the legs represented medially and superiorly and the head laterally. Other than the detailed localization of each part of the body, the size of the receiving area of the cortex for each part of the body is in proportion to the number of receptors in each part. You may have already determined through the exercise suggested on page 320 that the face, lips, fingers and toes are more sensitive, indicating that there are more receptors per unit volume. If you look at Figure 5.35, you will see that there is more representation of these areas in the cortex than the less sensitive areas.

Remember that fibers from the thalamus not only project to the postcentral gyrus, but also project to other areas of the brain. Also, the neurons from the postcentral gyrus communicate with many other ar-

eas. In this way, the sensations are linked to past experiences, learning, and memory. Just posterior to the sensory cortex is the sensory association area. This transforms raw sensations into meaningful ones, based on past learning.

Other than the sensory pathways described above, there are many other sensory, ascending pathways. Some other major sensory tracts include those carrying proprioceptive impulses to the cerebellum, the anterior and posterior spinocerebellar tracts. Although the sensations carried by these tracts do not reach consciousness, they are important for maintaining posture, balance, and motor coordination.

The Brain and Brain Divisions

The brain, similar to the spinal cord, consists of neurons and neuroglia. As a result of the larger number of neurons and greater, complex interconnections, the brain can do a variety of things, with the ability to alter responses according to past experiences. The brain contains 98% of the body's neural tissue and weighs about 1.4 kg (3 lb).

The brain is the upper, enlarged end of the spinal cord. It consists of four principal parts: the cerebrum, the cerebellum, the diencephalon, and the brainstem (Figure 5.36). The brainstem connects the spinal cord to the other principal structures and is divided into three parts (from inferior to superior): the medulla oblongata, the pons, and the midbrain (Figures 5.36 and 5.37). Superior to the brainstem is

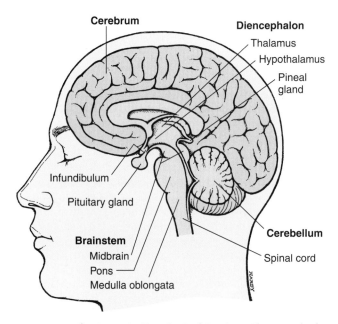

FIGURE 5.36. The Brain (In Situ; Sagittal Section). Showing the location of the four principal parts: cerebrum, diencephalon, brainstem, and cerebellum.

EFFECTS OF LESIONS IN THE SENSORY AREA

Injury to the sensory cortex results in deficits, not complete loss, of the ability to sense in the part represented by the cortex. The sensations most affected are fine touch, proprioception—position sense, and ability to discriminate size and shape of objects if using the affected part. Temperature and pain sensations are least affected.

Dyslexia

This disorder is related to damage to the interpretive area, where comprehension and word use is affected. Children with this condition have difficulty reading and writing; however, the other intellectual functions may be normal or above normal.

the diencephalon. The thalamus and the hypothalamus are important components of the diencephalon. The cerebrum lies over and around the diencephalon and can be divided into two large, **cerebral hemispheres.** Located posterior and inferior to the cerebrum is another enlargement called the **cerebellum.**

The two cerebral hemispheres are separated into right and left hemispheres by a long, deep depression known as the **longitudinal fissure,** and the hemispheres are connected to each other by the **corpus callosum,** which contains nerves that run across from one hemisphere to the other.

The brain is divided into many **lobes** named by the skull bone they underlie. The boundaries of the lobes are also determined by specific sulci. The **frontal lobe** is separated from the **parietal lobe** by the **central sulcus.** The **lateral sulcus,** which runs somewhat transversely, separates the frontal from the **temporal lobe.** The **occipital lobe,** located posteriorly, is separated from the parietal lobe by the **parieto-occipital sulcus.** Each lobe can be considered to have somewhat specific functions; however, the brain is too complex and the activities of the brain too interlinked for functional boundaries to be drawn between lobes. The locations of areas that have specific functions are described briefly below.

The gyrus located posterior to the central sulcus, is called the **postcentral gyrus.** This is the region where sensory impulses are relayed and is also known as the **primary sensory cortex.** The sensations of vision, hearing, taste, and smell relay to other areas of the cortex. Vision sensations reach the occipital lobe (**primary visual area**), and the auditory and smell sensations are relayed to the temporal lobe (**primary auditory area** and **primary olfactory area**). The taste sensations are relayed to the lateral and inferior part of the postcentral gyrus in the parietal cortex (**primary gustatory area**). Anterior to the central sulcus is the **precentral gyrus,** which initiates motor commands to the motor neurons in the brainstem and the spinal cord, and is known as the **primary motor cortex.** These neurons and the pathway taken by the fibers to the motor neuron is the **pyramidal system.**

In addition to the primary cortex, there are **association areas** for motor and sensory function that help interpret sensations. If the association areas are damaged, a person will perceive the sensation, but will not be able to understand it. For example, if the visual association area is damaged, the person may be able to see a picture of a cup but not understand what it is. Motor association areas are needed to relay the proper instructions to the primary motor cortex, to bring about smooth, coordinated movements in the right sequence. The details of the control of posture and movement are discussed later.

The white mater of the brain contains three different types of fiber tracts (see Figure 5.38). Some axons interconnect areas of the cerebral cortex in the same hemisphere and are known as **association fibers.** Others, the **commissural fibers,** interconnect the two hemispheres; others run between the cortex and other structures such as the cerebellum, brainstem, and spinal cord and are known as **projection fibers.** Some important projection fibers that bring sensory impulses to and take motor impulses from the brain run close together in the **internal capsule** region. Because of the close proximity of fibers to and from different parts of the body in this region, a blockage to blood flow in the internal capsule can cause extensive damage to the opposite side of the body.

INTEGRATIVE CENTERS

Prefrontal Lobe

The brain also has areas that integrate and process various sensory information and then perform complicated and complex motor activities and analytic functions (Figure 5.37). The prefrontal areas integrate information from sensory association areas and perform various intellectual functions. Based on past experience, this area is able to predict the conse-

Concussion

Concussion refers to an immediate but temporary loss of consciousness often described as dazed or "star-struck" and is associated with a short period of loss of memory. It is a result of sudden movement of the brain within the skull as occurs after blunt impact or sudden deceleration.

Apparently, goats, rams, and woodpeckers can tolerate impact velocity and deceleration a hundred times more than that experienced by humans!

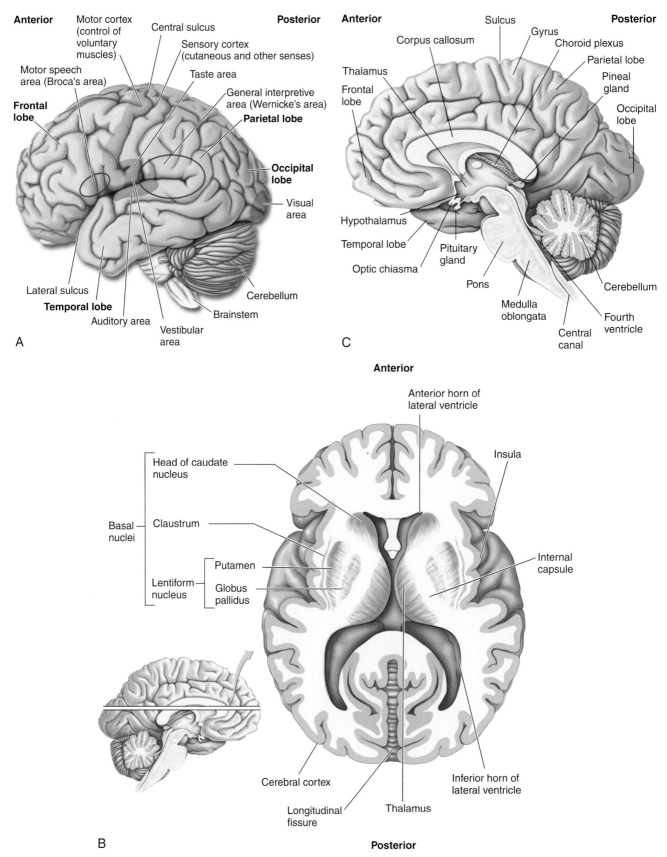

FIGURE 5.37. The Brain: Different Views and Sections. **A,** Lateral View; **B,** Transverse Section; **C,** Sagittal Section

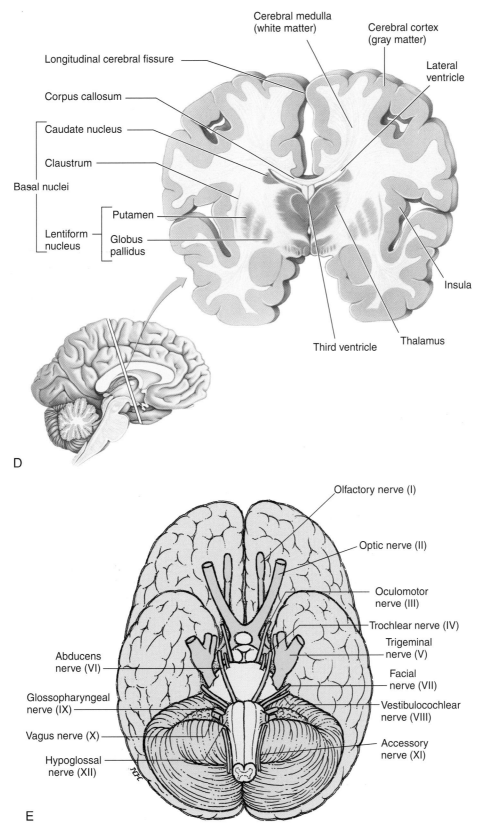

Cerebral medulla (white matter)

Cerebral cortex (gray matter)

Longitudinal cerebral fissure

Lateral ventricle

Corpus callosum

Caudate nucleus

Claustrum

Basal nuclei

Putamen

Lentiform nucleus

Globus pallidus

Insula

Third ventricle

Thalamus

D

Olfactory nerve (I)

Optic nerve (II)

Oculomotor nerve (III)

Trochlear nerve (IV)

Trigeminal nerve (V)

Facial nerve (VII)

Vestibulocochlear nerve (VIII)

Accessory nerve (XI)

Abducens nerve (VI)

Glossopharyngeal nerve (IX)

Vagus nerve (X)

Hypoglossal nerve (XII)

E

FIGURE 5.37., cont'd The Brain: Different Views and Sections. **D,** Coronal Section; **E,** Inferior View

(continued)

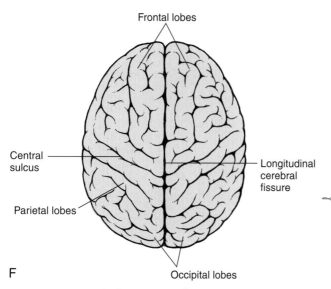

FIGURE **5.37.**, cont'd The Brain: Different Views and Sections. **F,** Superior View

quences of different responses. Frustration, anxiety, and tension may be generated.

General Interpretive Area or Wernicke's Area

The **General Interpretive** or **Wernicke's area** located in the left hemisphere (Figure 5.37A), is important in integrating visual and auditory memory. Injury to this area affects the ability to understand and interpret what is seen or heard. Individual words may be understood but, when words are put together, the meaning may not be interpreted.

Speech Center

This center, **Broca's area**, is located near the Wernicke's area, in the same hemisphere along the precentral gyrus. This center regulates respiration and the various muscles required for speech.

RIGHT AND LEFT HEMISPHERE SPECIALIZATIONS

Left hemisphere. In most people, the general interpretive areas and the speech centers exist in the left hemisphere. Therefore, this hemisphere is responsible for skills related to language, such as reading, writing, and speaking. Analytical tasks are also per-

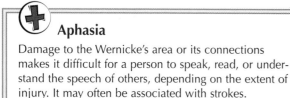

Aphasia

Damage to the Wernicke's area or its connections makes it difficult for a person to speak, read, or understand the speech of others, depending on the extent of injury. It may often be associated with strokes.

formed here. Hence, the left hemisphere is known as the **categorical hemisphere.**

Right hemisphere. This hemisphere helps analyze sensory information, such as facial recognition, emotion interpretation, music, art, and smell differentiation and is known as the **representational hemisphere.**

The distribution of the described functions varies individually; however, in the majority of both right- and left-handed individuals, the left hemisphere is the categorical hemisphere.

THE LIMBIC SYSTEM

The limbic system (see Figure 5.39) is a collection of nuclei and tracts involved with creation of emotions, sexual behavior, fear, rage, motivation, and processing

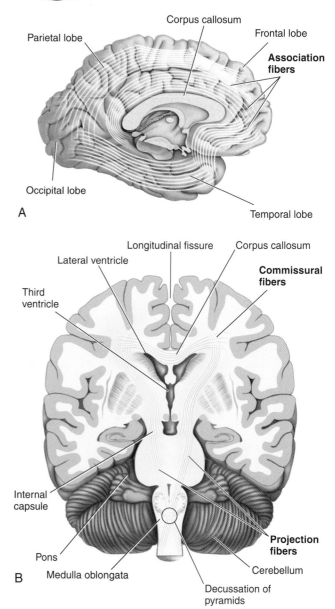

FIGURE **5.38.** Types of Fiber Tracts in the White Mater of Brain. **A,** Sagittal Section; **B,** Coronal Section

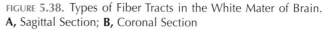

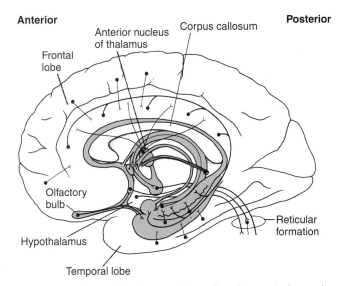

Anterior   **Posterior**

Anterior nucleus of thalamus

Corpus callosum

Frontal lobe

Olfactory bulb

Reticular formation

Hypothalamus

Temporal lobe

FIGURE 5.39 The Limbic System. The colored areas indicate the components of the limbic system

of memory. These components of the limbic system are primarily located as a border at the point where the cerebrum is connected to the midbrain. This includes the rim of gyri around the corpus callosum, some parts of the temporal lobe, hypothalamus, thalamus, and olfactory bulbs, among other regions.

Emotions

Emotions have both physical and mental components; for example, it requires awareness of the sensation and its meaning; the association with past memories; and the urge to act on the emotions and the physical changes that accompany it, such as increased heart rate and blood pressure. Hence, the limbic system is complex and has connections with many areas, such as the thalamus (sensory relay station) and hypothalamus (which links emotions to the autonomic and endocrine system). The paucity of connections with the cortex, which is responsible for voluntary control, is the reason for the inability to turn emotions on and off.

Sexual Behavior

The limbic system, along with the hypothalamus, is responsible for sexual behavior. Although copulation is a result of various reflexes integrated in the spinal

FEARLESS ANIMALS

Monkeys with lesions in certain areas of the limbic system approach snakes without fear, pick them up, and even eat them!

cord and brainstem, the behavior that accompanies it is regulated by the limbic system and hypothalamus. In humans, however, it is further conditioned by social and psychic factors.

Fear and Rage

Fear and rage are emotions regulated by the limbic system and hypothalamus. The physiologic changes that accompany them, such as pupillary dilation, cowering, and sweating, are caused by the autonomic system; however, the limbic system is required for initiating the response. Both fear and rage are protective responses to threats in the environment. Again, these emotions are conditioned by social factors and sex hormones.

Motivation

Experiments in which electrodes have been implanted in certain areas of the brains of animals and humans, with the ability of the experimental animals/humans to stimulate the area using these electrodes, have produced interesting findings. If the electrode is implanted in certain areas, pleasure is produced, and the animals/humans tends to stimulate the area repetitively and continuously. Other areas have been identified that, on stimulation, produce emotions such as fear and terror. These experiments have shown that the body has reward or approach systems and punishment or avoidance systems, which are part of the limbic system and play an important role in motivation.

The neurotransmitters secreted in this system have been identified, and drugs that act on the receptors, production/destruction of these neurotransmitters have an effect on mood and emotion.

THE THALAMUS

The thalamus is a paired structure, located superior to the brainstem on the sides of the third ventricle (Figure 5.37B, C, and D). It is a collection of many nuclei. The thalamus is the principal relay point for sensory information that comes from the spinal cord, brainstem, cerebellum, and parts of the cerebrum. From here, the information is relayed to the sensory cortex. The thalamus does perceive some crude sensations of pain, temperature, and pressure (i.e., in the absence of the cerebral cortex, it is possible to perceive some crude sensations but the cerebral cortex is needed for proper perception).

The thalamus consists of four major groups of nuclei. The **anterior** is connected to the limbic system and deals with emotions. The **medial** nuclei provide a conscious awareness of emotional states. The **ventral** nuclei relay sensory information from the rest of the body to the cortex and also monitor communication between the motor cortex and association areas. The **posterior** nuclei relay sensory information from the eye and ear to the cortex.

In addition to these functions, the thalamus is needed for acquisition of knowledge (cognition) and memory and for planning of movement. (Detail of its other connections and functions are beyond the scope of this book).

THE HYPOTHALAMUS

The hypothalamus (Figures 5.36 and 5.37C, D) is located close to the thalamus and lies just above the pituitary gland. It also has many collections of neurons—nuclei. It is closely associated with the limbic system. In addition, the hypothalamus has important regulatory functions:

- It controls skeletal muscle contractions that accompany various emotions, such as changes in facial expression and muscle tone.
- It coordinates the activities of the centers that control respiration, heart rate, blood pressure, and digestion that are located in the pons and medulla.
- It secretes various stimulatory and inhibitory hormones into the blood, which are transported to the pituitary gland located close to the hypothalamus, where they regulate pituitary hormone secretion (Figure 6.4). Certain neurons located in the hypothalamus manufacture antidiuretic hormone and oxytocin in their cell bodies. Axons from these cell bodies project into the posterior pituitary and secrete the hormones into the blood in vessels perfusing this region.
- It has centers, such as feeding centers and thirst centers, that modify emotions and behavior to fulfill such basic needs. Neurons located in the hypothalamus monitor blood glucose levels and blood volume and alter behavior accordingly.
- It has numerous connections with the rest of the brain and is a link between voluntary, endocrine, and autonomic functions. It controls and inte-

MNEMONICS

Many mnemonics have been devised to help someone remember the number and names of the cranial nerves. You can device your own. Here's one for a start: Oh, Once One Takes The Anatomy Final, Very Good Vacations Are Heavenly!

grates the activities of the autonomic nervous system. For example, even the thought of stressful situations increases heart rate and blood pressure and produces many other physiologic changes similar to the fight-or-flight reaction.
- It has certain nuclei responsible for maintaining body temperature. Neurons located here monitor the core body temperature and produce such changes as sweating, shivering, and vasodilation or constriction in cutaneous blood vessels by regulating the vasomotor centers and other centers located in the medulla and pons.
- It plays a major role in the establishment of sleep patterns.

THE BRAINSTEM: MIDBRAIN, PONS, AND MEDULLA

Together these three regions are known as the **brainstem** (Figure 5.37A, C, E). They lie between the brain and the spinal cord, with the midbrain closer to the cerebrum and the medulla closer to the spinal cord. The brainstem contains gray (nuclei) and white matter (tracts). Collections of neurons (nuclei) located here control basic vegetative functions such as heart rate, blood pressure, and respiratory rate. Other nuclei give rise to the various cranial nerves. Numerous ascending and descending tracts synapse and/or pass through the brainstem.

Nuclei located in the midbrain coordinate muscles in relation to received visual and hearing input. For example, movement of the eyeballs and turning of the head, neck, and trunk as one follows an object or hears a loud noise are regulated here. Midbrain nuclei that receive input from the vestibular apparatus (located in the inner ear; see **page 364**) and other sensory areas help the body to alter the posture to maintain balance.

✓ Massage and the Hypothalamus

A relaxation massage, by reducing stress, has the potential to affect almost all parts of the body via the hypothalamus. A reduction of sympathetic nervous system activity and, thereby, slowing heart rate, reducing blood pressure, and lowering muscle tone are some physiologic changes produced by a relaxation massage.

Cranial Nerves

Cranial nerves are part of the peripheral nervous system, which is connected to the brain. Twelve pair of cranial nerves arise from the ventrolateral aspect of the brain (Figure 5.37E). The cranial nerves are numbered according to their position in the longitudinal axis of the brain, beginning at the cerebrum. Each nerve is named, the name being related to the appearance or function. Similar to the spinal nerves, the cranial nerves may carry sensory fibers, motor fibers, or both; some carry fibers with autonomic function.

The sensory nerves synapse at the brainstem or join the ascending sensory tracts from the rest of the body to reach the thalamus and cerebral cortex. In addition to sensory nerves that carry sensations such as pain, temperature, touch-pressure, some cranial nerves carry impulses generated by special sense organs located in the eye (vision), ear (hearing and balance), nose (smell), and tongue (taste).

The motor nerves, such as those in the spinal cord, have numerous synapses and serve as the final common pathway for muscles of the head and neck. The blood vessels, glands, and smooth muscles of the eye (for dilation of pupils) are supplied partly by the autonomic component of some of the cranial nerves.

The nerves and their functions are listed in Table 5.4, and the nerves relevant to massage are discussed further.

Table 5.4

The Cranial Nerves and Their Functions

Cranial Nerve (number)	Cranial Nerve	Primary Function
I	Olfactory*	*Special sense:* smell
II	Optic	*Special sense:* vision
III	Oculomotor	*Motor:* controls four of six eye muscles that move the eyeball
		Autonomic: also carries autonomic fibers that control the dilation of pupils and convexity of the lens, regulating the amount of light reaching the retina. Also, by altering the convexity of the lens, objects both near and far can be seen clearly.
IV	Trochlear	*Motor:* controls one of the eye muscles that helps you look upward
V	Trigeminal*	It has three main branches (hence, the name)
		Sensory: carries general sensations from the face, nose, mouth, and pharynx
		Motor: muscles of mastication
VI	Abducens	*Motor:* controls one of the eye muscles that help you look to the side
VII	Facial*	*Special sense:* taste from anterior two-thirds of tongue
		Motor: muscles of facial expression; stapedius (muscle in middle ear that dampens sound)
		Autonomic: regulates secretion from tear glands; mucous glands of nose, and two of three salivary glands
VIII	Vestibulocochlear*	*Special sense:* hearing (cochlear branch); balance (vestibular branch)
IX	Glossopharyngeal	*Special sense:* taste from posterior third of tongue
		Sensory: carries general sensations from pharynx and palate
		Motor: pharyngeal muscles
		Autonomic: regulates secretion of saliva from the parotid salivary gland; carries impulses from baroreceptors and chemoreceptors in/near the carotid arteries
X	Vagus*	*Special senses:* taste sensations from receptors in the pharynx
		Sensory: general sensations from pharynx, external ear, pinna
		Motor: muscles of the palate and pharynx
		Autonomic: sensory and motor fibers from/to various organs of the digestive, respiratory, and cardiovascular systems in the thorax and abdomen; also carries impulses generated by the baroreceptors and chemoreceptors in/near the aortic arch
XI	Accessory	Also known as the spinoaccessory nerve because some of fibers originate from the upper spinal segments
		Motor: muscles of the neck and upper back (i.e., sternocleidomastoid, trapezius, and various muscles of the palate, pharynx and larynx
XII	Hypoglossal	*Motor:* controls muscles of the tongue

*discussed further in text

OLFACTORY NERVE (CRANIAL NERVE I)

Sense of smell and taste are considered visceral sensations because they are related to gastrointestinal functions. The flavor of most food is a result of a combination of taste and smell; a person with a cold often complains of diminished taste as a result of a depression of the sense of smell. The receptors for both smell and taste are chemoreceptors (i.e., they are stimulated by chemicals). However, the sense of smell is different in that it is the only sensation that does not relay to the thalamus. Also, there is no direct communication with the sensory cortex.

The Olfactory Mucous Membrane

The receptors for smell are located in the nasal mucosa, in a small area about 5 cm² (0.8 in²) in the roof of the nasal cavity and upper portion of the nasal septum (see Figure 5.40). There are about 10–20 million receptor cells here. Each receptor is the end of a neuron; this region is obviously the closest the nervous system gets to the external world. The axons of the neurons go through the cribriform plate of the ethmoid bone and enter the paired projections of the brain—the olfactory bulb and tract. They synapse at the olfactory bulb from which other neurons convey the impulses to the olfactory cortex.

The olfactory cortex consists of two major areas of the brain—the medial olfactory area and the lateral olfactory area. The medial area lies in the middle of the brain, superior and anterior to the hypothalamus and is responsible for reflexes such as licking the lips

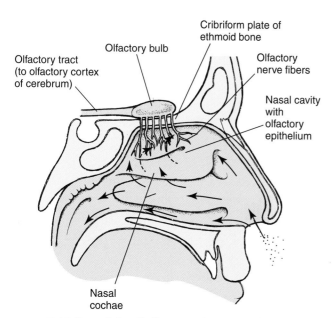

FIGURE 5.40 Part of the Skull—Sagittal Section: The Olfactory Nerves

Aromatherapy

Because the olfactory mucosa is easily accessible and yet so close to the brain, aromatherapy has a great potential to directly affect the functioning of the nervous system. Because of the wide nervous connections, emotions, memories, and moods, the autonomic system via the hypothalamus and many other functions can be impacted. However, there is a great need for research in this fascinating area.

and salivation that occur with response to the smell of food. The lateral olfactory area is located in the base of the brain, spreading to the temporal lobe, and is part of the limbic system with its many connections. Connections with the cortex of the opposite side allow for transfer of memories from one side to the other. Other neurons have connections with the frontal lobe via the thalamus and help with conscious perception and discrimination of smell. The recognition of delectable and detestable food, based on past experience, is a function of the lateral olfactory area. Because of the wide connections, smell has the ability to trigger memories; strong odors can trigger a seizure in individuals with epilepsy.

Stimulation of Olfactory Receptors

Olfactory receptors are stimulated by substances dissolved in the mucus covering the nasal epithelium. The substance binds to the receptor, which then opens sodium channels, with resultant depolarization and initiation of action potentials. Small substances, with 3–20 carbon atoms; volatile substances (substances that evaporate easily); and those relatively soluble in water and lipids have strong odors that are easily smelled. We can distinguish between 2,000 to 4,000 odors; the physiologic basis is not fully known. These receptors adapt quickly (i.e., the perception of the odor decreases with time). This is beneficial, especially when one is caught in the midst of disagreeable odors! The direction of the smell is identified by the slight difference in the time the smell stimulates the receptors on each side.

In many species of animals, there is a close relationship between smell and sexual function. In many species, behavioral and other physiologic changes are produced in animals of the opposite sex by air-transported hormones. These hormones are known as **pheromones** and certain fatty acids present in large amounts at ovulation in female vaginal secretions have been identified as pheromones.

The nose is innervated by the trigeminal nerve, which carries general sensations (e.g., touch, pressure, pain, temperature) to the brain. They may be stimulated by irritating odors, and the characteristic

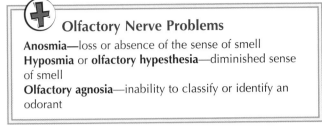

Olfactory Nerve Problems

Anosmia—loss or absence of the sense of smell
Hyposmia or **olfactory hypesthesia**—diminished sense of smell
Olfactory agnosia—inability to classify or identify an odorant

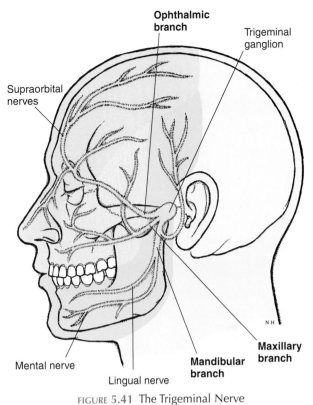

FIGURE **5.41** The Trigeminal Nerve

smell of such substances as peppermint, menthol, and chlorine is partly a result of the stimulation of pain fibers carried by the trigeminal nerve.

TRIGEMINAL NERVE (CRANIAL NERVE V)

The touch, pressure, and other sensations triggered during a facial massage are carried by the trigeminal nerve. This nerve, as the name suggests, has three major branches (see Figure 5.41). The **ophthalmic branch** carries sensations from the eye, nasal cavity, skin on the forehead, upper eyelid, eyebrow, and part of the nose. The **maxillary branch** carries sensations from the lower eyelid, upper lip, gums, teeth, cheek, nose, palate, and part of the pharynx. The **mandibular branch** carries sensations from the lower gums, teeth, lips, palate, and part of the tongue. In addition, this nerve controls the muscles of mastication: the temporalis, the masseter, and the pterygoids. The sensory impulses ultimately reach the facial area of the sensory cortex, and the motor reach the respective area of the motor cortex.

FACIAL NERVE (CRANIAL NERVE VII)

The facial nerve (see Figure 5.42) arises from the pons and contains nerves fibers that have many different functions (Table 5.4). The major motor function of the facial nerve is control of the muscles of facial expression. When the nerve is affected, the muscles of the face become weak, with sagging eyelids; difficulty closing the eyelids tightly, pursing the lips, and blowing out the cheeks; and drooping of the side of the mouth.

Taste Sensations

The taste receptors are located in the walls of tiny projections (papillae) in the tongue and the mucosa

of the epiglottis, palate, and pharynx. Similar to smell, these are chemoreceptors, stimulated by substances dissolved in the saliva. Specialized cells, the **taste buds,** surround the receptors. About 50 nerves innervate each taste bud, and there are about 10,000 taste buds.

The facial nerve carries taste sensations from the anterior two-thirds of the tongue, the glossopharyngeal from the posterior one-third, and the vagus nerve from the other areas. From the medulla, the neurons cross over to the other side and reach the cerebral cortex via the thalamus.

In humans, there are five basic tastes: sweet, sour, bitter, salt, and umami. In general, acidic substances taste sour, those containing sodium ions taste salty, and most sweet substances are organic. Umami taste is described as 'meaty' or 'savory'.

Temporomandibular Joint Syndrome

Often, pain in the temporomandibular joint is referred to other regions supplied by the trigeminal nerve. This is one reason why the symptoms of temporomandibular joint syndrome are so varied.

Trigeminal Nerve Problem

Trigeminal neuralgia is a condition caused by irritation of the trigeminal nerve, and it is characterized by excruciating, intermittent pain along the distribution of the nerve on one or both sides. The pain may be triggered by any touch or movement, such as chewing, eating, and swallowing. In some people, even a draft of air and exposure to heat or cold may trigger an attack.

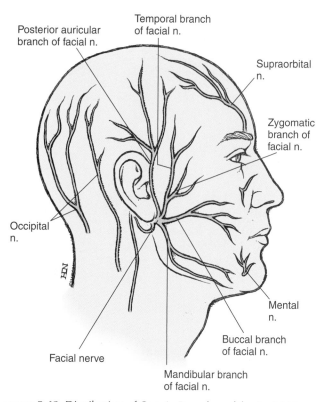

Posterior auricular branch of facial n.

Temporal branch of facial n.

Supraorbital n.

Zygomatic branch of facial n.

Occipital n.

Mental n.

Facial nerve

Buccal branch of facial n.

Mandibular branch of facial n.

FIGURE **5.42** Distribution of Certain Branches of the Facial Nerve (Cranial Nerve VII). The branches to the tongue (taste fibers), salivary, nasal mucosal, and lacrimal glands are not shown.

VESTIBULOCOCHLEAR NERVE (CRANIAL NERVE VIII)

This nerve has two major divisions: the **vestibular nerve** and the **cochlear nerve.** The vestibular nerve conveys sensations from the vestibular apparatus (described on **page 364**). This organ is stimulated by linear and rotational accelerations of the body and is responsible for equilibrium and balance. After the nerve reaches the medulla, it has extensive connections with the cerebellum. Its connections with cranial nerves III, IV, and VI help the body adjust eye movements according to the position of the body. Its other connections help the body increase or decrease the tone of different muscle groups to maintain balance.

The cochlear branch carries hearing sensations. The cochlea has many receptors, each stimulated by a specific wavelength. In this way, the pitch of the sound is detected. The intensity of the sound is determined by the number of action potentials produced in each receptor. The neurons from the cochlea synapse with others in the medulla, and the impulses ultimately reach the temporal lobe where sound is interpreted. Similar to the representation of the body in the primary sensory and motor cortex, there is a representation in the temporal lobe for various tones.

VAGUS (CRANIAL NERVE X)

This nerve has an extensive distribution and is the primary parasympathetic nerve that supplies most of the viscera in the thorax and abdomen (see Figure 5.43). Because it also controls the muscles of the larynx and pharynx, lesions in this nerve can result in hoarseness, difficulty swallowing, and regurgitation of food through the nose. The parasympathetic effects can be deduced from Table 5.5 on **page 372.**

✚ Facial Nerve Lesions

The signs and symptoms of facial nerve lesions differ according to which neuron has been affected. Facial nerve lesions can occur in two ways. One, the motor neuron that goes to supply the muscle (the final common pathway) can be affected anywhere along its path to the muscle. This neuron is known as *the lower motor neuron.* Two, the neuron from the motor cortex (precentral gyrus) that synapses with the final common pathway (lower motor neuron) that is responsible for voluntary control of the muscles may be affected. This is known as the *upper motor neuron.*

Similar to the spinal nerves, the *lower* motor neuron on one side supplies the muscles of the same side. The *upper* motor neuron of one side, however, crosses to the opposite side in the medulla. Therefore, the left motor cortex controls the muscles of the right side and the right cortex controls the muscles of the left side.

In the facial muscle, the lower motor neurons innervating the muscles of the upper part of the face have synapses with the upper motor neuron of both sides. Based on this anatomic structure and connections, lesions of upper and lower motor neuron of the facial nerve present differently.

Lower motor neuron lesion: Because the facial nerve is affected after it leaves the brainstem in this condition, all the muscles supplied by the facial nerve of that side become weak and atrophic. This will also depend on where the nerve is affected. If it is affected after it has exited the skull, taste sensations are intact because the damage is after the branch to the tongue has left. Bell's palsy is a condition in which there is sudden onset of paralysis of the muscles on one side of the face, supplied by the facial nerve. It is a result of inflammation of the nerve after it has exited the brain. Most often, there is spontaneous recovery within a few weeks.

Upper motor neuron lesion: Here, the nerve directly supplying the muscle is intact and the nerve from the cortex is affected. If the left cortex of a person is affected, she or he has weakness of the muscles of the lower part of the face on the opposite side. The muscles of the upper part are all right because neurons from both the right and left cortex synapse with the lower motor neurons innervating these muscles.

✚ Damage to Nerve VIII

Problems with the cochlea or the cochlear nerve result in loss of hearing (nerve deafness). Hearing may also be reduced if the sound is not conducted properly to the cochlea. This may happen if the external auditory canal is blocked by wax or the air pressure in the middle ear has not been equalized to that of the atmosphere. The later is caused by opening and closing the eustachian tube that connects the pharynx and the middle ear. This is why hearing is often diminished when a person has a sore throat or cold.

Lesions in the vestibular nerve result in **vertigo.** Vertigo is a feeling of movement, either of the individual or the world around the individual. It is often accompanied with nausea, vomiting, and increased heart rate. If severe, the person is unable to stand or walk as a result of defective balance. Another symptom is an abnormal, rapid movement of the eyeball known as nystagmus.

Control of Posture and Movement

The contraction of skeletal muscles ultimately depends on the pattern and discharge rate of the lower motor neurons supplying the muscle. These motor neurons, the final common pathway, are bombarded by impulses from thousands of neurons that synapse with it in the spinal cord and brainstem. Many synapses are from neurons in the same segment. Some neurons that synapse are from the segments above and below. There are other neurons that descend from the brainstem and cerebral cortex. It is the integrated activity of all these inputs that regulate posture and make coordinated movements possible.

The activity of the input achieves three functions: (1) they produce voluntary movement; (2) they initiate adjustments to the posture to provide stability when parts move; and (3) they coordinate various muscle groups to make movements precise and smooth.

The **motor cortex** of the brain plans the patterns of voluntary activity and conveys it to the **final common pathway** via the **corticospinal** and **corticobulbar** tracts. The **cerebellum** coordinates and makes the movements smooth as the activity planned by the motor cortex, visual input, input from the inner ear, as well as input from proprioceptors are conveyed to it. The **basal ganglia** help maintain muscle tone and participate in automatic movements. Constant feedback from the muscle and joints help the basal ganglia and part of the cerebellum adjust the commands sent by the cortex.

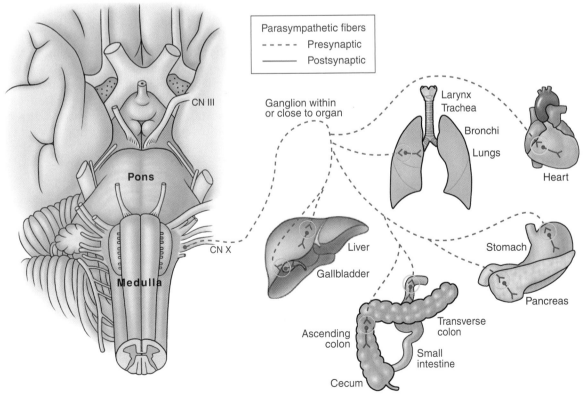

FIGURE 5.43 Organs Supplied by the Vagus Nerve

GENERAL PRINCIPLES OF THE CONTROL OF VOLUNTARY MOVEMENTS

The commands for voluntary movement originate in the cortical association areas (see Figure 5.44). The movements are planned in the cortex, as well as the basal ganglia and part of the cerebellum. The commands are then relayed via the corticospinal tracts (from the cortex to the spinal nerves) and the corticobulbar tracts (from the cortex to the cranial nerves) to the lower motor neuron that supplies the muscle. As the movement occurs, receptors in the muscle—the muscle spindle, Golgi tendon organ, joint receptors, and those in the skin—are stimulated. This feedback information is relayed back via sensory nerves to the cerebellum and the motor cortex and the movements are adjusted to make them smooth and precise.

The neurons from the cerebellum project to the brainstem, from which they descend to the lower motor neurons via the rubrospinal, reticulospinal, tectospinal, and vestibulospinal tracts.

THE MOTOR CORTEX

The motor cortex is located in the precentral gyrus. Similar to the sensory cortex, the various parts of the body are represented in the cortex, with the feet at the superior aspect of the gyrus and the face on the inferior and lateral aspect (see Figure 5.45). The facial area is represented in both sides; however, the rest of the body is represented on one side, with the left cortex representing the right half of the body and the right cortex the left half. Again, similar to the sensory cortex, the size of cortical representation is in proportion to the number of motor units going to the muscle. This, in turn, correlates with the skill with which the part is used for fine, precise, voluntary movements. For example, although the hands are

Amyotrophic Lateral Sclerosis (ALS)

Also known as Lou Gehrig's disease, ALS affects the motor neurons present in the cerebral cortex and the spinal cord. Because these nerves supply muscles, voluntary control of muscles is lost in various regions of the body and the muscles atrophy.

small, the cortical representation is large. The lips, pharynx, and tongue required for speech also have a large representation.

The corticospinal tracts and the corticobulbar tracts originate from the motor cortex. However, there are many other areas of the brain in the parietal lobe and elsewhere that participate in motor function.

Motor Pathway

The neurons responsible for voluntary control project from the motor cortex to the nerves supplying the muscles in question via **direct, pyramidal,** or **corticospinal/corticobulbar pathways.** They are called pyramidal pathways because the axons form pyramidlike bulges, the **pyramids,** in the medulla. Axons of neurons originating in the cortex descend to the medulla (see Figure 5.46). As they pass near the thalamus, all the fibers lie close together in the region of the **internal capsule.** The sensory tracts are also in close proximity in this region.

On reaching the medulla, most fibers of the corticospinal tract cross over to the opposite side, descend as the **lateral corticospinal tract,** and synapse with the respective motor neuron. The neurons in the corticospinal tract are the **upper motor neurons.** Some axons descend on the same side as the **anterior corticospinal tract** and cross over at the spinal segment

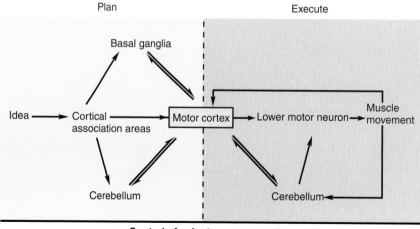

Control of voluntary movement

FIGURE 5.44 Control of Voluntary Movement

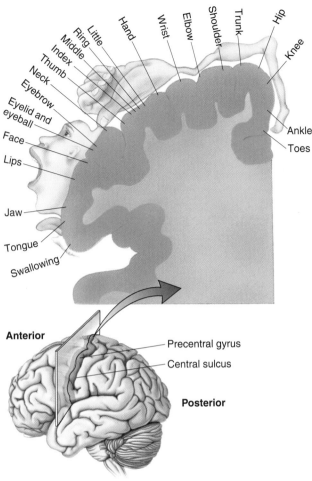

FIGURE 5.45 The Motor Cortex. Representation of the right half of the body in the left cerebral cortex (coronal section). Note that there is a similar representation of the left half of the body in the right cerebral cortex.

where they synapse with **lower motor neurons** (the neurons that directly supply the muscles). In this way, axons from one side control the muscles of the opposite side of the body. Just like the corticospinal tracts, the axons of upper motor neurons that control skeletal muscles in the head form the **corticobulbar tracts.** They synapse with lower motor neurons that exit via the cranial nerves.

In addition to the direct or pyramidal pathways, there are **indirect** or **extrapyramidal motor pathways.** These tracts are complex and involve impulses

Akinesia

Akinesia is the inability to initiate changes in activity and to perform ordinary voluntary movements rapidly and easily. Bradykinesia and hypokinesia are lesser degrees of impairment.

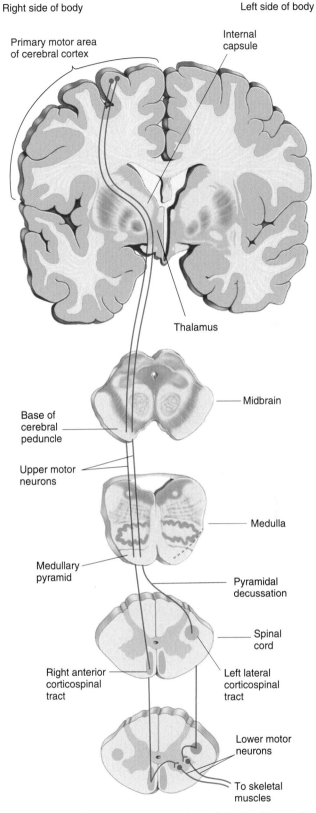

FIGURE 5.46 Schematic Representation of Major Motor (Descending) Pathways

Epilepsy

Epilepsy is a group of disorders characterized by chronic, repeated, periodic changes in nerve function caused by abnormalities in the electrical activity of the brain. Each episode of abnormal neural function is called a **seizure.** The episode may be in the form of convulsions when there is abnormal motor activity or in the form of abnormalities in other neurologic functions such as sensations, emotions, and cognition.

from the basal ganglia, limbic system, cerebellum, thalamus, and reticular formation, etc. Some tracts are the rubrospinal, tectospinal, reticulospinal, and vestibulospinal tracts.

LESIONS AND MUSCLE TONE

If there is a lesion in the lower motor neuron, the muscle it supplies atrophies (becomes smaller). There is loss of muscle tone, resulting in **flaccidity.** No reflexes can be elicited because the muscle cannot be stimulated.

If there is a lesion in the upper motor neuron, the presentation is different because the lower motor neuron is intact. Also, the presentation will depend on which upper motor neuron is affected.

In a normal person, some descending tracts inhibit stretch reflexes and others stimulate; however, the inhibitory effect is more prominent. If the corticospinal tract (has stimulatory effect) alone is injured, the muscle tone is diminished (**hypotonic**) and there is muscle weakness (**paresis**) rather than complete loss of movement.

If the extrapyramidal tracts are injured, the inhibitory effect on the lower motor neuron is removed and the muscle tone is increased (**hypertonic/spastic**) and the reflexes are exaggerated. There is little muscle atrophy.

If the cerebellum or its projections are injured, there is incoordination of movement.

OTHER POSTURE-REGULATING SYSTEMS

As can be seen in Figures 5.44 and 5.46, the posture regulating mechanisms are multiple and controlled

Physiological Explanation of Situations That May Be Encountered In Practice When Working With People with Hyperactive Muscles

Clasped-Knife Effect or Lengthening Reaction
Occasionally, when treating individuals with spastic muscles and trying to stretch the muscle, the muscle seems to resist and give alternately. For example, if the elbow is passively flexed, there is immediate resistance as a result of the stretch reflex in the triceps muscle. Further stretch activates the inverse stretch reflex and causes the triceps to suddenly relax, reducing the resistance.

Clonus
Occasionally, when treating individuals with spastic muscles, sudden stretch of the muscle may result in regular, rhythmic contractions that are startling. This reaction is known as **clonus** and is partly a result of the hyperactive muscles being subjected to alternating activity of stretch reflex and reverse stretch reflex.

Mass Reflex
In persons with chronic paraplegia, excitatory or inhibitory effects may spread up and down the spinal cord, producing discharge of many neurons. For example, a mild painful stimulus may cause not only a withdrawal reflex but also urination, defecation, sweating, and blood pressure fluctuations. This is known as the mass reflex. Sometimes, this reflex is taken advantage of to initiate urination or defecation in paraplegics.

at many levels. At the spinal cord level, sensory stimuli produce simple reflex responses.

- At the medullary level, antigravity reflexes are regulated (i.e., changes in tone of different groups of muscles according to the effects of gravity).
- At the midbrain level, locomotor reflexes are present (i.e., walking movements can occur).
- At the hypothalamus limbic system level, changes in motor function in relation to emotions are produced.
- At the cerebral cortex level, initiation of movements and movements in relation to memory and conditioned reflexes occur.

Lesions in any of these levels result in retention of the reflexes and function mentioned *below* the level.

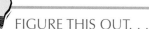

FIGURE THIS OUT. . .

If the right half of the spinal cord was cut transversely at the upper thoracic region, how will the sensations of the body be affected below the level of the cut?

FIGURE THIS OUT. . .

If the right half of the spinal cord is cut transversely at the upper thoracic level, how will it affect the motor function of the body?

BASAL GANGLIA

Deep to the cerebral cortex, there are many collections of gray mater on both sides. The **basal ganglia,** or **basal nuclei,** are a group of these gray areas. The basal ganglia (Figure 5.37B) include the **caudate nucleus, putamen, globus pallidus,** the **subthalamic nucleus,** and the **substantia nigra.**

The basal ganglia have numerous connections. A major input is from various parts of the cerebral cortex and the thalamus. The different regions of the basal ganglia are extensively interconnected too. The basal ganglia, in turn, send efferents to the cortex via the thalamus and other areas (see Figure 5.44).

The major function of the basal ganglia is its role in planning and programming movement. Its role can be better examined in animals and people with lesions in this region. Basal ganglia lesions are characterized by involuntary movement. Some movements and dysfunctions are described in Symptoms and Signs of Lesions in the Basal Nuclei.

CEREBELLUM

Another important region involved in posture and movement is the cerebellum (Figures 5.36, 5.37, and 5.44). The cerebellum is required for learning and performing rapid, coordinated, and skilled movements. It is a structure that lies posterior to the brainstem and numerous tracts enter and leave it in the brainstem. An important input is from proprioceptors located over

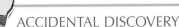

ACCIDENTAL DISCOVERY

A drug dealer in northern California supplied some clients with a homemade preparation of "synthetic heroin," which was unknowingly contaminated with a chemical that specifically destroys dopamine-secreting neurons in the basal ganglia. To his and everyone else's dismay, the clients developed Parkinson's disease dramatically and rapidly. Since then, the chemical has helped accelerate research in this area.

the body. It also receives input from the vestibular apparatus (see below). The motor cortex and basal ganglia send impulses through the pontine nuclei that inform the cerebellum of the motor plan. The cerebellum compares the motor plan with what is actually happening (feedback from proprioceptors, vestibular apparatus, and eyes) and smoothes and coordinates the movement by sending impulses to the motor cortex (via the thalamus) and the nuclei in the brainstem (see Figures 5.44 and 5.47).

Lesions of the cerebellum produce pronounced abnormalities when an individual begins to move. The individual has **ataxia**—incoordination as a result of errors in the rate, range, force, and direction of movement. The individual has a drunken gait and involuntary movements and tremors when she or he intends to do something. Typically, every movement is performed in slow motion, as if every component of the movement has been dissected out and done one

Signs and Symptoms of Basal Nuclei Lesions (Basal Ganglia)

Athetosis—continuous, slow, writhing movement
Ballism—characterized by flailing, violent movements
Chorea—involuntary, rapid, dancing movements
Hemiballism—sudden onset of ballism on one side of the body
Parkinson's disease (paralysis agitans)—a syndrome in which neurons that interconnect different nuclei belonging to the basal ganglia degenerate as a result of various reasons. These neurons secrete dopamine as their neurotransmitter and drugs that depress dopamine activity, like certain tranquilizers, can precipitate the syndrome.

Symptoms of Parkinson's disease include difficulty in initiating voluntary movements. Normal movements, such as swinging the arms when walking and changes in facial expression, are conspicuously absent. The tone of both flexors and extensors are increased and passive movement of the limbs feel as if a lead pipe is being bent, and it is classically known as lead-pipe rigidity. Sometimes, the resistance gives somewhat at intervals and this is known as cogwheel rigidity. The person also presents with tremors at rest that tend to disappear with activity.

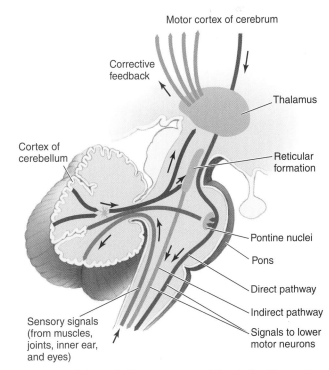

FIGURE **5.47** Schematic Representation of Cerebellar Connections

at a time. Cerebellar problems, however, do not affect the sensory system.

VESTIBULAR APPARATUS

This paired organ is part of the inner ear (see Figure 5.48) and sensations produced here are conveyed to the brain along with that of hearing via the vestibulo-cochlear nerve. Because it is directly related to equilibrium and balance, it is discussed in this section.

The vestibular apparatus, on each side, consists of three circular canals. Each canal lies perpendicular to each other and is enclosed in a bony labyrinth. To visualize this, place a half-open book, vertically on a table. Then each canal would lie along the two halves of the book, with one canal flat on the table. The canals are interconnected and filled with fluid. At the point where they meet, the canal is expanded to form the **ampulla,** which, in turn, is connected to fluid-filled structures called **utricle** and **saccule.** The ampulla of the canals, the utricle and saccule have receptors that respond to movement.

The receptors in the utricle and saccule are found in a small, thickened area called the **macula** (Figure

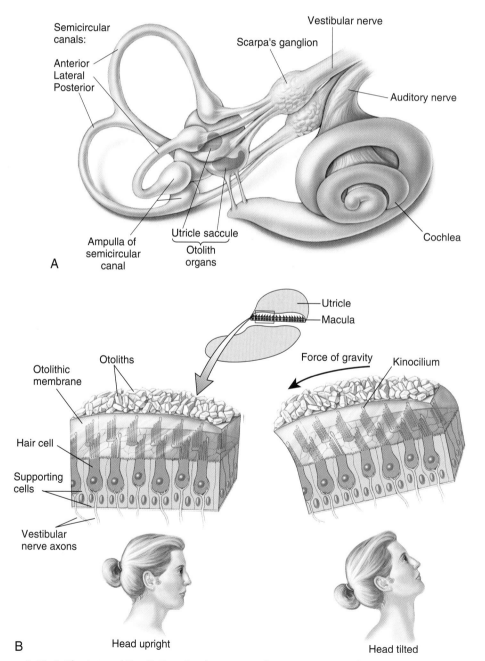

FIGURE 5.48 **A,** The Internal Ear. **B,** Details of receptors, showing position when the head is upright or tilted.

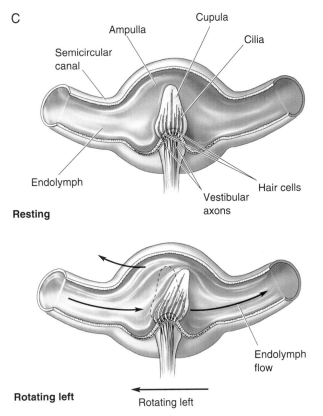

Resting

Rotating left
Rotating left

FIGURE **5.48., cont'd C,** Details of receptors (in crista) showing position when the head is resting or rotated.

5.48B). The receptors are in the form of hair cells with cilia, surrounded by a glycoprotein membrane, the **otolithic membrane.** Calcium carbonate crystals, known as **otoliths,** are found on top of the membrane. When the head is tilted, the otoliths move as a result of gravity and pull on the hair cells, resulting in changes in membrane potential and impulse formation. The receptors in the utricle and saccule respond when the head moves forward or backward—linear acceleration.

The receptors in the canals respond maximally when the head is rotated—rotational acceleration. These receptors are located in small, elevated regions in the ampulla known as **crista** (Figure 5.48C). Here, too, the receptors are in the form of hair cells, but they are covered by a gelatinous mass known as the **cupula.** Every time the head is moved, the fluid in the semicircular canals is set in motion. Depending on which direction of the head is turned, fluid in specific semicircular canals of the two sides move, causing the cupula to move in turn and generate impulses in the receptors.

The impulses travel to the brainstem where some descend as the vestibulospinal tract that affects lower motor neurons. Certain impulses enter the cerebellum to give information about head movement. Certain neurons take information to the cranial nerves that supply the eye to help the eye adjust to the movement; others take information to the motor cortex. In

Motion Sickness

Rapid, repetitive stimulation of the vestibular apparatus produces motion sickness, which is characterized by nausea, vomiting, and giddiness.

this way, the body is able to increase and decrease tone and maintain balance and equilibrium.

Because fluid has inertia, it continues to move even after stopping a rotational movement. This is the reason why individuals continue to feel giddy when they stop after turning rapidly. If the eyes were watched closely, rapid movements would be observed after stopping the movement (i.e., the eye movement persists for as long as the fluid continues to move in the canal).

The vestibular apparatus is important for orientation in space. Orientation of the body is aided by visual input, input from proprioceptors, and from touch and pressure receptors.

MOTOR SYSTEM LESIONS

Cortex and Corticospinal (Pyramidal) Lesions

Lesions of the cortex or corticospinal tract (e.g., stroke) result in muscle weakness without atrophy. Atrophy may ensue later because of disuse. The weakness is more in the extensors than the flexors in the upper limb, and so the upper limbs tend to be flexed. In the lower limb, it is the opposite, with the extensors being stronger. Stretch reflexes like the knee jerk tend to be brisk. There is dorsiflexion of the foot if the plantar response is elicited (positive **Babinski's sign**). Because the tracts cross over at the medulla, the opposite half of the body is affected—**hemiplegia.** If the lesion is in the brainstem area, the functioning of cranial nerves that arise from there is also affected.

Babinski's Sign

When the pyramidal system is injured, primitive reflexes, such as the withdrawal reflexes in the leg, become exaggerated. In infancy, if the lateral aspect of the foot is scratched, the big toe dorsiflexes, the other toes fan out, and the leg is withdrawn by flexing. Once proper nerve myelination occurs, as in adults, the same reflex produces plantar flexion of all toes. If the lateral corticospinal tract is injured, the reflex produces a response as in infants. This sign is called the Babinski's sign and is one test to determine the site and extent of spinal cord lesions.

Spinal Cord Lesions

Spinal Shock

As soon as the spinal cord is injured or cut, it is followed by a period of spinal shock when all spinal reflex responses are depressed. This lasts for about two weeks in humans. The cause of spinal shock is uncertain.

With time, the spinal reflexes below the cut become exaggerated and hyperactive. It could be a result of many reasons. One reason is the removal of the inhibitory effects of the higher motor centers. Also, the neurons become hypersensitive to the excitatory neurotransmitters. In addition, the spinal neurons may sprout collaterals that synapse with excitatory input. Whatever the reason, the stretch reflexes are exaggerated and muscle tone increases. The first reflex response that comes back is a slight contraction of the leg flexors and adductors in response to some painful stimuli.

The extent of disability depends on the level of the spinal cord that has been injured. It must be remembered that although the spinal cord has all the segments—8 cervical, 12 thoracic, 5 lumbar, 5 sacral, and 1 coccygeal—the length of spinal cord is shorter than the vertebral column and ends at level L1 and L2. Hence, injury below the second lumbar vertebra may affect only the muscles and dermatomes innervated by the sacral and coccygeal nerves.

If spinal cord injury occurs above the third cervical spinal segment, other than the loss of voluntary movements of all the limbs, respiratory movements are affected as the phrenic nerve arising from C3, 4, 5 supplies the diaphragm. Loss of movement of all four limbs is known as **quadriplegia.** If the lesion is lower, only the lower limbs are affected, and this is termed **paraplegia.** If the nerves to only one limb are affected, it is referred to as **monoplegia.**

Other Complications of Spinal Cord Injuries

One common complication among people with spinal cord injuries is **decubitus ulcer.** Because voluntary weight shifting does not occur, the weight of the body compresses the circulation to the skin over bony prominences, producing ulcers. These ulcers heal slowly and are prone to infection.

As a result of disuse, calcium from bones are reabsorbed and excreted in the urine. This increases the incidence of calcium stones forming in the urinary tract. Paralysis of the muscles of the urinary bladder, in addition to stone formation, result in stagnation of urine and urinary tract infection.

When the spinal reflexes return, they are exaggerated. For example, in a person with quadriplegia, the slightest of stimuli can trigger the withdrawal reflex and the stimulated limb flexes with flexion/extension

responses from the other three limbs. With time, as a result of prolonged and repeated flexion, scar tissue may form in the limb and the limb becomes fixed in one position, known as **contractures.**

The function of the autonomic system below the level of lesion is also affected. Voluntary control is lost if the lesion is above the sacral segments, and reflex contractions of a bladder and rectum occur as soon as they get full. Bouts of sweating and blanching of the skin as a result of vasoconstriction of blood vessels may occur. Wide swings in blood pressure can occur as a result of imprecise blood pressure regulation.

Even though sexual reflexes are complex, with integration at various levels, manipulation of the genitals in males can produce erection and even ejaculation.

Mass Reflex

Below the level of the injury, afferent stimuli can travel from one level to the other and even a slight stimulus to the skin can trigger many reflexes, such as emptying the bladder and rectum, sweating, and blood pressure changes. This is known as the **mass reflex.** People with chronic spinal injuries use this reflex to give them some degree of control over urination and defecation. They can be trained to initiate these reflexes by stroking or pinching the thigh triggering the mass reflex intentionally.

RETICULAR ACTIVATING SYSTEM AND AROUSAL MECHANISMS

The various sensory impulses reach the cerebral cortex for perception and localization, as already explained. En route, these nerves send collaterals to the **reticular activating system** (RAS), a network of neurons located in the brainstem. This system is largely responsible for the conscious, alert state of the body.

The reticular formation, or RAS, is a network of small neurons located at the center of the medulla and midbrain. It is a complex network with varied functions and is the site where the cardiac, vasomotor, and respiratory centers are located. The reticular formation also communicates with sensory pathways and plays a role in motor reflexes. Only its function in arousal and sleep are elaborated here.

Coma

Coma is a state of unconsciousness from which a person cannot be aroused by even the most intense external stimuli. Usually it is a result of trauma that affects the reticular activating system. Ingestion of drugs or poisons or chemical imbalances associated with certain diseases may also cause coma

The reticular formation has input not only from the general sensory tracts, but also from taste, smell, visual, and hearing sensations. Fibers from the reticular formation go to every part of the cortex, some via the thalamus, and it is the activity of these fibers that is largely responsible for the electrical activity of the cortex. When one is asleep, the reticular activating system is in a dormant state. But it becomes active when there is any form of sensory input and the electrical activity of the brain increases—the arousal reaction. Many theories have been presented to explain sleep. It is believed that sleep may be a result of fatigue of the various synapses in the brain. Secretion of certain chemicals in the brain has also been thought to induce sleep.

Sleep consists of different levels with two components: **nonrapid eye movement (NREM) sleep** and **rapid eye movement (REM) sleep.** The different levels of sleep can be identified by the characteristic appearance of waves in **electroencephalograph** (EEG) recordings.

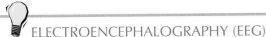

ELECTROENCEPHALOGRAPHY (EEG)

The EEG is an examination to study the electrical activity of the brain. By using electrodes on the scalp, the electrical activity is magnified and recorded. It is used to identify such conditions as epilepsy, brain tumor, cerebrovascular disease, and brain injury.

LEARNING AND MEMORY

Learning is the ability to acquire new skills or knowledge, and **memory** is the ability to retain what is learned. Many areas of the brain, including the association areas, parts of the limbic system, thalamus, and hypothalamus, are believed to be involved in these processes. Although there are no complete explanations for how we learn or how memory is stored, it has been shown that neurons have the ability to change in response to stimuli from internal and external environments. This ability, referred to as **plasticity,** is associated with changes in production of specific proteins by neurons and formation of new dendrites and new synapses and neuronal circuits. Interestingly, it has been shown that areas of the cerebral cortex that are not used become thinner and those areas used extensively become larger.

MENINGES, CEREBROSPINAL FLUID, AND ITS CIRCULATION

The spinal cord and brain are delicate structures that need protection. They are so delicate that the brain can be scooped out of the skull with a spoon. They

DRUGS THAT AFFECT THE CNS

Analgesics (pain killers)—relieve pain at the site of origin or along the CNS pathway (e.g., morphine, codeine, aspirin, ibuprofen)
Anticonvulsants—prevent spread of impulses in the CNS (e.g., dilantin)
Psychotropics (mood changers)—directly alter CNS function; resulting in change of mental state/mood, such as antidepressants (imipramine), antipsychotics (chlorpromazine), antianxiety drugs (Librium, Valium), caffeine, and alcohol.
Sedatives and hypnotics (downers)—depress CNS activity; they may promote sleep and reduce anxiety (e.g., barbiturates, benzodiazepines [Valium], benadryl, alcohol)
Stimulants—facilitate CNS activity (e.g., caffeine, amphetamines, diet pills, Actifed)

are protected, to a large extent, by the body covering—the vertebral column and the tough connective tissue sheaths—the **meninges** (the structure of the meninges is described on **page 322**).

The dura mater in the cranial cavity, unlike that in the spinal region, is a double-layered structure with the outer layer adhering to the periosteum and the inner layer following the contours of the brain. In some regions of the cranial cavity, the two layers are separated to enclose the **dural sinus** (see Figure 5.49) containing venous blood. This blood eventually drains into the internal jugular vein. In some regions of the cranial cavity, the dura also forms thick septae that separate major structures on the surface of the brain. For example, a thick layer of dura, the **falx cerebri,** separates the right and left cerebral hemispheres and the **tentorium cerebelli** separates the cerebrum from the cerebellum.

The arachnoid and the pia mater are similar in structure to that around the spinal cord (**see page 322**).

For further protection, the CNS floats in a cushion of fluid known as the **cerebrospinal fluid** (CSF). This fluid is manufactured from blood by specialized secretory structures, the **choroid plexus,** located inside the brain. The CSF then flows through four

Contrecoup Injury

The CSF protects the brain from everyday trauma; however, a severe blow can cause cerebral damage. The brain on the opposite side of the blow may be injured as it continues to move as a result of inertia, even when the skull stops moving, and hits the bone on the other side. This is known as contrecoup injury.

A blow to the nose, resulting in fracture, may cause CSF to leak through the nose.

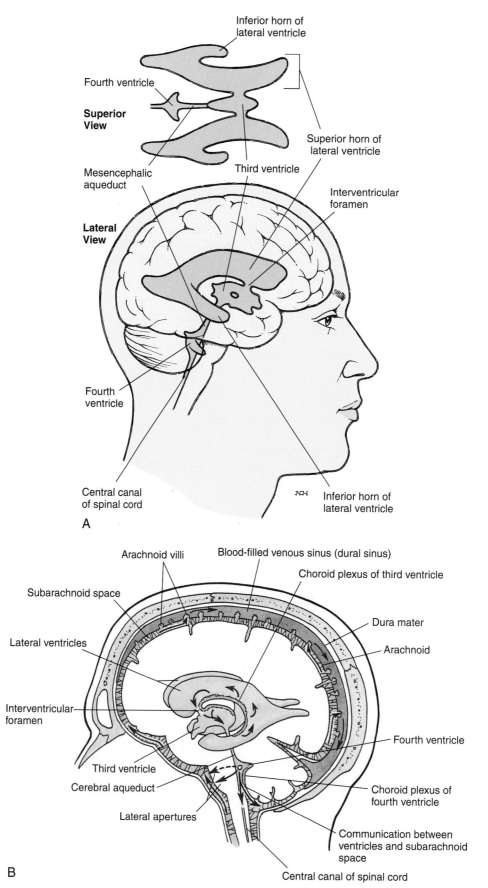

FIGURE 5.49 The Circulation of Cerebrospinal Fluid. **A,** Location of the ventricles; **B,** Flow of cerebrospinal fluid

widened chambers and narrower channels located inside the brain and exit into the subarachnoid space through openings located in the brainstem. From the subarachnoid space, the CSF flows into the large veins draining the brain (Figure 5.49B).

The four widened chambers inside the brain are known as **ventricles** (Figure 5.49A). The two **lateral ventricles** are large and located in the cerebrum. They extend from the frontal lobe anteriorly to the occipital lobe. In the region of the parietal lobe, an inferior extension of the cavity projects into the temporal lobe.

The lateral ventricles communicate with another cavity, the **third ventricle,** that is located in the midline between the thalamus and hypothalamus. The third ventricle narrows inferiorly and opens into another widened area, the **fourth ventricle,** that is located in the pons and medulla anterior to the cerebellum. Three openings located in the fourth ventricle allow the CSF to flow into the subarachnoid space.

The CSF is a clear, watery fluid; the volume is about 150 mL (5 oz). The composition is similar to that of plasma without the proteins and cells. The normal circulation of CSF and its volume and pressure is a balance between the rate at which it is produced by the choroid plexus and absorbed into the veins.

BLOOD SUPPLY TO THE BRAIN

Please refer to **page 483** for the arterial supply and **page 485** for the venous drainage.

The Autonomic Nervous System

For the proper functioning of all the cells in the body, the internal environment must be maintained within a narrow range: The temperature of the body, pH, oxygen levels, volume of blood, blood pressure, intake of food, digestion and absorption of food and water, and excretion of waste products must be monitored and regulated. All these levels are largely maintained without us being conscious of it. The **auto-nomic nervous system** (ANS) is responsible for this activity by coordinating the functions of almost all systems of the body.

The ANS, similar to the somatic nervous system, is organized on the basis of a reflex arc and consists of afferent nerves that relay impulses from the viscera to the central nervous system, where they are integrated at various levels. Efferent nerves from the central nervous system carry impulses to the visceral effectors, such as smooth muscles, cardiac muscles, and glands, inhibiting or stimulating them.

The autonomic nerves are slightly different in structure than the somatic nerves. The somatic motor nerves reach the effector—the skeletal muscle directly from the central nervous system. Nerves belonging to the ANS always synapse and communicate with another neuron that lies outside the CNS before they reach the effectors (see Figure 5.50).

The region of the synapse, which lies outside central nervous system, is known as the **autonomic ganglion.** The neuron that reaches the ganglion from the CNS is referred to as the **preganglionic fiber.** The neuron that synapses with the preganglionic fiber and leaves the ganglion to reach the effector is referred to as the **postganglionic fiber.** Each preganglionic fiber diverges and synapses with at least 8–10 postganglionic fibers. That is why the effects of the autonomic system are diffuse and not as precise and specific as the effects of the somatic nervous system.

The autonomic system is divided into two divisions, the **sympathetic** and **parasympathetic.** Usually, the two systems have opposing effects. For example, if the sympathetics excite a target organ, the parasympathetics inhibit it. However, this is not always true; sometimes the two divisions may work independently, with the structure innervated by one division or the other. At other times, both divisions may have the same type of effect, with each division controlling one part of the complex process.

The dual innervation gives the body greater scope for varying organ functions. For example, the heart rate is maintained at about 72 beats/minute as a result of the inhibitory impulses from the parasympathetic and stimulatory impulses from the sympathetic. It has been shown experimentally that if the action of the vagus nerve (parasympathetic input) is removed with only the sympathetics acting, the heart rate increases to about 150–180 beats/minute. If the effect of both the sympathetics and parasympathetics are removed, the heart beats at 100 beats/minute. This indicates that a **sympathetic tone** and a **vagal tone** exist in the heart. So, the heart rate can be increased by reducing the parasympathetic impulses or increasing the sympathetic impulses. Like the heart, such dual innervation and action is seen in other systems, such as the digestive tract.

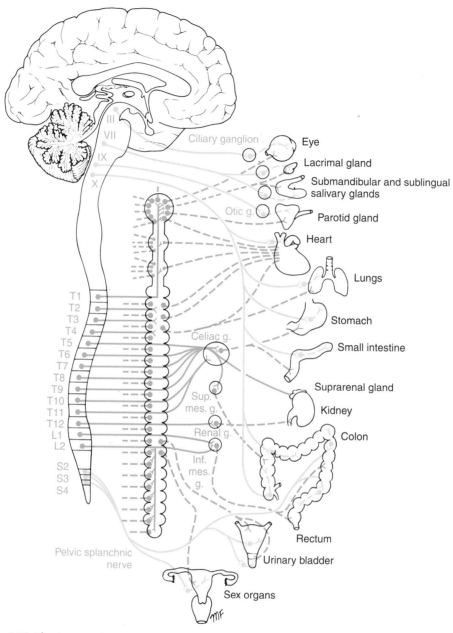

FIGURE 5.50 The Autonomic Nervous System. The sympathetic division is shown in red, the parasympathetic division in blue. The solid lines indicate preganglionic fibers, the dotted lines the postganglionic fibers.

THE SYMPATHETIC DIVISION

The cell bodies of neurons belonging to the sympathetic division arise from the region of the thoracic and lumbar region of the spinal cord and leave the spinal cord with the first thoracic to the first and second lumbar spinal nerves. This is the reason why this division is also referred to as the **thoracolumbar outflow** (Figure 5.50). The preganglionic fibers, after leaving the spinal cord with the spinal nerves, separate from the spinal nerves to reach the paravertebral ganglionic **sympathetic chain.** The sympathetic chain, which has a beaded appearance, is located on either side of

BIOFEEDBACK

Through the various levels of autonomic control, conscious thoughts can alter autonomic function. However, the physiologic changes initiated by the autonomic system are not sensed by the individual. Biofeedback tries to bridge this gap. By using special equipment, the person is made aware of physiologic changes as and when they take place by using visual or auditory signals. In this way, the person can learn to re-create the thought or mood that brought about the desired change. Biofeedback has been used to influence heart rate, blood pressure, control of micturition, and defecation.

the vertebra and consists of the cell bodies of the post-ganglionic fibers and the nerve ending of preganglionic fibers. It may also contain interneurons. Each ganglion of a sympathetic chain innervates a particular body segment or group of segments.

The postganglionic fibers leave the sympathetic chain and reach the visceral effectors. Some of these nerves rejoin the spinal nerves and travel with them to target organs located in the area supplied by the spinal nerves (see Figure 5.17, page 325). For example, the sympathetic nerve that travels with spinal nerve T10 will go to supply the sweat glands and blood vessels located in the region of the umbilicus. Some postganglionic fibers from the chain pass to target organs via the various sympathetic nerves.

The postganglionic fibers to the head travel along with the blood vessels supplying target organs. In many areas, the sympathetic postganglionic fibers mingle with the parasympathetic preganglionic fibers and form networks or plexus before they reach the target organ. Many autonomic plexus, such as the cardiac plexus, pulmonary plexus, esophageal plexus, and mesenteric plexus, exist in the thoracic and abdominal cavity.

THE PARASYMPATHETIC DIVISION

The preganglionic fibers of the parasympathetic division arise from the cranial and sacral parts of the nervous system, and this division is, therefore, referred to as the **craniosacral outflow** (Figure 5.50). The parasympathetic division to the head (cranial component) reaches the target organs via the oculomotor (III), facial (VII), and glossopharyngeal (IX) cranial nerves. The supply to the thorax and upper abdomen reaches the target organs via the vagus (V) cranial nerves (see Figure 5.43, page 359). Nerves from the sacral region supply the pelvic viscera via the pelvic branches of sacral spinal nerves S2–S4. The preganglionic fibers from the cranial and sacral region synapse with short, postganglionic fibers located close to or in the target organs that they supply.

NEUROTRANSMITTERS OF SYMPATHETIC AND PARASYMPATHETIC DIVISIONS

The communication between the preganglionic and postganglionic fibers and between the postganglionic fibers and the target organ is by neurotransmitter secretion. The principal neurotransmitter secreted in the region of the ganglion in both the divisions is acetylcholine. The neurotransmitter secreted by most of the postganglionic fibers of the sympathetic division is norepinephrine (noradrenaline). The neurotransmitter secreted by the postganglionic fibers of the parasympathetic division is acetylcholine.

Based on the neurotransmitter secreted, the autonomic nervous system can be divided into **cholinergic** (acetylcholine secreting) and **noradrenergic** (noradrenaline secreting) **divisions.** Obviously, all preganglionic fibers and the postganglionic fibers of the parasympathetic system belong to the cholinergic division. As an exception, postganglionic sympathetic fibers that supply sweat glands and those that supply the blood vessels of skeletal muscles, producing vasodilation, are also cholinergic. The postganglionic fibers of the sympathetic system are noradrenergic. Other neurotransmitters, such as dopamine, are secreted by interneurons located in the ganglia.

The effect the neurotransmitter has on a target organ depends on the type of neurotransmitter receptor possessed by the cells of the organ. For example, the effect of postganglionic parasympathetic fibers may be stimulatory or inhibitory depending on the receptor. In general, postganglionic sympathetic fibers are excitatory (see Table 5.5).

Receptors of the Sympathetic System

There are two main classes of sympathetic receptors: **alpha (α) receptors** and **beta (β) receptors.** Each have further subtypes: alpha-1 and alpha-2 receptors; beta-1 and beta-2 receptors. A few examples are given to explain how these receptors alter the effects.

Alpha-1 receptors are present in the smooth muscle of peripheral blood vessels. If the sympathetics are stimulated, norepinephrine reacts with these receptors and the smooth muscles contract, with resultant vasoconstriction and reduction of blood flow. However, alpha-2 receptors present in the junction between parasympathetic nerves and their target tissue inhibit the activity of the parasympathetics, enhancing the effect of the sympathetics. At the same time, beta-1 receptors present in the skeletal muscles are stimulated to increase the metabolic activity. In the heart, the beta-1 receptors increase the rate and force of contraction. Beta-2 receptors present in the smooth muscle of the bronchi have an inhibitory effect. When they are stimulated by norepinephrine released by the postganglionic sympathetic cells, the bronchi relax and increase their caliber, allowing more air to enter the lungs. In this way, the same neurotransmitter norepinephrine is able to produce varied effects in different organs, based on the type of receptor the organ possesses.

When the neurotransmitter is released by the nerve ending, it is quickly destroyed by the enzymes present in the vicinity. Thus, their effects last for a short time. However, the epinephrine and norepinephrine released by the adrenal medulla are not removed as fast, as the blood and most tissues have relatively low concentration of the enzymes.

Table 5.5

The Effect of Sympathetic and Parasympathetic Divisions on Various Structures

Structure	Parasympathetic System Response	Sympathetic System Response
Skin		
Sweat glands	Secretion (generalized)	Increased secretion (locally)
Arrector pili muscle	None (not innervated)	Contraction, erection of hairs
Skeletal Muscles	Increased force of contraction	Secretion
Eye		
Radial muscle of iris		Contraction (pupils dilate)
Sphincter muscles of iris	Contract (pupils constrict)	
Ciliary muscle	Contract (lens bulge for near vision)	Relax (lens become thinner for far vision)
Lacrimal (tear) glands	Secretion	Secretion
Cardiovascular System		
Heart	Decrease in heart rate and force of contraction	Increase in heart rate and force of contraction
Blood Vessels to:		
Skin	Dilation	Constriction
Skeletal muscle	Dilation	Dilation (and constriction depending on receptors)
Heart (coronary)	Dilation	Dilation (and constriction depending on receptors)
Gut		Constriction
Veins		Constriction
Respiratory System		
Bronchial muscles	Contraction	Relaxation
Bronchial glands	Stimulation of secretion	Inhibition
Digestive System		
Salivary glands	Watery secretion, profuse	Thick, viscous secretion
Motility and tone	Increase	Decrease
Sphincters	Relaxation	Contraction
Secretions	Stimulation	Inhibition(?)
Liver	Glycogen Synthesis	Glycogen breakdown; glucose synthesis and release
Pancreas	Increased exocrine and endocrine (insulin) secretion	Decreased exocrine secretion
Adipose Tissue	None (not innervated)	Breakdown and release of fatty acid
Urinary System		
Kidney	Increased urine production	Decreased urine production
Urinary bladder		
Detrusor muscle	Contraction	Relaxation
Sphincter	Relaxation	Contraction
Reproductive System		
Male sex organs	Erection	Ejaculation
Uterus	Variable	Variable

As mentioned earlier, the postganglionic sympathetic fibers innervating the sweat glands and the smooth muscle of blood vessels to skeletal muscles and brain secrete acetylcholine. Activation of these fibers results in increased secretion of sweat and dilation of blood vessels in the skeletal muscle.

THE SYMPATHETIC SYSTEM AND THE ADRENAL MEDULLA

The adrenal medulla, located deep to the adrenal cortex of the adrenal gland, is actually a sympathetic ganglion. It has preganglionic sympathetic fibers reaching it. The cells of the adrenal medulla are postganglionic neurons (embryologically) that have lost their axons and secrete the neurotransmitter directly into the bloodstream. The adrenal medulla secretes adrenaline (epinephrine) and noradrenaline (norepinephrine).

GENERAL PATTERN OF RESPONSE PRODUCED BY THE SYMPATHETIC AND PARASYMPATHETIC SYSTEMS

Table 5.5 compares the effect of the sympathetic and parasympathetic divisions on various organs. In general, the sympathetic division prepares a person to either flee or fight—the **fight-or-flight response.** To list some of the effects it has on various organs, think of a situation in which you are hiding from a predator. Your body responds by making you more alert. Activities such as digestion and urination are slowed and blood flow to the skeletal muscles is increased. Your heart beats faster, and you start breathing rapidly. You feel a trickle of sweat down your back (and, if you were an animal, your hackles would rise), your hair stands on end, you feel warm, and your mouth goes dry. Your pupils dilate and, if your blood pressure were measured, it would surely be high. This summarizes some of the effects of the sympathetic system.

The parasympathetic system generally produces a **rest-and-digest** response. In brief, it increases secretion and smooth muscle activity along the digestive tract, relaxing the sphincters; produces contraction of the urinary bladder and relaxation of the sphincters such as occurs during urination; and is largely responsible for sexual arousal and stimulation of sexual glands. Pupils constrict and hormones that promote the absorption and utilization of nutrients by peripheral tissue increase. The parasympathetic system is often referred to as the anabolic system because it leads to increased nutrient content in the blood and increased absorption that supports growth, cell division, and creation and storage of energy.

Receptors of the Parasympathetic System

Similar to the sympathetics, the effect of the parasympathetic postganglionic fibers on a target organ depends on the type of receptors present in the cells. Two types of receptors—**nicotinic** and **muscarinic**—have been identified. The nicotinic receptors are present in the parasympathetic and sympathetic ganglions (Remember that acetylcholine is secreted here?) and in the neuromuscular junction (recollect that acetylcholine is secreted by motor neurons to skeletal muscles). The muscarinic receptors are located in target organs supplied by postganglionic parasympathetic fibers. The terms nicotinic and muscarinic are based on the effects of nicotine, a powerful toxin obtained from a variety of sources, including tobacco, and muscarine, a toxin present in poisonous mushrooms. If a large quantity of nicotine is ingested, it produces symptoms in accordance to the presence of nicotinic receptors; for example, vomiting, diarrhea, sweating, high blood pressure, rapid heart rate and sweating (sympathetic effects). By stimulating skeletal muscles, convulsion may also occur.

The symptoms of muscarine poisoning produce symptoms that are almost all a result of parasympathetic effects, including vomiting, diarrhea, bronchi constriction, low blood pressure, and slow heart rate.

Knowledge of receptors and the actions and distribution of parasympathetics and sympathetics is important for all health care professionals. Almost all drugs used in conditions such as asthma, hypertension, common cold, constipation, diarrhea, and many others, have been developed and are being used based on this knowledge. Adverse effects of these drugs can be logically derived if one knows which receptors they affect and whether the drug imitates or opposes the sympathetic/parasympathetic systems.

CONTROL OF AUTONOMIC FUNCTION

Although the term autonomic implies automatic function without much interference, the autonomic sys-

Antihypertensives

In general, antihypertensive drugs reduce blood pressure by relaxing the smooth muscles of blood vessels. This is done by reducing the activity of the sympathetic nervous system, by affecting the areas in the brain that regulate the system, or by giving drugs that reduce the availability of the neurotransmitters secreted by the sympathetic nerve endings. These drugs have the potential to produce adverse effects as a result of excessive suppression of the sympathetic system.

tem can be influenced and regulated (see Figure 5.51). Similar to the somatic motor system, the autonomic system has many levels of regulatory control. At the lowest level, are the visceral reflexes. Similar to the reflex arc in the somatic motor system, the visceral reflex arc consists of a receptor that senses the stimuli and continues as the sensory (afferent) neuron. The sensory neuron conveys the impulse to the spinal cord or brainstem and enters along with the dorsal spinal and cranial nerves. Here, they synapse with a motor (efferent) neuron. In the autonomic system, this is the cell body of the preganglionic fiber. There may be interneurons interspersed between the synapses here. Also, other neurons from the brain, hypothalamus, or other areas may synapse with the preganglionic fiber, altering and influencing the reflex. The preganglionic fibers leave the spinal cord/brainstem ventrally to innervate the target organs.

There are many kinds of reflexes in the viscera. Short reflexes control simple motor responses such as motility of short segments of the gut. The synapse(s) between sensory and motor neurons may be located in a ganglion. Long reflexes tend to control the activity of a whole organ. Many visceral reflexes exist in the body, including the micturition reflex, defecation reflex, and swallowing reflex.

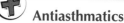

Antiasthmatics

Many different drugs may be used to prevent or reduce the severity of an asthmatic attack. One group acts by relaxing the smooth muscles of the bronchi. Because relaxation of the bronchi is initiated by the sympathetic nervous system, drugs that resemble the neurotransmitters secreted by the sympathetic nerve endings work well (e.g., noradrenaline).

The levels of activity in the sympathetic and parasympathetic divisions are controlled by centers located in the brainstem, which have an effect on specific visceral functions. For example, there are networks of neurons in the medulla such as those that control: (1) the heart rate and force of contraction—the cardiac center, (2) the caliber of blood vessels—the vasomotor center, (3) the swallowing center, (4) the coughing center, (5) the respiratory center, (6) and defecation and urination. The pons, too, has networks such as the respiratory center. The centers in the medulla and pons are, in turn, subject to regulation by the hypothalamus.

The hypothalamus can be considered the headquarters for the autonomic system. It must be remembered that the hypothalamus has numerous nervous connections. For example, it has connections with the limbic system, which is related to emotions, etc.; it communicates with the thalamus, the sensory relay station; it also connects with the cerebral cortex. Thus, activities in any region with which it communicates can influence its own function and that of the autonomic system. Think of all the physiologic changes that take place when you are angry or stressed. Your heart rate goes up, your muscles become tense, and your blood pressure rises. The trigger for your anger or stress could be something or someone around you, but the physiologic changes that occur are deep inside you. By reducing stress, perhaps by massage or changing your outlook on life, the functions of the internal organs can be influenced via the autonomic system and its higher levels of control.

Age-Related Changes in the Nervous System

The nervous system changes that occur with age do not interfere too much with day-to-day routines. Personality changes occur only if there are specific neurologic diseases. With age, there is a steady loss of neurons in the brain and spinal cord. Because the neurons do not reproduce, they are replaced by sup-

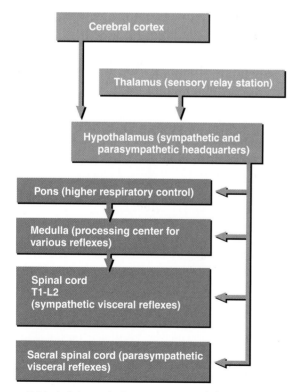

FIGURE 5.51 A Schematic Representation of the Levels of Autonomic Control. Note that not all communications between the various levels are shown.

porting cells. There is a reduction in synaptic connections and neurotransmitter synthesis and secretion. Combined, this results in diminished reflexes and slower reaction time. The learning ability may be less, with some failing of short-term memory and integration of sensory input. However, thinking and cognition are intact.

One important change that occurs is in relation to proprioception. Balance in an individual is maintained by the integration of input from vision, vestibular apparatus, joint position sense, touch-pressure sensations, and hearing. If incorrect or insufficient input is received and if the input is not well synthesized, dizziness, light-headedness, and falls may occur.

Some studies have shown that the threshold is increased for sensations such as pain, touch, and vibration.

VISION

There is a general decrease in vision in most individuals older than age 55, requiring glasses for reading or distance. The elasticity of the lens decreases, making it difficult for it to bulge when near objects are to be seen. The protein in the lens gets altered, making the lens less transparent. Color discrimination diminishes with age, especially differentiating greens and blues. This is probably a result of problems related to filtering these wavelengths through the yellowed opaque lens.

HEARING

There is a gradual, progressive loss of hearing for high frequency tones and the ability to discriminate spoken words.

TASTE AND SMELL

Atrophy of neurons may result in diminished sense of taste and smell.

AUTONOMIC NERVOUS SYSTEM

Changes in muscle and gland response to the autonomic nervous system have a profound effect on autonomic reflexes such as baroreceptor reflexes and vascular changes in accordance to environmental temperature. Therefore, the incidence of hypothermia and hyperthermia are higher in older individuals.

IMPLICATION FOR BODYWORKERS

Patience is required because reflexes and movements are slow. The sight and hearing of the person should also be considered and communication altered accordingly. Use of hot and cold packs should be done with care as temperature regulation is impaired. The therapist should watch for orthostatic hypotension when changing the client's position.

Bodyworkers and the Nervous System

The beneficial effects of bodywork on the nervous system is undisputed, but are too complex and difficult to explain in terms of anatomy and physiology, with many aspects still a mystery. Also, the effects are hard to quantify because they seem to vary from person to person. The effects of massage techniques on the nervous system have been described in detail on **page 75.** The role of various therapies in chronic pain reduction is discussed on **page 344.**

Manipulative techniques produce changes in function in a variety of ways. An array of stimuli, such as cutaneous receptors, smell, sight, and sound, are used by bodyworkers to affect the nervous system. Changes throughout the nervous system could be reflex effects, such as relaxation of muscle, vasodilatation, and changes in blood flow; psychological effects, such as those that occur in the mind, emotions, or behavior; and psychoneuroimmunologic effects, such as those produced by alteration in hormone levels and immune functions even as the mind is affected.

Research indicates that the relaxation produced, with the lowered blood pressure, heart rate, and respiratory rate, is primarily a result of stimulation of the parasympathetic nervous system.[5] Interestingly, research[6,7] on the effect of aromatherapy has shown characteristic changes in recordings of brain wave patterns on using essential oils believed to be stimulatory or relaxing. For example, wave patterns diminished (indicating relaxation) on using the relaxing oil marjoram and increased (indicating stimulation) on using oils such as lemon. There is evidence that massage can reduce anxiety and depression in children with behavioral problems[8,9] and others.[10-17] Massage is certainly an effective way of reducing stress levels.[5] Sleep patterns have also been shown to be affected by massage.[18]

Therapeutic manipulation seems to reduce pain by interrupting the pain-spasm-pain cycle.[5] It reduces pressure on nerves by initiating a relaxation of local muscles, increasing blood flow, and removal of chemicals that stimulate pain receptors. These techniques have been shown to result in the release of endorphins, the natural painkillers. By stimulating large, myelinated touch and pressure nerve fibers, such techniques result in the inhibition of impulses through the pain pathway (gate control theory).[3] Much of the effects of massage are also a result of stimulation of proprioceptors (muscle spindles, Golgi tendon organs, and joint receptors). Careful stimulation of these receptors can reflexively cause relaxation or contraction of stimulated muscles, antagonistic muscles, and even the muscles of the opposite side (by eliciting the stretch reflex, tendon reflex, crossed-extensor reflex; see **pages 334-337**). In those with paralysis, such reflexes may help alter tone of the paralyzed muscles. However, care should be taken when massaging such clients to prevent stimulation of the mass reflex that is accompanied by many autonomic responses (see **page 366**). Release of trigger points also helps interrupt the pain-spasm-pain cycle. In addition, the rapport of the bodyworker with the client and the relaxing colors, aroma, and music also play an important part.

Given the array of stimuli that bodyworkers seem to use to produce the desired effect on the client, it is important for them to consider the sensitivity of the client to various forms of stimuli.

REFERENCES

1. Porth CM. Pathophysiology—Concepts of Altered Health States. 6th Ed. Baltimore: Lippincott Williams & Wilkins, 2002.
2. International Association for the Study of Pain. Web site: http://www.iasp-pain.org. Accessed: November, 2002
3. Melzack R, Wall PD. Pain mechanism: A new theory. Science 1965:150;971–979.
4. Melzack R. From the gate to the neuromatrix. Pain 1999; 6(Suppl.):S121–S126.
5. Cochran-Fritz S. Physiological effects of therapeutic massage on the nervous system. Int J Alternative Complementary Med 1993;11(9):21–25.
6. Diego MA, Jones NA, Field T, Hernandez-Reif M. Aromatherapy reduces anxiety and enhances EEG patterns associated with positive mood and alertness. Int J Neuroscience 1998;96:217–224.
7. Diego M, Jones NA, Field T, et al. Aromatherapy positively affects mood, EEG patterns of alertness, and math computations. Int J Neuroscience 1998;96:217–224.
8. Scafidi F, Field T, Wheeden A, et al. Cocaine exposed preterm neonates show behavioral and hormonal differences. Pediatrics 1996;97:851–855.
9. Field T, Lasko D, Mundy P, et al. Autistic children's attentiveness and responsivity improved after touch therapy. J Autism Dev Disorders 1986;27:329–334.
10. Field T, Sunshine W, Hernandez-Reif, M. et al. Chronic fatigue syndrome: Massage therapy effects on depression and somatic symptoms in chronic fatigue syndrome. J Chronic Fatigue Syndrome 1997;3:43–51.
11. Rowe M, Alfred D. The effectiveness of slow-stroke massage in diffusing agitated behaviors in individuals with Alzheimer's disease. J Gerontol Nurs 1999;25:22–34.
12. Field T, Quintino O, Hernandez-Reif M, Koslovsky, G. Adolescents with attention deficit hyperactivity disorder benefit from massage therapy. Adolescence 1998;33:103–108.
13. Field T, Grizzle N, Scafidi F, Schanberg, S. Massage and relaxation therapies' effects on depressed adolescent mothers. Adolescence 1996;31:903–911.
14. Onozawa K, Glover V, Adams, D, et al. Infant massage improves mother-infant interaction for mothers with postnatal depression. J Affective Disord 2001;63:1–3.
15. Field T, Ironson G, Scafidi F, et al. Massage therapy reduces anxiety and enhances EEG pattern of alertness and math computations. Int J Neuroscience 1996;86:197–205.
16. Hernandez-Reif M, Field T, et al. Multiple Sclerosis patients benefit from massage therapy. J Bodywork Movement Ther 1998;2:168–174.
17. Field T, Morrow C, Valdeon C, et al. Massage therapy reduces anxiety in child and adolescent psychiatric patients. J Am Acad Child Adolesc Psychiatry 1992;31:125–130.
18. Scafidi F, Field, Schanberg S. Effects of tactile/kinesthetic stimulation on the clinical course and sleep/wake behavior of preterm neonates. Infant Behav Dev 1986;9:91–105.

SUGGESTED READINGS

Bray R. Massage: Exploring the benefits. Elderly Care 1999;11(5): 15–16.
Clemente CD. Gray's Anatomy. 30th Ed. Baltimore: Williams & Wilkins, 1985.
Day JA. Effect of massage on serum level of beta-endorphin and beta-lipotropin in healthy adults. Phys Ther 1987;67:926–930.
Duncombe A, Hopp JF. Modalities of physical treatment. Phys Med Rehabil: State of the Art Reviews 1991;5(3).
Field T, Schanberg S, Kuhn, C. et al. Bulimic adolescents benefit from massage therapy. Adolescence 1998;33:555–563.
Harrison JR. An introduction to aromatherapy for people with learning disabilities. Mental Handicap 1995;23(1):37–40.
Hernandez-Reif M, Field T, Krasnegor J, Theakston T. Low back pain is reduced and range of motion increased after massage therapy. Int J Neuroscience 2001;106:131–145.
Longworth JCD. Psychophysiological effects of slow stroke back massage in normotensive females. Adv Nurs Sci 1982;4:44–61.
McArdle WD, Katch FI, Katch VL. Exercise Physiology: Energy, Nutrition and Human Performance. 5th Ed. Baltimore: Lippincott Williams & Wilkins, 2001.
McKechnie AA, Wilson F, Watson N, Scott D. Anxiety states: A preliminary report on the value of connective tissue massage. J Psychosom Res 1983;27:125–129.
Morhenn, VB. Firm stroking of human skin leads to vasodilatation possibly due to the release of substance P. J Dermatol Sci 2000;22:138–44.
Premkumar K. Pathology A to Z. A Handbook for Massage Therapists. 2nd Ed. Calgary: VanPub Books, 1999.
Scull CW. Massage—Physiological Basis. Arch Phys Med 1945;26: 159–167.
Shulman KR, Jones GE. The effectiveness of massage therapy intervention on reducing anxiety in the work place. J Appl Behav Sci 1996;32:160–173.
Tortora GJ, Grabowski SR. Principles of Anatomy and Physiology. 9th Ed. New York: John Wiley & Sons, 2002.
Van de Graaf KM, Fox SI. Concepts of Human Anatomy & Physiology. 5th Ed. New York: McGraw-Hill, 1999.
Yates J. Physiological effects of therapeutic massage and their application to treatment. Massage Therapists Association of British Columbia, 1989.

Review Questions

Matching

A. *Match the following neurons with the correct (and best) description:*

a. _____ This neuron conducts impulses to the spinal cord and brain.

b. _____ This neuron carries impulses to skeletal muscles.

c. _____ This neuron lies between two or more neurons.

d. _____ This neuron takes impulses to the CNS from the organs.

e. _____ In this type, the cell body lies to one side, with a single process leading off from one side of the body.

f. _____ This neuron conducts impulses away from the spinal cord and brain.

1. unipolar neuron
2. afferent neuron
3. efferent neuron
4. interneuron
5. visceral afferent
6. somatic efferent

B. *Match the different neuroglia with their functions:*

a. _____ form thin sheaths around the axon of neurons in the PNS that serve as insulation

b. _____ produce, circulate, and monitor the cerebrospinal fluid

c. _____ surround the collections of cell bodies of neurons (ganglions) lying outside the CNS

d. _____ maintain the blood-brain barrier

e. _____ form thin sheaths around the axon of neurons in the CNS that serve as insulation

f. _____ engulf dead cells and cellular remnants in the CNS

1. ependymal cells
2. astrocytes
3. microglia
4. oligodendrocytes
5. Schwann cells
6. satellite cells

C. *Match the different receptors with their description:*

a. _____ receptors concerned with the internal environment

b. _____ receptors that give information about the body in space at any given instant

1. teleceptors
2. exteroceptors
3. proprioceptors
4. chemoreceptors
5. nociceptors
6. interoceptors

c. _____ receptors stimulated by a change in the chemical composition of the environment

d. _____ receptors concerned with events at a distance

e. _____ receptors that respond to pain

f. _____ receptors concerned with events near at hand

D. *Match the following pain theories with their description:*

a. _____ Pain receptors share endings or pathways with other sensory modalities, and the kind of impulses in the same neuron determines if the sensation perceived is pain or another sensation.

b. _____ A special mechanism at the spinal segment in which all sensory neurons enter the cord; modifies pain sensations with possibilities of interaction between pain and other sensations.

c. _____ Pain is a separate sensory modality that is perceived when specific pain receptors are stimulated and transmitted to pain centers located in the brain.

1. specificity theory
2. pattern theory
3. gate-control theory

E. *Match the following structures to their function:*

a. _____ sensory relay station

b. _____ smoothes and coordinates movement by comparing the motor plan with what is actually happening (feedback from proprioceptors)

c. _____ secretes various stimulatory and inhibitory hormones into the blood

d. _____ responsible for the conscious, alert state of the body

1. limbic system
2. thalamus
3. hypothalamus
4. basal ganglia
5. cerebellum
6. vestibular apparatus
7. reticular formation
8. brainstem

e. _____ involved with creation of emotions, sexual behavior, fear and rage, motivation, and processing of memory

f. _____ planning and programming of movement; lesion in this region causes Parkinson's disease

g. _____ orientation of the body in space; detects sensations such as acceleration, deceleration, and rotation

h. _____ passage where ascending and descending tracts synapse and/or pass through

Sequence of Events

1. The sequence of events involved in the process of action potential production is given below. Arrange the steps in the correct order of occurrence.
   a. positively charged sodium rushes in, rapidly depolarizing the neuron
   b. when the stimulus is given to the neuron, some depolarization occurs in the area of the stimulus
   c. the resting membrane potential is about -70 mV
   d. if depolarization reaches threshold level (i.e., about -60 mV), voltage-gated sodium channels open
   e. Na-K pump actively pumps sodium out and brings potassium in using ATP for energy, bringing the ionic concentrations back to normal
   f. this depolarization is propagated to the rest of the cell
   g. during rapid depolarization, voltage-gated sodium channels close and voltage-gated potassium channels open
   h. sodium does not move into the cell as rapidly as before, but positively charged potassium moves out, making the inside negative until it reaches the resting potential

2. The sequence of events involved in the process of impulse transmission across a synapse is given below. Arrange the steps in the correct order of occurrence.
   a. neurotransmitters in the synaptic vesicles are released into the synaptic cleft by exocytosis
   b. ions move into the postsynaptic neuron along the concentration and electrical gradient, causing changes in membrane potential
   c. neurotransmitters become attached to the receptors on the cell membrane of the postsynaptic neuron
   d. when a stimulus arrives at the end of the axon of a presynaptic neuron, the synaptic vesicles fuse with the cell membrane
   e. the attachment of the neurotransmitters to the receptors results in opening of channels

3. The route of circulation of CSF is given below. Arrange the steps in the correct order.
   a. it flows through four, widened chambers and narrower channels located inside the brain
   b. it flows into the large veins, draining the brain
   c. it exits into the subarachnoid space through openings located in the brainstem
   d. CSF is manufactured from the blood by the choroid plexus located inside the brain

True–False

(Answer the following questions T, for true; or F, for false):

1. A decrease in body temperature makes the neurons more excitable.

2. Impulses are conducted faster in myelinated neurons.

3. Impulses travel faster in those neurons that have thicker axons.

4. Neurons have the capacity to regenerate.

5. It is possible for neurons to recover if the pressure applied to a neuron is released after a few hours.

6. If the cut ends of an axon are placed in close contact with each other, chance of recovery is high.

7. Damaged neurons in the CNS recover more easily than those in the PNS.

8. Neurons rely on aerobic metabolism for their survival.

9. All sensations enter the spinal cord ventrally.

10. Body parts with more sensory receptors per unit area can discriminate two stimuli placed close to each other better than those regions with less sensory receptors.

11. Each sense organ or sensory receptor can convert many forms of energy into action potentials in the sensory nerves.

12. Each sensation has a discrete pathway to the brain.

13. The sensation perceived and the ability to localize which part of the body it originated from is determined by the particular part of the sensory cortex activated by the impulse.

14. Differences in sensation intensity are determined by changes in the frequency of action potentials.

15. A typical spinal nerve may carry motor, sensory, and autonomic nerve fibers.

16. The muscle spindle is a receptor that detects changes in joint movement.

17. Muscle spindles are innervated by both sensory and motor nerve fibers.

18. Muscle spindles are the receptors involved in stretch reflexes.

Short-Answer Questions

1. What are the physiologic changes caused by heat application in the treatment of acute pain?
2. What are the physiologic changes caused by cold application in the treatment of acute pain?
3. What are the beneficial effects of massage in the treatment of chronic pain?
4. What is a dermatome?
5. What are the age-related changes that occur in the nervous system? What are the implications for the bodyworker?

Completion

1. Compare acute and chronic pain by completing the following table:

	Acute Pain	**Chronic Pain**
Defined as:	Pain of less than 6 months	
Accompanied by autonomic responses:		Not usually
Presence of tissue injury:	Yes	
Correlation between intensity of pain and pathology:	Well correlated	
Type of treatment:	Removal of cause; rest; ice; compression; elevation	

2. A flowchart, showing the structures involved and the process of voluntary muscle control, is given below. Identify the structures involved by completing the flowchart.

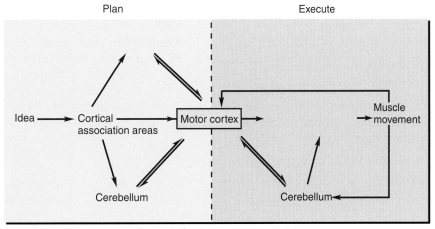

Control of voluntary movement

3. *Identify major nerves arising in the brachial plexus, the spinal segments from which they arise, and their distribution by completing the following table.*

Spinal Segment	Nerve	Distribution Motor	Sensory
C5–C6	Axillary		Skin of shoulder; shoulder joint
C5–C7		Flexor muscles of the arm (biceps; brachialis; coracobrachialis)	Skin over lateral surface of the forearm
C5–T1	Radial	Extensor muscles of the arm and forearm	
	Median		Skin over anterolateral surface of the hand
C8–T1		Flexor muscles of the forearm	

Fill-In

a. The major nerve plexus in the body are the cervical, _____, _____ and _____ .

b. Three examples of neurotransmitters are _____, _____, and _____.

c. The two major subdivisions of the autonomic system are the _____, and the _____.

d. The response produced by the _____ division can be described as the fight-or-flight response.

e. The neurotransmitter secreted by the ends of most postganglionic sympathetic fibers is _____, and that secreted by the postganglionic parasympathetic fibers is _____.

f. The hormones secreted by the adrenal medulla are _____ and _____.

g. The sympathetic division is also known as the _____ outflow because the nerves enter and exit in this region of the spinal cord.

h. The parasympathetic division is known as the _____ outflow.

Identify

Identify the cranial nerves involved in each of the following cases:

a. Following a head injury several months ago, this person has difficulty identifying various smells.

_____

b. She has a lopsided smile, with one-half of her face not having much movement.

_____

c. When swimming under water, he is unable to determine the surface from the bottom because his sense of direction of movement is deficient.

_____

d. She cannot feel the touch when the left side of her face is massaged.

_____

e. He has difficulty moving his tongue from side to side following his stroke.

_____

Case Studies

1. Mr. Gupta had an accident when working in the lumber industry. His right leg was caught under a falling tree, just below the knee. Fortunately, he had no broken bones or crushed muscles; however, he did have some bruises and pain. He first noticed that the sensations were diminished in the lateral aspect of his calf region and leg and the dorsum of his foot when he came for massage. He did not have trouble moving his leg.
   A. Why is the sensation diminished in Mr. Gupta's leg?
   B. What type of nerve could be affected?
   C. If, in addition, he had difficulty plantar flexing and everting the foot, what do you think may have happened?

2. If Mr. Gupta injured his spinal cord at the lumbar level, with the injury completely severing the spinal cord transversely, would he have the same symptoms?

A. What additional signs and symptoms, if any, do you expect to see?

3. Mr. Grant had a stroke two years ago. A blood clot had lodged in a major artery in the left side of the brain, with resultant damage to the left side of his cerebral cortex. He had the same problem as Mr. Gupta, together with many other signs and symptoms.
   A. Can you think of some of the other problems Mr. Grant could have?
   B. If the problem was on the left side of the brain, why do signs and symptoms occur on the right side?

4. As part of the community outreach program at the massage school, students were sent to the local senior citizen's home. Mr. Snell, who had Parkinson's disease, was Sheila's patient. Mr. Snell greeted Sheila with tight lips, and she could not determine if he felt pain or pleasure because he had a masklike face. His constant shaking initially alarmed her; however, she became used to it.
   A. What is Parkinson's disease?
   B. Which part of the brain does it affect?
   C. Why do people with Parkinson's disease have tremors?
   D. Why is their face expressionless?

5. Mrs. Dawson's face seemed completely uncoordinated after she had Bell's palsy. Her mouth was lopsided. The right side of her mouth seemed to disobey and pull down rather than up when she smiled. When she blinked, her eyes seemed to rebel and blink asynchronously. Mrs. Dawson had great faith in her clinician and was unperturbed. As her face was massaged, she said "My doctor said that, in most people, Bell's palsy goes away by itself in a few weeks or months."
   A. What is Bell's Palsy?
   B. Which nerve is affected?
   C. What structures are supplied by this nerve?

6. The students also needed to work at a home for cerebral palsy patients as part of their massage therapy program. This huge building housed many children with cerebral palsy, and the massage students had to work along with the physiotherapists. Mary, one of the therapists, loved the children and resolved to work at the home as a volunteer after getting out of school.

   Working here was a challenge because each child presented differently. For example, the muscles of some children were flabby and flaccid, and Mary could move their limbs with no effort. However, other children had limbs that were so stiff and contracted, with fingers

clenched, that Mary did not even try to pry open the fingers or straighten the limbs. When Mary gently tried to straighten a limb, occasionally, it would start moving uncontrollably in jerks. Oh, how it startled her the first time that happened. But the physiotherapist close by assured her that the child's reaction was clonus.
   A. Why did the limbs feel different?
   B. What are lower motor neuron and upper motor neuron lesions?

7. Corri had been sitting in the sauna for about a half hour. She had won a trip for two to Hawaii in a contest held by her local massage therapy association, and this was her first day there. Rather than walk to the beach, she opted to laze in the indoor swimming pool and sweat it out in the sauna.

   When she got up to leave, her heart was beating fast and everything began to swim and darken before her eyes. She fell to the floor with a thud. "Oh, I should have known that this would happen. I stayed in here for too long," she thought as she lost consciousness.
   A. What do you think happened to Corri?

Answers to Review Questions

Matching

A.
1. e   2. a   3. f   4. c   5. d   6. b

B.
1. b   2. d   3. f   4. e   5. a   6. c

C.
1. d   2. f   3. b   4. c   5. e   6. a

D.
1. c   2. a   3. b

E.
1. e   2. a   3. c   4. f   5. b   6. g
7. d   8. h

Sequence of Events

1. c, b, d, a, f, g, h, e

2. d, a, c, e, b

3. d, a, c, b

True–False

1. F
2. T
3. T

4. F
5. T
6. T
7. F
8. T
9. F
10. T
11. F
12. T
13. T
14. T
15. T
16. F
17. T
18. T

Short-Answer Questions

1. see **page 245**
2. see **page 246**
3. see **page 246**
4. see **page 320**
5. see **page 374**

Completion

1. **See page 344.** a. Acute pain is usually accompanied by autonomic responses such as blood pressure and heart rate changes; in chronic pain, there may be signs of tissue injury and the intensity of pain may not correlate with physical findings. Many treatment options, such as drugs; surgery; biofeedback; aromatherapy; and massage therapy can be used for treatment of chronic pain and the effectiveness of therapy is individual.
2. See Figure 5.44 on **page 360.**
3. See Table 5.2 on **page 327.**

Fill-In

a. brachial, lumbar, sacral
b. adrenaline, noradrenaline, acetylcholine, nitric oxide, dopamine, serotonin
c. sympathetic, parasympathetic
d. sympathetic
e. noradrenaline, acetylcholine
f. adrenaline, noradrenaline
g. thoracolumbar
h. craniosacral

Identify

a. olfactory nerve
b. facial nerve
c. vestibulocochlear nerve
d. trigeminal nerve
e. hypoglossal nerve

Case Studies

1. A. From the description, it appears Mr. Gupta has lost all cutaneous sensations. The cutaneous branch of the nerve has been affected.
   B. On looking at the dermatomal pattern (Figure 2.6), it can be seen that the lateral part of the calf, leg, and dorsum of the foot is supplied by nerves from L5 and S1.
   C. From Table 5.3, it can be noted that the tibial nerve supplies the muscles that plantar flex the foot. Because the lesion is only in a cutaneous branch of the nerve, the muscles supplied by the nerve are unaffected in B. In C, both branches to the muscle, as well as the cutaneous branches, are affected. (See **page 339** Pathways of Cutaneous Sensations; **page 330 and 333** for major nerves of lumbosacral plexus; **page 316** for the sensory nervous system; **page 226** for muscles that move the foot and toes; **page 69** for inflammation; and **page 341** for pain.)
2. A. (see references in Case 1; **page 365** for motor system lesions). At the lumbar level: The nerves entering and leaving the level will be damaged. As a result, all sensations at the level of injury will be lost and all motor function at the level of injury will be lost (i.e., the muscles supplied by the nerve cannot be moved voluntarily, there will be no reflex movement; the muscles will be atrophied with loss of tone).

   Below the level of the lesion, on both sides: loss of all sensations; loss of voluntary control; reflexes would be exaggerated; tone is likely to be increased (because the inhibitory control from the brain has been removed. Reflexes are present as the motor and sensory nerves are intact, only the connection with the brain is lost). No changes would be seen above the level of the lesion.
3. A. The signs and symptoms will depend on the extent of the damage—whether both sensory and motor cortex have been affected and, specifically, which region of the brain.
   B. Because the pyramidal pathway crosses lower in the brainstem region, the left side of the cortex controls the right half of the body. Therefore, Mr. Grant would have difficulty controlling and coordinating the right half. Reflexes would be exaggerated and tone would be usually increased. Sensations will be diminished/lost on the right half if the left sensory cortex is affected. The exact region will depend on which part of the sensory cortex. (See page 365 for motor system lesions;

page 483 for arterial supply to head and face; page 359 for control of posture and movement; page 360 for motor pathway; and page 339 for sensory pathway.)

4. A. See page 359 for control of posture and movement; and page 363 for basal ganglia

5. A and B. Bell's palsy is a problem with the facial nerve as it exits the cranial cavity. Therefore, only the motor branches of the facial nerve are affected with loss of voluntary control. C. The muscles of facial expression are supplied by the facial nerve. (See page 357 for facial nerves and page 203 for muscles responsible for changes in facial expression.) The facial nerve also carries taste sensations from part of the tongue (these sensations are not affected in Bell's palsy because the branch to the tongue leaves the facial nerve before it exits the cranial cavity).

6. A. In cerebral palsy, the cerebral cortex is affected. The region affected varies by individual. This is why the muscles are flaccid in some individuals and rigid in others. Because the upper motor neuron is affected, the inhibitory effects may be lost, resulting in exaggerated reflexes and clonus. If the joint is fixed in a particular position for a long period, contractures result—replacement of muscle tissue with fibrous tissue (See page 334 for muscle spindle; page 359 for control of posture and movement; and page 362 for definition of clonus.)

B. Lower motor neurons directly reach the skeletal muscle fibers from the brain and spinal cord. Upper motor neurons are neurons from the brain that communicate with the lower motor neuron.

7. A. Because Corri stayed in the sauna for a long time, her core temperature would have increased, triggering her temperature regulatory mechanisms to bring the temperature down. Increased sweating and dilation of cutaneous blood vessels, enabling cooling of blood by exposure to the periphery, are some mechanisms that come into play. When Corri stands up, less blood reaches her brain as a result of a large volume of blood flowing through the dilated vessels and the effect of gravity tending to pool blood in the lower limbs. (See page 369 for autonomic nervous system; page 487 for regulation of the cardiovascular system; and page 65 for temperature regulation.)

Coloring Exercise

Label the structures in the given diagrams, and color the structures, using the color code.
1. Color the neuron yellow, the nucleus black, and the myelin sheath brown. Label the following: a. dendrite; b. axon; c. nucleus; d. node of Ranvier; e. myelin; and f. collateral axon. On the diagram, draw arrows to indicate the direction of impulse conduction.

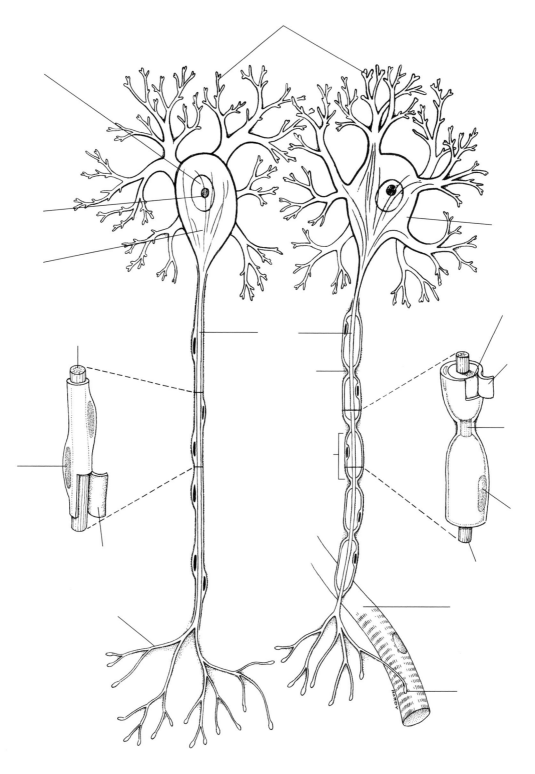

2. The outline of the anterior and posterior view of man is shown, with the outline of areas of referred pain. Referring to the diagram on **page 344,** use different colors to shade each area and label the organ that produces pain in those areas.

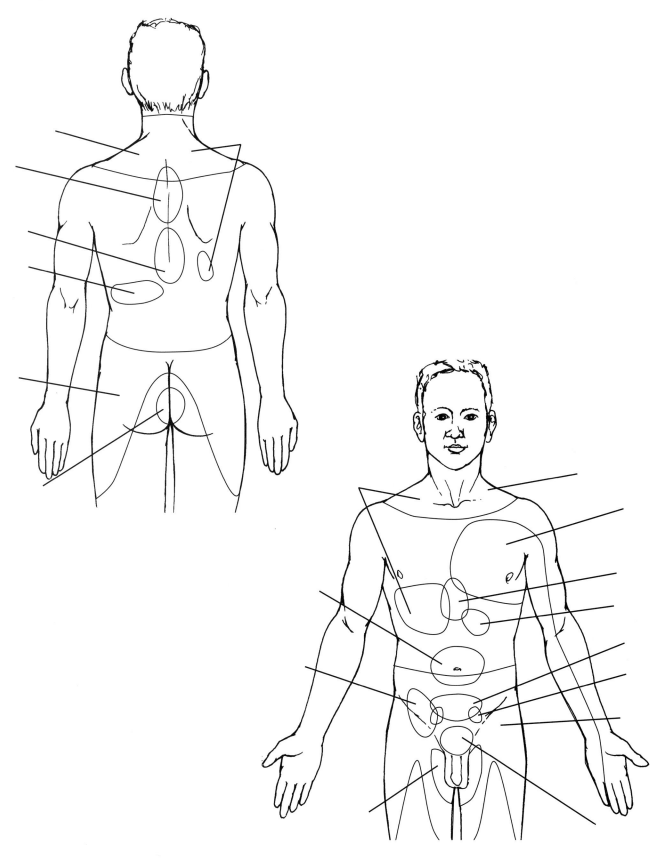

3. The structure of a synapse is given. Outline the cell membrane brown. Color the cytoplasm of the presynaptic and postsynaptic neuron yellow; the synaptic vesicles red; the synaptic cleft green; the receptors blue; and the acetylcholinesterase pink. Name the structures against the label lines.

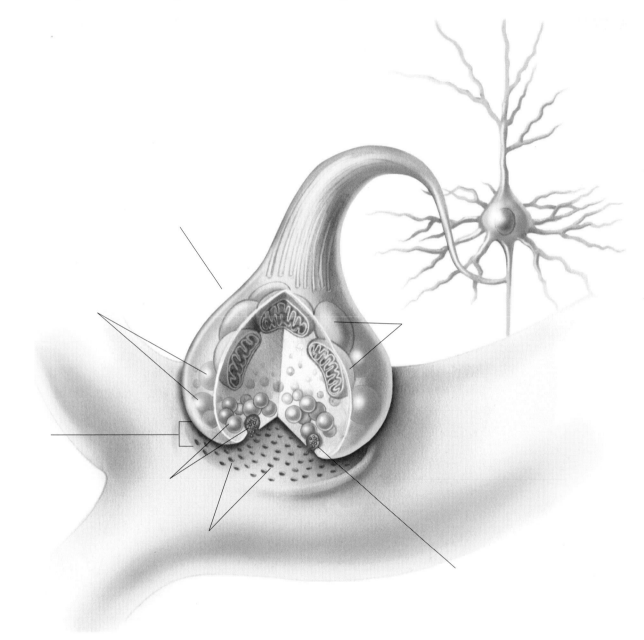

4. On the diagram of the transverse section of the spinal cord, color the gray mater light brown; the white mater yellow; and the central canal blue. Label the spinal nerve; spinal ganglion; posterior root of spinal nerve; anterior horn; central canal; lateral horn; posterior median sulcus; anterior median fissure; posterior horn; posterior white column; anterior white column; and lateral white column.

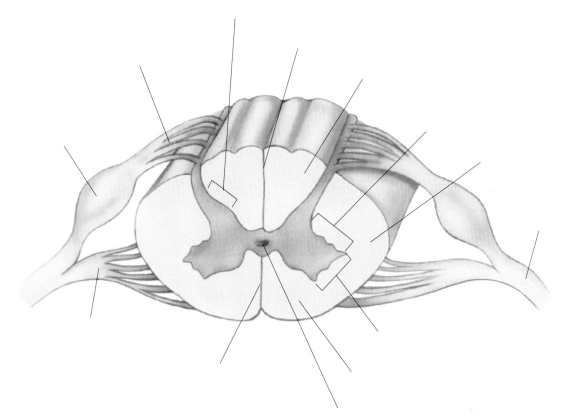

5. This is a diagram of a monosynaptic reflex (biceps jerk). Shade the white mater of the spinal cord yellow, the gray mater light brown; the bones gray; the muscles reddish brown, and the tendons yellow. Outline the sensory neuron green and the motor neuron dark blue. Also color the hammer. Label the dendrite of sensory neuron; cell body of sensory neuron; axon of sensory neuron; synapse; axon of motor neuron; cell body or motor neuron; the effector (muscle); receptor (muscle spindle); and draw an arrow in the direction of the expected limb movement.

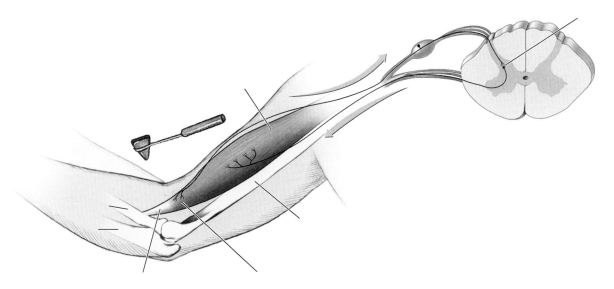

6. The lateral view of the brain is shown. Shade the frontal lobe pink; the parietal lobe yellow; the occipital lobe green; the temporal lobe light blue; the cerebellum brown; and the brainstem dark blue. Color the precentral gyrus red and postcentral gyrus orange. Shade the general interpretive area purple; the auditory area dark green; the motor speech area black. Label the brainstem; cerebellum; lateral sulcus; central sulcus; sensory area; motor area; postcentral gyrus; precentral gyrus; parietal lobe; frontal lobe; occipital lobe; temporal lobe; auditory area; motor speech area; and general interpretative area.

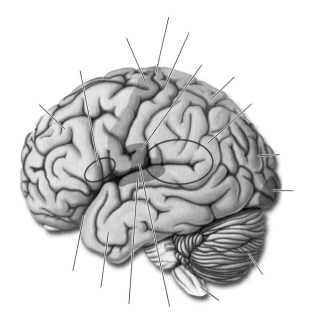

7. The sagittal section of the brain is given. Color the corpus callosum orange; the pituitary gland purple; the pons red; the medulla oblongata pink; the cerebellum green. Shade all other areas light brown. Label the medulla oblongata; pons; location of the thalamus; hypothalamus; and optic chiasma. Name the location and functions of the limbic system; thalamus, hypothalamus; basal ganglia; cerebellum; corpus callosum; and choroid plexus of third ventricle.

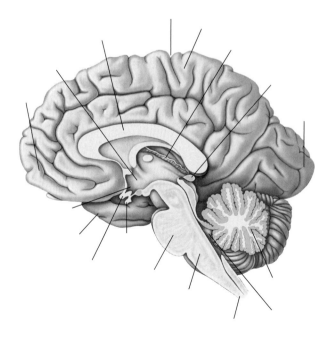

8. Color the spinal nerve yellow; the white mater of the spinal cord yellow; and the gray mater gray. Shade the dura mater green; the subarachnoid mater orange, and the pia mater blue; and color the bones light brown. Label the dura mater; pia mater and arachnoid mater, and number them 1–3, according to the order of appearance from superficial to deep. Also label the spinal nerve; lumbar vertebra; and vertebral foramen.

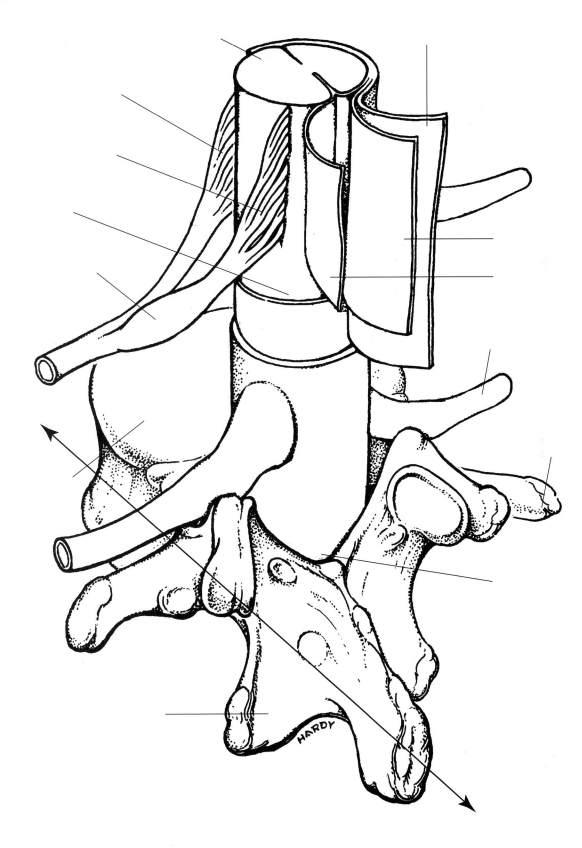

9. The Figure outlines various organs and the sympathetic nerve supply. Color each organ, using your choice of color. Outline the preganglionic neurons blue and the postganglionic neurons red. Name each organ; beside each organ, write the action of sympathetic stimulation. For example, eye (dilation of pupil) and lungs (dilation of bronchioles).

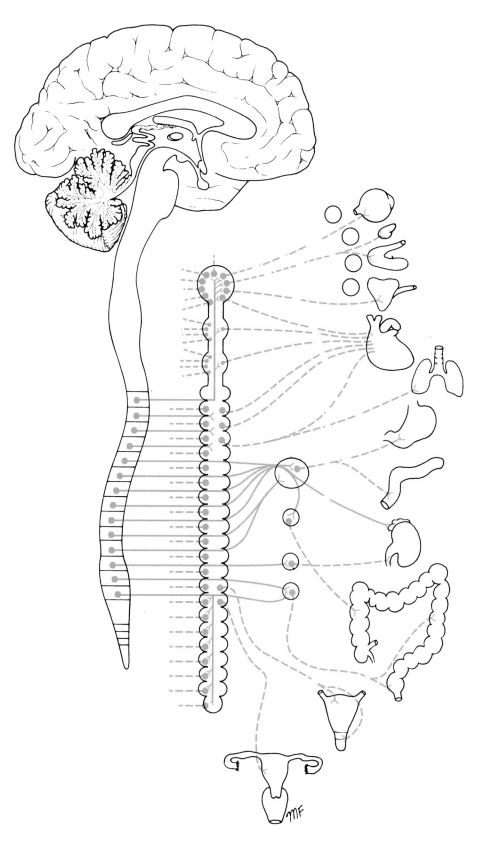

CHAPTER 6

Endocrine System

Objectives On completion of this chapter, the reader should be able to:

- Compare and contrast endocrine and exocrine glands.
- List the functions of the endocrine system.
- Define hormones.
- Describe, briefly, the chemical structure of hormones.
- Describe the action of local hormones.
- List the three types of stimuli that produce hormonal secretion.
- Describe, briefly, how hormones affect cell functions.
- Describe the mode of transport of hormones.
- Explain how hormones are destroyed.
- Describe, with examples, positive and negative feedback mechanisms.
- Identify the endocrine glands.
- Identify the location of each endocrine gland.
- Describe the regulation of hormonal secretions of various endocrine glands.
- Name the hormones liberated by each endocrine gland and describe their major functions.
- Describe the body changes that occur when there is hyposecretion or hypersecretion of the hormones secreted by each endocrine gland.
- Name the function(s) of hormone(s) secreted by cells in those tissue and organs with endocrine function.
- Define stress.
- Explain how the stress response is produced.
- Describe the stress response produced in various systems of the body.
- Describe the changes that occur to the endocrine glands with aging.
- Explain the role of massage in stress.
- Describe the effects of massage on the endocrine system.

The endocrine system is closely related to the nervous system in function. Similar to the nervous system, the endocrine system helps coordinate and regulate the activities of the cells, tissue, and organs and maintain homeostasis. While the nervous system generally has a rapid effect and shorter duration of action, the actions of the endocrine system are generally slow and have a longer duration of action.

This chapter describes the endocrine glands and the hormones they secrete. It explains the functions of the hormones and how they are regulated. Knowledge of hormone function will enable the therapist to fully understand the various signs and symptoms exhibited by clients with endocrine disorders. General hormonal properties are discussed first, followed by descriptions of the individual endocrine glands.

General Properties of Hormones

The glands of the body are classified as being **exocrine** or **endocrine,** according to the type of secretion (see Figure 1.22). Exocrine glands secrete into ducts, which, in turn, are connected to body cavities, lumen of organs (e.g., salivary gland), or to the outside of the body (e.g., sweat glands). Glands are considered endocrine if they secrete chemicals into the interstitial fluid around them. These chemicals then diffuse into the circulation and have an effect on structures *away* from the gland. The chemicals secreted by endocrine glands are known as **hormones.** Hormones, therefore, are chemical messengers released by one tissue into the interstitial fluid that have an effect on other tissues.

Many hormones have been identified and many are still being identified. Each endocrine gland may secrete one or more hormones. Recently, other organs, such as the heart, have been found to have endocrine function. The gastrointestinal tract also secretes numerous hormones, with hormones from one part of the gut affecting smooth muscle activity and secretion of glands located further away. If so many hormones are secreted into the circulation and all cells are exposed to all of them, how do hormones affect specific tissues?

RECOGNITION OF HORMONES BY CELLS

All cells are exposed to all hormones in the circulation; however, each cell has **receptors** on the cell membrane, cytoplasm, or nucleus that recognize and respond to only specific hormones (see Figure 6.1).

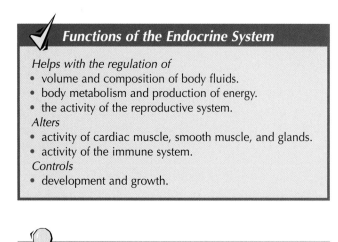

Functions of the Endocrine System

Helps with the regulation of
- volume and composition of body fluids.
- body metabolism and production of energy.
- the activity of the reproductive system.

Alters
- activity of cardiac muscle, smooth muscle, and glands.
- activity of the immune system.

Controls
- development and growth.

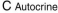

ENDOCRINOLOGY

The study of the structure, function, and disorders of endocrine glands and tissue.

Receptors are proteins or glycoproteins that are analogous to a key that can fit only a specific lock. Cells may have receptors for more than one hormone. Thus, more than one hormone can have a simultaneous effect on a cell. Cells that have receptors for a particular hormone are known as the **target cells** for that hormone. Because cells have receptors for more than one type of hormone, cell operations can be varied and modified, according to the different hormones that affect them at one time.

Individual target cells also have the ability to reduce or increase the number of receptors for a particular hormone. Usually, each cell may have as many as 2,000 to 10,000 receptors for a specific hormone. Receptors, being proteins or glycoproteins,

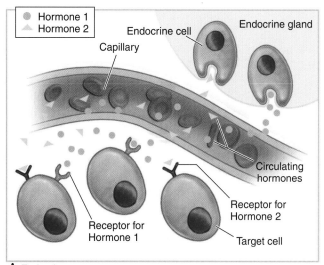

A Endocrine

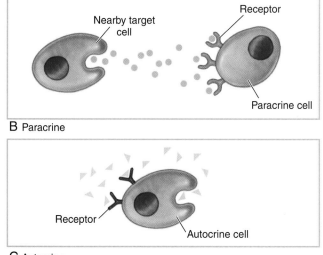

B Paracrine

C Autocrine

FIGURE 6.1. Recognition of Hormones by Cells. **A,** Circulating hormones (endocrine secretion); **B,** Local hormones (paracrine secretion); **C,** Local hormones (autocrine secretion)

are constantly manufactured and destroyed. If a specific hormone excessively stimulates the cell, the number of receptors may be reduced (**down-regulation**). If the hormone stimulating the cell is deficient, the cell manufactures more receptors (**up-regulation**).

Transported by blood, hormones can affect more than one tissue at the same time. For example, hormones secreted by the ovaries have an effect on the uterus, vagina, breasts, and brain, etc. Tissue response to hormone stimulation is usually slow to appear and may persist for days.

A striking similarity between the endocrine and nervous system is that both act on a target cell by releasing chemicals that bind to receptors. In fact, some of the chemical messengers used in the nervous system are the same as those used by the endocrine system. For example, the nerves of the autonomic nervous system secrete epinephrine (adrenaline) and norepinephrine (noradrenaline)—the same chemicals secreted as hormones into the circulation by the adrenal gland.

CHEMICAL STRUCTURE OF HORMONES

Chemically, hormones may be derivatives of amino acids, chains of amino acids (peptides), glycoproteins (proteins to which a carbohydrate group is attached), or derivatives of lipids (steroids). The more recently discovered hormones—the eicosanoid hormones—are derivatives of arachidonic acid and nitric oxide, yet, another hormone, is a gas. The hormones adrenaline, noradrenaline, and dopamine are derivatives of amino acids; insulin is a polypeptide; the male and female sex hormones are derivatives of lipids; and prostaglandins and leukotrienes are eicosanoids.

The chemical structure of the hormone determines if it is lipid-soluble or water-soluble. Steroids and thyroid hormones are lipid-soluble, while other hormones are water-soluble. The chemical structure of hormones also determines, to some extent, how long the hormone stays in the circulation before it is destroyed. After secretion into the blood, the lipid hormones, for example, bind to proteins, enabling them to remain longer in the circulation than the peptide hormones.

> ### ✔ Special Characteristics of Hormones
> - Hormones affect only those cells that have receptors for them.
> - Cells may have receptors for more than one hormone.
> - Being transported by blood, hormones can affect more than one tissue at a time.

STIMULI FOR HORMONE SECRETION

An endocrine gland releases a particular hormone in response to three different types of stimuli. Some hormones are released when there is an alteration in the concentration of a specific substance in the body fluids. For example, the parathyroid gland responds to a fall in calcium levels in the blood.

Some hormones are released only when the specific endocrine gland receives instructions from another endocrine organ. For example, the ovaries secrete estrogen when they are "instructed" by hormones from the pituitary. Other hormones are released when nerves stimulate the gland; for example, the release of adrenaline by the adrenal gland when stimulated by sympathetic nerves. The release of some hormones is regulated by its own circulating level.

CIRCULATING AND LOCAL HORMONES

Hormones are classified as circulating or local hormones, depending on how far away they act. Typically, hormones secreted by endocrine glands enter the circulation and have an effect on cells far away. Local hormones are those that affect neighboring cells or the cells that originally secreted the hormone (Figure 6.1). Hormones affecting neighboring cells are known as **paracrine hormones;** hormones affecting the cells from which they were secreted are known as **autocrine hormones.**

TRANSPORT AND DESTRUCTION OF HORMONES

Hormones are typically released where there is an abundant blood supply. Once released, the hormones quickly enter the circulation. The water-soluble hormones dissolve in and are carried by the plasma. Most of the lipid-soluble hormones bind to special plasma proteins (**transport proteins**) and are transported in a bound form. When hormones are bound to proteins, they are destroyed at a slower rate and, therefore, have the capacity to exert their effects on cells for a longer time. Also, the bound hormones are a ready-made reserve that can replenish the free (unbound) lipid-soluble hormones. It is the free hormones that diffuse out of the capillaries and actually affect target cells.

The freely circulating hormones are quickly inactivated and are functional for a short period—a few minutes to an hour. Hormones are inactivated when they enter the interstitial fluid and are bound to target cells receptors, when they are absorbed by liver and kidneys cells that break them down, or when they are broken down by enzymes in the plasma or interstitial fluid. In patients with liver or kidney failure, the hormones are not destroyed as rapidly and signs and symptoms of hormone hypersecretion may be observed.

HORMONE ACTIONS

On reaching the target cells, hormones are bound to receptors. Receptors may be present in the plasma membrane, cytoplasm, or nucleus. Lipid-soluble hormones easily move across the plasma membrane to bind with receptors present in the cytoplasm or nucleus of target cells and initiate responses. Water-soluble hormones cannot easily pass through the plasma membrane. Instead, they bind to receptors present in the plasma membrane of the cells. On binding, they trigger other enzymes (**second messengers**) located inside the cell to produce the physiologic reaction.

On binding to a cell receptor, hormones bring about many different types of responses. Some hormones stimulate the synthesis of enzymes not already present in the cytoplasm by activating specific genes in the nucleus. Some hormones affect the production rate of certain enzymes or structural proteins. Some hormones can alter the action of enzymes by changing their shape or structure. Thus, hormones can alter the physical structure or the biochemical properties of the cell. Effects such as alteration of cell permeability, degree of smooth muscle contraction, change in cardiac muscle contraction, and secretions by cells can be produced.

The effect of hormones on cells depends on the quantity of hormones in the fluid, the number of receptors in the target cell, and the influence of other hormones released at the same time. When a high quantity of hormones is released or there are more receptors in the target cell, the physiologic response is vigorous. Some hormones require the action of another hormone before they can produce a cell response. The second hormone is said to have a **permissive effect.** Sometimes, two hormones produce a greater physiologic response than they would if acting alone; each hormone is said to have a **synergistic effect.** Often, one hormone opposes the effect of another hormone; this is called an **antagonistic effect.**

Control of Endocrine Glands

Each hormone released by the endocrine glands has its own mechanism that controls the level in plasma. Most endocrine gland secretions are controlled by a **negative feedback mechanism** (see Figure 6.2A). For example, the secretion of hormones by the endocrine gland is triggered by a stimulus. The hor-

mone secreted reduces the activity of the stimulus and this, in turn, reduces the secretion of the hormone. This type of control is similar to the reflexes in the nervous system. Sometimes, like a polysynaptic

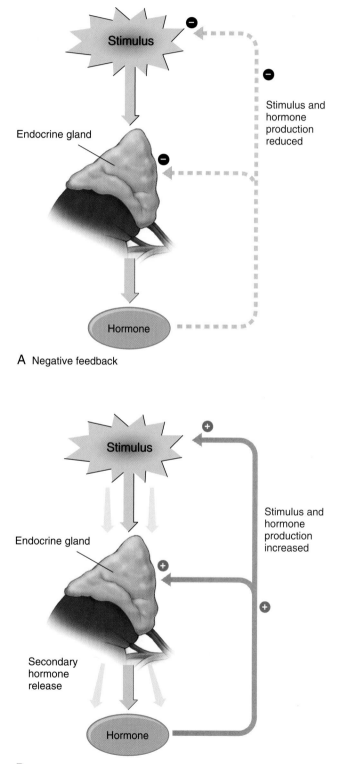

FIGURE 6.2. Schematic Representation of Feedback Mechanisms. **A,** Negative Feedback Mechanism. **B,** Positive Feedback Mechanism

reflex, there are many steps involved in the control of endocrine secretion.

Rarely, secretions are controlled by a positive feedback mechanism (see Figure 6.2B) in which the hormone secreted increases the activity of the stimulus.

The Endocrine Glands

Classically, the endocrine system includes the **hypothalamus, pineal, pituitary, thyroid, parathyroid,** and **adrenal glands;** the **pancreas** (the islets); and the male **testis** and female **ovaries** (see Figure 6.3). Other tissue and organs with endocrine function include the heart, kidney, thymus, liver, placenta, and the digestive tract.

THE HYPOTHALAMUS

The hypothalamus, as the name suggests, is located in the brain below (hypo) the thalamus (see Figures 6.3 and 6.4). It is a large collection of neurons that have been divided into different groups or nuclei, according to their functions. The hypothalamus has a rich blood supply and extensive connections with different parts of the brain, such as the limbic system, cerebral cortex, thalamus, reticular activating system, sensory input from internal and external structures, and retina. Other than its endocrine function which will be described later, the hypothalamus regulates body temperature; hunger; thirst; sexual behavior; defensive reactions, such as fear and rage; sleep; and activities of the autonomic nervous system.

The close relationship between the nervous and endocrine systems can be appreciated fully in the hypothalamus, which is a part of the nervous system as well as the endocrine system.

The hypothalamus executes its endocrine effects through the pituitary gland and communicates with the pituitary gland via blood vessels and nerves (Figure 6.4). The blood, after flowing through the hypothalamus, flows to the *anterior* pituitary, and hypothalamic hormones regulate the secretion of pituitary hormones. Neurons connect the hypothalamus with

Causes of Endocrine Disorders

Endocrine disorders develop as a result of underproduction (hyposecretion) or overproduction (hypersecretion) of hormones. Disorders may be a result of abnormalities in the endocrine gland itself, the endocrine or neural regulatory mechanism or in the target tissue.

The symptoms of specific endocrine disorders can be easily predicted if a student has knowledge of the endocrine organs and their functions.

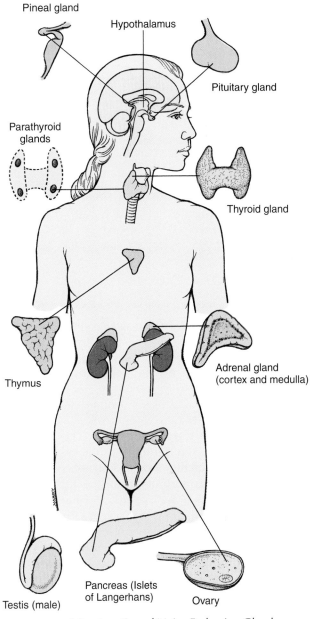

FIGURE 6.3. Location of Major Endocrine Glands

the *posterior* pituitary. The cell bodies of these neurons lie in the hypothalamus; the axons descend to the pituitary, transporting the hormones **vasopressin** and **oxytocin** from the cell body to the nerve endings. The hormones are released into the blood in the posterior pituitary.

Hypothalamic Hormones

The hypothalamus controls the secretion of pituitary hormones; numerous hypothalamic releasing and inhibiting hormones have been identified. Some stimulate while others inhibit the pituitary gland (see Table 6.1). With the pituitary, the hypothalamus gland has an important role in regulation of growth and devel-

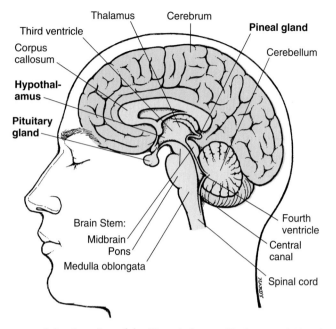

FIGURE **6.4.**   Location of the Hypothalamus, Pituitary, and Pineal Glands

opment, metabolism, and maintenance of homeostasis in the body.

The thyroid-stimulating hormone (TSH) (thyrotropin) of the pituitary is controlled by the **thyrotropin-releasing hormone** (TRH). The reproductive hormones of the pituitary—follicle-stimulating hormone (FSH) and luteinizing hormone (LH)—are controlled by the **gonadotropin-releasing hormone** (GnRH), also known as the luteinizing hormone-releasing hormone (LHRH). Prolactin, the pituitary hormone that regulates breast milk production, is controlled by **prolactin-inhibiting hormone** (PIH) and **prolactin-releasing hormone** (PRH). Growth hormone secretion by the pituitary is controlled by the **growth hormone-releasing hormone** (GH-RH) and **growth hormone-inhibiting hormone** (GH-IH), also

called somatostatin. The pituitary secretion of adrenocorticotropic hormone (ACTH) (corticotropin) is controlled by **corticotropin-releasing hormone** (CRH).

The Significance of the Control of the Pituitary Gland by the Hypothalamus

The control by the hypothalamus of the pituitary gland is one example of the regulation of the endocrine system by the nervous system—**neuroendocrine regulatory function** (see Figure 6.5 and the section on Stress, page 412). It highlights the integration between the two systems. The nervous system receives ongoing information about the conditions in the internal (inside the body) and external (outside the body) environments via the sensory organs. Based on this information, it brings about somatic movements and also adjusts the rate of hormone secretion.

For example, the nervous system (the hypothalamus and its nervous connections), based on the increasing number of daylight hours in spring, stimulates the gonads (testis and ovaries) of birds and mammals via GnRH and starts the breeding season. It is claimed that ovulation in Eskimo women ceases in winter and resumes in spring. In some other species, the sight of the male performing the mating dance increases GnRH production, ultimately resulting in ovulation. It is well known that emotion, stress, and travel can alter a woman's menstrual cycle.

Because the hypothalamus has so many major functions, hypothalamus problems can present in many ways, such as precocious puberty (early attainment of puberty), obesity, abnormalities of temperature control, anorexia, bulimia, and emaciation.

THE PITUITARY GLAND (HYPOPHYSIS)

The pituitary gland is a small, oval gland that lies in a bony recess called the sella turcica (Figure 3.12) in the

---

Table 6.1

The Hormones of the Hypothalamus, Anterior Pituitary, and Glands and Tissues Affected

Hypothalamus hormones	TRH	GnRH	PIH/PRH	GH-RH/GH-IH	CRH
Pituitary hormones	TSH	FSH and LH	Prolactin	Growth hormone	ACTH
Gland/ Tissue	Thyroid	Ovaries/ Testes	Breasts	Various tissues	Adrenal cortex

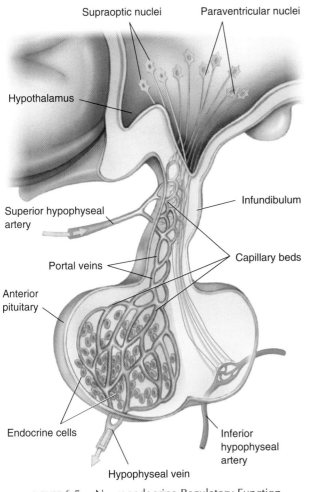

FIGURE 6.5. Neuroendocrine Regulatory Function

To Ponder:

Given the various functions of the hypothalamus, do you think that massage can affect the functioning of the hypothalamus in some way? If yes, how?

---

sphenoid bone at the base of the skull. The gland, which is about the size of four peas (1–1.5 cm or 0.39–0.59 in), lies inferior to the hypothalamus connected by nerves and blood vessels (Figure 6.5). The pituitary gland is divided into three lobes—**anterior, intermediate,** and **posterior.** Because each lobe secretes different hormones, the lobes can be considered as three separate endocrine organs that together secrete a total of 14 or more hormonally active substances.

Anterior Lobe (Adenohypophysis)

The anterior lobe is connected to the hypothalamus by special blood vessels known as the portal hypophyseal vessels. It secretes six established hormones—**TSH,**

ACTH, LH, FSH, prolactin, and **growth hormone.** The function of each of these hormones is self-explanatory. TSH controls thyroid gland secretions, ACTH controls the secretions of the adrenal cortex of the adrenal gland, LH affects the corpus luteum formation in the ovaries, and FSH affects ovarian follicle development. Note that LH and FSH also have an important role in male reproductive function. Prolactin is one of the hormones needed for milk production, and growth hormone, together with many other hormones, affects growth. In addition, the anterior pituitary also secretes **ß-lipotropin,** which contains the amino acid sequences of **endorphins** and **enkephalins (see page 399).**

Cells that secrete the hormones manufacture and store the hormones in vesicles. When stimulated, the cells secrete the stored hormones into the blood where they circulate throughout the body to reach the target organs.

Thyroid Stimulating Hormone (TSH) (Thyrotropin)

Alterations of the circulating levels of TSH regulate the secretion of hormones from the thyroid gland. TSH levels are, in turn, controlled by TRH of the hypothalamus (Table 6.1). By negative feedback mechanism, increasing levels of thyroid hormone in the circulation reduce TRH and TSH secretion (see Figure 6.6). Within a few hours of secretion, TSH is rapidly removed from circulation by the kidney and liver. Prolonged thyroid stimulation by TSH can result in an enlargement of the thyroid called a **goiter** (see Abnormalities of Thyroid Secretion). Abnormalities of TSH secretion by the pituitary can, therefore, present as hyposecretion or hypersecretion of the thyroid (see Thyroid Gland, page 401).

Adrenocorticotropic Hormone (ACTH)

The cells in the adrenal cortex that produce glucocorticoids have receptors for ACTH. Binding of ACTH to these receptors results in steroid synthesis. The level of steroids regulates ACTH secretion (see Figure 6.7)

 Pituitary Tumors

Tumors arising in the pituitary grow upward because the gland is surrounded by bone. As a result, the tumor presses on the optic chiasma, which is closely related to this region. One of the early symptoms is loss of vision.

Hormone hypersecretion by the pituitary gland can overstimulate the other endocrine glands it controls. For example, increased secretion resulting from tumors in the pituitary can cause the thyroid to secrete excessive thyroxine and produce symptoms of hyperthyroidism.

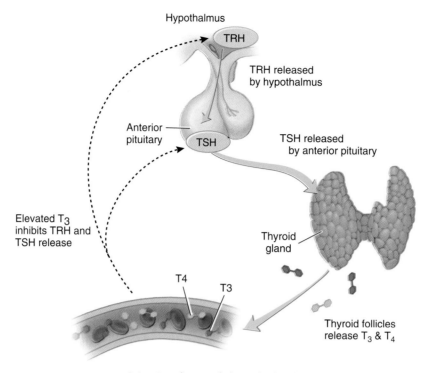

Hypothalamus

TRH

TRH released
by hypothalamus

Anterior
pituitary

TSH

TSH released
by anterior pituitary

Elevated T_3
inhibits TRH and
TSH release

Thyroid
gland

T4

T3

Thyroid follicles
release T_3 & T_4

FIGURE 6.6.   Regulation of Thyroid Gland Secretion

by negative feedback mechanism. (See page 403, Adrenal Cortex for the function of steroids.)

Luteinizing Hormone (LH) and Follicle-Stimulating Hormone (FSH)

LH stimulates ovulation and formation of corpus luteum from female ovarian follicles and stimulates male testosterone secretion. FSH stimulates the growth of female ovarian follicles and the formation of sperm (spermatogenesis) in males. Absence of pituitary hormones can result in atrophy of the testis and ovaries (see page 431 on menstrual cycle for more details).

Prolactin

Prolactin initiates and maintains breast milk secretion after the breasts have been primed by the hormones estrogen, progesterone, glucocorticoids, human growth hormone, thyroxine, and insulin. It also inhibits the effects of FSH and LH on the ovaries and is probably responsible for the slow onset of menstrual cycles in lactating women. Although prolactin is required for milk production, the *ejection* of milk is initiated by the hormone oxytocin. The role of prolactin in males is not fully understood.

Abnormal prolactin levels can result in milk production (**galactorrhea**), even in the absence of pregnancy and absence of menstruation (**amenorrhea**).

Hypersecretion of prolactin has been associated with impotence in men.

Growth Hormone

Growth hormone is a protein hormone that, as the name suggests, affects growth. It increases the formation of cartilage in bone and increases height in young children in whom the epiphysis is not fused. Other than affecting growth, this hormone increases glucose levels in blood and collagen formation.

The effects of growth hormone on growth, cartilage, and protein anabolism depend on its interaction with other **growth factors** (proteins) called **somatomedins** produced by the liver, skeletal muscle, cartilage, bone, and other tissues. A variety of growth factors have been identified, such as *insulinlike growth factor, nerve growth factor, epidermal growth factor, ovarian growth factor,* and *fibroblast growth factor* (depending on the tissue and organ they affect). Growth factors cause cells to grow and multiply by increasing the uptake of amino acids and decreasing the breakdown of proteins. Growth factors increase the breakdown of fat from adipose tissue; the fatty acids released are used for energy production. They decrease the uptake of glucose by cells, sparing glucose for utilization by nervous tissue. They also stimulate the release of glucose from the liver into the blood by the breakdown of liver glycogen.

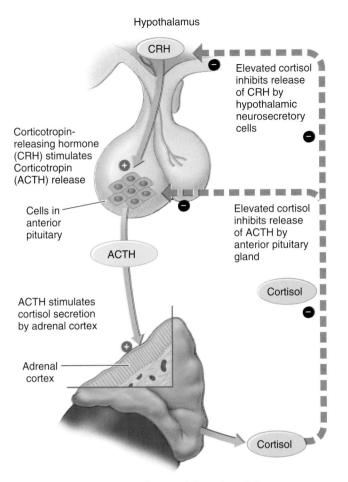

Hypothalamus

CRH

Elevated cortisol inhibits release of CRH by hypothalamic neurosecretory cells

Corticotropin-releasing hormone (CRH) stimulates Corticotropin (ACTH) release

Cells in anterior pituitary

ACTH

Elevated cortisol inhibits release of ACTH by anterior pituitary gland

Cortisol

ACTH stimulates cortisol secretion by adrenal cortex

Adrenal cortex

Cortisol

FIGURE **6.7.** Regulation of the Adrenal Cortex

Other than growth hormone, individual growth is affected by thyroid hormones, sex hormones, steroids, and insulin. Genetic factors and adequate nutrition also play an important role in growth.

Growth hormone secretion is primarily controlled by growth hormone-inhibiting hormone (GHIH) and growth hormone-releasing hormone (GHRH) of the hypothalamus, which are then regulated by glucose levels in the blood. Other factors also affect growth hormone secretion, such as levels of fatty and amino acids; increased activity of the sympathetic nervous system; and hormones, such as glucagon, insulin, estrogen, and cortisol.

Hormones and Growth

Normal growth requires the interaction of many hormones. Other than growth hormone, thyroid hormones, insulin, parathyroid hormone, vitamin D, and gonadal hormones (estrogens in females and androgens in males) are some important hormones required for growth.

Intermediate Lobe

The intermediate lobe is rudimentary in humans and appears to secrete hormones in insignificant levels. In humans, some of the cells migrate to the anterior pituitary and secrete the hormones **melanocyte-stimulating hormone** (MSH) and **endorphins.** The physiologic function of MSH in humans is not known; however, in lower animals, such as fish, reptiles and amphibians, it results in darkening of the skin. The darkening of the skin when these animals are placed in a dark background is another example of a neuroendocrine reflex, in which nerves from the eye alter endocrine secretions in accordance to the external environment.

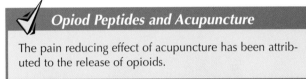

Opiod Peptides and Acupuncture

The pain reducing effect of acupuncture has been attributed to the release of opioids.

In mammals, treatment with MSH increases synthesis of melanin and darkens the skin of humans in 24 hours. Because ACTH has some MSH activity, abnormally high levels of ACTH can result in darkening of skin creases and other areas of the body.

Endorphins are small peptides found, in addition to the pituitary gland, in many parts of the body, including the nervous system. With other peptides—enkephalins and dynorphins—endorphins were identified when scientists discovered that brain cells had receptors for morphine, a synthetic painkiller. These peptides are thought to be the natural painkillers of the human body and are, therefore, known as opioid peptides or endogenous opioids. Two hundred times more potent than morphine as analgesics, these peptides have been linked to memory and learning, pleasure sensations, body temperature control, regulation of hormones that affect onset of puberty, sexual drive and reproduction, and disorders such as depression and schizophrenia.

Posterior Lobe (Neurohypophysis)

The posterior pituitary does not have its own secretory cells. Instead, it has the endings of axons whose cell bodies lie in the hypothalamus (Figure 6.4). These axons secrete **oxytocin** and **vasopressin** (antidiuretic hormone [ADH]) into the capillary network located in this region. The hormones secreted by the posterior pituitary are typically **neural hormones**—hormones secreted into the circulation by nerve endings.

Disorders Associated With Abnormalities of Growth Hormone Secretion

Hypersecretion

Abnormally high levels of growth hormone in children can lead to **gigantism** (see Figure). When the epiphysis of bones in adults are fused, abnormal increase in growth hormone leads to bone and soft tissue deformities, such as large hands and feet and protrusion of the lower jaw. This condition is known as **acromegaly** (see Figure).

Hyposecretion

In children, hyposecretion of growth hormone results in **dwarfism** (see Figure). The child is of short stature, with slow epiphyseal growth and larger than normal adipose tissue reserves. Normal growth can be restored by the administration of growth hormone.

   Presently, purified human growth hormone is being produced by genetically manipulated bacteria. Easy availability has led to many using growth hormone under questionable circumstances, such as for an "antiaging" product or to enhance growth in children who are short but otherwise healthy. Although growth hormone can slow the loss of bone and muscle mass that occurs with aging, the adverse effects that may result from long-term use in adults is not known. In children, although the child may grow faster, body fat content is drastically reduced and sexual maturation may be delayed.

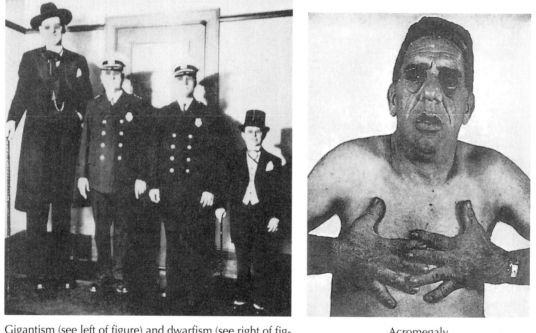

Gigantism (see left of figure) and dwarfism (see right of figure); two men of normal stature appear in between. Reproduced with permission from Thibodeau. Anatomy and Physiology. 3rd Ed. Mosby, 1996; p. 16. Thibodeau GA & Patton KT. Mosby-Yearbook Inc. St. Louis, MO.

Acromegaly

Oxytocin

The primary target organs of oxytocin are the uterus and breasts (see Figure 6.8). In mammals, nipple stimulation results in the generation of impulses in sensory nerves located in and around the nipples. These impulses communicate with the nerve cells in the hypothalamus that manufacture oxytocin. Oxytocin, released by the axons of these nerve cells into the capillaries in the posterior pituitary, is transported to the breasts where it stimulates contraction of smooth muscle cells. The smooth muscle cells (**myoepithelial cells**) located around the ducts of the breast contract and eject the milk that has already been produced. This is known as the **milk ejection reflex,** or **milk let-down reflex,** and is an example of a neuroendocrine reflex.

   In addition to its action on the breasts, oxytocin causes contraction of the smooth muscle of the uterus. In late pregnancy, the uterus becomes more sensitive to oxytocin as a result of an increase of oxytocin receptors on the smooth muscle cells (up-regulation). Stretching of the cervix by the descending fetus results in an increase in impulses in the sensory nerves located in this region. These sensory nerves communicate with the hypothalamus and increase production of oxytocin. During labor, as the fetus further dilates

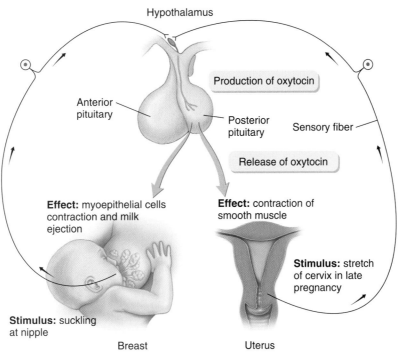

FIGURE **6.8.**   Regulation and Effect of Oxytocin

the cervix, further increase in oxytocin levels result, producing strong contractions of the uterus. This continues until the fetus is expelled and is one of the few situations in the body where positive feedback occurs. Oxytocin, however, is not the only hormone or mechanism involved in labor.

Oxytocin may also play a part in the transport of sperm up the reproductive tract at intercourse and the feeling of sexual pleasure during and after intercourse. In men, oxytocin stimulates the contraction of the vas deferens and the prostate glands before ejaculation occurs. In animal experiments, this hormone has been linked to parental bonding with offspring.

Vasopressin or Antidiuretic Hormone (ADH)

A major function of vasopressin is to conserve water by acting on the kidney; hence, the name antidiuretic hormone. Vasopressin acts on the collecting ducts of the kidney (see page 613), making them more permeable to water. The water moves into the interstitial region from the ducts, reducing urine volume and increasing urine concentration. In the absence of vasopressin, more dilute urine is formed. ADH also decreases the loss of water through sweat.

Vasopressin in large doses causes contraction of the smooth muscle of the arterial walls and a rise in blood pressure. This regulatory mechanism is particularly useful when blood pressure drops after hemorrhage. Circulating vasopressin is rapidly removed by

the kidneys and the liver; the half-life of vasopressin is about 18 minutes.

Vasopressin secretion is triggered by stimulation of **osmoreceptors** located in the hypothalamus. These receptors respond to changes in osmotic pressure in the blood. When the osmotic pressure in plasma is increased, the extracellular fluid volume is decreased, as a result, vasopressin levels increase to reverse the situation (see Figure 6.9).

THE THYROID GLAND

The thyroid is a butterfly-shaped gland located in the anterior aspect of the neck, inferior to the larynx (see

---

✚ Abnormalities of Vasopressin (ADH) Secretion

If vasopressin is deficient, **diabetes insipidus** (*diabetes,* overflow; *insipidus,* tasteless) results. Diabetes insipidus may result from hyposecretion of ADH from the pituitary (neurogenic diabetes insipidus) or reduced response of the kidney to ADH (nephrogenic diabetes insipidus). The symptoms include **polydipsia** (excessive thirst) and **polyuria** (passage of large amounts of dilute urine). Urine output increases tremendously—to as much as 20 liters (normal, 1–2 liters). Dehydration is another symptom of diabetes insipidus and may cause death if a person with this condition is deprived of water even for a day or so.

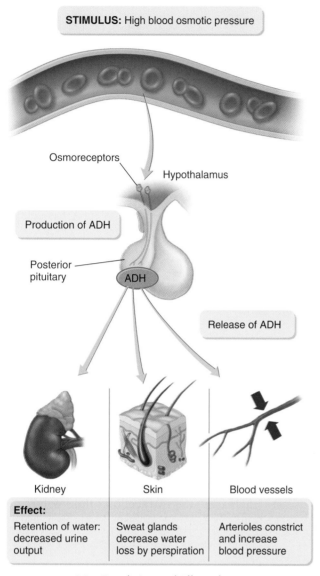

FIGURE **6.9.**   Regulation and Effect of Vasopressin

Figure 6.10). It covers the second to fourth tracheal rings and is surrounded by a capsule. Posteriorly, the capsule encloses the four, small parathyroid glands (discussed later). The thyroid has two lobes located on either side of the trachea. The gland becomes visible when it is enlarged.

The thyroid's main function is to maintain the metabolism level in the body. Therefore, the thyroid is needed to regulate lipid and carbohydrate metabolism and for normal growth and function. The formation and secretion of thyroid hormones is controlled by thyroid-stimulating hormone (TSH) from the pituitary. TSH levels are, in turn, regulated by the thyroid hormone levels by negative feedback mechanism. TSH secretion is also regulated by the releasing hormone secreted by the hypothalamus (Figure 6.6). When TSH levels are reduced in the plasma, the thy-

roid gland atrophies and its function is depressed. If TSH stimulation is prolonged, the thyroid gland enlarges and hypertrophies, forming a **goiter** (see box on page 405).

The principal hormones secreted by the thyroid are **thyroxine** (T_4), **triiodothyronine** (T_3), and **calcitonin.**

Iodine is required for the formation of T_3 and T_4, and iodine from the plasma is actively absorbed by thyroid gland. The hormones are manufactured by the cells that line spherical sacs **(thyroid follicles)** and stored in the follicles in the form of a colloid **(thyroglobulin).** The thyroid gland is the only endocrine gland that stores large quantities of hormones. When required, the hormones are secreted into the blood where most of them are transported bound to plasma proteins. It takes many days for thyroid hormones to be removed from the circulation by the liver, kidneys, and other tissues. Most of the iodine from the hormones is recycled and reused for forming the hormones.

The main hormone action is to increase oxygen consumption (increase metabolism) by most of the cells, with the exception of the brain, uterus, testis, lymph nodes, spleen, and anterior pituitary. They also affect growth and development. Thyroid hormones increase the metabolic rate by stimulating cells to use oxygen to form ATP. When ATP is produced, heat is produced and body temperature increases **(calorigenic effect** of the thyroid). Other effects include an increase in protein synthesis, a breakdown of carbohydrates and fat, and excretion of cholesterol. In addition, thyroid hormones enhance the action of adrenaline and noradrenaline. Together with other hormones, such as growth hormone and insulin, thyroid hormones speed growth of the body, especially nervous tissue. The actions of these hormones can be better illustrated by studying individuals with hyperthyroidism and hypothyroidism **(see Abnormalities of Thyroid Secretion on page 404).**

Calcitonin

Calcitonin is a hormone secreted by cells that lie between or outside the follicles. It causes an increase in the deposition of calcium and phosphates in bones by reducing resorption and facilitating deposition **(see page 91).** This is accomplished by inhibiting the action of osteoclasts. As a result of the bone-building effect of calcitonin, it is used to treat osteoporosis.

PARATHYROID GLANDS

The four, tiny, parathyroid glands are embedded in the posterior aspect of the thyroid gland (see Figure 6.10). **Parathormone** or **parathyroid hormone** (PTH) is se-

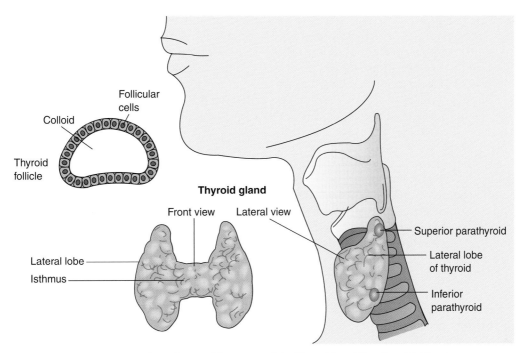

FIGURE **6.10.**   Location and Structure of the Thyroid and Parathyroid Glands

creted by the parathyroid glands. This hormone plays an important role in calcium metabolism.

The net effect of parathormone is to increase calcium levels in the blood by increasing absorption of calcium from the gut and the bones and reducing calcium excretion in the urine. An increase in bone resorption is a result of stimulating osteoclastic activity (**see page 89**). Parathormone also stimulates vitamin D (another hormone that participates in calcium metabolism) formation in the kidney.

Abnormalities of Parathormone Secretion

Excessive secretion of parathyroid hormone, as may happen in tumor formation, causes demineralization and the resultant weakening of bones and a tendency to form kidney stones.

Hypoparathyroidism leads to lower blood levels of calcium. As a result, neurons and muscles spontaneously depolarize, leading to muscle twitching and spasm. This condition is called **tetany.** If inadvertently removed during thyroid gland surgery, it can result in a sudden drop in blood calcium levels, cessation of respiratory muscle contraction, and death.

ADRENAL GLANDS

The paired adrenal glands are located on the superior and medial aspects of the kidney, similar to pyramid-shaped cap. As a result of their anatomic location, they are also known as **suprarenal glands.** They are found at the level of the twelfth rib, or T_{11}–T_{12} vertebral levels, and are firmly attached to the kidney by a thick connective tissue capsule that surrounds them. The adrenal glands are in close contact with the diaphragm (superiorly) and large arteries and veins (medially). Anteriorly, the adrenal glands are covered by the parietal peritoneum and are, therefore, considered to be retroperitoneal. As with other endocrine glands, they have a rich blood supply.

The adrenal gland is actually a compilation of two separate endocrine glands—the outer **adrenal cortex** and the inner **adrenal medulla** (see Figure 6.11).

Adrenal Cortex

Essential for life, the outer adrenal cortex secretes hormones that have widespread effects of carbohydrate, protein, and fat metabolism and in electrolyte balance. More than 24 hormones, collectively known as **adrenocortical steroids** or **corticosteroids,** are secreted. However, only a few are secreted in physiologically significant amounts. The adrenal cortex is considered to have three zones. The outer zone—**zona glomerulosa**—secretes **mineralocorticoids,** of which **aldosterone** is principal. As the name suggests, the mineralocorticoids have a major effect on the levels of minerals, such as sodium and potassium, in the body fluids. The middle zone, or **zona fasciculata,** secretes **glucocorticoids.** These hormones affect glucose metabolism. The principal glucocorticoids are cortisol (hydrocortisone), cortisone, and corticosterone. The innermost zone of the cortex is the **zona reticularis,** which secretes small quantities of **androgens,** or **sex hormones.** The principal hormones are dehydroepiandrosterone and androstenedione.

All of the steroids in the adrenal cortex are derived from cholesterol. By the action of various enzymes located here, cholesterol is converted to the respective hormones through complex chemical reactions. Congenital absence of certain enzymes can lead to abnormalities and accumulation of precursors, as the chemical reactions cannot proceed beyond a certain point. To understand the signs and symptoms that accompany adrenal cortex malfunction, it should be understood that all steroids share the functions of others. For example, mineralocorticoid, although its major function is electrolyte balance, also has some glucocorticoid and androgenic functions. Similarly, glucocorticoids have some mineralocorticoid and androgenic function.

Mineralocorticoids

The target organ of aldosterone is the kidney. Aldosterone reduces the excretion of sodium in the urine by stimulating reabsorption from the kidney tubules into blood. Water is reabsorbed by osmosis along with sodium. Potassium, however, is lost in exchange for sodium. Thus, aldosterone is important in conserving

Abnormalities of Thyroid Secretion

Problems related to the thyroid may be a result of various causes. Problems with the feedback control of thyroid secretion can play a role. Thyroid abnormalities may develop as a result of hypothalamus malfunctioning (TRH secretion), pituitary secretion (TSH), or changes in the availability of iodine. Thyroid problems can be a result of autoimmune reactions. Antibodies may be formed against the thyroid and either hyperthyroidism or hypothyroidism may result.

Hyperthyroidism
In hyperthyroidism, if food intake is not increased as the metabolic rate is increased, the body's protein and fat stores are used up and the person loses weight. There is associated muscle weakness, partly the result of the breakdown of muscle protein. However, the muscles react more vigorously with increased hormones. Hyperthyroidism is associated with a fine muscle tremor caused by the increased sensitivity of the nerves that control muscle tone.

As a result of the increase in metabolic rate, more heat is produced and there is a rise in body temperature. This triggers the body mechanisms that regulate heat. The blood vessels in the periphery dilate to dissipate heat, there is increased sweating, and the person becomes intolerant to heat—all typical signs of hyperthyroidism. There is also a rise in heart rate and cardiac output, partly as a result of its effect on increasing the sensitivity of the heart to adrenaline and noradrenaline.

The effect on metabolism raises the vitamin requirements; vitamin deficiency is often associated with hyperthyroidism. Although thyroid hormones do not increase the metabolism of the uterus, they are required for normal functioning of the reproductive system. Menstrual irregularities are associated with thyroid abnormalities. Excessive thyroid hormones make the person irritable and restless. In short, the signs and symptoms of hyperthyroidism or thyrotoxicosis are that of overactivity of the sympathetic nervous system—anxiety, nervousness, rapid heart rate, sweating, tremor, and diarrhea.

Sometimes the metabolic rate of the hyperthyroid individual accelerates out of control and the person has a rapid heart rate, high fever, and other symptoms of high metabolism. This situation is termed **thyrotoxic crisis** or **thyroid storm** and requires immediate medical intervention.

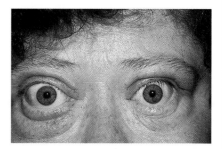

Grave's Disease (note exophthalmos)

Graves' Disease
Graves' disease is a thyroid gland disorder in which excessive thyroid hormones are produced. Its cause is believed to be a result of autoimmunity. All hyperthyroidism symptoms, together with protrusion of the eyes (**exophthalmos**) (see Figure) are observed. Exophthalmos may be caused by swelling of the eye muscles within the bony orbit or inflammatory reactions caused by accumulation of immune complexes, connective tissue and fluid behind the eye.

Hypothyroidism
Conversely, if the thyroid hormones are decreased, a variety of proteins and polysaccharides tend to accumulate in the skin. The body retains water and gives the individual a puffy appearance (**myxedema**) (see Figure). Metabolism is lowered and the person is lethargic, with a reduced heart rate and intolerance to cold. Thyroid hormones have a significant effect on brain development in young adults. Synapses in the brain are formed abnormally, with defective myelination. Deficiency of thyroid hormones in young newborns and children results in short stature and mental retardation (**cretinism**) (see Figure). Muscle weakness, cramps and stiffness are often seen in individuals with hypothyroidism.

⊕ Abnormalities of Thyroid Secretion—cont'd

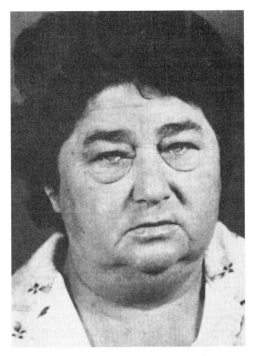

Hypothyroidism in an Adult (myxedema)

To avoid situations in which thyroid swelling is a result of iodine deficiency (iodine deficiency goiter) (see Figure), iodide is added to table salt. Individuals with hyperthyroidism are treated with antithyroid drugs, which work by affecting the enzymes required for forming the thyroid hormones. In severe cases, radioactive iodine may be given to destroy thyroid tissue or surgery may be performed. Naturally occurring antithyroid agents exist in such foods as cabbages, turnips, and rutabagas. If ingested in large quantities, the levels may be sufficient to reduce hormone production and goiter formation.

Goiter

Goiter (see Figure) is the term given to denote enlargement of the thyroid gland. It may be associated with hyperthyroid, hypothyroid, or euthyroid states. Usually, enlargement is a result of excessive TSH secretion or proteins that resemble TSH. At times, the goiter may be a result of benign or malignant tumors.

Endemic goiter is the result of chronic iodine deficiency in the diet. It occurs mainly in inland mountainous regions, such as the Alps, Andes, and Himalayas and inland regions of Asia and Africa, away from coastal waters or where there is reduced iodine in the soil. With the routine addition of iodine to table salt, endemic goiter incidence has reduced.

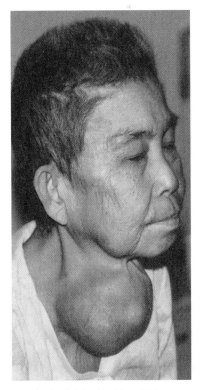

An Individual With a Goiter

Cretinism (left). A normal child of the same age (right). Reproduced with permission from Wilkins. Clinical Endocrinology I. Grune & Statton, 1960.

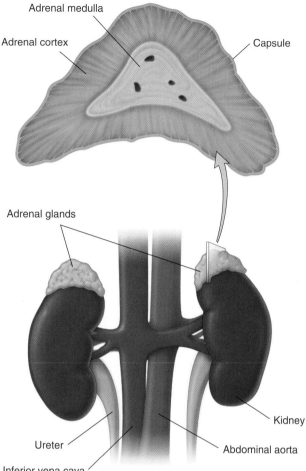

Adrenal medulla

Adrenal cortex

Capsule

Adrenal glands

Kidney

Ureter

Abdominal aorta

Inferior vena cava

FIGURE 6.11.   Location and Structure of the Adrenal Glands

a number of metabolic reactions. They are also required for vascular smooth muscles to respond normally to sympathetic stimulation. They have an anti-insulin effect and increase the level of glucose in the blood and reduce the uptake of glucose by all tissue other than the brain and the heart.

Another powerful effect of glucocorticoids is the anti-inflammatory effect. Glucocorticoids inhibit the activities of white blood cells and other components of the immune system. Lymph nodes and the thymus are atrophied. They reduce the rate of white cell migration into injured areas and prevent mast cells from releasing products, such as histamine, that are responsible for inflammation. As a result of this steroid effect, synthetic steroids are often used to reduce inflammation, especially in chronic inflammatory conditions; for allergies; and to reduce adhesions. Steroids are, therefore, used as ointments, eyedrops, tablets, and injections. However, steroids slow the healing of wounds by inhibiting fibroblastic activity. Because they retard the immune system and lower defenses, the incidence of infection is increased in individuals on steroids.

Other glucocorticoid effects include effects on the nervous system. Glucocorticoid deficiency results in personality changes, such as irritability, apprehension, and the inability to concentrate. Glucocorticoids, like mineralocorticoids, cause retention of sodium and water.

Androgens

Androgens liberated by the adrenal cortex exert a masculinization effect. They promote growth and protein formation. These androgens are less potent than testosterone, the androgenic hormone secreted by the testis. In adult men, excess androgens accentuate the male characteristics; however, in young boys, it can cause premature development of male

salt and water. Aldosterone is particularly important when the extracellular fluid volume is reduced and the blood pressure drops, as in dehydration. Apart from its effect on the kidneys, aldosterone reduces sodium and water loss via sweat glands, salivary glands, and the digestive tract. The hormone angiotensin II stimulates aldosterone secretion (see page 411).

Glucocorticoids

Glucocorticoid secretion is stimulated by ACTH from the pituitary. ACTH is regulated by CRH from the hypothalamus. By negative feedback, glucocorticoids alter the levels of ACTH and CRH.

Glucocorticoids have a glucose-sparing effect (i.e., they increase the formation of glucose and glycogen). Fatty acids and proteins are used for metabolism instead of glucose. Adipose tissue is broken down and fatty acids are released into the circulation. In the absence of glucocorticoids, water, carbohydrate, protein, and fat metabolism are abnormal and exposure to even minor stresses can result in collapse of the individual and death. Glucocorticoids are required for

Abnormalities of Mineralocorticoid Secretion

The secretion of aldosterone is sometimes reduced (**hypoaldosteronism**) as a result of low angiotensin II levels. This produces loss of excessive sodium and water in urine associated with low blood volume and low blood pressure. Because sodium is required for normal impulse conduction in the nervous and muscular tissues, these tissues are also affected.

Conversely, if there is excessive secretion of aldosterone (**aldosteronism**), there is sodium and water retention with loss of potassium in the urine and increased blood volume and blood pressure. The loss of potassium can present as muscle weakness and cardiac and kidney problems.

✚ Abnormalities of Adrenal Cortex Secretion

Glucocorticoid actions can be fully studied in individuals with high systemic levels of steroids. This condition is known as **Cushing's syndrome** (see Figure). Conditions which produce excessive glucocorticoid as a result of excessive ACTH secretion are known as **Cushing's disease.** As a result of excess protein breakdown, the individuals are protein depleted. The skin and subcutaneous tissue are thin and muscles are poorly developed. Wounds heal slowly, and the skin bruises easily. As a result of the androgenic effects of glucocorticoids, as well as the accompanying increase in adrenal androgen secretion, females often tend to grow facial hair and have acne. Body fat is characteristically distributed in the trunk (truncal obesity), the back of the neck (buffalo hump), and around the face (moon face). As a result of the anti-insulin effect of steroids, individuals on steroids tend to develop diabetes mellitus.

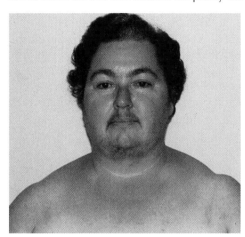

A Female With Cushing's Syndrome

Bone formation is reduced and resorption is increased, resulting in osteoporosis. Its effect on the nervous system can result in lack of sleep and other mental disorders.

Adrenocortical insufficiency is called **Addison's disease.**

At times, there is excessive androgen secretion. This condition is known as **adrenogenital syndrome.** In females, significant physical changes occur. The clitoris enlarges and resembles a penis. The hair distribution changes to resemble that of a male, with growth of beard, and the voice deepens. Deposition of proteins in the skin and muscle gives a typical masculine appearance (see Figure). If this occurs in boys before puberty, there is rapid development of the male sexual organs and creation of male sexual desires.

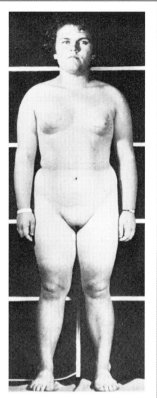

A Female Patient With Adrenogenital Syndrome

---

sexual characteristics such as growth of beard, pubic, and axillary hair and external genitalia (**adrenogenital syndrome**). In females, facial hair, baldness, receding hairline, small breasts, heavy arms and legs, and enlarged clitoris are some of the findings.

Adrenal Medulla

The adrenal medulla is actually a sympathetic ganglion. Axons of the sympathetic neurons (preganglionic fibers) from the T_5–T_{10} level of the spinal cord end in the adrenal medulla, where they synapse with the cells that secrete **adrenaline** (epinephrine), **noradrenaline** (norepinephrine), and **dopamine.** These hormones are not essential for life, but they prepare an individual to face emergency situations. Together, the three hormones are known as **catecholamines** because of their biochemical makeup. During an emergency when the sympathetic nervous system is stimulated, the preganglionic nerves to the adrenal medulla stimulate the medullary cells to secrete the hormones into the circulation. Because the effects of the hormones are similar to sympathetic stimulation, the hormones are said to be **sympathomimetic.**

These hormones have many actions: They increase the breakdown of glycogen from the liver and skele-

tal muscle and mobilize free fatty acids, making glucose and fatty acids available to tissue. They increase the metabolic rate, increase the rate and force of the contraction of the heart and, thereby, the blood pressure. They increase the blood flow to the heart, liver, and skeletal muscles and also dilate the bronchi. They increase the alertness of the individual. In short, they are largely responsible for the fight-or-flight response.

PINEAL GLAND

The pineal gland is located in the posterior portion of the roof of the third ventricle in the middle of the brain (Figure 6.4). It was originally thought to be the

✚ Abnormalities of Adrenal Medullary Secretion

Rarely, tumors called **pheochromocytoma** develop in the adrenal medulla. There is intermittent release of large quantities of adrenaline into the circulation, with development of intermittent fight-or-flight response. Rapid and irregular heart rate, high blood pressure, sweating, headache, and blurred vision are observed.

seat of the soul. This gland secretes **melatonin,** a hormone that is derived from serotonin (a modified amino acid, also known as 5-hydroxytryptamine). Shown to have connections with neurons from the eye, the pineal gland is believed to function as a timing device that keeps internal events synchronized with the light-dark cycle of the environment. Melatonin levels are increased during the night and reduced during the daylight. The fluctuation in the levels is believed to be responsible for sleep and many other actions, which are still obscure.

It is thought that melatonin participates in determining the onset of puberty by reducing the secretion of GnRH from the hypothalamus. Melatonin may be involved in the daily changes in physiologic processes that follow a regular pattern.

ENDOCRINE FUNCTION OF THE PANCREAS

The pancreas (see **Chapter 11**) has both exocrine and endocrine functions. While the exocrine function produces enzymes secreted into the gut to help with digestion, the endocrine function secretes hormones into the circulation. Specialized cells, known as the **islets of Langerhans** or **pancreatic islets,** are scattered throughout the pancreas and secrete at least 4 peptides with hormonal activity. There are four types of cells in the islets, each secreting a different hormone. Two of the hormones, **insulin** (secreted by the beta or B cells) and **glucagon** (secreted by the alpha or A cells), are involved with the regulation of carbohydrates, proteins, and fat metabolism. The third, **somatostatin** (secreted by delta or D cells), plays a role in regulating the secretions by the islets. The function of the fourth, **pancreatic polypeptide** (secreted by F cells), is still not settled.

Light and Behavior

Light and dark cycles have many effects on the central nervous system. One condition associated with changes in light exposure is **Seasonal Affective Disorder** (SAD). Seasonal affective disorder is a periodic major depression that manifests at specific seasons. Studies show that some people in the Northern Hemisphere experience swings in moods and activity according to seasons, feeling most energetic from June to September and least energetic from December to March. The opposite effects are observed in those living in the Southern Hemisphere. SAD has been linked to fluctuating levels of melatonin as a result of melatonin secretion being regulated by sunlight. Exposure to sunlamps emitting a full spectrum of light is a successful treatment option.

Insulin

Insulin is anabolic in that it increases the storage of glucose, fatty acids, and amino acids. It is known, therefore, as the "hormone of abundance." The target cells for insulin have specific receptors on the cell membrane that bind to insulin. The number of receptors and their affinity for insulin are affected by such factors as exercise, food, other hormones, and plasma insulin levels. Exposure to increased insulin decreases the receptor concentration and the affinity of the receptors for insulin and exposure to less insulin has the reverse effect. The number of receptors increases in starvation and decreases in obesity; thus, the cells adapt to the plasma levels.

Effects of Insulin

The actions of insulin are complex. Insulin increases the storage of carbohydrates, proteins, and fats. Its actions can be conveniently divided into rapid actions (within seconds), intermediate actions (within minutes), and delayed actions (within hours). Insulin rapidly increases glucose uptake by almost all tissue. The glucose that enters the cells is rapidly converted into storage forms. Insulin speeds the uptake by increasing the number of glucose transporters (proteins that transport glucose) in the cell membrane.

The intermediate actions of insulin include stimulation of protein synthesis and inhibition of degradation of proteins. Within hours, insulin causes an increase in the manufacture of enzymes required for the various metabolic processes. Insulin also increases the uptake of amino acids by cells and speeds protein synthesis. Formation of fat from fatty acids (lipogenesis) is also accelerated.

Regulation of Insulin Secretion

The primary stimulus for insulin secretion is an increase in blood glucose levels. In addition, insulin secretion is stimulated by acetylcholine (a neurotransmitter secreted by parasympathetic nerves), glucagon, hormones from the gastrointestinal tract that are released when there is digestion and absorption of proteins and carbohydrates, among others. The control of secretion of insulin and glucagon are closely related.

Glucagon

Glucagon is secreted by the A cells of the pancreas. This hormone increases glucose output from the liver and increases breakdown of lipids and formation of glucose from amino acids, increasing the blood glucose level. Glucagon secretion is increased by many

✚ Disorders of Insulin Secretion

Diabetes Mellitus

Insulin deficiency or **diabetes mellitus** (*diabetes,* overflow; *mellitus,* honey sweetened) is a common and serious pathologic condition. The term diabetes refers to conditions where the urine volume is increased. Two conditions—diabetes mellitus, in which the urine tastes sweet and diabetes insipidus, in which the urine is tasteless—were identified by early Greek and Roman physicians. While the former refers to insulin deficiency, the latter refers to a deficiency of antidiuretic hormone (ADH) (vasopressin) from the posterior pituitary. Today, the term diabetes is a synonym for diabetes mellitus. There are two types of diabetes—**type I** (insulin-dependent diabetes; juvenile diabetes) and **type II** (non-insulin-dependent diabetes; maturity-onset diabetes).

Signs and Symptoms

Diabetes mellitus is characterized by *polyuria* (increased urine), *polydipsia* (thirst), and *polyphagia* (hunger). As a result of the reduced entry of glucose into cells and increased liberation of glucose into the circulation by the liver, plasma glucose levels are increased while glucose levels are decreased intracellularly—literally "starvation in the midst of plenty." Protein entry into muscle is also decreased and breakdown of fat is increased.

The glucose levels in diabetes increase significantly, especially after meals. It also takes a longer time for the glucose levels to reach normal levels (if at all) as compared with a person without diabetes.

The oral glucose tolerance test, which monitors changes in plasma glucose levels after intake of glucose, is used for diagnosis. Normally, the fasting plasma glucose level is 115 mg/dL and the level of glucose 2 hours after ingestion of 75 grams of glucose is less than 140 mg/dL. Diabetes is said to be present if the 2-hour value and one other value are more than 200 mg/dL (see Figure). In a normal person, all the glucose filtered by the glomeruli of the kidney is reabsorbed without loss of glucose in the urine. In patients with diabetes, when the plasma glucose levels are high, the kidney is unable to reabsorb all the filtered glucose. This glucose is, therefore, lost in the urine (*glycosuria*). Because glucose is osmotically active, it draws water into the kidney tubules and large volumes of urine results (*polyuria*). Loss of water leads to dehydration and thirst (*polydipsia*). As a result of glucose loss in the urine, the person always feels hungry and the intake of food is increased (*polyphagia*).

The protein and fat inside the cells are broken down for energy. Protein depletion leads to wasting and poor resistance to infection. In addition, microorganisms thrive in the sugar-rich body fluids. Wound healing is also slow. The increase in fat catabolism results in accumulation of breakdown products, such as acetoacetate and β-hydroxybutyrate (together known as **ketone bodies**). These products make the plasma acidic and, if levels are high, it can lead to unconsciousness. Thus, both hypoglycemia and chronic hyperglycemia can lead to unconsciousness (coma) and death.

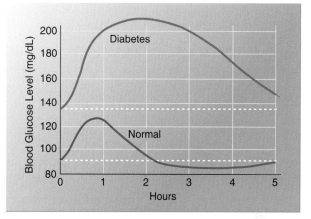

Glucose Tolerance Test. The graph shows glucose blood level changes with time

In diabetes, plasma cholesterol levels are also elevated and individuals with diabetes are prone to hypertension and other cardiovascular problems. Diabetes can produce complications in almost all body systems. The retina of the eye can be affected, leading to blindness. Effects on the kidney can lead ultimately to kidney failure. The function of nerves, especially those of the autonomic nervous system, can lead to various dysfunctions. By speeding the development of atherosclerosis—thickening of the blood vessels—blood flow can be affected, leading to formation of chronic ulcers and gangrene (particularly in the leg). Foot ulcers are common in patients with diabetes. Ulcers may become so severe that amputation may be required. Lesions are mainly a result of the reduced blood supply, impaired pain sensation, and slow healing that complicates diabetes.

The incidence of stroke and myocardial infarction (heart attack) is higher in patients with diabetes as a result of atherosclerosis development.

Diabetes is sometimes seen during pregnancy and is referred to as **gestational diabetes.** Mothers with gestational diabetes are at higher risk for complications of pregnancy and fetal death and abnormalities.

Continued

✚ Disorders of Insulin Secretion—cont'd

Insulin Excess

Hypoglycemia, or decrease in the plasma level of glucose, is the major biochemical change that occurs with insulin excess. The symptoms are a result of the effect of hypoglycemia in the brain. The brain uses glucose in appreciable quantities for metabolism. It does not have much reserve and, therefore, has to be supplied with glucose on a continual basis. The areas of the brain, such as the cortex whose metabolic rate is high, are affected first when glucose levels drop. The early symptoms are dizziness, irritability, personality changes, confusion, headache, weakness, and hunger. Soon, the person has convulsions and goes into a coma. If hypoglycemia is prolonged, irreversible changes occur in the brain. Because hypoglycemia is a potent stimulus for the sympathetic system, increasing levels of adrenaline and noradrenaline produce excessive sweating, pallor, tremors, palpitations, and nervousness. It is, therefore, important for glucose to be administered immediately.

Signs and symptoms of hypoglycemia can be easily precipitated in individuals with diabetes if they have not eaten enough food, have increased the dosage of antidiabetic drugs or insulin, or exercised more than usual.

Insulin levels in the blood are regulated by many factors. The major control is negative feedback by plasma glucose levels. Many hormones secreted in the gut play a part in regulating insulin levels. In addition, sympathetic stimulation increases insulin secretion. Many drugs given for diabetes act by stimulating islet cells to secrete insulin. Individuals in whom islet cell response is inadequate are given insulin injections.

The entry of glucose into skeletal muscle is increased by exercise. Exercise also increases the affinity of the insulin receptors in muscle and the rate of absorption of injected insulin. That is why exercise can precipitate hypoglycemia in a person being treated with insulin. It is important for diabetic individuals on insulin to reduce the insulin dose and/or increase their food intake when they exercise.

---

factors, including sympathetic stimulation, exercise, infection, and stress. Decreased secretion occurs when the blood glucose levels increase or when insulin secretion is stimulated.

Somatostatin

This hormone is secreted by D cells of pancreatic islets. Somatostatin serves to regulate the secretion of hormones from other pancreatic cells. Somatostatin inhibits the secretion of both insulin and glucagon and reduces the absorption of nutrients from the gut.

Pancreatic Polypeptide

The exact function of this hormone is unknown. It has been shown to slow down the secretion of pancreatic digestive enzymes and absorption of food in humans.

TESTIS, OVARIES, AND PLACENTA

Please refer to **page 393** for details of hormones secreted by the testis, ovaries, and placenta.

THE ENDOCRINE FUNCTION OF THE KIDNEYS

The kidneys secrete three hormones—**calcitriol, erythropoietin,** and **renin.** Calcitriol is important in calcium ion homeostasis; the other two hormones are involved in the regulation of red blood cell formation, blood pressure, and blood volume.

Calcitriol

Calcitriol is a steroidal hormone secreted in response to parathyroid hormone. Calcitriol is formed from a precursor vitamin D_3 or cholecalciferol, which is absorbed from the diet or formed in the skin. In the skin, cholecalciferol is formed from 7-dehydrocholesterol by the action of sunlight. Cholecalciferol is absorbed from skin and the diet and is transported to the liver by the blood where it is converted into an intermediate product and released into the circulation. This intermediate product is converted by the kidneys into calcitriol. Vitamin D indicates this entire group of steroids—calcitriol, cholecalciferol, and the intermediate product (**see Chapter 2, Integumentary System for more details**).

Vitamin D production is modified mainly by changing levels of calcium and phosphates in the plasma.

Erythropoietin

Erythropoietin is the hormone responsible for maintaining normal hemoglobin levels. When a person bleeds heavily or if the oxygen levels in the blood are reduced, the hemoglobin synthesis and production of red blood cells by the bone marrow is enhanced. Conversely, if the hemoglobin level is increased by blood transfusion, the body adapts by reducing the production of hemoglobin. These responses are a result of the hormone erythropoietin.

Renin

The action of renin is to convert the peptide angiotensinogen present in the plasma into angiotensin I. Angiotensinogen is manufactured in the liver and secreted into the plasma. Angiotensin I is converted into a more active form—angiotensin II—by enzymes located in the endothelium of blood vessels. This conversion mainly occurs in the lungs as the blood passes through.

$$\text{Angiotensinogen} \xrightarrow{renin} \text{Angiotensin I} \xrightarrow{lungs} \text{Angiotensin II} \rightarrow \text{vasoconstriction}$$

Angiotensin II is a potent hormone that produces constriction of arterioles, with a rapid increase in blood pressure. In addition, it stimulates the production of aldosterone from the adrenal cortex, stimulates the brain to directly increase blood pressure, and increases water intake—all measures toward maintaining blood pressure and volume.

Renin is produced by cells located in the afferent arterioles of the kidney. Secretion by these cells is triggered by falling pressure in the arterioles (as in hypotension and hemorrhage). Rising levels of angiotensin II have a negative feedback effect on these secretory cells.

THE ENDOCRINE FUNCTION OF THE HEART

The cells of the atria of the heart contain secretory granules that secrete a hormone called **atrial natriuretic peptide** (ANP) and is released when the plasma sodium level is increased and/or the volume of the extracellular fluid is increased. The target organ of this hormone is the kidney, where it promotes sodium excretion (the opposite effect of aldosterone), lowers the blood pressure, and reduces the sensitivity of smooth muscles of blood vessels to vasoconstrictor substances. It also reduces the secretion of vasopressin. ANP secretion is increased directly by stretch of the atrial wall.

THYMUS

The thymus gland is described further under the lymphatic system (**see Chapter 9**). This gland is located posterior to the sternum, in the mediastinum. It is large in infants and children; however, it reduces in size after puberty. The thymus is important for immunity and contains lymphocytes in various stages of development. Lymphocytes processed in the thymus, known as T lymphocytes, migrate to various parts of the body.

The gland is considered to have endocrine function because it secretes many hormones (**thymosins**) that stimulate the synthesis and development of lymphocytes.

DIGESTIVE TRACT

Numerous hormones secreted by the digestive tract control smooth muscle activity and secretions in the digestive tract. For example, the hormone **gastrin** is secreted by the stomach when peptides and amino acids are present in the chyme. This results in increased gastric secretion and motility. Similarly, the arrival of lipids and carbohydrates in the duodenum stimulates secretion of the hormone **cholecystokinin** (CCK) and **gastric inhibitory peptide** (GIP). Both hormones slow the motility of the stomach and gastric secretion to allow more time for lipids to be digested and absorbed in the intestines. Many such hormones have been identified in the digestive tract. Please refer to more advanced textbooks for details.

THE ENDOCRINE FUNCTION OF ADIPOSE TISSUE

Several new hormones continue to be identified. **Leptin** is one such hormone secreted by adipose tissue. When glucose and lipids are absorbed by adipose tissue, leptin is secreted. One of the functions of leptin is to affect neurons in the nervous system, producing a sense of satisfaction and suppression of appetite. Leptin also facilitates the secretion of GnRH and gonadotropin synthesis, which could be the cause of later puberty onset in thin girls and menstrual cycle irregularity in women with low body fat content.

✚ Hypertension and Kidneys

Rarely, hypertension can be caused by narrowing of one renal artery. The narrowing causes the kidney to secrete renin, which then produces a rise in blood pressure. This type of hypertension is known as **renal** or **Goldblatt hypertension.** In these cases, hypertension can be cured by widening the artery.

Drugs that reduce renin production and angiotensin II levels in the plasma are one type of antihypertensive drugs used to control high blood pressure.

Stress

Any condition that threatens homeostasis is a form of stress. Stress has been defined in many ways and means different things to different people. To some, it implies excessive demands made on them, leading to tension and emotional upset. To others, stress is anything that upsets their psychological status. Hans Selye, a famous endocrinologist and a pioneer of stress research, defines stress as the nonspecific response to any demands made on the body.

Stressors

The events and/or environmental agents that produce a stress response are referred to as **stressors.** There can be many types of stressors—physiologic, psychological or sociologic. They may originate from inside the body or from outside the body. The body's response to physiologic stressors, such as change in temperature, is different than the response to psychological stressors. Physiologic stressors produce a response that is *specific* to the type of stress and the response is quick and temporary. However, the body responds with a lesser degree of specificity—the *general* response—when it is stressed psychologically or stressed for a longer period.

The Stress Response

The general response is a pattern of physiologic and hormonal adjustments that are observed whatever the stress may be. This is known as the **general adaptation syndrome** or the **stress response.** Classically, the stress response is divided into three phases—**the alarm phase, the resistance phase,** and **the exhaustion phase** (see Figure). During the alarm phase, there is an immediate response to stress primarily caused by the sympathetic nervous system. The body mobilizes the energy reserves and there is the fight-or-flight response (see Figure). In addition to the action of epinephrine, renin secretion increases (producing increased blood pressure). Secretion of ADH and aldosterone also increase, resulting in water and sodium retention.

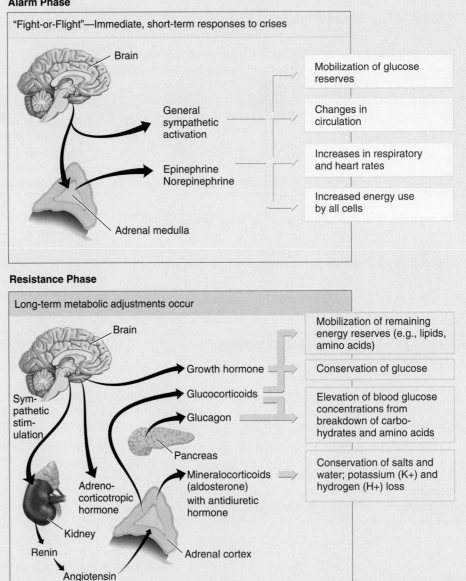

Alarm Phase

"Fight-or-Flight"—Immediate, short-term responses to crises

Brain

General sympathetic activation

Epinephrine Norepinephrine

Adrenal medulla

Mobilization of glucose reserves

Changes in circulation

Increases in respiratory and heart rates

Increased energy use by all cells

Resistance Phase

Long-term metabolic adjustments occur

Brain

Sympathetic stimulation

Growth hormone

Glucocorticoids

Glucagon

Pancreas

Adreno-corticotropic hormone

Kidney

Renin

Angiotensin

Mineralocorticoids (aldosterone) with antidiuretic hormone

Adrenal cortex

Mobilization of remaining energy reserves (e.g., lipids, amino acids)

Conservation of glucose

Elevation of blood glucose concentrations from breakdown of carbohydrates and amino acids

Conservation of salts and water; potassium (K+) and hydrogen (H+) loss

Exhaustion Phase

Vital systems collapse

Causes include:

- Exhaustion of lipid reserves
- Inability to produce glucocorticoids
- Failure of electrolyte balance
- Cumulative structural and functional damage to vital organs

The Alarm Phase, Resistance Phase, and Exhaustion Phase

Continued

Stress—cont'd

The person enters the resistance phase if the stressor persists for longer than a few hours. In this phase, glucocorticoids are the primary hormones, supported by epinephrine, growth hormone, glucagon, and thyroid hormones. With the help of these hormones, the body mobilizes lipid and protein reserves to maintain blood glucose levels. This is because the neural tissue has a high demand for glucose to produce energy. The adipose tissue responds by releasing stored fatty acids. The muscles respond by breaking down protein and releasing amino acids. The liver responds by manufacturing glucose from other carbohydrates, fats, and proteins. Blood volume is maintained by the hormones ADH and aldosterone.

In addition to the responses described above, other hormonal functions are pronounced. For example, the anti-inflammatory effect of glucocorticoids slows healing and makes the individual susceptible to infection. The fluid retaining effect of ADH and aldosterone result in higher blood pressure and blood volume.

The exhaustion phase begins when the homeostatic mechanisms break down at the end of the resistance phase. The hallmark of this phase is the collapse of vital systems. The resistance phase ends faster when poor nutrition, emotional and physical trauma, chronic illness, or damage to key organs is present.

The stress response is, therefore, an integration of activities in many systems. The autonomic, endocrine, immune, and musculoskeletal systems are all involved. All these responses are integrated in the central nervous system in a complex manner, and the central nervous system serves as the link between the stressor and the response of the body. The purpose of this response is to adapt to the stress and maintain homeostasis. The schematic diagram shows the relationship between the different regions of the brain and their role in the stress response (see Figure).

The roles of the various regions of the nervous system are described to give an understanding of how stress can influence almost all activities of the body.

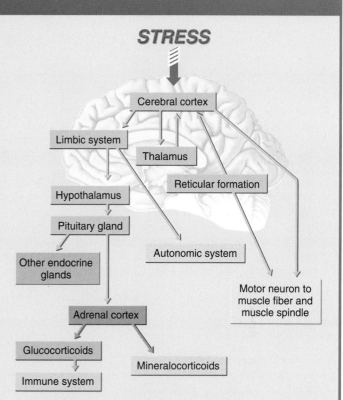

Relationship Between Regions of the Brain and Stress

Role of the Cerebral Cortex
This region determines the stressor. The stressor may vary from individual to individual. It may be taking an examination, giving an impending speech, being overcrowded, or meeting deadlines. Of course, it could be internal, too, such as exposure to extreme cold or cancer. Major outcomes are increased attention, arousal, and alteration in sleep.

Role of the Thalamus
The thalamus is the sensory relay station; all neurons carrying all sensations (except smell) reach the thalamus, where they are distributed to other parts of the brain.

Role of the Limbic System
The collections of neurons belonging to this system are responsible for the emotional components of response, such as rage, fear, and excitement. The limbic system has connections to the hypothalamus. In this way, it can influence the activities of the endocrine and autonomic nervous systems.

Role of Hypothalamus
The hypothalamus has many functions (**see Chapter 5**). Thirst centers, hunger centers, and sexual activity centers, among others, are all located in the hypothalamus. In addition, it produces hormones that influence the secretions of the pituitary gland. Stress, by having an effect on the hypothalamus, has widespread impact on the rest of the body.

Manifestations of Stress in Various Systems
The Musculoskeletal System

One manifestation of stress is the tensing of muscles. Prolonged tension causes neck stiffness, backache, headaches, and clenching of teeth. This occurs to some extent by the increased activity of the reticular activating system/reticular formation. This region (**see page 366**) has input from various parts of the body. In fact, all ascending tracts have a branch to this region. Neurons from the reticular formation descend to the motor neurons (alpha and gamma) and stimulate them, resulting in an increase in tone.

Continued

Role of the Cerebral Cortex

The Autonomic Nervous System

The response of the autonomic nervous system can be described as the fight-or-flight response (**see Chapter 5**) as a result of an increase in sympathetic nervous system activity. Some manifestations are pupil dilation, increased heart rate and blood pressure, increased respiratory rate, decreased gut motility, dry mouth, and sweating.

The Endocrine System

Many hormones come into play during stress. The hypothalamus causes hormonal secretion. The hypothalamus has numerous connections with the cortex and limbic system, among others, and situations perceived as stressful have an effect on the hypothalamus. As observed in **Figure 6.5, page 397,** the hypothalamus controls the pituitary. The pituitary gland regulates hormone secretion from the thyroid gland, adrenal cortex, ovaries, and testis. One hormone secreted by the adrenal cortex is cortisol, which is important in responses to stress.

Cortisol maintains blood glucose levels, facilitates fat metabolism, effects protein and collagen synthesis, and reduces immune system activity and inflammatory response. Some other functions are the effects on bone calcification, blood cells production, gastric acid secretion, and central nervous system (CNS) function modulation. Increased cortisol secretion in stressful situations reduces the immune reaction. The anti-inflammatory effect of cortisol can also slow healing.

Stressful situations inhibit thyroid hormones and conserve energy in this way. The reproductive hormones and growth hormones are also reduced. This is evidenced by menstrual cycles irregularity observed in women in times of stress.

Other hormone secretions, such as ADH, renin, and aldosterone, are also affected by stress.

The Immune System

The immune system is suppressed during stress. The exact mechanism is not known. It is probably the result of the effect of hormones such as cortisol that influence immunity. Because of the diminished response, the individual is prone to infections and cancer.

Factors Affecting Adaptation to Stress

One of the remarkable effects of changes—both internal and external—is the body's ability to adapt. The single purpose of all the body systems is to maintain the internal environment—homeostasis. There are innumerable control systems that detect change and modify organ activity accordingly to nullify the change, using feedback loops. Fortunately, the body has the capacity to adapt to stress. When a person tries to cope with stress, he or she has to be aware of the various factors that affect adaptation, allowing the effects of these factors to be negated. Think of various measures that can be taken to nullify the effects of the factors mentioned below.

Previous Experience and Learning

An individual, placed in a different, unaccustomed situation, experiences stress, together with its responses.

Physiologic Reserve

The stress response depends on the ability of systems to increase or decrease function according to needs. If the ability of an organ to respond to demands is diminished, it is hard for the body to maintain the internal environment, even with small demands, and dysfunction and disease ensue.

Rate of Change

The body is better able to adapt if changes are gradual. Sudden changes, along with a diminished physiologic reserve, can have dramatic negative effects on the body.

Genetic Endowment

The effect of stress on the body is also determined by genetic makeup. A person's genetic makeup is responsible for how well the different organs adapt and respond to stressful situations.

Age

The ability to adapt is diminished with age.

Health Status

Individuals who are mentally and physically fit are able to adapt to stress much more easily than others. It is well known that those who are motivated to live survive the worst onslaughts made on their mind and body.

Nutrition

Deficiencies or excesses of nutrition can impair the ability to adapt.

Sleep-Wake Cycles

Studies show that sleep is important for restoring energy and regenerating tissue. Irregular cycles of sleep and wakefulness can reduce immunity and physical and psychological function.

Psychosocial Factors

Psychological stress can be combated by a supportive social network. Circumstances that require life pattern change can be stressful, making individuals more susceptible to disease.

Age-Related Changes in the Endocrine System

Changes occur in both the production of hormones and in the receptors in target tissue that bind these hormones. Some hormonal levels are increased, while others remain unchanged or are decreased. For example, the sex hormones (testosterone in males and estrogen in females) are decreased, with resultant atrophy of the reproductive organs; insulin, thyroid hormones, and cortisol secretion remain normal, while FSH and LH are increased. Refer to page 442 for changes that occur with menopause.

Endocrine System and Massage

Massage may have indirect effects on the endocrine system through the nervous system. The therapist should be familiar with conditions of hyposecretion and hypersecretion of the various glands and take suitable precautions.

Diabetes mellitus is a common disorder likely to be seen in clients. A complication of diabetes is the development of hypoglycemia, which may happen when the glucose level drops below normal levels. Hypoglycemia is characterized by giddiness, weakness, pallor, and profuse sweating, followed by unconsciousness. Prompt administration of fruit juice or another carbohydrate can revive the person and this should be done before calling for help. Because diabetes has the potential to affect every system in the body, a careful history is required. For example, peripheral neuropathy is a complication of diabetes and clients will have reduced sensory perception in the extremities.

Please refer to pathology books specific for bodyworkers for precautions to be taken for all other conditions (**see page 415**).

STRESS AND BODYWORKERS

The study of stress and how the body responds reveals how people respond to what happens around them, their social setting, and their environment, all of which can affect the inner working of the body. Conversely, it gives us an idea of how therapeutic technique, such as massage, can affect the body, even at the molecular level (the secretion of hormones and immune processes).

Massage can help relieve stress in many ways. The soothing touch helps relax muscles that are tensed. The rapport of the therapist with the client is also important. The relaxing atmosphere of the clinic, the calming effect of the music, and the slow rhythmic strokes can reduce the activity of the sympathetic nerves and the fight-or-flight reaction that occurs with stress. By negating the effects of stress, massage can have a direct effect on the hypothalamus-pituitary-adrenal cortex axis and stimulate immune responses and healing.

Although massage has many positive effects on stress, the therapist should understand that it is the individual and the individual alone who actually adapts to stress. The therapist is just one component of the management process.

SUGGESTED READINGS

Braunwald E, Fauci AS, Kasper DL, et al. Harrison's Principles of Internal Medicine. 15th Ed. New York: McGraw-Hill, 2001.

Linde B. Dissociation of insulin absorption and blood flow during massage of a subcutaneous injection site. Diabetes Care 1986;6:570–574.

Premkumar K. Pathology A to Z. A Handbook for Massage Therapists. 2nd Ed. Calgary: VanPub Books, 1999.

Smyth A. SAD, Seasonal Affective Disorder: Who Gets It, What Causes It, How to Cure it. London: Thorsons, 1990.

Wilson JD, Foster DW (eds). Williams' Textbook of Endocrinology. 8th Ed. Philadelphia: WB Saunders, 1992.

Zang F. An introduction to keeping fit-massage. J Tradit Chin Med 1994;14(2):152–156.

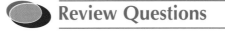 **Review Questions**

Multiple Choice

1. All of the following hormones are secreted by the anterior pituitary gland EXCEPT
   A. prolactin.
   B. thyroxine.
   C. growth hormone.
   D. thyroid-stimulating hormone.

2. All of the following hormones have an effect on the breasts EXCEPT
   A. estrogen.
   B. oxytocin.
   C. prolactin.
   D. aldosterone.

3. Which of the hormones may be the cause of Seasonal Affective Disorder?
   A. Melatonin
   B. Melanin
   C. Aldosterone
   D. Epinephrine

4. Which of the hormones causes an increase in the basal metabolic rate?
   A. Prolactin
   B. Thyroxine
   C. Erythropoietin
   D. Renin

5. Which of the following organs is involved in the destruction of hormones?
   A. Large intestine
   B. Skin
   C. Liver
   D. Pituitary gland

6. What is the function of insulin?
   A. Increase glucose uptake by cells
   B. Increase urine formation
   C. Speed glucose excretion by the liver
   D. Increase calcium deposition in bone

7. A decrease in secretion of antidiuretic hormone will result in
   A. diabetes insipidus.
   B. Grave's disease.
   C. diabetes mellitus.
   D. adrenogenital syndrome.

8. Cushing's syndrome is characterized by all of the following EXCEPT
   A. moon face.
   B. buffalo hump appearance.
   C. decrease in inflammatory response.
   D. exophthalmos.

9. In general, hormonal secretion may be stimulated by all of the following EXCEPT
   A. nerves.
   B. alteration in the concentration of a specific substance.
   C. instructions from another endocrine organ.
   D. genetic makeup.

10. In the stress response following injury, all of the following occurs EXCEPT
    A. discharge in parasympathetic nerves.
    B. increased metabolic rate.
    C. release of adrenaline.
    D. retention of fluid.

Fill-In

1. The hormones secreted by the adrenal medulla are _____ and _____.

2. The hormones of the pituitary gland, which regulate the ovaries and testis, are _____ and _____.

3. Two hormones that have an effect on the breast are _____ and _____.

4. Antidiuretic hormone is also known as _____.

True–False

(Answer the following questions T, for true; or F, for false):

1. Hormones that are fat-soluble may enter the target cells before acting in a specific manner.

2. Cells may have receptors for more than one hormone.

3. Hormones affect only the cells that have receptors for them.

4. The secretion of antidiuretic hormone would be increased after drinking 2 liters of water.

5. Calcitonin promotes bone resorption.

6. Deficiency of thyroid hormones from birth causes low mental ability.

7. In uncontrolled diabetes mellitus, the large volume of urine excreted is principally a result of the lack of secretion of antidiuretic hormone.

8. In a normal person, the secretion of insulin is depressed by high blood glucose levels.

9. Hypothalamus functions include regulation of the pituitary gland, hunger, and thirst.

Matching

Match the hormone (1–7) that is secreted in response to the condition (a–g) given on the right. Write the correct letter next to the appropriate number.

1. Erythropoietin
2. Aldosterone
3. Oxytocin
4. Thyroxine
5. Thyroid-stimulating hormone
6. Insulin
7. Parathormone

a. Decrease in blood calcium levels
b. Increase in blood glucose levels
c. Lack of iodine in the diet
d. Decrease in blood volume
e. Exposure to cold
f. Dilatation of the cervix during labor
g. A decrease in partial pressure of oxygen in the atmosphere (e.g., high altitude)

Short Answer Questions

1. What physical changes are you likely to see in a female client who has been on corticosteroids for a long time?
2. What is meant by negative and positive feedback mechanisms? Give an example of each.
3. What is a neuroendocrine reflex? Give one example.
4. Define hormones.
5. List the major endocrine glands of the body.
6. Which endocrine glands are located in the
   a. head.
   b. neck.
   c. thorax.
   d. abdomen.

Case Studies

Mr. Armstrong is 50 years old and slightly overweight. He is known to have diabetes mellitus. On one occasion, he came to the clinic for massage and complained of excessive sweating and dizziness.

A. Which of the hormones is deficient in diabetes mellitus?
B. What is the endocrine gland that secretes the deficient hormone? Where is the gland located?
C. What may be the cause of excessive sweating and dizziness?
D. What are the signs of decreased blood glucose levels?
E. List a few important questions that the therapist needs to ask when taking a history from a client with diabetes mellitus?

Coloring Exercise

Color each endocrine gland, using a different color for each. Label the endocrine glands and write the name(s) of the hormones each secretes next to each gland in brackets.

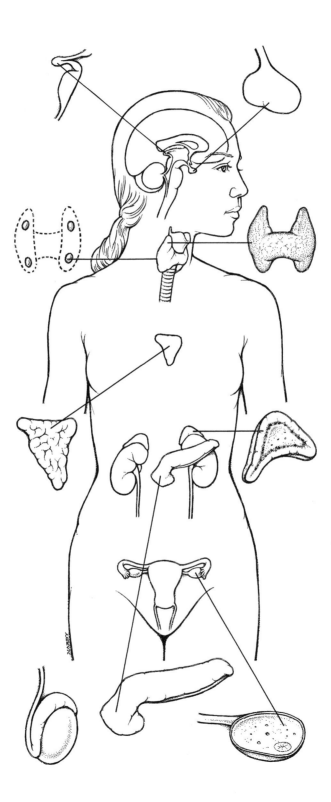

Answers to Review Questions

Multiple Choice

1. B	2. D	3. A	4. B	5. C
6. A	7. A	8. D	9. D	10. A

Fill-In

1. epinephrine, norepinephrine
2. FSH, LH
3. Oxytocin, prolactin (estrogen, progesterone, growth hormone, cortisol, and thyroxine are other hormones that affect the breast)
4. vasopressin

True–False

1. True
2. True
3. True
4. False. It would decrease secretion
5. False. It helps deposit calcium in bones, which is why it may be used to treat osteoporosis
6. True
7. False. The increase in urine volume is a result of glucose being lost in the urine. Glucose draws water into the renal tubules by osmosis, causing polyuria
8. False. Insulin secretion is increased.
9. True

Matching

1. g
2. d
3. f
4. e
5. c
6. b
7. a

Short-Answer Questions

1. There will be symptoms of Cushing's syndrome. **See page 407** for description of a person with Cushing's syndrome.
2. Negative feedback mechanism is a response where the stimuli cause an increase in secretion of a specific hormone. The increase in hormone level results in negating the stimuli (e.g., an increase in blood glucose levels causes secretion of insulin. Insulin increases uptake of glucose by cells, reducing the blood glucose levels). In positive feedback mechanisms, a stimuli causes an increase in secretion of a specific hormone. The in-crease in hormone level results in further increasing the stimuli (e.g., when the cervix is dilated during labor, nerves sense the dilatation and stimulate the pituitary to secrete oxytocin, which causes the muscles of the uterus to contract and push the baby further down, resulting in further dilatation of the cervix).

3. A neuroendocrine reflex results in secretion of hormone by an endocrine gland following stimulation of nerves (e.g., the secretion of oxytocin following dilatation of the cervix in labor).
4. Hormones are chemicals secreted by endocrine glands, which have an effect on structures located away from the secreting gland.
5. Pineal, hypothalamus, pituitary, thyroid, parathyroid, thymus, pancreas, adrenal gland, testis, and ovary. The heart, kidney, adipose tissue, placenta, and gastrointestinal tract also have endocrine function.
6. a. Pineal, hypothalamus, pituitary gland
   b. thyroid, parathyroid
   c. thymus
   d. pancreas, adrenal gland, ovary

Case Study

A. In diabetes mellitus, insulin is deficient.

B. Insulin is secreted by the endocrine part of the pancreas, the islets of Langerhans. The pancreas is located retroperitoneally in the abdomen, in relation to the duodenum.

C. Mr. Armstrong may be having a hypoglycemic attack. Because hypoglycemia is a potent stimulus for the sympathetic system, increasing levels of adrenaline and noradrenaline produce excessive sweating, pallor, tremors, palpitations, and nervousness. It is, therefore, important for glucose to be administered immediately.

D. The typical signs of hypoglycemia are dizziness, irritability, personality changes, confusion, headache, weakness, and hunger. Soon, the person has convulsions and goes into a coma. If hypoglycemia is prolonged, irreversible changes occur in the brain.

E. In a client with diabetes mellitus, it is important to find out what kind of treatment is being given the client. If insulin is given, details of when insulin was last given are required. Massage over the insulin site may increase absorption of insulin into blood and precipitate a hypoglycemia attack. Signs and symptoms of hypoglycemia can be easily precipitated in diabetic individuals if they have not eaten enough food; increased the dosage of antidiabetic drugs or insulin, or exercised more than usual. It is important for the therapist to have details regarding when food was last eaten, if activity has increased more than usual before the massage, or if changes have been made to the dosage. The therapist should question diabetes complications, such as slow healing, peripheral neuropathy (may have reduced sensation in the periphery), associated hypertension, and history of stroke and angina and take suitable precautions.

Reproductive System

Objectives **On completion of this chapter, the reader should be able to:**

- Explain the process of sex differentiation and development.
- Describe the changes that occur at puberty in males and females.
- Describe the components of the male reproductive system.
- Give the functions of each component.
- Identify the different parts of the male external genitalia.
- Describe the nervous and hormonal mechanisms that regulate male reproductive functions.
- Describe the components of the female reproductive system.
- Give the functions of each component.
- Describe the phases and events of the menstrual cycle.
- Identify the different parts of the female external genitalia.
- Describe the physiologic basis of the different contraceptive methods available.
- Describe the major physiologic changes that occur in pregnancy and lactation.
- Describe the physiologic changes that occur during menopause.
- Describe the age-related changes in the reproductive system.
- Describe the possible effects of massage on the reproductive system.

*T*he reproductive system is of major importance for the propagation of the species. It is the only system, in the absence of which, the body can continue to function. However, even if the body can function without many of the reproductive organs, deficiencies in this system have a tremendous impact on the physiologic, psychological, and social aspect of a person's life.

To add another dimension, the fields related to the reproductive system have recently become greatly advanced and more complex. The advancements in in vitro fertilization, human cell cloning, the ova and sperm marketing, and same-sex marriages are just some of the issues linked with ethical dilemmas.

Given the impact this element has in everyday life, although it is important for every individual to have a good understanding of this system, it is even more im-

portant for those in health-related fields. This chapter focuses on the basic structures and functions of the reproductive system, fetal development, and changes that occur during pregnancy and lactation.

Genetic Sex, Fetal Development, and Puberty

The reproductive system includes those organs and structures that are involved directly or indirectly with the formation, functional maturation, nourishment, storage, and transport of the male and female reproductive cells. Its genesis is at the chromosomal level.

GENETIC SEX

The differences between the two sexes depend on the presence of a single chromosome—the **Y chromosome**—and two endocrine structures, the **testis** and the **ovaries.** The hormonal secretions from the testis are responsible for the development of the male external genitalia and male sexual behavior.

The sex of the individual is determined genetically by two chromosomes (X and Y), called the **sex chromosomes.** Each individual has two sex chromosomes—**XX** (female) or **XY** (male)—and 22 other

pairs of chromosomes, called **autosomes.** When the ovaries in the mother and the testis in the father manufacture reproductive cells (the **ova** and **sperm,** respectively), only one of the sex chromosomes is present in each of the cells. This is because cell division occurs by meiosis (**see page 31**). Each ovum from the female contains one X chromosome (in addition to 22 autosomes). Of the sperm, some contain one Y chromosome and others contain one X chromosome (in addition to 22 autosomes). Therefore, when the ova and sperm come together during fertilization, two types of combinations can occur—XX (genetic female) and XY (genetic male). The fertilized ovum has 23 pairs of chromosomes (22 autosomes plus two sex chromosomes).

FETAL DEVELOPMENT

As the embryo develops in the mother after fertilization, there is no differentiation of the sexes for the first six weeks. In the seventh or eighth week, the genetic males start developing testis in a region close to the adrenal glands inside the abdomen. The testis starts secreting hormones that cause the development of the male internal and external genitalia. In genetic females, the absence of Y chromosomes and lack of male hormones is responsible for the development of the female internal and external genitalia.

In addition to affecting the formation of genitalia, male hormones affect the brain and are responsible for the male pattern of sexual behavior and hormonal activity of the hypothalamus. In the absence of male hormones, female patterns develop.

PUBERTY

As mentioned, the burst of male hormones in male fetuses affects the brain (hypothalamus), changing the pattern of hormonal secretion and behavior. In both sexes, the **gonads** (ovary and testis) remain dormant until they are activated by secretions from the pituitary to bring about the final maturation of the reproductive system. This period of final maturation is known as **adolescence.** It is also known as **puberty.** However, physiologically, puberty is the period when the endocrine and gamete-producing functions of the gonads have first developed to where reproduction is possible. The age at puberty has decreased over the years. In recent years, puberty tends to occur between the ages of 8 and 13 in girls and 9 and 14 in boys.

In females, adolescence begins with the development of breasts and axillary and pubic hair, followed by the first menstrual period (**menarche**). The physiologic changes that occur with the menstrual cycle are described later.

Abnormalities of Sexual Development

Abnormalities at the Genetic Level

Abnormalities of sexual development can be produced by genetic and hormonal mechanisms. Genetically, on rare occasions during division in the ovary, both sex chromosomes may go to one gamete, while the other has no sex chromosomes. If fertilization occurs in this case, there are four different ways for the gametes to combine and form a zygote (the product of ova and sperm combination).

- 44XO (*22 other chromosomes and zero sex chromosomes from ova + 22 other chromosomes and one X chromosome from sperm*)
- 44XXX (*22XX from ova and 22X from sperm*)
- 44YO (*22 other chromosomes and zero sex chromosomes from ova and 22Y from sperm*)
- 44XXY (*22XX from ova and 22Y from sperm*).

A zygote with 44YO dies in the uterus. A person with 44XO chromosome is short in stature and develops with female external genitalia and absent or rudimentary ovaries. Maturation does not occur at puberty. This is called **Turner's syndrome** or **gonadal dysgenesis.**

Those with XXY pattern (the most common sex chromosome disorder) develop as males with male genitalia. There is a high incidence of mental retardation in these individuals. This syndrome is known as **Klinefelter's syndrome.**

The XXX (**superfemale**) pattern is not associated with any characteristic abnormalities.

Abnormalities Resulting From Hormones

Some abnormalities can develop as a result of hormonal imbalances. For example, if female fetuses are exposed to male hormones, especially during the eighth to thirteenth weeks of pregnancy, they may develop genitalia that looks like that of a male. Conversely, in male fetuses, abnormalities in testis and testosterone secretion can cause development of female genitalia. This syndrome is known as **pseudohermaphroditism.** In this case, although the genetic makeup and the gonads are of one sex, the genitalia are of another. Many such genetic male individuals grow up as females until puberty when they seek medical advice for lack of menstruation and this syndrome is then detected.

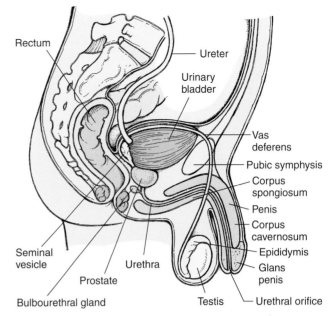

FIGURE **7.1.**   Male Reproductive Organs—Sagittal Section

The body changes that occur at puberty in males are enlargement of the external and internal genitalia, voice changes, hair growth, mental changes, and changes in body conformation and skin. The penis increases in length and width and the scrotum becomes pigmented and rugose (wrinkled). All internal organs increase in size. The larynx enlarges, with thickening of the vocal cords and deepening of the voice. Body hair, in general, increases and hair begins to appear on the face, axilla, chest, and pubis. Mentally, the person becomes more interested in the opposite sex. There is a predisposition to acne as the sebaceous gland secretions thicken and increase.

The Male Reproductive System

The male reproductive system consists of the **gonads** (testes) that produce gametes and hormones; the **ducts** that receive and transport the gametes; the **accessory glands** that secrete fluid into the ducts for the nourishment and maintenance of the gametes; and the external structures associated with the reproductive system, collectively known as the **external genitalia** (see Figure 7.1).

THE TESTIS

Each testis, shaped like a flattened egg, is about 5 cm (2 in) long, 3 cm (1.2 in) wide, and 2.5 cm (1 in) thick. The testis hangs inside the **scrotum**—a pouch that lies posterior to the penis and anterior to the anus. In the fetus, the testis develops inside the abdominal cavity close to the kidney. As the fetus develops, the testis descends (anteriorly and inferiorly), pushing through the anterior abdominal wall, into the scrotum. As it moves down, it is accompanied by the supplying blood vessels, lymphatics, and nerves. In addition, it is covered by remnants of the peritoneum and abdominal wall through which it passed during its descent. Normally, the testis has descended by the seventh month of development and is positioned in the scrotum at birth.

The Scrotum

The scrotum (see Figure 7.2) consists of a thin layer of skin and underlying fascia. The fascia has a layer of smooth muscle known as **dartos,** which is responsible for the wrinkles seen in the skin. Deep to the dermis, there is a layer of skeletal muscle known as the **cremaster muscle.** The contraction of this muscle causes the testis to be pulled closer to the body when cold. Relaxation of the muscle causes the testis to move away from the body. Thus, the temperature of the testis is maintained about 1.1°C (34°F) below that of the body—the temperature required for normal sperm production.

Internally, the scrotum (see Figure 7.2) is divided into two chambers. The division can be seen on the external surface as a thickening in the midline. A testis lies in each of these chambers or cavities. Due to the partition, infection or inflammation in one cavity does not easily spread to the other. The testis is separated from the inner surface of the scrotum by a space lined by serous membrane. The membrane, known as the **tunica vaginalis,** is a remnant of the peritoneum through which the testis pushed during development. The tunica vaginalis reduces the fric-

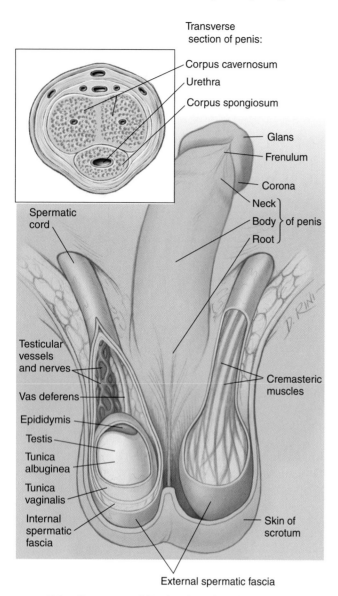

Transverse
section of penis:

Corpus cavernosum
Urethra
Corpus spongiosum

Glans
Frenulum

Corona
Neck
Body } of penis
Root

Spermatic
cord

Testicular
vessels
and nerves

Cremasteric
muscles

Vas deferens

Epididymis

Testis

Tunica
albuginea

Tunica
vaginalis

Internal
spermatic
fascia

Skin of
scrotum

External spermatic fascia

FIGURE 7.2. Scrotum and Testis—Anterior View (A transverse section through the penis is also shown)

Microscopic Structure of the Testis

tion between the testis and the scrotum. If inflamed, this cavity can be filled with fluid, producing a condition known as **hydrocele.**

Microscopic Structure of the Testis

Deep to the tunica vaginalis, a layer of thick collagen fibers called the **tunica albuginea** covers the testis. This layer extends into the testis, partitioning it into many **lobules.** Tightly coiled, slender tubules, known as **seminiferous tubules,** lie inside each of the lobules. Each tubule averages about 80 cm (31.5 in); together, end to end, the tubules extend to more than a kilometer long (0.6 mile). The sperm are manufactured inside the tubules, and sperm in different stages of development can be seen inside a cross-section of the tubules (see Figure 7.3B).

The formation process of sperm is known as **spermatogenesis.** Spermatogenesis (Figure 7.3B) begins in the outermost cell layer in the tubule and more mature sperm can be seen closer to or in the lumen. The seminiferous tubule is isolated from the general circulation by the **blood-testis barrier.** This barrier is maintained by the **Sertoli cells** or **sustentacular cells.** The Sertoli cells located in the outermost layer of the seminiferous tubules are joined together by tight junctions and regulate the composition of fluid in which the sperm is suspended. The Sertoli cells, in addition, provide nutrition to the sperm and also secrete important hormones needed for sperm maturation. The blood-testis barrier is important in preventing the immune system from attacking the sperm.

Leydig cells, specialized cells that secrete the male hormones, lie between the tightly coiled seminiferous tubules.

The Mature Sperm (Spermatozoa)

Each sperm (Figure 7.3B) has a rounded head and a long flagellum. The head houses the nucleus with densely packed chromosomes. The head is covered by a cap (**acrosomal cap**), which contains the enzymes required for digesting the outer layer of the ova at the time of fertilization. The flagellum helps the sperm propel forward with a rapid, corkscrew motion. Because the sperm does not have energy reserves, it relies on the surrounding fluid for survival.

Epididymis

The seminiferous tubules drain into a network of ducts, which, in turn, are continuous with a highly coiled structure known as the **epididymis.** The epididymis lies along the posterior border of the testis and consists of a coiled tubule about 7 meters (7.7 yd) long. This tubule continues as the **vas deferens** or **ductus deferens** from the inferior portion of the testis. The epididymis monitors and adjusts the composition of the tubular fluid. It also removes damaged sperm and dead cells. In addition, it stores the sperm and facilitates its maturation. The sperm are moved along the reproductive tract by peristaltic

Undescended Testis

Rarely, the testis does not descend into the scrotum by birth. This condition is known as **cryptorchidism.** In most instances, descent occurs a few weeks after birth. Descent of the testis is important because the slightly lower temperature in the scrotum facilitates sperm formation. Undescended testis can result in sterility. Also, serious abnormalities in the testis, if present (e.g., cancer), can remain undetected.

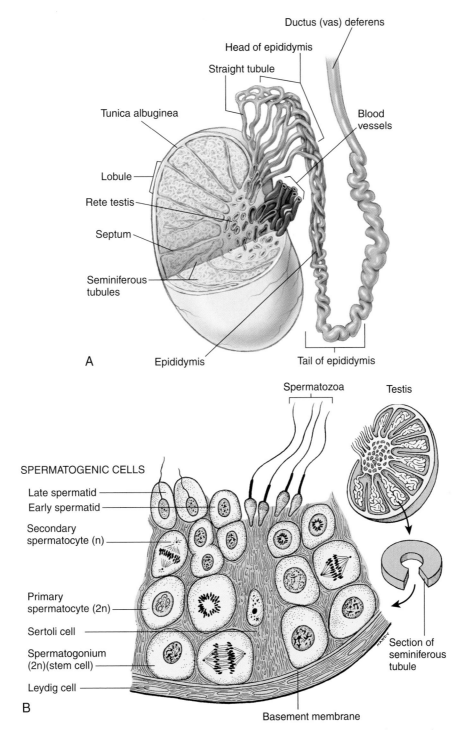

FIGURE 7.3.   The Testis. **A,** Sagittal section. **B,** Transverse section through a portion of a seminiferous tubule

contractions of the smooth muscle in the walls of the tubule.

THE VAS DEFERENS

The vas deferens is a tube about 45 cm (1.5 ft) long. It begins at the inferior, posterior aspect of the testis and ascends superiorly and enters the inguinal canal. The vas deferens, together with the blood vessels,

lymphatic vessels, nerves, muscles, and connective tissue fascia that surrounds it in this region, is known as the **spermatic cord** (Figure 7.2). The spermatic cord consists of structures that accompany the testis as it descends from the abdomen early in life. It extends from the deep and inferior aspect of the anterior abdominal wall—the **deep inguinal ring**—to the testis. The structures, after entering the deep inguinal ring, pass through the inguinal canal, exit through the **superficial inguinal ring** (superficial aspect of the anterior abdominal wall), and descend superficially to reach the testis (the route taken by the testis as it descends). In males, as a result of the presence of the spermatic cord, this region of the anterior abdominal wall is weaker. In situations where the pressure in the abdominal cavity is chronically increased, the contents of the abdomen tend to push through this weak point, a condition known as **inguinal hernia.** In females, only a nerve and a ligament of the uterus pass through this canal and inguinal hernia rarely occurs.

After passing through the deep inguinal ring, the vas deferens passes posterior to the urinary bladder toward the superior and posterior margin of the **prostate gland.** At this point, the vas deferens enlarges slightly to form the **ampulla.** The duct from the accessory gland (**seminal vesicle**) joins it here to form the **ejaculatory duct.** This duct passes through the prostate gland and empties into the **prostatic urethra.**

The urethra extends from the urinary bladder to the tip of the penis. It is about 20 cm long (7.9 in) and passes through the prostate (prostatic urethra), connective tissue in the perineum (**membranous urethra**), and the penis (**penile urethra**).

ACCESSORY GLANDS

The seminal vesicle, together with the prostate and bulbourethral gland, form the accessory glands. These glands function to provide the nutrients required by the sperm for motility, to activate the sperm, to help propel the sperm along the reproductive tract, and to counteract the acidity of the urethral and vaginal contents. The secretions of the glands and the contraction of smooth muscles are regulated by the autonomic nervous system.

Seminal Vesicles

The two seminal vesicles are located on the posterior aspect of the urinary bladder (Figure 7.1), embedded in the connective tissue between the bladder and the rectum. The two glands contribute about 60% of the semen fluid. The fluid contains fructose (nutrient), prostaglandins (stimulates contraction of smooth muscles), and fibrinogen (which helps the fluid to form a temporary clot in the vagina), among other substances.

Prostate Gland

The prostate gland is a muscular, rounded organ of about 4 cm (1.6 in). It surrounds the urethra as it leaves the bladder and consists of 30 to 50 compound

Enlarged Prostate

In men older than 50 years, the prostate tends to enlarge as androgen secretion decreases. This is known as **benign prostatic hypertrophy.** Sometimes, the enlarged prostate obstructs the urethra passing through it, producing difficulty in micturition, stagnation of urine in the bladder, urinary tract infection and, in severe cases, kidney failure. The obstruction produced by the enlarged prostate can be treated by surgically removing part of the prostate.

tubuloalveolar glands that open into the urethra. The fluid secreted by the prostate is acidic and contains, among others, an antibiotic that prevents urinary tract infection. Its secretion makes up 25% of the volume of semen.

The Bulbourethral Glands

The two bulbourethral glands (**Cowper's glands**) are situated at the base of the penis. They secrete thick, alkaline mucus, which helps to neutralize the acidity and provide lubrication.

SEMEN

During **ejaculation** (**see page 434**), the propulsion of sperm from the urethra to the exterior, about 2–5 mL (0.07 oz) of **semen** (**ejaculate**) is expelled. Each milliliter of ejaculate contains about 20–100 million sperm/milliliter. The fluid from the seminiferous tubules contributes 5% of the semen, and the accessory glands provide the rest. Thus, the fluid component of the semen is a mixture of secretions from the seminiferous tubule and the accessory glands.

PENIS

The penis is the tubular organ through which the urethra passes before it opens into the exterior. The penile urethra serves as a common passage for urine as well as ejaculate. The penis helps to introduce the ejaculate into the vagina of the female.

The penis consists of a maze of vascular channels in three cylindrical columns—two **corpus cavernosa**

Semen Analysis

Semen is analyzed in individuals who have infertility. In addition to the sperm count, the motility and appearance of the sperm are studied. Normally, more than 60% of sperm are motile.

and one **corpus spongiosum** (Figures 7.1 and 7.2). The latter surrounds the penile urethra. The columns are surrounded by thick, elastic connective tissue and smooth muscle. The blood flow through the channels varies according to the state of sexual arousal. **See page 434** for details of the physiology of sexual intercourse. The penis is divided into the **root, body, neck,** and **glans.** The root is the portion attached to the body wall, inferior to the pubic symphysis, and consists of the **bulb** of the penis (the expanded portion of the corpora spongiosum) and the **crura** (the two, separated portions of the corpora cavernosa). The bulb of the penis is attached to the perineal muscles and fascia and is surrounded by the skeletal muscle (**bulbospongiosus).** The crura are attached to the pubic rami and are surrounded by the **bulbocavernosus** muscle. The bulbospongiosus and bulbocavernosus help with ejaculation. The body (shaft) is the movable portion and the glans is the enlarged distal end. The neck is the narrow portion between the shaft and the glans. The thin, delicate fold of skin that overlies the tip of the penis is known as the **prepuce.** In many males, the prepuce is surgically removed by a procedure known as **circumcision.**

ENDOCRINE FUNCTION OF THE TESTIS

The male sex hormones are known as **androgens.** The major hormone secreted by the interstitial cells (Leydig cells) of the testis is **testosterone.** Testosterone is a steroid hormone and, like all steroids, is derived from cholesterol. The adrenal cortex also contributes to the concentration of androgens in the plasma.

At the time of fetal development, as mentioned, testosterone has an effect on the brain, resulting in the male pattern of behavior. It also stimulates the development of the internal male genitalia. Later, testosterone develops and maintains the male secondary sex characteristics (described on **page 423**). It also has a growth-promoting and protein-building effect. The androgens increase the synthesis and decrease the breakdown of proteins. The synthetic anabolic steroids, often misused in sports, capitalize on this function.

Control of Testosterone Secretion

Testosterone secretion is controlled by follicular stimulating hormone (FSH) and luteinizing hormone (LH) from the anterior pituitary (see Figure 7.4). FSH and LH are, in turn, controlled by gonadotropin releasing hormone (GnRH) secreted by the hypothalamus. FSH is required for sperm manufacture. LH mainly functions to stimulate production of testosterone. The level of testosterone in the plasma has a

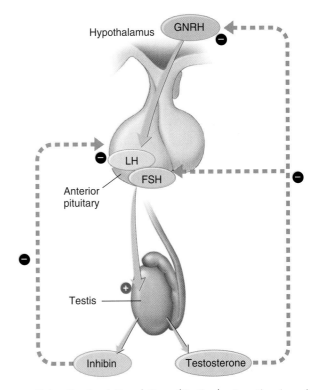

FIGURE 7.4. Feedback Regulation of Testicular Function (−ve indicates inhibitory effects; +ve stimulatory effects)

negative feedback effect on the hypothalamus and pituitary.

The cells of the testis also produce another hormone known as **inhibin,** which helps to regulate the secretion of FSH.

The Female Reproductive System

The function of the female reproductive system is to produce sex hormones, functioning gametes (ova), and to support and protect the developing embryo. The major organs are the **ovaries** (gonads), **uterine tubes** (fallopian tubes or oviducts), the **uterus,** the **vagina, accessory glands** (see Figures 7.5 and 7.6), and the components of the **external genitalia** (see Figure 7.7). The **breasts (mammary glands)** are also considered part of the female reproductive system.

THE OVARIES

The two ovaries are almond-shaped organs, about 5 cm (2 in) long, 2.5 cm (1 in) wide, and 8 mm (0.3 in) thick, located near the lateral walls of the pelvic cavity. The ovaries are held in place by ligaments that

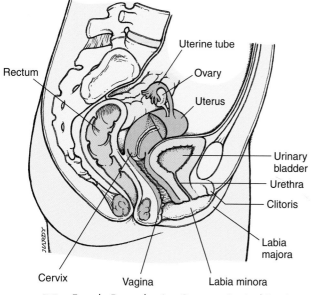

Rectum

Uterine tube

Ovary

Uterus

Urinary bladder

Urethra

Clitoris

Labia majora

Cervix   Vagina   Labia minora

FIGURE 7.5.   Female Reproductive Organs—Sagittal Section

connect them to the uterus **(ovarian ligament)** and the pelvis **(suspensory ligament).** The surface of the ovary is nodular and has ova **(primordial follicles)** in various stages of development. At the time of birth, there are about 2 million immature ova in the ovaries. Many of the ova degenerate; at puberty, there are only about 400,000 remaining. The immature ova **(oocytes)** lie dormant in the ovary until they are stimulated by a sudden surge in the hormone FSH at puberty. Every month thereafter, some of the oocytes undergo further development. This is known as the ovarian cycle (the **ovarian cycle** is discussed further under the section on Menstrual Cycle, **page 431**).

THE UTERINE TUBES (FALLOPIAN TUBES; OVIDUCT)

Each muscular uterine tube is about 12 cm (4.7 in) long. One end is free and opens into the pelvic cavity and the other end is continuous with the superior and lateral aspect of the uterus. The free end of the tube, the **infundibulum,** is expanded and funnel-shaped, with fingerlike projections known as **fimbriae.** The fimbriae are in close contact with the ovary, especially at ovulation. The fallopian tube is

lined with ciliated epithelium, which help move the ovum toward the uterine cavity.

THE UTERUS

The nonpregnant uterus (see Figure 7.6) is a pear-shaped organ about 7.5 cm (3 in) long and 5 cm (2 in) wide (at the widest diameter). It lies suspended between the urinary bladder anteriorly and the rectum posteriorly. The upper portion of the uterus is normally bent forward (anteflexed), lying over the superior and posterior aspect of the urinary bladder. Part of the superior portion of the uterus is covered by the peritoneum.

The uterus can be divided into the anatomic regions—the **body** and the **cervix.** The body is the largest region of the uterus. The part of the body of the uterus above the attachment of the uterine tubes is known as the **fundus.** Inferiorly, the body becomes narrower and continues down as the **cervix.** The cervix is the region of the uterus that projects into the vagina.

The Uterine Walls

The uterus has a thick, muscular wall, consisting of three layers. The outer layer is the **perimetrium,** which is actually part of the peritoneum covering the superior aspect. Deep to the perimetrium is the muscular **myometrium.** The third and innermost layer is the **endometrium,** a glandular mucosa lining the uterine cavity. The myometrium consists of smooth muscle arranged in longitudinal, oblique, and circular layers. It forms 90% of the uterine wall and is responsible for the powerful contractions that occur at the time of labor. The endometrium is the inner lining that undergoes cyclical changes influenced by hormones. It has an abundant blood supply and nu-

---

ANIMALS AND OVULATION

Did you know that cats, rabbits, minks, and some other animals ovulate only after copulation? Sensory nerves from the genitalia, eyes, and ears reach the hypothalamus, which then stimulates the pituitary to secrete LH. The increase in LH levels in the blood causes ovulation.

Pelvic Inflammatory Disease and Ectopic Pregnancy

Pelvic inflammatory disease is a condition in which there is inflammation and infection in the pelvis. The uterine tubes may be affected and scar tissue may form, predisposing the individual to conditions such as infertility and ectopic pregnancy. **Ectopic pregnancy** is the term given to a condition in which the fertilized ovum implants in regions other than the uterine cavity.

The movement of ova along the scarred uterine tube may be slower than normal and fertilized ova may be retained in the tube, embedding in the walls of the tube and eventually causing it to rupture. Such a pregnancy is referred to as **tubal pregnancy.** A tubal pregnancy is dangerous because it can cause profuse bleeding in the abdominal cavity.

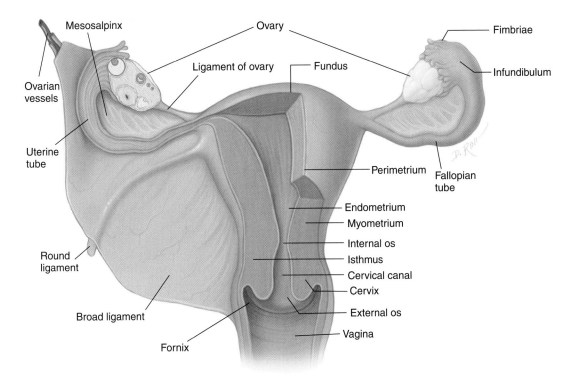

FIGURE **7.6.**   The Wall of the Uterus

merous glands that help support the growing fetus at the time of pregnancy.

The Uterine Cavity

The uterine cavity is somewhat triangular in shape, with the base of the triangle located superiorly. The openings of the fallopian tubes are located in the two upper angles. The lower end of the cavity narrows to a portion known as the uterine **isthmus.** The isthmus is continuous with the opening of the cervix, which projects about 1.5 cm (0.6 in) into the vagina. The passage in the middle of the cervix is known as the **cervical canal.** The two ends of the cervical canal are known as the **internal** (opens into the uterine cavity) and **external os** (opens into the vagina).

Blood Supply and Innervation

The uterus has an extensive blood supply. Blood is supplied by the **uterine arteries,** which are branches of the internal iliac arteries. The blood leaves the uterus via the **uterine veins** and drains into the internal iliac veins.

Sensory nerves from the uterus reach the spinal cord at the T11 and T12 level. Hence, spinal nerves T10–L1 are targeted for anesthetic block (if necessary) during labor. The uterus is also supplied by both sympathetic and parasympathetic nerves; there-

fore, the activities in the uterus are controlled by both nervous and endocrine systems.

Uterine Support

The ovaries, uterine tubes and the uterus are held in place inside the abdomen by ligaments that connect them to the surrounding walls.

Laterally, the peritoneum covers the fallopian tube and becomes continuous with the walls of the pelvis. The sheet of peritoneum lateral to the uterus is known as the **broad ligament** and serves to support the uterus. Another pair of ligaments—the **uterosacral ligament**—runs from the lateral surface of the uterus to the anterior aspect of the sacrum, holding the uterus in place and preventing it from sliding anteriorly and inferiorly. The **round ligaments** run from the lateral aspect of the uterus, just below the uterine

✚ Uterine Prolapse

In certain women, the ligaments and other structures supporting the uterus may become weak with a resulting shift of uterus position. The uterus tends to descend downward into the vagina and, in extreme cases, the cervix of the uterus may project through the vagina into the perineal region. This is known as **uterine prolapse.**

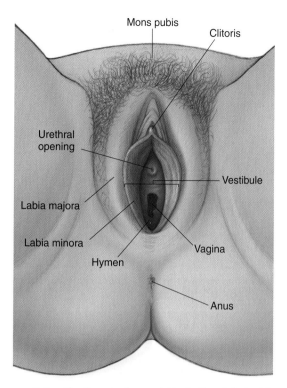

FIGURE 7.7. The Female External Genitalia—Inferior View

tube toward the lateral wall of the pelvis into the inguinal canal, preventing the uterus from sliding posteriorly. Another pair of ligaments, the **lateral ligaments,** runs from the lower end of the uterus near the vagina to the lateral wall of the pelvis, preventing inferior movement of the uterus. The skeletal muscles and the fascia covering the pelvic outlet further help support the uterus.

THE VAGINA

The vagina is a muscular, extensible elastic tube about 10 cm long (3.9 in), which extends from the cervix to the external genitalia. The cervix protrudes into the vagina. The part of the vagina surrounding the cervix is the **fornix.** In women who have not had intercourse, a thin epithelial fold—the **hymen**—partially or fully covers the opening of the vagina. Skeletal muscles similar to that present in the male, the **bulbospongiosus,** extend along the sides of the vagina and help constrict the opening. The vagina is lined by stratified squamous epithelium and houses many harmless bacteria, whose acidic secretions prevent harmful organisms from thriving there.

The Perineum

The perineum denotes the region between the thighs and buttocks that houses the external genitalia and anus in both sexes. The perineum extends to the pubic symphysis anteriorly, to the ischial tuberosities laterally, and to the coccyx posteriorly.

THE EXTERNAL GENITALIA

The region of the external genitalia (see Figure 7.7) is known as the **vulva** or **pudendum.** Adipose tissue over the pubic symphysis produces a bulge known as

the **mons pubis.** Folds of skin cover the sides of the openings; the outermost thicker fold, with coarse hair (in adults), is known as the **labia majora.** Inner to this is the thinner, smooth, hairless fold known as the **labia minora.** The space enclosed by the labia minora is known as the **vestibule.** There are three major openings in the perineum. The most anterior opening is the urethra, with the vaginal opening posterior to it. The anal opening is the most posterior opening. Superior to the urethral opening is the **clitoris,** the structure that is embryologically equivalent to the male penis. The clitoris is a small cylindrical mass of tissue that is erectile. As in males, it is capable of enlarging in size when stimulated.

Glands in the External Genitalia Region

Many glands are found in this region that help keep the vestibule moist and provide lubrication. The **paraurethral** or **Skene's glands** are located near the urethral opening and the **lesser** and **greater vestibular (Bartholin's) glands** are found near the vaginal

FEMALE CIRCUMCISION

In many cultures, parts of the clitoris are removed, with resultant scarring of the external genitalia. Much controversy exists over this practice.

entrance. In addition, sebaceous and sweat glands located in the labia majora help with the function.

Breasts

The glandular portion of the breast is known as the **mammary gland.** The two mammary glands are modified sudoriferous (sweat) glands. The breasts are positioned over the second to sixth ribs and lie superficial to the pectoralis major, part of the serratus anterior and external oblique muscles. Medially, the breasts extend to the lateral margin of the sternum. Laterally, the breasts follow the anterior border of the axilla. The **axillary process** of the breast extends upwards and laterally toward the axilla close to the axillary vessels.

In nonpregnant individuals, the breasts (see Figure 7.8) are largely made up of fat and connective tissue, scattered with immature glands. During pregnancy, under the influence of many hormones, the glands enlarge and occupy the major portion of the breast. The glands consist of 15 to 20 compartments, or **lobes,** which are separated by fat tissue. Between the lobules, **suspensory ligaments (Cooper ligaments)** extend from the skin to the deep fascia over the pectoralis major, supporting the breast. Each lobe has many smaller compartments (**lobules**) that are collections of milk-secreting glands known as **alveoli.** The alveoli are lined by secretory cells and surrounded by spindle-shaped smooth muscle cells called **myoepithelial cells.** Contraction of these cells helps expel the milk toward the nipples. The alveoli open into larger ducts, which join with more ducts and eventually form about 15 large **lactiferous ducts** that open out through the **nipple.** Just before the ducts open into the nipple, they are enlarged into the **lactiferous sinus (ampulla)** where a larger volume of milk can be held before they are expelled. The nipple is a cylindrical part containing some erectile tissue. Surrounding the nipple is a circular pigmented area known as the areola. The color of the areola varies according to the complexion of the woman. During pregnancy, the areola becomes darker and enlarged in area. See **page 441** for regulation of the breasts, lactation, and changes that occur during pregnancy.

THE MENSTRUAL CYCLE

After puberty, the female reproductive system, unlike that of the male, undergoes cyclical changes that can be regarded as periodic preparation for fertilization and pregnancy. This cyclical change is known as the **menstrual cycle** (see Figure 7.9). The most conspicuous of these changes is the vaginal bleeding that occurs with the shedding of part of the inner lining of the uterus (**menstruation**). The duration of the cycle is variable. Typically, the cycle lasts for 28 days, with day

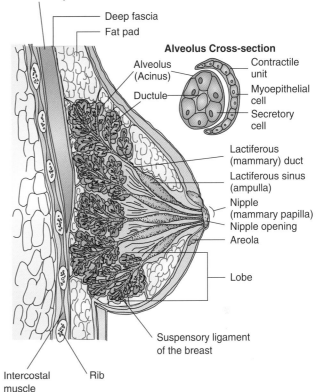

FIGURE **7.8.** The Structure of the Mammary Gland—Sagittal Section

1 denoted as the first day of menstruation and day 28 as the day before menstruation of the next cycle. Although the menstrual cycle has effects throughout the body, only those changes occurring in the ovary, fallopian tube, uterus, vagina, and breast are described here. The changes in the cycle are a result of the ebb and surge of sex hormone levels in the plasma.

Ovarian Cycle and Fate of the Ova

At the beginning of every cycle, a cavity filled with fluid forms around the **oocytes (primordial follicles)** in the ovary (Figure 7.9). Soon, one of the follicles rapidly increases in size while the others regress. This is the dominant follicle. Certain cells in the follicle secrete the hormone **estrogen.** About 14 days before the start of the next cycle, the enlarged follicle ruptures and the ovum is extruded into the abdominal cavity. This process is known as **ovulation.** The ovum is picked up by the fimbriae of the uterine tubes and transported into the uterus. If fertilization occurs, the fertilized ovum embeds in the uterine cavity wall. If unfertilized, it is expelled from the uterus into the vagina and then outside the body at the time of menstruation.

After ovulation, the ruptured follicle in the ovary fills up with blood. The cells lining the follicle rapidly

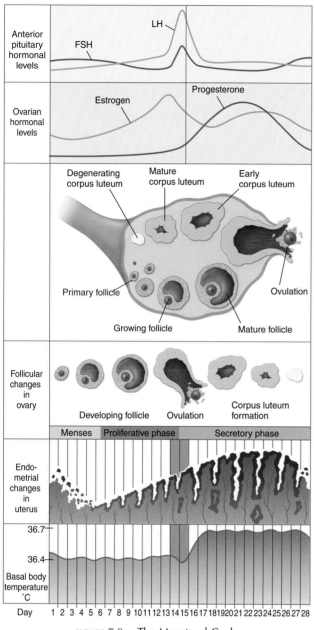

FIGURE 7.9. The Menstrual Cycle

After ovulation, as the remnants of the follicle are replaced by luteal cells, the rest of the menstrual cycle is known as the **luteal phase.** This phase is also known as the **progestational phase** because of the high level of progesterone at this time.

Changes in the Uterus

At the beginning of the menstrual cycle, the uterine cavity has only the remnants of the deep layer of the endometrium. From the fifth to the fourteenth days, the endometrium rapidly increases in thickness, and the uterine glands lengthen. This phase of the cycle is referred to as the **proliferative phase.** After ovulation, the endometrium becomes highly vascularized. The glands coil and secrete a clear fluid. Hence, this phase (from the fourteenth to twenty-eighth days) is known as the **secretory phase.** If the ovum is not fertilized, the endometrium becomes thinner and areas of cell death (necrosis) begin to appear in the endometrium. Blood vessels go into spasm and some bleeding is seen. The inner lining of the endometrium sloughs off and this collection of dead cells, together with the blood, is the **menstrual flow.**

Normal Menstruation

Normally, the menstrual blood contains 75% arterial and 25% venous blood. It contains tissue debris from the endometrial lining together with prostaglandin and fibrinolysin (an enzyme that prevents clotting); therefore, clots are not seen in the menstrual flow (unless the flow has been excessive). Usually, menstruation lasts from 3–5 days (range, 1–8 days). The volume of blood can range from slight spotting to 80 mL (2.7 oz). Flows greater than that are considered abnormal.

Functionally, the uterus restores the endometrium from the previous menstruation during the proliferative phase and prepares to embed the fertilized ovum during the secretory phase. The length of the secretory phase is remarkably constant at 14 days from the day of ovulation to the beginning of the next menstrual cycle. This is used to determine the day of ovulation in females. For example, if an individual has regular cycles of 32 days duration, the day of ovulation is likely to be on day 18 of the cycle (i.e., 32 − 14 = 18).

At times, especially the first year after menarche (first menstrual period) and the last few years of menopause (the time when menstrual cycles cease), ovulation does not occur in every cycle. These are known as **anovulatory cycles.**

Changes in the Cervix

The cervical mucosa and its secretions also undergo cyclical changes. The mucus secreted is thinner (less

multiply and yellowish, lipid-rich cells known as the **luteal cells** replace the clotted blood. The follicle is now known as the **corpus luteum.** The luteal cells secrete the hormones **estrogens** and **progesterone.** If pregnancy occurs, the corpus luteum persists and menstruation does not occur until delivery as a result of continuous estrogen and progesterone secretion. If there is no pregnancy, the corpus luteum degenerates by about 12 days after ovulation and is eventually replaced by scar tissue.

The phase from the 1st day of menstruation to the day of ovulation is known as the **follicular** or **preovulatory phase.** Since follicular enlargement is brought about by estrogen secretion, this phase is also known as the **estrogenic phase.**

THE FERTILE PERIOD

The ovum lives for approximately 72 hours after it has been expelled from the ruptured ovarian follicle and is probably viable for less than half this time. The sperm live for approximately 48 hours. Therefore, the fertile period is approximately 120 hours, probably much shorter. It is calculated that there is little chance of conception before day 9 and after day 20 (in a 28-day cycle). However, there are documented cases of pregnancy occurring from having isolated intercourse on every day of the cycle! This indicates that methods of contraception other than avoiding intercourse during the time of ovulation have to be resorted to for greater reliability.

In women with infertility complaints, an easy method for determining if ovulation has occurred is to check the characteristics of the vaginal epithelium in the secretory phase of menstrual cycle.

viscous) and more alkaline during the follicular phase. These changes promote survival and motility of the sperm. During the secretory or luteal phase, the secretions become thicker. Some individuals use the changes in the consistency of the cervical secretion to determine the approximate time of ovulation.

Changes in the Vagina

The cells in the vagina also undergo cyclical changes. During the later part of the cycle, the epithelium becomes thicker and is infiltrated with white blood cells. The mucus secretion becomes thicker during this phase.

Changes in the Breast

During the proliferative phase, the ducts of the mammary gland increase in number and size. In the later half of the cycle, the lobules of the glands increase in size. The blood flow is increased and fluid tends to accumulate in the interstitial tissue. This is responsible for the tenderness, swelling, and pain experienced by individuals about 10 days before the start of the next cycle. All of these symptoms disappear at the start of menstruation.

✓ Sitz Bath

Sitz bath is the immersion of the pelvis in water. Hot, cold, or alternating hot and cold water may be used. The individual sits with the knees bent, allowing the buttocks and pelvic area to be covered with water. Sitz bath helps relieve painful symptoms and pelvis congestion.

Changes in Body Temperature

In addition to the previously mentioned changes, the basal body temperature also fluctuates. At the time of ovulation, the temperature (taken orally or rectally in the morning before rising from bed) is raised by about 0.5°C (32.9°F). This, along with other cyclical changes, can be used to determine the time of ovulation.

Menstrual Cycle Regulation

All changes that occur during the menstrual cycles are a result of the changing levels of hormones secreted by the hypothalamus, pituitary, and ovaries (see Figure 7.10).

The Role of the Hypothalamus

The hormones secreted by the pituitary are controlled by **gonadotropin-releasing hormone (GnRH)** of the hypothalamus. The hypothalamus is primed early in life by the presence or absence of testosterone in the fetus (Testosterone secretion from the testicular cells is determined by the presence of the Y chromosome.) In the absence of the Y chromosome (and consequent absence of testosterone), the hypothalamus begins to secrete hormones in the cyclical female pattern.

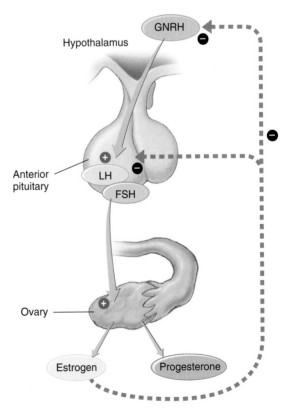

FIGURE 7.10.   Feedback Regulation of Ovarian Function (− indicates inhibitory effects; + stimulatory effects)

Because of the connections of the hypothalamus with the rest of the nervous system, hormones secreted by it can be altered according to changes detected by the nervous system in the external environment. For example, regular menstrual periods often disappear when young girls move away from home (boarding school amenorrhea). The fear of pregnancy, at times, can inhibit menstruation. Other than being affected by neural mechanisms, the hypothalamus is affected by the plasma levels of sex hormones by negative feedback mechanisms.

The Role of the Pituitary Gland

The pituitary secretes two hormones, **follicle-stimulating hormone** (FSH) and **luteinizing hormone** (LH). FSH stimulates the growth of ovarian follicles. LH is responsible for the final maturation of the follicles and estrogen secretion from the ovary. A sudden increase in levels of plasma LH results in ovulation. LH also causes the development of the ruptured ovarian follicle into the corpus luteum (in the later part of the cycle) and secretion of the hormones estrogen and progesterone by the corpus luteum.

The Role of the Ovaries

As previously mentioned, the ovaries secrete the female sex hormones **estrogen** and **progesterone.** The secretion of estrogen peaks twice during the menstrual cycle; once just before ovulation and once in the middle of the luteal phase.

Estrogen

The hormone estrogen affects many organs. It facilitates the growth of the ovarian follicle and increases the motility of the fallopian tubes. It increases the size of the uterus and excitability of the uterine smooth muscles. It also sensitizes the uterus to the hormone oxytocin at the time of labor. Being from the same steroidal family, it has the properties of other steroids, such as fluid and salt retention in the body. In the breast, estrogen is largely responsible for the increase in size at puberty. Estrogen accelerates the growth of long bones and closure of epiphysis at puberty and decreases the rate of bone resorption. Estrogens tend to lower the levels of cholesterol in the blood. This may be one of the reasons for the lower incidence of cardiovascular disease, such as atherosclerosis, in women.

Progesterone

Progesterone is a hormone secreted mainly by the corpus luteum. The primordial follicles also secrete small amounts. During pregnancy, the placenta secretes this hormone. The principal organs affected by this hormone are the brain, uterus, and breasts. It is responsible for the cyclical changes that occur in the luteal phase of the menstrual cycle and for the slight increase in body temperature at the time of ovulation. Together with estrogen, progesterone is used in varying doses to prevent ovulation (oral contraceptives).

Relaxin

The ovaries secrete a hormone called **relaxin.** This hormone is also secreted by the placenta in pregnant women. Relaxin relaxes the pubic symphysis and other pelvic joints and softens and dilates the uterine cervix at the time of pregnancy.

THE PHYSIOLOGY OF SEXUAL INTERCOURSE (IN BRIEF)

The sexual function in males and females are regulated by a complex interplay between the sympathetic, parasympathetic, central, and peripheral nervous systems. During arousal, thoughts, as well as sensory stimulation, stimulate the parasympathetic nerves to alter blood flow and glandular secretions in the genitalia.

In Men

Process of Erection

When sexually aroused, **erection** or stiffening of the penis occurs by stimulation of afferent nerves from the genitalia, as well as by nerves from the brain that responds to erotic psychic stimuli. These nerves stimulate the efferent nerves located in the lumbar region of the spinal cord. Stimulation of the parasympathetic nervous system causes the arterial blood vessels to dilate and the smooth muscles to relax, filling the vascular channels with blood. At the same time, veins in the penis are compressed. This blockage in outflow adds to the turgor of the penis. The subsequent tensing of the skin over the penis further increases the sensitivity of the sensory receptors.

Process of Ejaculation

The rhythmic stimulation of the sensory receptors during intercourse results in sympathetic stimulation and contraction of the smooth muscles of the reproductive tract to push the semen into the urethra. At the same time, the sphincter guarding the urinary bladder contracts, preventing urine from being expelled. This process is known as **emission.** Soon, the skeletal muscles—ischiocavernosus and bulbospongiosus—located in the perineum contract, expelling the semen. This process is known as **ejaculation.** The associated pleasurable sensation experienced is known as **orgasm.**

In Women

In women, similar phases occur. The parasympathetic nerves increase blood flow to the genitalia. Local glands are stimulated to increase their secretions to help with lubrication. Erection of the clitoris helps increase the sensitivity of the area to stimuli. The rhythmic stimulation of the clitoris and vagina, together with other stimuli (touch, smell, auditory), leads to orgasm. Orgasm in females is accompanied by peristaltic contractions of walls of the vagina and uterus and the pelvic muscles.

CONTRACEPTION (STRATEGIES FOR BIRTH CONTROL)

There are many methods of contraception available, each with its own advantages and disadvantages. When selecting a contraceptive, the convenience, as well as the failure rate (chances of becoming pregnant), have to be taken into account.

Permanent Methods of Contraception

If a more permanent type of contraception is desired, **sterilization** can be performed. This is a surgical procedure in which the continuity of the reproductive passage of sperm and ova is disrupted, preventing fertilization. In males, the vas deferens on each side is cut, tied, and blocked as it ascends close to the scrotum as part of the spermatic cord before it enters the abdominal cavity. This procedure, known as **vasectomy,** is simple and can be performed in minutes in a physician's office. In females, the fallopian tubes are blocked by a procedure known as **tubal ligation.** This involves opening the abdominopelvic cavity, locating the tubes, and producing discontinuity of the passage. This procedure is more complicated than vasectomy. The failure rate for these two procedures ranges from 0.02% to 0.45%.

✚ Vasectomy

Vasectomy is a surgical procedure in which the vas deferens continuity is stopped by bilateral ligation.

Some men who have had vasectomy develop antibodies against the spermatozoa. This may affect the fertility of the individual if the patency of the vas deferens is restored at a later date. Rarely, a tender nodule (sperm granuloma) may develop at the site of ligation. This is a result of a chronic inflammatory reaction at the site. The symptoms usually disappear with analgesics. Other rare complications of vasectomy include postoperative edema, intrascrotal bleeding, and infection. Rarely, recanalization of the vas deferens may spontaneously occur.

✓ Sexually Transmitted Diseases

Sexually transmitted diseases (STDs) are diseases transferred from one person to another, usually by sexual intercourse. There are many bacterial, viral, and fungal infections included in this category. They may result in conditions such as pelvic inflammatory disease, infertility, genital lesions, and even death. Some common STDs are: gonorrhea, syphilis, herpes, genital warts, and chancroids.

Temporary Contraception Methods

Other contraceptive methods can be used on a less permanent basis. **Oral contraceptives** are pills that contain varying quantities of the hormones progesterone and/or estrogen. The hormones are adjusted to prevent ovulation. The pills are taken 5 days after the start of menstruation and continued for 3 weeks. Following this, the pills taken are placebos or contain small quantities of hormones. Thus, despite the prevention of ovulation, regular menstrual cycles are achieved. More than 20 brands of oral contraceptives are available, each with a different dosage of estrogen and progesterone. The brand most suitable for each individual has to be determined by a physician. Recently, **skin implants,** containing progesterone and progesterone injections, are available that provide birth control for a more prolonged period. The failure rate for oral contraceptives ranges from 0.32% to 1.2%.

Intrauterine devices (IUDs) are in the form of a small, plastic/copper loop, T or 7 (shapes) that can be inserted into the uterine cavity. The exact mechanism of action is still uncertain, but it is believed that the uterine secretions/atmosphere is altered to prevent the implantation of the fertilized ovum. Not commonly used in the United States, it is a popular form of contraception in other countries. The failure rate ranges from 5% to 6%.

Some methods work as **barriers** between the ova and the testis. The *condom* (rubber) is used as a sheath over the penis at the time of intercourse. This prevents the spermatozoa from reaching the female reproductive tract. As it can also prevent the transmission of sexually transmitted diseases, including AIDS, its use has increased tremendously. The failure rate has been estimated as between 6% to 17%.

In the female, similar barriers like the *diaphragm* and *cervical cap* can be used. The diaphragm is inserted deep in the vagina, covering the superior portion of the vagina and the cervix. The cervical cap is smaller and covers only the cervix. Often, these barriers are combined with *creams* that are spermicidal. The failure rate ranges from 5% to 8%. The failure rate is less if the barrier and spermicide are used together.

Another method, although its failure rate is as high as 25%, is the **rhythm method.** With this method, the person abstains from intercourse during the days ovulation may occur. The various indicators of ovulation already described (e.g., changes in basal body temperature, consistency of the cervical mucus, calculation of day of ovulation if periods are regular) are used to estimate time and duration of abstinence.

Pregnancy

This section gives an overview of fetal development, the maternal changes that occur during pregnancy, and the physiology of labor and lactation.

DEVELOPMENT OF THE FETUS

The development of the fetus involves the division and differentiation of cells and the changes that occur in the fertilized ovum to produce and modify the anatomic structures. This process begins at the time of **fertilization** or **conception.** Although all human beings go through the same developmental processes, individual distinct characteristics are a result of the genetic makeup of the chromosomes in the sperm and ova.

Pregnancy Test

The human chorionic gonadotropin (HCG) can be detected in the maternal blood soon after implantation. The tests for early pregnancy detection show positive if this hormone is present in the urine/blood of the pregnant woman.

Fertilization

The process of fertilization involves the fusion of the contents of the sperm and ova to make up a **zygote** with 46 chromosomes. This typically occurs in the fallopian tube, which implies that the sperm has to travel the long distance between the vagina and the fallopian tube. The sperm are helped along by the movement of the flagella, contractions of the uterine wall, and the cilia in the tubal epithelium. Although about 200 million sperm are introduced into the vagina, only about 100 reach the ova. Despite the fact that ultimately only *one* sperm is required for this process, the enzymes located on the head of the sperm are required to penetrate the layer of cells from the ovarian follicle that surrounds the ova. The moment one sperm penetrates the cell membrane of

the ovum, rapid changes occur in the cell membrane to prevent other sperm from entering. From this time, the zygote rapidly multiplies and differentiates until a 3–4 kg (6.6–8.8 lb) infant is formed at the end of 9 months.

In Vitro Fertilization

In vitro fertilization is the process by which the mature ova is removed, fertilized with a sperm, and implanted in the uterus.

Gestation

The time spent in **prenatal** (time in the uterus) development is known as the **period of gestation.** The gestation period is about 38 weeks, calculating from the estimated date of fertilization (approximately two weeks from the first day of the last menstruation). This period, for convenience, is divided into 3 **trimesters** of 3 months each.

The First Trimester and Formation of Placenta

About 4 days after fertilization, the dividing, fertilized mass of cells (now known as the **blastocyst**) reaches the uterine cavity where it **implants** (attaches) in the endometrium of the uterus. The cells closest to the endometrium undergo rapid changes, eroding the maternal capillaries to form the **placenta** (see Figure 7.11). The endometrium also changes and, together with the fetal cells, forms the pancake-shaped placenta. Thus, the fetal blood, although not mixing with the mother's blood, comes in close contact with it. Eventually, the fetus moves away from the placenta, only connected to it by blood vessels—two umbilical arteries and one umbilical vein. This is the **umbilical cord.** The umbilical arteries carry deoxygenated blood from the fetus, and the umbilical vein carries oxygenated blood from the placenta to the fetus.

The amniotic fluid cushions the developing fetus. The cavity where this fluid is located is known as the **amniotic cavity.** The amniotic fluid regulates fetal body temperature, serves as a shock absorber, and

Developmental Abnormalities and Risk Factors

Because important developments occur particularly in the first trimester, exposure of the developing fetus and mother to toxins, drugs, viruses, and radiation, etc. can result in major developmental abnormalities.

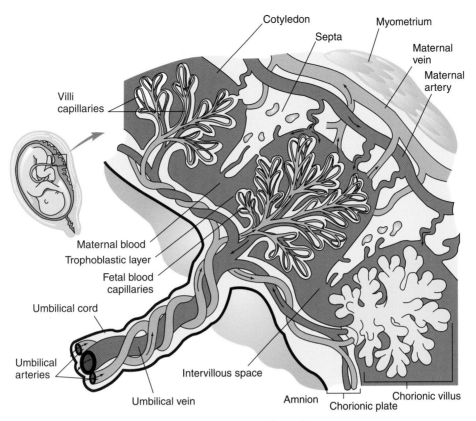

FIGURE 7.11. Structure of the Placenta

<table>
<tr><td colspan="2">

➕ **Amniocentesis**

When genetic abnormalities are suspected in certain individuals, the amniotic fluid is withdrawn by a needle to study the genetic makeup of fetal cells present in the fluid. This process is known as **amniocentesis.**
</td></tr>
</table>

prevents the fetal tissue from adhering to the maternal tissue. The fluid is initially derived from the mother's blood. Later, the fetus contributes to its formation. This fluid is referred to as the bag of waters, which ruptures at labor. (Please refer to more advanced textbooks for details of fetal development.)

Functions of the Placenta

The placenta has many functions. It serves as the respiratory, gastrointestinal, and excretory system for the fetus. Oxygen from the maternal blood diffuses into the fetal blood while the carbon dioxide diffuses in the opposite direction. Nutrition required by the fetus is brought by the uterine blood vessels to the placenta to be transported into the fetal circulation. The placenta also stores carbohydrates, fats, proteins, calcium, and iron, which can be released into the fetal circulation as and when required.

Waste products, such as urea, are removed from the fetus via the placenta. In addition, the placenta has endocrine functions. It secretes many hormones such as **human chorionic gonadotropin** (HCG), prolactin, relaxin, progesterone, and estrogen. The hormone HCG resembles LH and is responsible for maintaining the endometrium in the secretory phase during pregnancy. In addition, HCG keeps the corpus luteum in the ovary functional, secreting progesterone for 3 to 4 months of gestation, at which time the placenta takes up this function.

✓ ***Estimated Daily Dietary Requirements in Pregnancy***

Proteins	100 g	410 kcal
Fats	100 g	920 kcal
Carbohydrates	300 g	1,230 kcal
Other:		
Phosphorus	1.9 g	
Calcium	1.5 g	
Iron	15 mg	
Vitamin A	6,000 I.U.	
B complex	25 mg	
Vitamin C	100 mg	
Vitamin D	600 I.U.	

The placenta also serves as a protective barrier; not allowing most microorganisms to pass through. Certain antibodies (IgG antibodies) can cross the placenta and protect the fetus from certain diseases. The placenta also contains enzymes that are capable of converting biologically active molecules into less active, water-soluble forms. In this way, the placenta prevents harmful substances from reaching the fetus. Unfortunately, certain viruses, such as those causing AIDS, German measles, herpes, chickenpox, measles, encephalitis, and poliomyelitis, can cross the placenta. Many drugs and other substances, such as alcohol, ingested by the mother can cross the placenta. Of these, a number are capable of causing fetal birth defects.

Abnormal Implantation of Placenta

At times, the placenta may grow close to the cervical opening. As pregnancy progresses or when the cervix dilates late in pregnancy, severe bleeding may occur. This condition is known as **placenta previa.**

The time between the start of the third week to the end of the eighth week is referred to as the **embryonic period,** and the developing organism is called the **embryo.** Before the embryonic period, the developing structure can sustain itself. The embryo, however, depends on its mother for sustenance. From the eighth week, the embryo is called a **fetus.** The **fetal period** extends from the beginning of the ninth week to birth. At the end of 38 weeks, the fetus is considered **full-term.**

The Second and Third Trimester

By the end of the first trimester, the rudiments of all the major organ systems have formed. During the second trimester, the fetus rapidly grows in size and development of the major organ systems is complete. By the third trimester, the organs are ready to function. In the third trimester about 2.6 kg (5.7 lb) weight is gained by the fetus.

OTHER USES OF PLACENTA AND UMBILICAL CORD

The placenta is a source of hormones and blood. The tissue from the placenta can be used for covering burns and speeding healing. The veins from the placenta and umbilical cord are used for blood vessel transplants. Because the blood from the cord contains stem cells, these cells can be harvested and stored for future use.

Common Symptoms Associated with Pregnancy

First Trimester:
- Nausea and vomiting (morning sickness): probably a result of increased hormonal levels in the blood; the symptoms usually disappear by week 16
- Frequent urination
- Constipation: may be a result of lowered gut motility and the pressure of the uterus on the gut.
- Lower blood pressure: associated with feeling of faintness, especially after prolonged standing
- Breast changes: sense of increased fullness; tenderness
- Musculoskeletal changes: aching feet, pain over symphysis pubis, and sacroiliac joint, etc., as a result of increased weight bearing, shift in center of gravity, and laxity of joints
- Alteration of taste and smell
- Mood swings: Irritability, anxiety, depression.

Second Trimester:
- Sensation of fetal movement: between 18 and 21 weeks
- Edema
- Hypotension when supine
- Shortness of breath
- Backache
- Varicose veins and hemorrhoids as a result of pressure on abdominal veins
- Pigmentation: darkening of freckles; butterfly distribution of pigmentation over the nose and cheeks (chloasma); darkening of the region of the linea alba (linea nigra)
- Stretch marks: tissue overlying rapidly enlarging structures (e.g., breasts; abdomen)
- Heartburn: relaxation of the esophageal sphincter and the increase intra-abdominal pressure as a result of the growing fetus may precipitate this.
- Vaginal discharge: increase in vascularity in the perineal region induces increase in vaginal discharge. The warmth and moisture in this region encourages growth of microorganisms.

Third Trimester:
- Edema; compression syndromes, such as thoracic outlet syndrome; carpel tunnel syndrome, etc., secondary to edema
- Backache; sacroiliac sprain; leg cramps; costal margin pain
- Frequent urination; incontinence
- Fatigue
- Insomnia; restlessness

Postpartum Changes:
- Symptoms associated with postsurgical recovery, e.g., cesarean section; episiotomy(incision in the perineum made just before birth to prevent tearing of tissue)
- Soreness and tenderness of breasts
- Mood changes: postpartum blues (postpartum depression is more serious and involves feelings of extreme anxiety, hopelessness, and sadness that last for more than a few weeks)

MATERNAL CHANGES IN PREGNANCY

The fetus is solely dependent on the mother for its nutrition, waste removal, and respiratory functions. During pregnancy, major changes have to be made in the various organ systems of the mother to adapt to the new demands. Initially, the demands are minimal; however, as the fetus grows, the demands greatly increase. First, changes occur in the reproductive organs and breasts. Second, the metabolic functions are increased to provide sufficient nutrients to the fetus. Third, hormones secreted by the placenta produce their own effects.

Weight Changes

An average of 10 kg (22 lb) is gained by the mother during pregnancy. The weight of the fetus contributes about 3.63–3.88 kg (7.5–8.0 lb); the uterus, 0.90 kg (2 lb); placenta and membranes, 0.90 kg (2 lb); breasts, 0.68 kg (1.5 lb); with the remaining weight from fat and extracellular fluid.

Changes in Metabolism

The metabolism increases in proportion to the weight gain. Other than supplying the fetus its needs, the energy is utilized for the resultant increase in heart rate, respiratory rate, and liver function. The increase in metabolism is aided by the increase in thyroid hormone secretion caused by the thyroid stimulating hormone from the pituitary gland. Often, the thyroid gland hypertrophies as a result and may appear enlarged in about 70% of individuals.

Carbohydrate Metabolism

There is a demand by the fetus for an easily convertible source of energy. The mother tries to meet these demands by maintaining a higher level of glucose in the blood. As a result, there is less glucose storage in the muscle and liver as glycogen.

Protein Metabolism

Generally, there is less breakdown of protein during pregnancy. Blood amino acids are rapidly used by the

Terms

Neonatal period—time between birth and one month after birth
Infancy—from one month to two years of age
Childhood—from infancy to adolescence
Adolescence—period of sexual and physical maturation
Pediatrics—medical specialty that focuses on individuals from birth to adolescence

fetus for growth. Plasma proteins that help transport hormones are increased. To combat bleeding, the proteins required for clotting, such as fibrinogen, are also increased.

Fat Metabolism

Fat is the mother's main form of stored energy. Most of it is stored in the abdominal wall, back, and thighs.

Changes in Body Fluids

The sex hormones and adrenocortical hormones produced during pregnancy cause the mother to gain weight by fluid retention. There is an increase in the number of red blood cells, as well as plasma, in the blood. As a result, the blood volume increases as much as 1 liter (33.8 oz). This, in turn, increases the amount of blood pumped by the heart by 30%. At the time of labor, the mother loses about 200–300 mL (6.8–10 oz) of blood. The changes in the hormonal secretion soon after delivery bring the fluid levels close to normal.

The total amount of electrolytes (ions such as sodium, potassium, and calcium) in the blood is increased.

Respiratory Adjustments

The respiratory rate increases together with the volume of air inhaled with every breath (tidal volume).

Pregnancy and Heat Therapy

A warm footbath with 3–5 drops of essential lemon oil is relaxing at any time during pregnancy. Mild heat can be used over the back, gluteal, and neck regions to relieve aches. For those with edema, cold baths or wraps to the feet and legs may be beneficial. Figure-eight wraps may be used around the breasts to reduce pain and congestion.

Multiple Pregnancies

Twin pregnancies occur about 1 of 85 pregnancies. If it results from two ova being fertilized by two sperm in the same cycle, they are known as dizygotic/fraternal or nonidentical twins. These twins may be of the same or opposite sex. Monozygotic or identical twins are formed from a single zygote; therefore, they are of the same sex and genetically identical. If the zygote does not fully separate, conjoined twins (Siamese twins) are formed.

Triplets, quadruplets, and so on may be from one or more than one ovum. Often they result from maturation of many ova in one menstrual cycle, induced by drugs given to treat infertility.

High-Risk Pregnancies

A pregnancy that is complicated by conditions that put the mother and/or the fetus at risk for illness or death is termed a high-risk pregnancy. The condition may be present in the mother even before the pregnancy, induced during pregnancy, or the result of an abnormal physiologic reaction to pregnancy. Some of the conditions considered high-risk include:

- Diabetes (history of) or gestational diabetes
- Incompetent cervix (painless dilatation of cervix as pregnancy advances; predisposes to premature rupture of membrane and premature onset of labor)
- Maternal heart disease
- Multiple gestation
- Placenta previa
- Preeclampsia or toxemia of pregnancy
- Premature onset of labor (labor before 37 weeks of gestation)
- Premature rupture of membranes
- Vaginal bleeding
- History of repeated abortions
- Gestational diabetes in previous pregnancies
- History of repeated cesarean sections
- Older than 35 years
- Younger than 20 years
- Kidney disease

Flaring out of the ribs and increased movement of the diaphragm initiates this increase in volume. The anterior-posterior and transverse diameter of the chest increases by about 2 cm (0.8 in). As the fetus grows and occupies more space in the abdominal cavity late in pregnancy, the mother's breathing relies more on the movement of the ribs than the diaphragm. The diaphragm is elevated by about 4 cm (1.6 in) as a result of the abdominal contents, as well as the flaring out of the ribs. The changes in hormonal secretion often alter the caliber of the bronchi and, sometimes, mothers prone to asthma feel better during pregnancy. All these changes result in an increased intake of oxygen with improved supply to the fetus and a decreased level of carbon dioxide, which enables easier transfer of carbon dioxide from fetal to maternal blood.

Changes in the Cardiovascular System

Both the increase in maternal metabolism and the growth of the fetus place significant demands on this system. The increase in metabolism requires a parallel increase in blood supply to the lungs for gaseous exchange, to the kidneys for excreting the increased waste products, and to the skin to dissipate the increased heat produced. Also, blood supply to the placenta has to be increased as the fetus grows.

This demand is met by an increase in blood volume by retaining fluid. The total body water increases on an average by 5 liters (5.3 qt) towards the end of pregnancy. All this increases the workload of the heart. Both the heart rate and the volume pumped with each stroke (stroke volume) are increased. The heart increases in size and is located at a higher level as a result of the movement of the diaphragm.

The total number of red blood cells and hemoglobin content increases. Because the blood volume increases at a more rapid rate than the cells and hemoglobin, the hemoglobin levels may appear as less than normal. The number of platelets and white blood cells also increase significantly.

The blood pressure decreases early in pregnancy, with a slight decrease in systolic pressure and a marked decrease in diastolic pressure. The pressure decreases to its lowest level at midpregnancy, after which it gradually increases to reach its preconception level by 6 weeks after delivery. The change in blood pressure is mainly a result of the distensibility of the blood vessels.

Aromatherapy and Reproductive Conditions

Pregnancy
Essential oils that may induce uterine contractions should not be used during pregnancy. These oils include basil, bay, clary sage, cypress, fennel, frankincense, hyssop, jasmine, juniper, marjoram, myrrh, peppermint, rose, rosemary, and thyme. Tangerine, neroli, and lavender are oils that may be helpful during pregnancy. In general, those essential oils used should be diluted more than the recommended dosage during pregnancy.

Menopause
Fennel tea and ginseng root, taken as tea or in tablet form, have been helpful with menopausal symptoms of many women.

Dysmenorrhea
Antispasmodic essential oils, such as clary sage, chamomile, marjoram, peppermint, lavender, valerian, ginger, and nutmeg, may be used to prevent all forms of muscular spasms, including those of dysmenorrhea.

Some Pregnancy Symptoms That Require Physician Referral:

- Bleeding
- Difficulty walking
- Dizziness
- Irregular or rapid heart rate
- Pain
- Severe edema
- Shortness of breath
- Rapid weight gain
- Rupture of membrane

Exercise is recommended during pregnancy to improve posture, prepare the limbs for demands made during and after pregnancy, control pelvic floor musculature, facilitate cardiovascular fitness, and relaxation, among others. It is important for all pregnant women to be examined and evaluated by a physician before embarking on an exercise program. Proper warmup and cool down should be incorporated. When stretching, only one muscle group should be stretched. Pregnant women should avoid asymmetric stretching. Single-leg weight bearing; holding the breath, and exercises that cause pain should be avoided.

➕ **Labor and Surgical Procedures**

If there is a chance of the perineum tearing, the obstetrician may cut the perineal musculature to enlarge the vaginal passage. This procedure is known as **episiotomy.** If there are complications, the baby may be removed from the uterus by **cesarean section** (c-section). In this procedure, the abdominal wall and the anterior wall of the uterus are opened with an incision long enough to allow the passage of the baby's head.

The pressure exerted on the pelvic veins by the enlarged uterus causes vascular changes, especially in the lower limbs. Varicosities of veins and edema are common. These changes are more prominent during the day when the person is upright and gravity adds to the effect. In some individuals in a supine position, the uterus may press on the pelvic veins and reduce the volume of blood returning to the heart, with resultant fall in blood pressure and dizzy or unconscious spells.

Changes in the Gastrointestinal System

In general, appetite and thirst are increased. Toward the later part of pregnancy, the growing fetus exerts pressure on the gut, reducing the capacity for large meals. In the first trimester, the mother may be nauseous or may vomit. The increasing levels of progesterone tend to reduce the motility of the gut and reduces the relaxation of sphincters. As a result, relaxation of the sphincter in the lower end of the esophagus can produce regurgitation of food into the esophagus from the stomach and cause heartburn. The slower movement in the small intestine may aid better absorption of nutrients, while the slower activity of the large intestines aids better absorption of water. However, the latter may be responsible for the constipation often experienced by pregnant women.

Changes in Nutrient Requirements

The mother's requirements of vitamins and other nutrients increase by as much as 10% to 30%. The total energy required by the mother in the advanced stages of pregnancy is about 2,500 kcal/day (as compared with 2,100 kcal/day in a nonpregnant state). During lactation, the requirements increase to about 3,000 kcal/day.

Changes in the Renal System

The kidney increases in length by about 1 cm (0.4 in). As a result of the increase in waste production, the fluid filtered in the kidney (glomerular filtration) is significantly increased. In early and late stages of pregnancy, there is frequency of micturition. In early pregnancy, the enlarging uterus is still in the pelvis, compressing the bladder. In late pregnancy, the fetal head descends into the pelvis, irritating the bladder. The ureters appear to be dilated and the sphincter between the bladder and the ureter is more relaxed, resulting in reflux of urine into the ureter and predisposing the individual to urinary tract infection. As a result of fluid retention, the total urine volume excreted is less than that of nonpregnant individuals.

Changes in the Reproductive Organs

The breasts are fully developed by the end of the sixth month of pregnancy as a result of the action of many hormones, such as prolactin, oxytocin, estrogen, progesterone, thyroxin, growth hormone, and other hormones from the placenta. The glands begin to secrete, and the secretions are stored in the ducts.

Significant changes take place in the uterus. It increases in length from 7.6 cm (3 in) of a nonpregnant uterus to about 30.5 cm (12 in) at full term. At term, together with the contents and fluids, it weighs about 10 kg (22.1 lb)! Late in pregnancy, the elongated and hypertrophied smooth muscles contract spontaneously as a result of rising estrogen, oxytocin, and other hormonal levels. These contractions are irregular and nonpersistent and are indicators of false labor.

Hormones, such as estrogen and relaxin, soften the ligaments of the pelvic joints. This is to increase the capacity of the pelvis and to make it more mobile.

➕ **Diastasis Recti**

When there is separation of the rectus abdominus muscles in the midline (above, at, or below the umbilicus), the condition is known as diastasis recti. Pregnancy is one of the common causes of this condition. Herniation of abdominal contents, reduced protection of the fetus, and back pain are some complications.

LABOR

True labor commences at about 9 months (40 weeks) after the last menstrual period, resulting from the interaction of many factors. It is believed that both the fetus and the mother actively participate in the initiation of labor. For one, the stretching of the uterine wall and cervix by the enlarging fetus plays an important part. In addition, the concentration of progesterone secreted by the placenta begins to decrease, while estrogen concentration begins to rise toward term. The fetal and maternal pituitary secretes the hormone oxytocin in increasing amounts. Oxytocin stimulates smooth muscle contraction.

Soon, strong, rhythmic contractions and true labor begin. The contractions of the uterine musculature push the baby's head down into the pelvis, stretching the cervix and vaginal canal. The stretching of these structures stimulates sensory nerves that communicate with the pituitary to secrete more oxytocin by a positive feedback mechanism. This goes on until the baby is expelled from the uterus. The placenta and all the remnants are then expelled. The process of expulsion of the baby is known as **parturition.**

Traditionally, labor has been divided into three stages—**dilation, expulsion,** and **placental.** The dilation stage is from the beginning of labor to the time the cervix is completely dilated. This stage lasts for about 8 hours or longer. In this stage, the amniotic sac may rupture and the fluid may leak out.

During the expulsion stage, the rate of contractions occurs at about 2–3 minute intervals. It extends from the time of full cervical dilation to the expulsion of the baby and may last for about 2 hours.

During the placental stage, the uterus reduces in size and the placenta separates from the uterine wall to be expelled as the afterbirth. There is a loss of about 500–600 mL (17–20.3 oz) of blood at this time.

LACTATION

From the sixth month of pregnancy, the gland cells in the breast begin to secrete. The secretion in these early stages is known as **colostrum.** This secretion contains more protein than fat and is made up of protein immunoglobulins (antibodies) that help fight infection.

Human breast milk is largely made up of water (88.5 g/dL), lactose (6.8 g/dL), fat (3.8 g/dL), various ions such as sodium, potassium, chloride, calcium, magnesium, phosphorus, iron (very little), and vitamins. It also contains enzymes with antibiotic properties. It is shown that infants who are breast-fed have fewer infections than those who have been given formula from a bottle. This is because breast milk also contains immunoglobulins, lysosomes, neutrophils, and macrophages. A baby of normal size drinks about 850 mL, and the breasts secrete milk according to demand. Lactation may continue for 2 to 3 years after parturition if sucking occurs at regular and frequent intervals.

The reflex by which milk is secreted when an infant suckles the nipples is known as the **milk let-down reflex.** Here, the sensory nerves around the nipple are stimulated and, as a result of communication with the pituitary gland, result in oxytocin secretion. The bloodstream carries oxytocin to the breasts where it causes the myoepithelial cells (smooth muscle cells located around the mammary glands and ducts) to contract and expel the milk.

MILK LET-DOWN REFLEX

Milk let-down reflex often becomes a conditioned reflex, and oxytocin secretion is produced by visual cues or when the baby cries. Similarly, milk let-down reflex is inhibited by adrenergic stimulation—the fight-or-flight response. Hence, it is important for the nursing mother to be in a calm and quiet environment when she feeds her baby.

Effect of Lactation on the Mother

Breast-feeding reflexively inhibits the secretion of GnRH from the hypothalamus and gonadotropins from the pituitary and, thereby, ovulation. Breast-feeding can be considered a natural form of contraception. However, it is not an effective form of contraception in those who breast-feed infrequently, with wide intervals between feedings.

During lactation, the mother's diet has to be adequate because she uses large amounts of fat and protein to produce milk. In addition, if her calcium intake is insufficient, her parathyroid glands stimulate the absorption of calcium and phosphates from her bones, weakening them.

AGE-RELATED CHANGES IN THE REPRODUCTIVE SYSTEM

Menopause

Menopause is the time that ovulation and menstruation cease. It may be defined as the phase in the aging process of women that marks the transition from the reproductive stage of life to the nonreproductive stage. As a woman gets older, the ovaries become unrespon-

Reflexology and Symptoms

Reflexology has been effective in reducing premenstrual symptoms and duration of labor and providing symptomatic relief in those persons with pelvic inflammation and menstrual disorders, among others.

Hormone Replacement Therapy

Hormone replacement therapy (HRT) involves administration of a combination of estrogen and progesterone to menopausal women to decrease the symptoms and conditions associated with menopause. HRT has been of benefit in conditions such as hot flushes, reproductive organ atrophy, and osteoporosis. It helps enhance sexual response; alter mood, sleep, memory; enhance the feeling of well-being; and reduce the incidence of congestive heart failure in perimenopausal and postmenopausal women.

Some negative effects of HRT are menstrual bleeding, breast tenderness, headaches, tendency for thromboembolism, cardiovascular disease, hypertension, gall stones, and uterine cancer. The risk of breast and endometrial cancer associated with administration of estrogen alone is significantly reduced by using a combination of estrogen and progesterone. Women are prescribed HRT after taking family history and past and present medical history into consideration. It is important to consider the woman's risk for heart disease, osteoporosis, breast cancer, and other health problems, together with her personal feelings about taking hormones.

The most common hormones used are forms of estrogen, progesterone and, sometimes, testosterone. The hormones may be given in the form of pills, injection, through the vagina (vaginal rings, vaginal creams, suppositories), intrauterine devices, or by transdermal estrogen patches.

Recently, there has been an increasing interest on alternative therapies to HRT. These include natural products such as phytoestrogens (estrogenlike compounds found in plant products) and herbs. Several hundred plants have been found to exhibit estrogenic activity, including balm (*Melissa officinalis*); black cohosh (*Cimicifuga racemosa*); chaste tree, chasteberry (*Vitex agnus-castus*); ginkgo (*Ginkgo biloba*); ginseng (*Panax quinquefolius*); passionflower (*Passiflora incarnata*); St. John's wort (*Hypericum perforatum*); and valerian. Tofu, soy beans, lentils, and certain vegetables (broccoli, garlic, asparagus, and carrot, etc.) are dietary sources of phytoestrogens.

Testosterone replacement therapy is being suggested by some clinicians to enhance libido in older men.

sive to the gonadotropins (pituitary hormones) and, gradually, the sexual cycles disappear. The decline in function results in lower levels of estrogen and progesterone secretion. The reproductive organs slowly atrophy, together with the ligaments and supporting tissue as the hormonal stimulus decreases. Reduction of glandular secretion in the reproductive organs leads to excessive regional dryness. There is atrophy of the urethra, vaginal wall, and vaginal glands, with loss of lubrication. The glands in the breast also atrophy. However, menopause does not indicate the end of sexuality.

Menopause, also known as **climacteric,** usually occurs between the ages of 45 and 55 years (average, 52 years). In 8% of women, menopause occurs before the age of 40. A few years prior to menopause, the ovarian and uterine cycles become irregular. The cessation of menstruation is just one component in this transition period, which extends many years before and after the last cycle. It involves endocrine, physical, and psychological changes in the woman.

Menopause is often accompanied by psychological symptoms. As well, sudden sensations of warmth spreading from the trunk to the face (hot flushes) tend to appear. It is accompanied by increased perspiration, pulse rate, and vasodilatation. Although the cause is unknown, they tend to accompany sudden surges of LH secretion.

The risk of osteoporosis is higher after menopause. One reason is attributed to lower estrogen levels and many women, especially those at risk for developing osteoporosis, are routinely given low dose estrogen therapy after menopause. The risk of developing atherosclerosis is also high after menopause.

Other symptoms of menopause include headache, hair loss, muscular pains, insomnia, depression, weight gain, and mood swings.

Most women experience mild symptoms, although others experience unpleasant sensations. Many women undergo hormone replacement therapy (see Hormone Replacement Therapy) to alleviate osteoporosis and other symptoms.

In men, while the function of the testis diminishes slowly with age, there is no "male menopause" similar to that in women. Between the ages of 50 and 60, the level of testosterone decreases while FSH and LH levels increase. Sperm production may continue for a long time, but there is a gradual reduction in sexual activity.

In many elderly men, the prostate enlarges to two to four times its original size. This is known as **benign prostatic hyperplasia.** If the enlargement obstructs the urethra, the men experience obstructive symptoms, such as frequency of urination, hesitation, decreased force of the urine stream, and sensation of incomplete emptying.

MASSAGE AND THE REPRODUCTIVE SYSTEM

It is conceivable for massage to affect the functioning of the reproductive system, indirectly and directly, through its effects on the senses, autonomic nervous system, and the limbic system. Because the hypothalamus controls the secretions of the ovaries and testis via the pituitary gland, and the hypothalamus has close connections with various parts of the nervous system, massage can have some effects indirectly.

The tactile stimulation provided by massage increases the sensitivity of the body's sensory mechanisms. In addition, rhythmic and repetitive stimulation of certain areas, such as the gluteal region, thighs, and abdomen, has the potential to reflexly produce the physiologic changes in the genitals that occur during sexual arousal. This is because the lumbar and sacral nerve plexuses innervate all these areas.

The smooth muscles and glands of the reproductive system are controlled by the autonomic nervous system and massage affects these nerves. Massage primarily stimulates the parasympathetic nervous system that is responsible for "rest and digest." These nerves are also responsible for the sexual arousal response. Massage also affects the limbic system, the part of the nervous system that participates in emotions and sexual experiences.

It is important, therefore, for massage therapists to remember that the stimulation of the senses, parasympathetic nervous system, and the effects on the limbic system can produce a sexual response. Hence, both the client and the therapist must be capable of desexualizing the massage experience[1].

Massage therapy has positive effects in a number of conditions associated with the reproductive system. It improves mood; decreases anxiety and pain; decreases water retention symptoms in those with premenstrual syndrome[2]; and reduces aversion to touch and decreases anxiety and depression in women who had been sexually or physically abused.[3] In those with breast cancer, massage therapy has been shown to reduce anxiety, depression, and improve immune function.[4] Breast massage has been advocated for those with congestion, edema, lymphedema, premastectomy and postmastectomy surgeries, among others.[5] However, as touching the breasts has varying implications, breast massage requires special training and sensitivity.

Before treating a client, the therapist should always take a thorough history, including a history of menstrual cycles in female clients. Clients with complaints of unusual discharge from the genitals or breasts; swelling in the genital, inguinal, or breast regions; and irregularities in menstrual cycles should be encouraged to see their physician. It must be remembered that all body fluids, including those from the genital area are potential carriers of infections. Proper precautions should be taken while handling linen used in the clinic and all strategies for avoiding infection should be applied by the therapist.

Massage therapy is on the rise, especially during pregnancy, labor, and soon after childbirth. Massage decreases anxiety and levels of stress hormones during pregnancy.[6] There have been less complications during labor and postnatally in those women who had regular massage during pregnancy.[6]

Massage during labor decreases anxiety and pain, with a reduction in time of labor and hospital stay and lower incidence of depression postnatally.[6] Some women who received perineal massage during pregnancy claim that massage had positive effects on their preparation for birth and delivery.[7] The incidence of perineal trauma has also been decreased with massage.[8] Like breast massage, perineal massage is a specialized technique, accompanied by complex issues that need to be addressed.

There is growing evidence to show that massage not only has positive effects on the mother but also on the neonates.[9] For example, studies show that preterm infants gain more weight and infants who received massage therapy as newborns show greater weight gain and more optimal cognitive and motor development later.[9,10]

Massage certainly improves the overall sense of well-being and can help reduce some common complaints such as low back pain and of lower limb edema in pregnant women. It can help relax fatigued muscles that try to compensate for the shift in the center of gravity. Typically, a pregnant woman has a posture where the head is forward, chest is back, hip is tilted forward, the knees are locked, and the feet turned out. As a result, strain is placed on the neck and back muscles. In addition, the hormones secreted during pregnancy result in softening of the cartilage and ligament, increasing the tendency for joint instability and joint pain. Pregnant women who are confined to bed may benefit from the improved circulation, joint movement, and social contact that massage provides.

The client's position may need to be adjusted according to individual comfort. In the first trimester, women may be comfortable in the prone or supine position. In the third trimester, clients may feel more comfortable lying on the side or sitting up. This is because, in the supine position, the pressure of the fetus on the inferior vena cava may cause light-headedness, nausea, and backache and pressure on the descending aorta may impede blood flow to the placenta. Also, pressure on the diaphragm may produce shortness of breath. Some women may find a prone position comfortable if proper bolsters are available. For proper support, the therapist should use towels and pillows to fill any spaces. A pillow under the knees may help reduce back pressure when the client is in a half-reclining position.

When massaging a pregnant client, the therapist should focus on the neck, chest, lower back, hips, legs, and feet. Acupressure, acupuncture, reflexology, and other techniques can be incorporated to produce relaxation. Deep abdominal massage should be avoided throughout pregnancy. Deep massage and fascial techniques should be avoided over the low back, especially during the first trimester. As the joints are lax, joint mobilization techniques should be avoided throughout pregnancy and up to six months after delivery. Often, pregnant women complain of heartburn. In such cases, the massage should be scheduled at least 2 hours after the last meal to prevent regurgitation.

There are some conditions where massage should be avoided or given with great caution during pregnancy. In general, these mothers are identified as having "high-risk pregnancies" (See High-Risk Pregnancies, page 440). Individuals are considered high risk if they have had repeated abortions, have suffered from toxemia of pregnancy or had gestational diabetes in previous pregnancies, have had repeated cesarean sections, are older than 35 years or younger than 20 years, have heart disease, have kidney disease, expect multiple pregnancies, or are known to have any other complications. Fever, diarrhea, and a decrease in fetal movement over a 24-hour period are other general contraindications.

It is important to ensure that the pregnant client who has edema is not suffering from preeclampsia (a complication of pregnancy). Clients who appear visibly puffy, with rapid gain in weight and edema should be referred to their obstetrician. Also, pregnant clients who complain of bloody vaginal discharge, abdominal pain, a sudden gush of fluid from the vagina, severe headache, high fever, burning pain on passing urine, absence of fetal movement for more than a day, and excessive vomiting should promptly be referred to a medical professional.

Keep the temperature of the clinic slightly cooler than usual, as pregnant women tend to feel warm. It may be more convenient to use a space that is closer to a bathroom because pregnant women have a tendency to pass urine more frequently. One should ensure that there are enough pillows and supports to help position the woman comfortably. Assistance may be required while the client climbs on the table. Footstools come in handy on these occasions. It may be wiser to use a table at a lower level for clients who are in the late second or third trimester.

Ethical Issues

Many ethical issues have to be addressed while treating a client.[11,12] The most important of these is the proper draping techniques that need to be mastered and applied to avoid embarrassment and conflicts between the therapist and clients. Care should taken while massaging areas close to the external genitalia, lest the client is sexually aroused.[11]

Because of the intimate nature of massage therapy, the therapist can take some actions to create a more clinical yet relaxing atmosphere. The therapist can project a professional appearance by wearing a uniform or lab coat or overall during a therapeutic session. Care should be taken by the therapist to dress modestly, with hair in place. Using a clinic or office rather than the home for massage sessions is another suggestion. There should be zero tolerance for sexual misconduct. At the same time, respect for the client and his or her personal boundaries should be maintained. Effort should be made to maintain proper communication (both verbal and nonverbal) with the client at all times. Other measures include establish-

ing a professional healing space, using appropriate music, avoiding language that may be sexualized, obtaining informed consent, providing privacy while the clients dress and undress and, most of all, being aware of one's own sexuality.

Unfortunately, many individuals still indulge in "other" activities in the guise of massage, spoiling the reputation of certified professionals. Hence, it is important for massage therapists to report such individuals, to be active members of their local and national associations, and to visibly display their certifications and memberships in the work area.

REFERENCES

1. Redleaf A, Baird SA. Behind Closed Doors: Gender, Sexuality and Touch in the Doctor-Patient Relationship. Westport, CT: Auburn House/Greenwood, 1998.
2. Hernandez-Reif M, Martinez A, Field T, et al. Premenstrual syndrome symptoms are relieved by massage therapy. J Psychosom Obstet Gynecol 2000;21:9–15.
3. Field T, Hernandez-Reif M, Hart S, et al. Sexual abuse effects are lessened by massage therapy. J Bodywork Movement Ther 1997;1:65–69.
4. Chamness A. Breast cancer and massage therapy. Massage Ther J 1996;Winter.
5. Curtis D. Breast massage. Moncton: Curtis-Overzet Publications, 1999.
6. Field T, Hernandez-Reif M, Hart S, et al. Pregnant women benefit from massage therapy. J Psychosom Obstet Gynecol 1999;19:31–38.
7. Labrecque M, Eason E, Marcoux S. Women's views on the practice of prenatal perineal massage. Brit J Obstet Gynecol 2001;108:499–504.
8. Davidson K, Jacoby S, Brown MS. Prenatal perineal massage: preventing lacerations during delivery. J Obstet Gynecol Neonatal Nurs 2000; 29: 474–479.
9. Agarwal KN, Gupta A, Pushkarna R, et al. Effects of massage and use of oil on growth, blood flow, and sleep patterns in infants. Indian J Med Res 2000;112:212–217.
10. Field T, Scafidi F, Schanberg S. Massage of preterm newborns to improve growth and development. Ped Nurs 1987;13:385–387.
11. Ackermann D. Desexualizing the massage experience. American Massage Therapy Association. 2000. Available at: http//www.amtamassage.org/journal/su_00_journal/su_00_sexuality_desexualizing.html.
12. Humber JM, Almeder RF, eds. Biomedical Ethics Reviews: Alternative Medicine and Ethics. Totowa: Humane Press, 1983.

SUGGESTED READINGS

American Medical Association. Essential Guide to Menopause. New York: Pocket Books, 1998.
Hammond CB, Haseltine FP, Schiff I. Menopause: Biology and Pathobiology. San Diego: Academic Press, 2000.
Kinser C, Colby LA. Therapeutic Exercise: Foundations and Techniques. 2nd Ed. Philadelphia: FA Davis, 1990.
Lawless J. The Complete Illustrated Guide to Aromatherapy. Shaftesbury: Element Books, 1997. Shaftesbury, Dorset (U.K.).
Liisberg GB. Easier birth using reflexology. Tidsskrift for Jordemodre 1989;3.
Lobo RA, Kelsey J, Marcus R. Menopause: Evaluation, Treatment, and Health Concerns: Proceedings of a National Institutes of Health Symposium held in Bethesda, Maryland, April 21–22, 1988. New York: Alan R. Liss, 1988.

Oleson T, Flocco W. Randomized controlled study of premenstrual symptoms treated with ear, hand, and foot reflexology. Amer J Obstet Gynecol 1993;82(6) 906–911.

Premkumar K. Pathology A to Z. A Handbook for Massage Therapists. 2nd Ed. Calgary: VanPub Books, 1999.

Rattray F, Ludwig L. Clinical Massage Therapy: Understanding, Assessing, and Treating Over 70 conditions. Toronto: Talus, 2000.

Salvo SG. Massage Therapy Principles & Practice. Philadelphia: WB Saunders, 1999.

Review Questions

Multiple Choice

1. During pregnancy, all of the following occur EXCEPT
   A. The total number of red blood cells and hemoglobin content increases.
   B. Appetite and thirst increase.
   C. The motility of the small intestine increases.
   D. Respiratory rate and tidal volume increase.

2. During menopause, all of the following occur EXCEPT
   A. The ovaries become hypersensitive to the gonadotropins.
   B. The reproductive organs atrophy.
   C. Sudden sensations of warmth may occur, spreading from the trunk to the face.
   D. Levels of estrogen and progesterone decrease.

3. The reproductive organs that produce gametes and hormones are
   A. the vagina and penis.
   B. the accessory glands.
   C. the gonads.
   D. B and C are correct.

4. Before leaving the body, the sperm travel from the testis to the
   A. ductus deferens—epididymis—urethra—ejaculatory duct.
   B. epididymis—ductus deferens—ejaculatory duct—urethra.
   C. ejaculatory duct—epididymis—ductus deferens—urethra.
   D. epididymis—ejaculatory duct—ductus deferens—urethra.

5. In the male, the accessory glands are the
   A. epididymis, seminal vesicles, and vas deferens.
   B. prostate gland, inguinal canals, and epididymis.
   C. adrenal glands, bulbourethral glands, and seminal glands.
   D. seminal vesicles, prostate gland, and bulbourethral glands.

6. The spermatic cord is a structure that includes the
   A. ductus deferens, blood vessels, nerves, and lymphatics.
   B. vas deferens, prostate gland, blood vessels, and urethra.
   C. epididymis, ductus deferens, blood vessels, and nerves.
   D. A and C are correct.

7. Powerful, rhythmic contractions of the pelvic floor result in
   A. emission.
   B. erection.
   C. ejaculation.
   D. sperm production.

8. The three pairs of supporting ligaments that stabilize the position of the uterus and limit its range of movement are
   A. broad, ovarian, and suspensory.
   B. uterosacral, round, and lateral.
   C. endometrium, myometrium, and serosa.
   D. inguinal, lateral, and medial.

9. The most dangerous period in prenatal or postnatal life is the
   A. first trimester.
   B. second trimester
   C. third trimester.
   D. expulsion stage.

10. Organs and organ systems complete most of their development during the
    A. first trimester.
    B. second trimester.
    C. third trimester.
    D. stage of formation of placenta.

11. Blood flows to and from the placenta via
    A. paired umbilical veins and a single umbilical artery.
    B. paired umbilical arteries and a single umbilical vein.
    C. a single umbilical artery and a single umbilical vein.
    D. two umbilical arteries and two umbilical veins.

12. A cell from a normal male will contain _____ sex chromosomes, while a cell from a normal female will contain _____
    A. XX; XY.
    B. X; Y.
    C. Y; X.
    D. XY; XX.

Completion

Complete the following:

1. A pregnancy in which the embryo begins to develop outside of the uterus is called a(n) _____.

2. The middle layer of the uterus is called the _____.

3. The small body of erectile tissue homologous to the male glans penis is the _____.

4. Stretching of the cervix results in the release of _____ from the posterior pituitary gland at the time of labor.

5. Nutrition and excretion from the fetus are functions attributed to the _____.

6. The three gland(s) that secrete their products into the male reproductive tract are the _____, _____ and _____.

True or False

(Answer the following questions T, for true; or F, for false):

1. Breast milk release is a direct result of prolactin secretion.
2. Oxytocin is a hormone that stimulates the contraction of uterine smooth muscles.
3. The prostate gland is a paired gland.
4. Sperm accounts for 20% of the ejaculate volume.
5. Penile erectile tissue includes the corpus cavernosa and corpus spongiosum.
6. Both ejaculation and erection are reflex actions.
7. The prostate and seminal vesicles produce estrogens.
8. The mammary gland is synonymous to the breasts.
9. Ovulation typically occurs about 14 days prior to the beginning of the next menstrual cycle.
10. Vasectomy does not affect masculinity.
11. Breaking of the bag of waters refers to rupture of the amnion.
12. Male infertility may result from a sperm count of less than 40 million sperm/mL.

Matching

a. cremaster

b. fimbriae

c. seminiferous tubules

d. corpus luteum

e. clitoris

f. fornix

g. hymen

h. inguinal canals

i. prepuce

j. acrosome

1. The layer of skeletal muscle that contracts and pulls the testis closer to the body. _____

2. The shallow recess that surrounds the cervix as it protrudes into the vagina. _____

3. The fold of skin that surrounds the glans penis. _____

4. The fingerlike projections on the infundibulum that extend into the pelvic cavity. _____

5. The tip of the sperm that contains enzymes that play a role in fertilization. _____

6. The part of the male reproductive tract that manufactures sperm. _____

7. The endocrine structure formed after ovulation by degenerated follicular cells. _____

8. The narrow canals linking the scrotal chambers with the peritoneal cavity. _____

9. The female equivalent of the penis. _____

10. The thin epithelial fold that partially or completely blocks the vagina entrance prior to sexual activity. _____

Short Answer Questions

1. How is an individual's sex determined genetically?

2. What are the possible problems that may be encountered in the baby if the mother has had early exposure to sex hormones in pregnancy?

3. Why is it important for the mother to avoid radiation and exposure to drugs during the early months of pregnancy?

4. What are the physical changes seen in males and females at the time of puberty?

5. What are the functions of the testis?

6. What are the supports of the uterus in the abdominal cavity?

7. Why does menstruation occur?

8. What changes occur in the ovary and uterus during the different phases of the menstrual cycle?

9. What different contraceptive methods are available?

10. What changes occur in body fluids, respiratory, digestive, and cardiovascular systems during pregnancy?

11. What is menopause?

12. Why are postmenopausal women more at risk of developing osteoporosis?

13. What precautions should be taken by the therapist when treating a pregnant client?

14. What are some ethical issues that have to be addressed by the therapist?

15. What is the role of hormone replacement therapy in menopausal women?

16. What are the functions of estrogen?

Case Studies

1. Mary always had regular periods, but the length of her cycles is 40 days. She has been trying to conceive for a long time. Finally, Mary and her husband decided to seek medical help. Her doctor advised her to ensure that she and her husband had intercourse at the time of ovulation.
   A. If the first day of bleeding started on January 21, on what day is she likely to ovulate?
   B. What various methods can be used for detecting the time of ovulation?
   C. How can it be determined if Mary's husband is sterile?

2. Mr. McCullan was 56 years old. He had been having some difficulty passing urine during the past few months. His doctor, after a physical examination, mentioned that Mr. McCullan's prostate was enlarged.
   A. Where is the prostate gland located?
   B. What is the function of the prostate?
   C. How is the prostate related to the urethra?

3. Colleen, a new client, mentions to her therapist that she is pregnant. After three previous spontaneous abortions, she was excited that her pregnancy had continued until the fourth month this time. The therapist notices that Colleen has a puffy face and swollen feet.
   A. What are the normal symptoms associated with pregnancy in the first, second, and third trimester?
   B. Is the puffy face and swollen feet characteristic of normal pregnancy?
   C. List some conditions that are considered for a high-risk pregnancy.
   D. What are some signs and symptoms that require referral to a physician?

Answers to Review Questions

Multiple Choice

1. c	2. a	3. c	4. b	5. d	6. a
7. c	8. b	9. a	10. b	11. b	12. d

Completion

1. ectopic pregnancy
2. myometrium
3. clitoris
4. oxytocin
5. placenta
6. seminal vesicles, prostate, bulbourethral glands

True–False

1. False. Milk *release* is brought about by the hormone oxytocin
2. True
3. False
4. False. Only 5%
5. True
6. True
7. False. These accessory glands do not produce hormones
8. True
9. True
10. True. It only blocks the passage of sperm. Hormone production is not affected.
11. True
12. True

Matching

1. a
2. f
3. i
4. b
5. j
6. c
7. d
8. h
9. e
10. g

Short-Answer Questions

1. Genetically, an individual's sex is determined by the presence of XX (female) or XY (male) sex chromosomes.
2. If female fetuses are exposed to male hormones, especially during the 8th to 13th weeks of pregnancy, the genitalia may develop to look like that of a male. Conversely, in male fetuses, female hormone exposure can result in development of female genitalia. This syndrome is called pseudohermaphroditism.
3. Exposure to radiation and/or drugs can result in developmental abnormalities because the major organ systems develop during this period.
4. The body changes that occur at puberty in males are the enlargement of the external and

internal genitalia, voice changes, hair growth, mental changes, and changes in body conformation and the skin. The penis increases in length and width, and the scrotum becomes pigmented and rugose (wrinkled). All internal organs increase is size. The larynx enlarges, with thickening of the vocal cords and deepening of the voice. Body hair, in general, increases and hair begins to appear on the face, axilla, chest, and pubis. Mentally, the person becomes more interested in the opposite sex. There is a predisposition to acne because the sebaceous gland secretions thicken and increase.

In females, adolescence begins by the development of breasts and axillary and pubic hair, followed by the first menstrual period (menarche).

5. The functions of the testis are formation of sperm and production of androgenic hormones.

6. Laterally, the uterus is supported by the sheet of peritoneum (broad ligament); the uterosacral ligament, which runs from the lateral surface of the uterus to the anterior aspect of the sacrum, prevents the uterus from sliding anteriorly and inferiorly. The round ligaments, which run from the lateral aspect of the uterus just below the uterine tube toward the lateral wall of the pelvis into the inguinal canal, prevent the uterus from sliding posteriorly. The lateral ligaments run from the lower end of the uterus near the vagina to the lateral wall of the pelvis and prevent inferior movement of the uterus. The skeletal muscles and the fascia covering the pelvic outlet help further support the uterus.

7. If implantation of the fertilized ovum does not occur, the superficial layer of the endometrium sloughs off, leading to menstruation. The changing levels of the hormones estrogen and progesterone cause this to occur.

8. Please see Figure 7.9. Changes in the ovary: At the beginning of every cycle, a cavity filled with fluid forms around the oocytes (primordial follicles) in the ovary. Soon, one follicle rapidly increases in size, while the others regress. This is the dominant follicle. Some cells in the follicle secrete the hormone estrogen. At about 14 days before the start of the next cycle, the enlarged follicle ruptures and the ovum extrudes into the abdominal cavity. This process is known as ovulation. The ovum is picked up by the fimbriae of the uterine tubes and transported into the uterus. If fertilization occurs, the fertilized ovum embeds in the uterine cavity wall. If unfertilized, it is expelled from the uterus into the vagina and then outside the body at the time of menstruation.

After ovulation, the ruptured follicle in the ovary fills up with blood. The cells lining the follicle rapidly multiply and yellowish, lipid-rich cells known as luteal cells replace the clotted blood. The follicle is now known as the corpus luteum. The luteal cells secrete the hormones estrogen and progesterone. If pregnancy occurs, the corpus luteum persists and menstruation does not occur until delivery as a result of the continuous secretion of estrogen and progesterone. If there is no pregnancy, the corpus luteum degenerates by about 12 days after ovulation and is eventually replaced by scar tissue.

Changes in the uterus: At the beginning of the menstrual cycle, the uterine cavity has only the remnants of the deep layer of the endometrium. From the fifth to the fourteenth day, the endometrium rapidly increases in thickness and the uterine glands lengthen (proliferative phase). After ovulation, the endometrium becomes more highly vascularized. The glands coil and secrete a clear fluid (secretory phase). If the ovum is not fertilized, the endometrium becomes thinner and areas of cell death (necrosis) begin to appear in the endometrium. Blood vessels spasm and some bleeding are seen. The inner lining of the endometrium sloughs off. This collection of dead cells, along with the blood, is the menstrual flow.

9. Permanent methods: sterilization, vasectomy (males); tubal ligation (females); Temporary methods: oral contraceptives; intrauterine devices; barrier methods: condoms, diaphragm, cervical cap, spermicidal creams; rhythm method.

10. Changes that occur in body fluids: fluid retention, increased blood volume, increased amount of electrolytes; Respiratory system: rate and tidal volume increase, mother relies more on costal breathing and less on diaphragmatic movements, increased bronchial caliber, increased oxygen intake; Digestive system: increased appetite and thirst, during later part of pregnancy: reduced capacity for taking large meals, decreased gut motility, relaxation of sphincters; Cardiovascular system: increased blood supply to lungs, kidneys, skin, and placenta, increased heart rate and stroke volume, vascular changes in lower limbs such as varicosities.

11. Menopause is the time that ovulation and menstruation cease. It may be defined as the phase in the aging process of women that marks the transition from the reproductive stage of life to the nonreproductive stage.

12. A result of lower estrogen levels. Estrogen is one of the hormones required for proper calcium deposition in bones.

13. The therapist needs to take a good history: rule out high-risk pregnancies, check for symptoms such as abnormal weight gain, pain, vaginal bleeding, etc.; the client's position should be adjusted according to individual comfort and stage of pregnancy; techniques such as deep abdominal massage, fascial techniques over the back, and joint mobilization techniques should be avoided; the massage should be scheduled at least 2 hours after the last meal to avoid regurgitation.

14. To avoid conflict between therapist and client, proper draping techniques should be used; care when massaging areas close to the external genitalia; care to create a more clinical atmosphere; dress code; zero tolerance to sexual misconduct.

15. Hormone replacement therapy decreases the symptoms and conditions associated with menopause; it benefits conditions such as hot flushes, reproductive organ atrophy, and osteoporosis. It helps enhance sexual response, alter mood, sleep, and memory; enhances the feeling of well-being in perimenopausal and post-menopausal women. It has also been shown to reduce the incidence of congestive heart failure.

16. Estrogen facilitates ovarian follicle growth and increases fallopian tube motility. It increases the size of the uterus and excitability of uterine smooth muscles. It also sensitizes the uterus to the hormone oxytocin at labor. In the breast, estrogen is largely responsible for the size increase at puberty. Estrogen accelerates the growth of long bones and closure of epiphysis at puberty and decreases the rate of bone resorption. Estrogens tend to lower the levels of cholesterol in the blood.

Case Studies

1. **A.** She is likely to ovulate on February 16 (if this particular February has 28 days).
   B. Ovulation can be detected by measuring the basal body temperature; changes in the cervical secretion, thickening in the luteal phase, and uterine changes from proliferative to secretory phase are some methods that can be used to detect ovulation. Ovulation or presence of corpus luteum can be observed directly using laparoscopic techniques.
   C. Semen analysis can determine if the number, motility, and appearance of the sperm are normal. Normally, 20–100 million sperm are found per milliliter of semen and more than 60% of sperm are motile.

2. **A.** and **C.** The prostate gland is located inferior to the urinary bladder; it surrounds the prostatic part of the urethra.
   B. The prostate helps maintain the pH of the semen. It contains chemicals that prevent growth of microorganisms.

3. **A.** Common Symptoms Associated With Pregnancy
   First trimester: Nausea and vomiting, frequent urination, constipation, lower blood pressure associated with feeling of faintness, especially after prolonged standing, breast changes (sense of increased fullness, tenderness), musculoskeletal changes (aching feet, pain over symphysis pubis, sacroiliac joint) as a result of increased weight bearing, shift in center of gravity, and laxity of joints, alteration of taste and smell, mood swings (irritability, anxiety, depression).
   Second trimester: sensation of fetal movement between 18 and 21 weeks, edema, hypotension when supine, shortness of breath, backache, varicose veins and hemorrhoids resulting from pressure on abdominal veins, pigmentation: darkening of freckles; butterfly distribution of pigmentation over the nose and cheeks (chloasma); darkening of the region of the linea alba (linea nigra), stretch marks (tissues overlying rapidly enlarging structures—breasts and abdomen).
   Third trimester: edema; compression syndromes, such as thoracic outlet syndrome; carpel tunnel syndrome, etc., secondary to edema; backache; sacroiliac sprain; leg cramps; costal margin pain; frequent urination; incontinence, fatigue, insomnia; restlessness.
   B. The puffy face and swollen feet are not characteristic of normal pregnancy. It may be a result of preeclampsia or some other cause of edema may coexist.
   C. Some conditions that are considered as high-risk in pregnancy are diabetes, incompetent cervix, maternal heart disease, multiple gestation, placenta previa, preeclampsia, premature onset of labor, premature rupture of membranes, and vaginal bleeding.
   D. Some symptoms that require referral to a physician are bleeding, difficulty in walking, dizziness, irregular or rapid heart rate, pain, severe edema, shortness of breath, rapid weight gain, and rupture of membrane.

Coloring Exercise

Label the structures in the given diagrams, and color the structures, using your own color code.

O Uterus and fallopian tube
O Prostate
O Ovary
O Cervix
O Vagina
O Peritoneal cavity
O Urethra
O Epididymis and vas deferens
O Corpus cavernosum
O Corpus spongiosum

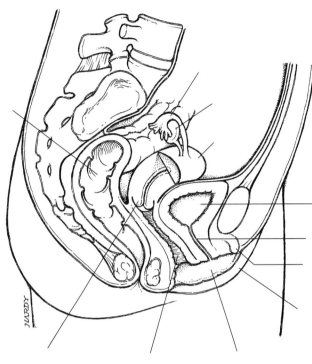

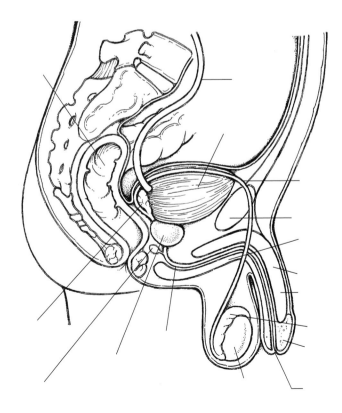

Cardiovascular System

Objectives

Blood

On completion of this chapter, the reader should be able to:

- List the functions of blood.
- Identify the composition of blood.
- List the cellular elements of blood.
- Discuss the origin, structure, and function(s) of each cellular element.
- Describe, in brief, the structure of hemoglobin.
- Describe the destruction process of red blood cells.
- Discuss the ABO and Rh blood grouping systems.
- Discuss the importance of blood grouping.
- Describe, in brief, the coagulation process of blood.
- Explain the process of clot lysis and its significance.
- Define thrombosis and embolism.
- List examples of anticoagulants.
- Describe plasma components and the function of its constituents.

Heart

- Describe the location and general features of the heart.
- Describe the function of each structure in the heart.
- Trace the blood flow through the different chambers and major blood vessels in the heart.
- Describe the components and function of the conducting system of the heart.
- Describe the blood supply to the heart and innervation of the heart.
- Mention the effects of nerves on heart activity.
- Describe the cardiac cycle events and the origin of heart sounds.
- Define stroke volume, cardiac output, venous return, blood pressure, systole, and diastole.
- List the factors that affect heart rate and cardiac output.

Blood Vessels

- Compare the structure and function of the different types of blood vessels.
- Identify the major arteries and veins of the body and the areas they supply/drain.
- Describe the hepatic portal system.
- Describe pulmonary circulation.
- Identify the location of superficial arteries.
- Describe the factors that affect blood pressure.
- Describe the regulation of blood pressure and blood flow.
- Identify the location and function of baroreceptors.

(continued)

- Describe the adaptation of the cardiovascular system to the effects of gravity, exercise, bleeding, and cardiac failure.
- Describe the cardiovascular changes that occur with aging.
- Discuss the possible effects of massage on the cardiovascular system.

The cardiovascular system, commonly known as the circulatory system, is an important communication and transport channel, and it is the only system with access to every living cell of the body. Similar to any complex communication channel, the cardiovascular system has networks, in the form of blood vessels, linking various tissue. The blood is the medium of communication. Because this is a fluid medium, it has to be pumped through the network—the heart is the pump.

This chapter describes the different components of the circulatory system. Blood composition and functions are initially discussed, followed by descriptions of the heart, blood vessels, and the mechanisms involved in maintaining pressure and flow. Finally, compensatory adjustments made by the system to certain challenges, such as effects of gravity and exercise, and the effects of aging and massage are addressed.

Blood

The blood is an example of connective tissue that is liquid. It is the body fluid that supplies oxygen, absorbed from the respiratory system, and nutrients, absorbed from the gastrointestinal tract, to the tissue. In the tissue, the oxygen and nutrients diffuse out of the blood vessels into the interstitial fluid that bathes the cells and, finally, across the cell membrane into the cell. Similarly, waste products, such as carbon dioxide, diffuse out of the cell into the interstitial fluid and then into the blood. The waste products and other products of metabolism are then carried to the lungs, kidneys, skin, and digestive tract for elimination.

Blood helps maintain the body temperature. It transports hormones and other agents that regulate the functioning of individual cells. It also helps regulate the pH of the body fluids. The composition of blood is important for regulating the volume of water in the body. Blood has a protective function because it contains white blood cells and proteins, such as antibodies and interferon, that help fight foreign agents.

HEMATOLOGY

Hematology is the study of blood and blood-forming tissue and associated disorders.

The blood contributes approximately 8% of the body weight. The volume of blood in an adult man is approximately 5–6 liters (5.3–6.3 qt) and, in an adult female, it is about 4–5 liters (4.2–5.3 qt). Blood is more viscous than water. The pH of blood is maintained between 7.35 and 7.45. The temperature of blood is about 38°C (100.4°F). The color of blood depends on hemoglobin content. When the hemoglobin is oxygenated, blood appears red—as in peripheral arteries. If the oxygen content is low, it appears blue—the color of blood in superficial veins.

Blood is made up of two major components: **cells,** the formed elements, and **plasma,** the liquid portion. If a small volume of blood is withdrawn and centrifuged, the cells (the heavier elements) will settle at the bottom of the centrifuge tube. The cells constitute about 45% of the blood's volume. The remaining 55% is the plasma, the liquid portion around the cells.

The formed elements of blood are the **red blood cells** (RBC), **white blood cells** (WBC), and **platelets.** The red blood cells make up about 99% of the volume of cells.

FORMATION OF BLOOD CELLS

Because many blood cells die within hours, days, or weeks, the body must constantly replace them. The total number of each cellular element is controlled by negative feedback mechanisms. The process of blood cell formation is called **hemopoiesis** or **hematopoiesis.**

The blood cells are formed from **pluripotent stem cells** found in the bone marrow. These stem cells are capable of multiplying. They also differentiate into precursor cells that can form all the formed elements of the blood. The **myeloid stem cells** give rise to the red blood cells, platelets, and white blood cells (all except lymphocytes). The **lymphoid stem cells** give rise to the lymphocytes; however, some of the lymphocytes complete their development in lymphoid tissue located outside the bone marrow.

A number of growth factors regulate the differentiation and multiplication of the stem cells. For example, **erythropoietin** (a hormone produced by the kidney) regulates red blood cell production. **Thrombopoietin,** a hormone produced by the liver, regulates the production of platelets. **Cytokines,** small glycoproteins produced in such different areas as the bone marrow, white blood cells, fibroblasts, and endothelial cells, also help regulate cell function and proliferation. Examples

Spherocytosis

In certain conditions, cells appear abnormal; for example, in **spherocytosis,** the red cells are rounded instead of biconcave. In such cases, the cells break up easily as they pass through the spleen. As a result, a person with spherocytosis is chronically anemic. The process of breaking up red cells is called **hemolysis.**

of cytokines include **colony-stimulating factors** and **interleukins.**

RED BLOOD CELLS

Red blood cells (see Figure 8.1), also known as **erythrocytes,** are packages that carry the oxygen-carrying protein pigment **hemoglobin** in the circulation. The red coloration is a result of the presence of hemoglobin. The red cells are biconcave and do not have a nucleus and other organelles. Hence, these cells cannot reproduce or perform complex metabolic activities as other typical cells. Under the microscope, they look like doughnuts because the central portion of the disk is indented. This shape and small size enables them to squeeze single file through the smallest blood vessels. The biconcave shape also allows the cell to swell without rupturing, if the surrounding environment becomes hypotonic.

There are about 5.4 million cells per cubic millimeter in males and about 4.8 million cells per cubic millimeter in females. Each of these cells has about 280 million hemoglobin molecules. Visualize the volume of blood that contains this number of red cells by identifying a millimeter on your tape measure.

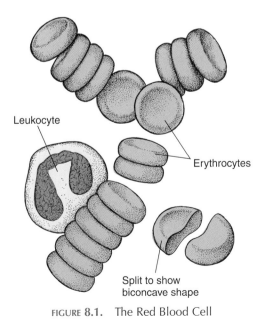

FIGURE **8.1.** The Red Blood Cell

Polycythemia, or Erythrocytosis

Polycythemia, or erythrocytosis, is a term that describes abnormally large numbers of red blood cells (RBCs) in the blood. It is usually a result of excess production of the hormone erythropoietin from the kidneys when there is an oxygen deficiency. People living in high altitudes exhibit this condition because the air has less oxygen than at sea level. The increased number of RBCs compensates for the reduced quantity of oxygen carried by each cell. Polycythemia may be observed in individuals with lung or heart problems that result in less oxygen perfusion of tissue.

The practice of **blood doping** has a similar basis. Weeks before a competitive event, athletes involved in sports that require increased endurance may remove some blood from their bodies and store it for future use. Meanwhile, the athletes' bone marrow replenishes the RBCs that have been removed. Just prior to the event, the stored RBCs (separated from the plasma) are reinfused into the athlete. The objective is to increase the oxygen-carrying capacity and, thereby, increase endurance and give an added edge over other athletes. Some athletes resort to the administration of erythropoietin to produce similar increases in RBC numbers. Unfortunately, the polycythemia produced increases blood viscosity and a tremendous workload for the heart.

Red Blood Cell Formation

The red blood cells are formed in the bone marrow, according to the needs of the body. The process of red cell formation is known as **erythropoiesis.** The kidneys monitor the blood and secrete a hormone called **erythropoietin** when the oxygen levels in the blood decrease below normal. Erythropoietin stimulates the marrow cells that manufacture red cells (also **see page 612.**) Other than erythropoietin, many other factors such as protein, iron, folic acid, and vitamin B_{12} are required for forming red cells and their hemoglobin content. Certain hormones, such as growth hormone, thyroxine, estrogen, and androgen, are also required.

The site of blood cell formation varies from age to age. In the fetus, the cells are formed in the liver and spleen. In children, the cells are formed in the marrow cavities of all bones. By age 20, the blood cells are manufactured in the upper end of the humerus and femur and in flat bones such as the sternum, and the pelvis, and vertebrae. In emergencies, however, other areas may revert to forming red cells. The marrow that is actively producing blood cells is red. Inactive bone marrow is infiltrated with fat and appears yellow.

Hemoglobin

Hemoglobin (Hb) (see Figure 8.2) is the most important component of red blood cells, and it has a great

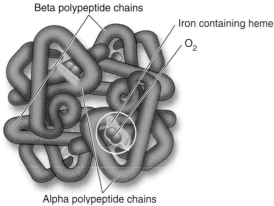

FIGURE **8.2.**   Structure of Hemoglobin

affinity for oxygen. Each hemoglobin molecule is a protein pigment that has a **heme** portion and a **globin** portion. The heme portion contains four iron ions in ferrous form to which four oxygen molecules becomes attached. The globin portion consists of four peptide chains (2 alpha and 2 beta polypeptide chains), the structure of which determines the property of hemoglobin (also **see box Hemoglobin Abnormalities**) Hemoglobin helps transport oxygen as well as carbon dioxide. In addition, it is a buffer, preventing rapid changes in the blood pH.

A more recent discovery is the role hemoglobin plays in blood pressure regulation. Hemoglobin attaches to nitric oxide gas (produced by tissues) and transports it to and from tissues. Nitric oxide produces vasodilation. Another form of nitric oxide—super nitric oxide—causes vasoconstriction. Hemoglobin thus affects blood pressure by transporting nitric oxide and super nitric oxide.

HEMOGLOBIN CONTENT

The content of hemoglobin in 100 mL of blood is approximately 16 grams. An easy way to measure red blood cells and thereby hemoglobin content is to centrifuge a small quantity of blood and estimate the percentage of volume that the blood cell sediment occupies. In a healthy person, this volume is equivalent to approximately 47%. This measurement is called the **hematocrit,** or the **packed cell volume** (PCV).

A reduction of red cells or hemoglobin content is known as **anemia.** Anemia is a condition in which the number of red blood cells per cubic millimeter is diminished or the volume of hemoglobin in 100 mL of blood and/or the packed cell volume of blood is less than the normal range. It may have various causes. Any condition that affects the production of hemoglobin/red blood cells, results in blood loss, and/or leads to rapid destruction of red cells can result in anemia. Iron-deficiency is just one cause of anemia.

Clinically, anemia presents as skin and mucous membrane pallor, shortness of breath, heart palpitations, soft systolic murmurs, lethargy, and fatigability.

Hemoglobin Abnormalities

Because of inheritance, the amino acid sequence in some hemoglobin peptide chains may be different in some people. These small sequence differences can alter the affinity of hemoglobin to oxygen or alter its properties. For example, in **sickle cell anemia,** the hemoglobin becomes insoluble when the oxygen levels in blood drop. The red cells become sickle-shaped (like a quarter moon) when the hemoglobin becomes insoluble. The cells are recognized as abnormal by the spleen and hemolyzed (broken down), resulting in anemia.

Red Blood Cell Death and Destruction

A normal red cell in circulation lasts for about 120 days. As the cells age, they become more fragile and are destroyed and removed by phagocytic cells as they squeeze through the network of capillaries in the spleen, liver, and bone marrow.

When the red cells are broken down, some of the contents, such as iron and protein, are recycled. Globin is broken down into amino acids that can be reused to form new proteins. The iron from the heme is removed and transported by a protein in the plasma known as **transferrin.** The iron detaches from transferrin on reaching tissue such as the liver, muscle cells, and spleen and become attached to iron storage proteins **ferritin** and **hemosiderin.** When needed, the iron is released from the storage proteins and transported in the blood to the bone marrow, where new red blood cells are formed.

The heme portion, without iron, is converted to a greenish-yellow pigment (**biliverdin**) and a yellow-orange pigment (**bilirubin**). The excessive production of bilirubin is responsible for the yellowish discoloration in jaundice.

Jaundice

When jaundice is mentioned, many individuals immediately associate it with hepatitis or liver disease. However, jaundice is only a sign that can be caused by any condition that results in excessive blood levels of bilirubin. You will realize this as you study the fate of bilirubin.

Jaundice in Newborns
Some newborns develop yellow discoloration soon after birth as a result of the formation of increased bilirubin by destruction of fetal hemoglobin. Fetal hemoglobin is different in structure and is destroyed and replaced by the adult type soon after birth. The immature liver is unable to cope with the rate of destruction; hence, the jaundice. Exposure to white light speeds the removal of bilirubin from the skin and mucous membranes, which is why jaundiced newborns are placed under white light.

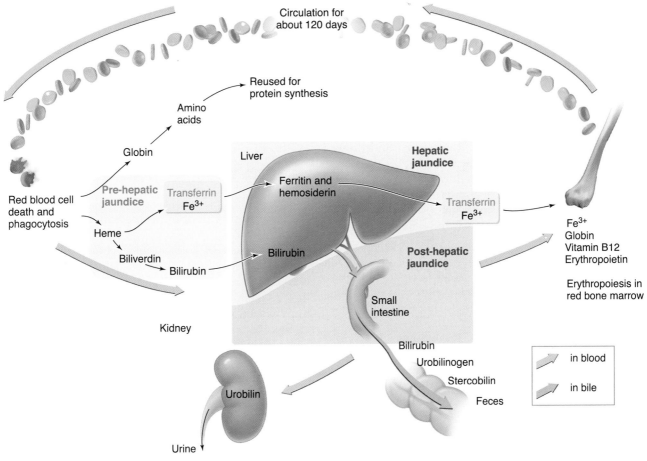

FIGURE 8.3.   Fate of Red Blood Cells

The Fate of Bilirubin

Bilirubin is carried in the blood from the macrophages in the spleen, liver, or red bone marrow to the liver, where it enters the liver cells and is converted into another form of bilirubin—**conjugated bilirubin.** Conjugated bilirubin is secreted by the liver cells into bile. (Bile is the yellow secretion formed by the liver, stored in the gall bladder, and secreted into the intestines when fat needs to be digested). As part of bile, bilirubin reaches the large intestine where it is converted by the bacteria in the intestine to **urobilinogen.** Some urobilinogen is reabsorbed into the blood and converted to the yellowish pigment **urobilin.** Urobilin is then excreted from the body in urine. The rest of the urobilinogen is excreted in the feces in the form of a brown pigment known as **stercobilin.** It is stercobilin that gives feces the characteristic color.

As can be observed, bilirubin is transported to many regions before it is excreted (see Figure 8.3). From the macrophages in the spleen, it goes via the blood to the liver; as part of bile to the gallbladder, bile ducts, and intestines. Any problems along this route can result in excessive blood levels of bilirubin. When the levels of bilirubin increase in the blood, it

spills over into connective tissue and the skin, mucous membrane, and white of the eye (sclera), producing a yellow discoloration. This yellow discoloration is called **jaundice** or **icterus.**

In summary, jaundice can result from increased red cell destruction by the macrophages in the spleen, liver, and bone marrow (**prehepatic jaundice**), as a result of liver disease (e.g., viral hepatitis or **hepatic jaundice**), or as a result of bile duct blockage (**posthepatic jaundice**). As you may have realized, not all conditions producing jaundice are infective.

BLOOD TYPES

The cell membrane of red blood cells contains a variety of glycoproteins and glycolipids (antigens) that can provoke antibody formation (**see page 524**). In the blood, these antigens are referred to as **agglutinogens;** the antibodies as **agglutinins.** Based on the presence of certain agglutinogens, blood is classified into different **blood groups,** such as ABO grouping and Rh grouping. Humans have more than 24 blood groups; however, ABO grouping and Rh grouping are the major groups. There may be many **blood types** in each group.

ABO Grouping

In the ABO group, there are two important antibody-provoking antigens—the **A** and **B agglutinogens.** Based on the *presence* or *absence* of these antigens, individuals are divided into 4 major blood **types—A, B, AB,** and **O.** Individuals with **type A** have the A antigen on the red blood cell membrane; individuals with **type B** have B antigen; individuals with **type AB** have both antigens on the cell membrane; and individuals with **type O** have neither antigen on the cell membrane. A and B antigens have been found in other tissue, such as salivary glands, saliva, pancreas, kidney, liver, lungs, testes, and semen.

In general, antibodies against antigens are inherited or developed upon exposure to the antigens (**see page 524**). In the blood, the antibodies (agglutinins) against A and B antigens are *inherited.* Therefore, individuals who are blood type A have antibodies against B antigen (anti-B antibodies) in their plasma; individuals with type B have antibodies against A antigen (anti-A antibodies); and individuals with type O have antibodies against both A and B antigens (anti-A and anti-B antibodies). Individuals with type AB do not have antibodies against A and B antigens because they possess both antigens (see Table 8.1).

Importance of Blood Grouping

Blood or blood components are often transferred from one person to another by a process known as **blood transfusion.** When a person is exposed to a wrong blood type, the antigens and antibodies react with each other. This results in **clumping** of red blood cells—the red cells are closely drawn to each other. The clumping of blood cells resulting from an antigen-antibody reaction is called **agglutination.** These red cell clumps can block capillaries and reduce blood flow to tissue, with serious consequences. In addition, all immune reactions (**see page 525**) are triggered with activation of the complement system, release of chemical mediators, and even anaphylaxis.

Table 8.1

Agglutinogens and Agglutinins of ABO Blood Groups

Blood Groups	Antigens on Red Cell Membrane (Agglutinogens)	Antibodies Present in Plasma (Agglutinins)
A	A	Anti-B
B	B	Anti-A
AB	A and B	None
O	None	Anti-A and Anti-B

The clumps are also hemolyzed (broken down) to release hemoglobin into the plasma. Free hemoglobin in the plasma can increase the viscosity of blood, block the glomeruli of the kidneys, and lead to kidney failure.

For example, agglutination of blood cells can happen if A type blood is transfused into a person of B type. This is because the B type person has existing antibodies against A antigen in the plasma. What do you think will happen if a person of O blood type is given the blood of an A group, B group, or AB group individual? Yes, there will be agglutination because the O group person already has antibodies against A and B antigen in their plasma. Now, identify what blood type can be given to a person belonging to AB blood group. Can blood type A be given? Yes, as the recipient plasma does not have antibodies against A antigen. Can blood group B be given? Yes—no antibodies against B antigen are present. What about O group? Yes—O group has no antigens. Because individuals with AB group can be given any type of blood, these persons are called **universal recipients.** However, because persons with group O cannot tolerate (or is incompatible with) any type of blood other than O (but can donate to individuals of any blood type), these persons are called **universal donors.** This is the basis of blood transfusion.

Cross Matching

Before blood is transfused, tests are performed to see if any agglutination occurs when the plasma of the recipient and red cells of the donor (and vice versa) are mixed. This test, called **cross matching,** is done even when blood types are known. Because there are several other blood group types, it is important to cross match blood before blood transfusion.

Some questions arise. What if the *donor* has antibodies against the red cells of the *recipient?* For example, what about the antibodies present in O group plasma if O group blood is given to a person of A group? Doesn't the O group blood have antibodies against A and B antigen? Will this not clump red cells of the recipient?

Yes, it can. However, because blood from the donor (about 400 mL (0.422 qt)) is given to the recipient slowly, the antibodies are diluted in the recipient's plasma (plasma volume is approximately 3.5l [3.7 qt]) before they can produce any reaction.

Rh Grouping

Rh system is another important blood grouping system, other than the ABO system discussed above. The **Rh factor** (or **Rhesus factor**) was named after the rhesus monkey, whose blood was first used to study this system, and it consists of many antigens (e.g., D, C, and E) on the red blood cell membrane. Of these, the D antigen is most important. When a person has the D antigen on the cell membrane she or he is said to be **Rh-positive** (Rh$^+$). If no D antigen is present, the individual is said to be **Rh-negative** (Rh$^-$). Unlike the ABO system in which antibodies are present against the antigens that are not present of the red cells, an Rh-negative individual does not have antibodies in the plasma against the Rh antigen. However, if those individuals are exposed to the Rh antigen, antibodies are eventually developed.

Importance of Rh Grouping

The Rh system gains importance in an Rh-negative mother if the father happens to be Rh positive. When the mother is pregnant with an Rh-positive fetus, small amounts of Rh-positive blood from the fetus may leak into the maternal circulation. This tends to happen especially at the time of delivery. If the mother is exposed to Rh-positive blood cells, she develops antibodies against the Rh antigen. Usually, the first fetus is not harmed by antigen-antibody reaction because the leakage tends to occur at the time of delivery and not many antibodies are developed by the mother. This is equivalent to the primary response described **on page 526.**

If the mother becomes pregnant again with an Rh-positive fetus, the antibodies that she has already developed can enter the fetal circulation and cause agglutination and hemolysis of fetal blood cells. This is called **hemolytic disease of the newborn** or **erythroblastosis fetalis.** If the reaction is severe, the fetus can die in the uterus; if less severe, the fetus can develop anemia, jaundice, or edema. Because the breakdown product of hemoglobin—bilirubin—can enter the fetal brain, neurologic problems can develop. (In an adult, barriers developed in the blood capillaries of the brain do not allow bilirubin to enter brain tissue).

Fortunately, injecting anti-Rh antibodies into the Rh-negative mother soon after delivery can prevent development of antibodies. These anti-Rh antibodies recognize Rh antigens if they enter the mother's circulation and destroy them before they can stimulate the mother's immune system.

One might wonder how blood grouping has any direct bearing on massage therapy. The basis of blood typing is an apt example of the basic concepts of immunity and how immunity is developed in an individual. The immune mechanisms involved in fighting off infection, recognizing foreign cells (as in transplantation), and benefits of immunization follow the same principles.

WHITE BLOOD CELLS (LEUKOCYTES)

The white blood cell, part of the immune system, provides the body with powerful defenses against infection and tumors. The white blood cells are divided into two types depending on whether they have granules in the cytoplasm. Those with granules are termed **granulocytes (polymorphonuclear leukocytes)** and those without are termed **agranulocytes.** The granulocytes have a lobed nucleus (see Figure 8.4), and the granules in the cytoplasm take on different colors if stained. Certain cells with small granules in their cytoplasm are called **neutrophils.** Those cells with granules that stain pink with acid dyes are called **eosinophils,** and those with granules that stain blue are called **basophils.** Each granulocyte subtype has specific functions.

There are two types of agranulocytes—**lymphocytes** and **monocytes.** They are involved in humoral and cell-mediated immunity and are described further **on page 524.**

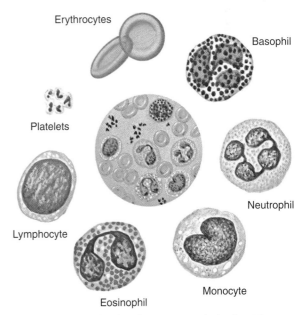

FIGURE 8.4.   White Blood Cells (WBCs) and Platelets. The normal range of white blood cells per cubic millimeter of blood is: Basophil (range, 0–150 or < 1%); Neutrophil (range, 1,800–7,300 or 50%–70%); Monocyte (range, 200–950 or 2%–8%); Eosinophil (range, 0–700 or 2%–4%); Lymphocyte (range, 1,500–4,000 or 20%–30%).

Granulocytes

The granulocyte granules contain substances that produce allergic and inflammatory reactions. For example, granules in basophils contain histamine and heparin, which are released when an individual has an allergic reaction. These substances, together with other chemicals, are responsible for symptoms such as redness, swelling, and watery nose seen in allergy. The eosinophils are also involved in allergic reactions and destruction of parasites.

As the granulocytes become older, the nucleus has more and more lobes. Because of the different shapes taken by the lobes, the granulocytes are also known as **polymorphs** or **polymorphonuclear leukocytes.**

The granulocytes have phagocytic properties. For example, the neutrophils seek out bacteria and ingest and kill them. Protein molecules on the bacteria surface help the neutrophils recognize them as foreign. The neutrophils extend limblike processes from the cytoplasm and engulf foreign agents into the cytoplasm (**phagocytosis**). They kill and digest the bacteria with the toxic enzymes present in the cytoplasmic granules. These cells are the *first line of defense* in bacterial infections.

Neutrophils can enter tissue spaces by squeezing between the endothelial cells of the capillaries (**diapedesis**) if there is infection or inflammation. Chemicals secreted by those neutrophils that have already reached the infection site, together with products released from injured cells, attract large numbers of neutrophils to the infection site (**chemotaxis**). The cells are produced in large quantities by the bone marrow at the time of infection because each cell only lives for about 6 hours.

Agranulocytes
Monocytes

Monocytes are large cells with a kidney-shaped nucleus that can also enter the tissue. The monocytes in the tissue spaces are called **tissue macrophages.** The macro-phages may be **wandering** or **fixed macrophages.** Wandering macrophages are defense cells that wander in the tissue, clearing up foreign and dead material. They are attracted to the site of infection by chemicals liberated by other white blood cells or injured tissue and, similar to the neutrophils, engulf and kill bacteria. They secrete up to 100 different substances, including those that affect lymphocytes and other cells. Fixed macrophages are monocytes that have the same function as wandering macrophages but remain in one tissue (e.g., in the spleen or liver). Monocytes play a key role in immunity.

Lymphocytes

Lymphocytes consist of cells with a large nucleus and scanty cytoplasm. Lymphocytes are formed in the bone marrow after birth. But some of the "mother" cells migrate to the lymph nodes, thymus, and spleen and production of lymphocytes also occurs in these regions (see **page 511.**)

White Blood Cell Formation

Similar to erythropoietin that regulates the production of red blood cells, specific factors regulate the production of white blood cells. These factors, called **colony-stimulating factors,** are secreted by macrophages, lymphocytes, fibroblasts, and endothelial cells, among others. They stimulate the production of specific white blood cells in the bone marrow.

An increase in white blood cells is known as **leukocytosis.** An increase is a normal response to infection, inflammation, strenuous exercise, and surgery. At times, the white blood cell count is lower than normal. This is known as **leukopenia.** Leukopenia may be caused by bone marrow deficiency following radiation and chemotherapy. An abnormal increase (cancerous) in white blood cells is referred to as **leukemia.**

PLATELETS

Platelets (Figure 8.4), also referred to as **thrombocytes,** are the smallest of formed elements in the blood and appear as dust particles under the microscope. Although small in size, they contain granules in the cytoplasm. Platelets are formed by large cells, called **megakaryocytes,** located in the bone marrow and are actually pinched off bits of cytoplasm from the megakaryocytes. Platelet formation is stimulated by the hormone **thrombopoietin.** The life span of platelets is about 5 to 9 days.

The major platelet function is to prevent blood loss. The platelets are sticky and collect at sites of injury inside blood vessels—**platelet aggregation.** The platelets then form a plug at the injury site and prevent blood loss. They secrete the contents of the granules at the injury site. Some of the platelet secretions are important in clot formation. The cytoplasm contains actin and myosin, the contractile proteins found in muscle. These proteins contract and help to pull the injured edges of the blood vessel together after the site of injury has been plugged in a process called **clot retraction.**

HEMOSTASIS

Hemostasis is the intrinsic process that the body uses to stop bleeding from an injured vessel. As soon as a vessel is cut or damaged, there is a reflexive **constriction of the vessel** triggered by chemicals such as serotonin that are present in platelet granules and the endothelium of blood vessels. The injured area attracts platelets, which then form a **platelet plug.**

In certain individuals, one factor required for clotting may be absent or reduced in quantity as a result of genetic defects. In these individuals, there is a tendency to bleed easily and for longer. One well-known bleeding disorder is **hemophilia.** In this condition, Factor VIII (antihemophilic factor) is reduced or absent. Because the genetic coding for this factor is present in an X chromosome, this abnormality is sex-linked and inherited from the mother. Because the gene is recessive, symptoms do not appear in the daughter if the other X chromosome is normal (females have two X chromosomes). However, the daughter can be a carrier of the gene and transmit it to a son. As there is only one X chromosome in males (males have one X and one Y chromosome), presence of the gene results in presentation of the disease in the form of bleeding.

Meanwhile, a series of events are triggered to form a **blood clot** in the region.

The semisolid blob of blood we know as a blood clot is actually a result of a series of complex enzymatic reactions. While we are thankful for its formation and prevention of blood loss, it causes alarm if it forms *inside* blood vessels or does not form when bleeding occurs. Therefore, the process of clot formation is complicated and must be so finely regulated that blood always stays fluid and clots only when bleeding occurs. The body has two opposing mechanisms in place—one that promotes clotting and one that prevents clotting.

THE CLOTTING MECHANISM

The fundamental reaction in the clotting process is the conversion of the soluble plasma protein **fibrinogen** into its insoluble form **fibrin.** For this conversion, many inactive substances in the blood must be

✔ *Excessive Clotting*

Although lack of clotting factors result in bleeding, predisposition to clotting poses its own problems. Formation of clots attached to the walls of blood vessels is called **thrombosis.** The clots are known as **thrombi** (singular–thrombus). The danger of thrombus formation is the possibility of dislodgment of bits of clot, or **emboli** (singular, embolus), which then can travel in the circulatory system, block major blood vessels, and cut blood supply to important organs. Emboli could cause stroke, myocardial infarction, and other conditions. Thrombosis tends to occur in areas where the blood flow is sluggish (e.g., in veins of legs after surgery or prolonged inactivity or in vessels that are injured or have irregular cholesterol plaques inside). It could also result from conditions such as atherosclerosis that facilitate coagulation of blood. Vigorous massage has the potential to dislodge thrombus.

activated. Thus, the clotting mechanism is a complex cascade of reactions that culminate in the formation of a mesh of insoluble fibrin threads. Red blood cells and other cells get caught in the mesh, giving the clot its red color.

Table 8.2 lists the various factors involved, together with their names, to give an idea of the number of factors involved in the clotting process. These factors include calcium, many inactive enzymes manufactured by the liver, and other molecules associated with platelets and injured tissue. The flowchart in Figure 8.5 shows the complex nature of the clotting mechanism that results in the final solid clot observed when a blood vessel is injured. One important requirement for the formation of some clotting factors by the liver is vitamin K.

Vitamin K is a fat-soluble vitamin manufactured by the normal flora inhabiting the large intestine. In conditions in which fat absorption is impaired, vitamin K deficiency may result, with uncontrollable bleeding.

ANTICLOTTING MECHANISMS

As in most systems in the body, there is a balance between the mechanisms that facilitate and mechanisms

Table 8.2

Clotting Factors

Factor	Name*
I	Fibrinogen
II	Prothrombin
III	Thromboplastin
IV	Calcium
V	Proaccelerin, labile factor, accelerator globulin
VII	Proconvertin, SPCA, stable factor
VIII	Antihemophilic factor, antihemophilic factor A, antihemophilic globulin
IX	Plasma thromboplastic component, Christmas factor, antihemophilic factor B
X	Stuart-Prower factor, Thrombokinase
XI	Plasma thromboplastin antecedent, antihemophilic factor C
XII	Hageman factor, glass factor
XIII	Fibrin-stabilizing factor, Laki-Lorand factor
HMW-K	High-molecular-weight kininogen, Fitzgerald factor
Pre-K	Prekallikrein, Fletcher factor
Ka	Kallikrein
PL	Platelet phospholipid

* Some factors may have more than one name because they were discovered by different people and later identified to be the same factor.

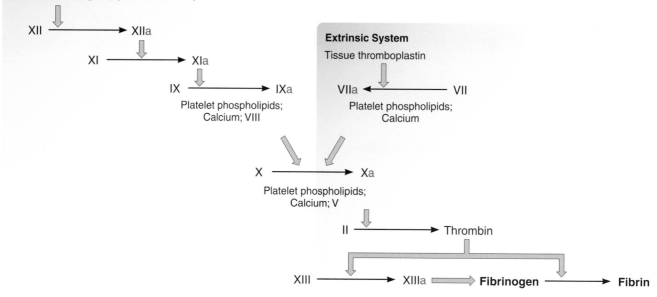

Intrinsic System

Exposure to collagen (injured vessel wall)

XII ——→ XIIa

XI ——→ XIa

IX ——→ IXa

Platelet phospholipids;
Calcium; VIII

Extrinsic System

Tissue thromboplastin

VIIa ←—— VII

Platelet phospholipids;
Calcium

X ——→ Xa

Platelet phospholipids;
Calcium; V

II ——→ Thrombin

XIII ——→ XIIIa ⟹ **Fibrinogen** ——→ **Fibrin**

FIGURE 8.5. The Clotting Mechanism. (the number indicates the factors involved; a = active form)

that inhibit a specific function. While the described clotting mechanisms facilitate, there are built-in mechanisms that inhibit the clotting process and dissolve the clots that do form. Both clotting and anticlotting mechanisms are equally important. A number of mechanisms are involved in the anticlotting process.

Anticlotting mechanisms include removal of clotting factors by the liver and reduction in the supply of clotting factors as they get used. Although some enzymes secreted by platelets potentiate aggregation of platelets, other enzymes in the blood vessel walls inhibit platelet clumping. **Antithrombin III** is a substance present in the plasma that inhibits the active form of clotting factors IX, X, XI, and XII. The endothelial cells and white blood cells secrete a substance called **prostacyclin,** which inhibits platelet adhesion and release. Mast cells and basophils secrete an anticoagulant **heparin.**

In addition, there are many other complex mechanisms that inhibit clotting. These **fibrinolytic** (breakdown of fibrin) **mechanisms** also rely on a cascade of reactions similar to the clotting mechanism illustrated. Some of the factors involved in preventing clotting have been isolated and are used to treat individuals with myocardial infarction.

Anticoagulants

Anticoagulants are often given to individuals with a tendency to form a thrombus. These anticoagulants inhibit vitamin K or stimulate the built-in system that prevents clotting inside blood vessels. A well-known

drug (also found naturally in the body), **heparin** facilitates the activity of antithrombin III, retarding thrombus formation. **Streptokinase,** an enzyme produced by bacteria, is fibrinolytic and often used as an anticoagulant. If blood must be stored outside the body, substances that remove calcium are introduced to prevent clotting. Because calcium is involved in muscle contraction, it is not feasible to prevent clotting by removing calcium from the blood when it is inside the body.

PLASMA

Plasma, the fluid portion of the blood comprises about 55% of the blood volume. Its composition is 91.5% water and 8.5% solutes. The solutes are protein (7%) and a variety of ions and substances that are transported from one part of the body to another (see Figure 8.6), including enzymes, hormones, gases, nutrients, waste

✚ Bleeding Time and Coagulation (clotting) Time

Normally, it takes about 1–9 minutes for a small skin wound to stop bleeding. Platelet deficiency prolongs **bleeding time.** The drug aspirin also prolongs bleeding time as it suppresses platelets.

If blood removed from a normal person is left undisturbed in a test tube, it takes about 3–15 minutes to form a clot. **Clotting time** is prolonged if any coagulation factor is deficient or absent.

products such as urea, uric acid, creatinine, ammonia, and bilirubin. Plasma occupies a volume of about 3,500 mL (3.7 qt) in a man weighing 70 kg (154 lb). The fluid that remains after blood is allowed to clot and the clot removed is known as **serum.**

Plasma Proteins

Plasma proteins are one of the major components of plasma. They consist of **albumin, globulin,** and **fibrinogen.** Most plasma proteins are manufactured in the liver. Some plasma proteins (immunoglobulins/antibodies) are made by specific lymphocytes.

The plasma proteins have varied functions. They serve to maintain the pH of the blood at 7.35-7.45. Some protein components are antibodies that recognize specific antigens. A few of the clotting factors are proteins. Some proteins serve as transport carriers for hormones, metals, amino acids, fatty acids, enzymes, and drugs. Because the protein molecules are large and the capillary walls are impermeable to them, substances escape filtration by the kidneys and stay longer in the blood when they are bound to proteins.

The protein fractions exert an osmotic force of about 26 mm Hg across the capillary wall (**see page 508**). This force tends to pull water into the blood from the surrounding fluid compartments, such as the interstitial compartment, and maintains the blood volume. In individuals with protein deficiency, the reduction of this force is responsible for the edema that develops. Example: individuals with kidney failure who lose protein in the urine, individuals with severe eating disorders with significantly reduced protein intake, individuals with malabsorption syndrome as a result of intestinal diseases, and individuals with liver disease in which protein manufacture is depressed.

Heart and Circulation

Each living cell in the body requires the correct temperature, adequate nutrients, and waste product removal for survival. This implies that the surrounding environment—the interstitial fluid—must be monitored and changed to suit its needs. The pumping action of the heart enables blood to constantly move through the body and change the composition of the interstitial fluid. The oxygen and nutrients used for cell metabolism are rapidly replenished by the blood, while waste products such as carbon dioxide and urea are quickly removed. The architecture of the heart and blood vessels are remarkably constructed to suit their function. Blood, pumped by the heart and transported by blood vessels, circulates through the lungs to replenish the oxygen used and dispose of the carbon dioxide produced. The kidneys remove other waste products as the blood circulates through. The nutrients are absorbed into the blood as it passes through the gastrointestinal tract.

AN OVERVIEW OF CIRCULATION

The heart is the pump that keeps the blood circulating. Blood leaves the heart and enters large blood vessels known as **arteries.** Large arteries on the right side of the heart take the blood to the lungs to dispose of carbon dioxide and to absorb oxygen. After passing through the lungs, the blood returns to the left side of the heart. This is known as **pulmonary circulation.** From here, the oxygenated blood is pumped into the large artery (**aorta**), which takes the blood to the rest of the body. It then returns to the right side of the heart. This is known as **systemic circulation.**

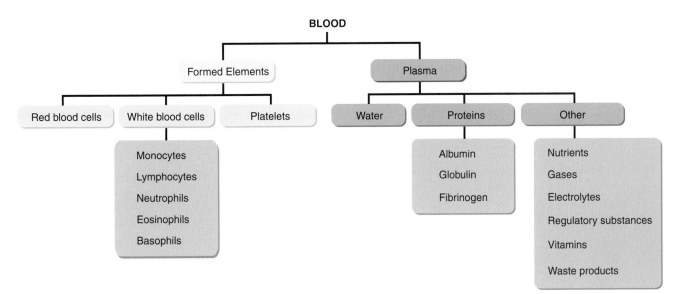

FIGURE 8.6.   The Components of Blood

The arteries conduct blood to different parts of the body. By the time they reach the cells in different organs, they branch repeatedly to form vessels known as **capillaries,** which have thin walls. It is only at the capillary level that an exchange of nutrients, gases, wastes, etc. between the interstitial fluid and blood takes place. The capillaries ultimately join to form the large **veins.** After perfusing the different parts of the body, the blood that is now deoxygenated returns to the right side of the heart via veins and it is again pumped to the lungs.

The Heart

The heart is an organ that is classically described to be the size of a clenched fist. It is located anteriorly, just behind the sternum. A major portion of the heart is situated towards the left side of the body.

The heart rests on the diaphragm, wedged between the two lungs (pleural cavities) in the **mediastinum** of the thorax. The mediastinum is the portion of the thoracic cavity located between the pleural cavities, and it

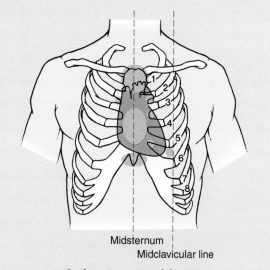

✔ Surface Anatomy of the Heart

The outline of the heart can be visualized by connecting the following points that can be located on the body surface.

Midsternum
Midclavicular line

Surface Anatomy of the Heart

Right border: from the third costal cartilage to the sixth costal cartilage, about 1 cm from the right margin of the sternum
Lower border: across the xiphisternal junction to the fifth left intercostal space, just medial to the midclavicular line (apex beat)
Left border: from the apex beat to the second intercostal space, 1 cm from the left margin of the sternum
Upper border: a line joining the upper point of the right and left borders

houses the heart, thymus, trachea, esophagus and large blood vessels.

The Pericardium

The heart is surrounded by a fluid-filled cavity known as the **pericardial cavity.** This cavity is lined by a membrane—the **pericardium.** The pericardium is a serous membrane, reinforced by dense connective tissue. The dense connective tissue is often referred to as the **fibrous pericardium,** and the serous membrane as the **serous pericardium.** The relationship of the heart to the pericardium (Figure 8.7C) is like a fist pushed into a partially filled balloon. In the latter, two layers separated by air will cover the fist, with one of the layers in close contact with the fist. In the case of the heart, the layer close to the heart is called the **visceral pericardium** or **epicardium.** The other layer is known as the **parietal pericardium.** Instead of air, this space is filled with the **pericardial fluid.** The point where the wrist would have entered the balloon is equivalent to the region where the large blood vessels enter and leave the heart. Although located superiorly, this region is known as the **base** of the heart. The inferior pointed tip of the heart (located to the left) is known as the **apex.**

The function of the pericardium is to prevent the heart from expanding too much and enlarging abnormally as could happen if too much blood returned to the heart. In addition, it helps hold the heart in position as the fibrous pericardium fuses with the diaphragm inferiorly and the outer wall of the blood vessels superiorly. The pericardial fluid, which is about 10–20 mL (0.01–0.02 qt), is a lubricant that reduces friction between surfaces as the heart beats.

Chambers of the Heart

The human heart has four chambers—the **right atrium, left atrium, right ventricle,** and **left ventricle.** The atria *receive* blood, while the ventricles *eject/expel* the blood. The right atrium communicates with the right ventricle, the left atrium with the left ventricle. In normal individuals, there is no direct communication between the chambers on the right side and the left side.

The location and boundaries of the four chambers can be identified on the surface of the heart. A deep groove filled with fat, the **coronary sulcus,** marks the boundary between the atria and ventricles (Figure 8.7). The coronary arteries and veins (blood vessels that supply the walls of the heart) run in this groove. Other depressions located anteriorly and posteriorly, the **anterior** and **posterior interventricular sulcus,** mark the boundary between the two ventricles (Figure 8.7).

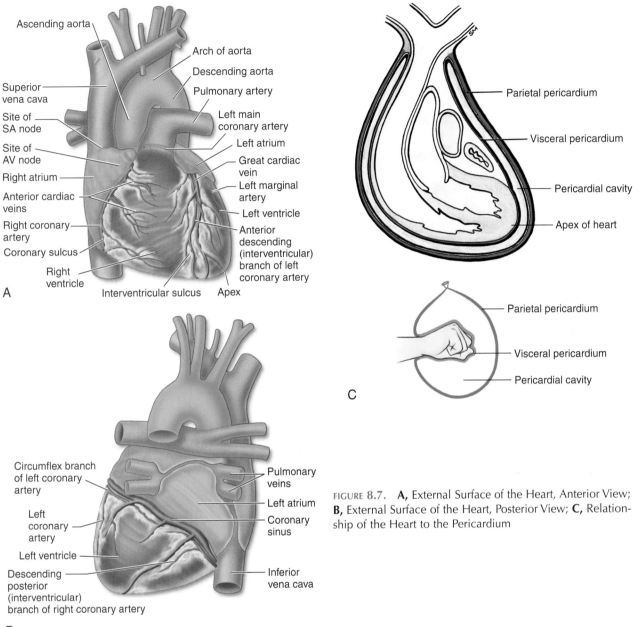

FIGURE 8.7. **A,** External Surface of the Heart, Anterior View; **B,** External Surface of the Heart, Posterior View; **C,** Relationship of the Heart to the Pericardium

The Right Atria

The two atria (see Figure 8.8) are separated by the **interatrial septum.** In the fetus, the two atria communicate with each other through an oval opening, the **foramen ovale,** shunting the blood from right to left because the lungs do not function and the placenta takes the place of lungs. This opening closes at birth when the baby takes its first breath and remains as an oval depression (**fossa ovalis**). The right atrium communicates with two large veins—the **superior vena cava** and the **inferior vena cava.** These veins drain blood from the upper and lower part of the body, respectively. The superior vena cava delivers blood to the atrium from the head, neck, upper limbs, and chest, and the inferior vena cava carries

blood from the rest of the trunk, the viscera, and the lower limbs. Blood from the heart walls is drained by coronary veins into a larger **coronary sinus** that opens into the right atrium. The inside wall of the right atrium is smooth, but has prominent muscular ridges.

Atrioventricular Valves

The atrium and ventricle on each side are separated by one-way valves known as **atrioventricular valves (AV valves).** The one on the right is the **tricuspid valve,** and the one on the left is the **mitral** or **bicuspid valve.** These valves have three and two **cusps,** respectively. Cusps are thin membranes or folds of fibrous tissue that are attached to the inner walls of the ventricles. When the cusps come together, blood cannot flow from the atrium into the ventricle. When the ventricle relaxes, the cusps are pulled apart, allowing blood to flow. The cusps are attached to the inner wall of the ventricle by thin, but tough, stringlike connective tissue known as the **chordae tendineae.** These are then connected to prominent muscular projections known as **papillary muscles.**

The valves open or close, according to the difference in pressure in the two chambers (see Figure 8.9). When the ventricle relaxes, the pressure drops below that of the atria and the valves open. The cusps point toward the ventricle and the chordae tendineae are relaxed. When the ventricle contracts, the pressure increases and the edges of the cusps are brought together, closing the opening between the two chambers. At the same time, the papillary muscles contract, pulling the chordae tendineae taut and preventing the cusps from everting into the atrium.

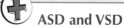

ASD and VSD

At times, the septum between the atrium (the interatrial septum) does not completely close, leaving a communication between the two atria and reducing the efficiency of the heart. This is referred to as a hole in the heart or, more specifically, **atrial septal defect (ASD).** Similarly, the interventricular septum may not close completely, allowing blood to pass between the ventricles. This is known as **ventricular septal defect (VSD).** As a result there is mixing of oxygenated and deoxygenated blood.

The Right Ventricle

The right atrium connects with the right ventricle. The right ventricle is separated from the left ventricle by the **interventricular septum.** The superior end of the ventricle tapers and opens into a large blood vessel—the **pulmonary trunk.** The opening is guarded by a valve

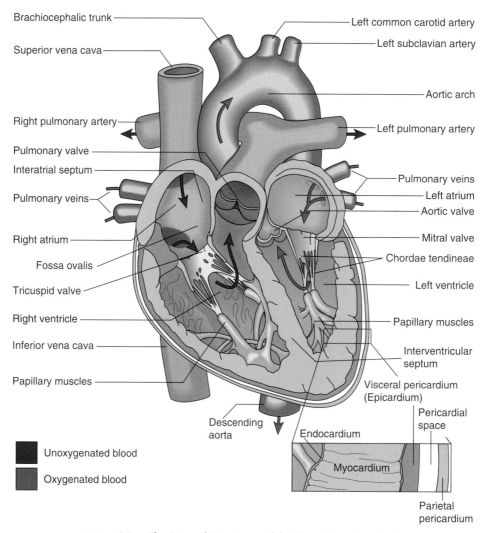

FIGURE **8.8.**   The Internal Structures of the Heart (Anterior view)

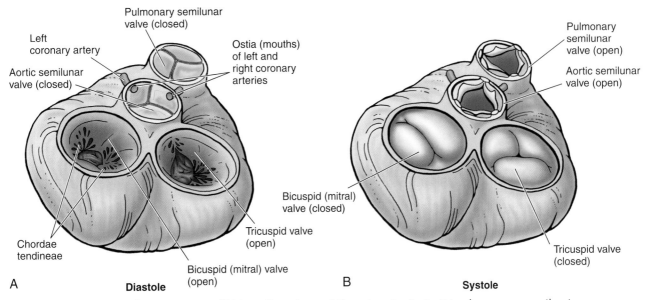

FIGURE **8.9.** The Movement of Valves (Superior and Posterior view). **A,** AV valves open; semiluminar valves closed; **B,** AV valves closed; semiluminar valves open

known as the **pulmonary semilunar valve.** This one-way valve has three moon-shaped cusps that open when the ventricle contracts and close when it relaxes, allowing blood to pass from the ventricle to the pulmonary trunk. The pulmonary trunk branches into the **right** and **left pulmonary arteries** soon after it leaves the ventricle. These arteries branch repeatedly after they enter the lungs, finally forming capillaries where gas exchange takes place (**see page 549**). The oxygenated blood from the pulmonary capillaries flows into the venules and then into the four **pulmonary veins.**

The Left Atrium

The four pulmonary veins (two left and two right) open into the posterior wall of the left atrium. Blood from the left atrium flows into the left ventricle. The opening between the atrium and ventricle, as with the right side of the heart, is guarded by the atrioventricular valve. This valve has only two cusps instead of three and is referred to as the **mitral** or **bicuspid valve** (*mitre*, a bishop's headpiece). This valve opens

when the ventricles relax and closes when the ventricles contract, allowing blood to flow one way, from the atrium to the ventricle. These valves, similar to those on the left, are attached to the walls of the ventricle by chordae tendineae and papillary muscles.

The Left Ventricle

The walls of the left ventricle are much thicker and more muscular than that of the right as they have to withstand a much higher pressure of blood. The higher pressure is needed here to push the blood through the systemic circulation. The wall of the right ventricle is much thinner as it only has to push blood into the lungs, which offer much less resistance. Unlike the various organs in the systemic circulation, the lungs are located close to the heart and not much pressure is required for blood to flow through them.

The blood from the ventricle is pumped into the largest of the blood vessels—the **aorta.** The opening into the aorta is guarded by the **aortic semilunar valve,** similar to that on the right. This one-way valve opens when the ventricle contracts and closes as it relaxes, allowing blood to pass from the ventricle to the aorta.

The Heart Wall

If the heart wall is cut, three distinct layers can be identified (see Figure 8.8). The outermost layer is the **epicardium** or **visceral pericardium** already described. Deep to it is the **myocardium** or muscular wall of the heart. The myocardium contains cardiac muscle tissue, blood vessels, and nerves. The muscles are arranged in

---

⊕ Rheumatic Fever

Rheumatic fever is an inflammation that may follow infection by streptococcal bacteria, characterized by fever, joint pain, stiffness, and rash formation. About 50% to 60% of those with rheumatic fever develop a more serious problem. They may develop heart inflammation and heart valve fibrosis, making the valves leaky or narrowing the opening. This reduces the efficiency of the heart and, if left untreated, may eventually lead to heart failure.

such a way that, when the muscle contracts, blood is squeezed out of the heart into the large blood vessels. The thickness of the heart wall varies according to the pressure it has to withstand. The atria are thin walled because they are exposed to low venous pressure. The wall of the right ventricle is also thin as a result of the low resistance offered by the lungs. The left ventricle has the thickest wall because it works the hardest.

The innermost layer of the heart is the **endocardium.** This layer also lines the heart valves. The endocardium consists of simple squamous epithelium that is continuous with the endothelium of the blood vessels.

Connective Tissue and the Fibrous Skeleton

For greatest efficiency, the atrium has to contract a little before the ventricle to allow time for the blood from the atrium to reach the ventricle before it contracts. This is accomplished because the muscles around the atrium and the ventricles are separated by a fibrous tissue ring. This connective tissue skeleton surrounds the valves, the aorta, and the pulmonary trunk, isolating the atrial and ventricular muscle. Although there is no direct connection between the muscles of the atrium and the ventricle, specialized tissue known as the **conducting system** pierce through the fibrous ring and convey impulses generated in the atrium to the ventricle.

In addition, the connective tissue fibers provide physical support for the cardiac muscle fibers, nerves, and blood vessels; help distribute the force of contraction and strength; prevent excessive stretching of the heart, and provide elasticity to help the heart return to its original size.

Cardiac Muscle

Cardiac muscle (**see Figure 4.18**) is striated similar to skeletal muscle. The contraction physiology is the similar to that of skeletal muscle; however, the structure of cardiac muscle is slightly different. Cardiac muscle fiber is shorter and broader than skeletal muscle fiber. It is branched, with a centrally located single nucleus. Individual muscle cells are interconnected by **intercalated disks.** These disks help convey the force of contraction and impulses from one cell to another. As a result, if an impulse is initiated in one of the cardiac muscle fibers, it is conveyed to all the muscles, and the heart contracts as a **functional syncytium** (i.e., as if one big muscle). Because the atria are separated from the ventricles by the fibrous tissue skeleton, the two atria contract as one functional syncytium, pushing the blood into the ventricle; the ventricles contract as another functional syncytium, pushing the blood into the arteries (pulmonary trunk and aorta).

The calcium in skeletal muscle is only derived from the sarcoplasmic reticulum; in cardiac muscle,

calcium is also obtained from the interstitial fluid surrounding the muscle. The contractility of the cardiac muscle is affected by hormones and ionic changes in the blood.

Action Potential in Cardiac Muscle

Another difference between cardiac muscle and skeletal muscle is the action potential—in the ventricular muscle it is about 30 times as long as the action potential in the skeletal muscle and lasts for about 250–300 milliseconds (see Figure 8.11A).

The resting membrane potential of the muscle fiber is about -90 mV. When the cardiac muscle fiber is stimulated, voltage-gated fast sodium channels present in the sarcolemma open, allowing sodium to rush into the cell (at rest, there are more sodium ions outside the cell). This produces **depolarization.** Soon after, the sodium channels close and voltage-gated calcium channels open, allowing positively charged calcium ions to enter. At the same time, there is a slow leak of potassium ions out of the cell. This results in a **plateau phase** that is responsible for prolonging the duration of the action potential. Note that this phase is absent in the action potential of skeletal muscles. Following the plateau phase, voltage-gated potassium channels open wider, allowing positively charged potassium to leak out and produce **repolarization.** This brings the membrane potential back to its resting state.

Excitation-Contraction Coupling

The action potential in the cardiac muscle leads to contraction. The mechanism is similar to that in skeletal muscle (**see page 181**). When the cell depolarizes, calcium levels rise inside the cytoplasm. The calcium attaches to troponin, which, in turn, triggers actin and myosin to slide past each other, causing a contraction.

✚ Heart Attack or Myocardial Infarction

This is a heart condition in which cardiac muscle cells die because of a lack of oxygen resulting from improper coronary circulation. The affected tissue does not function and it significantly reduces heart efficiency. The dead tissue area is known as an **infarct.** The outcome of myocardial infarction depends on the site of coronary blood vessel blockage. If the blockage is near the origin of the arteries, widespread damage occurs and the heart may stop beating. If the blockage involves one of the smaller arteries, less tissue is destroyed and the person may survive. The damaged tissue may trigger irregular heart rates.

Aspirin, if given in small doses, inhibits some of the platelet functions and, thereby, clot formation. This is why aspirin is given to individuals who have had stroke or myocardial infarction (heart attack)—to reduce the formation of thrombus.

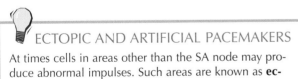

✚ Conduction Deficits

If any part of the conducting system is damaged, the normal heart rhythm is altered. If the SA node is damaged, the AV node takes over as the pacemaker, and the heart beats at a much slower rate. At times, damaged cells may begin to generate action potentials at a much faster rate than the SA node or AV node. These impulses override the nodes, making the heart beat irregularly and function less efficiently. Irregularities in heart rhythm are called **arrhythmia** and can be identified by ECG.

Refractory Period

The time interval in which a second contraction cannot be triggered is referred to as the **refractory period** of that muscle (see Figure 8.11). The cardiac muscle has a long refractory period compared with skeletal muscle because of the plateau phase of the action potential.

The longer duration of cardiac action potential (i.e., refractory period) is beneficial. For instance, if another impulse reaches the cardiac muscle during the first action potential, it cannot produce another contraction and prevents sustained (tetanic) contraction of the muscle. In the heart, if tetanic contractions were possible, it would have serious consequences because filling of blood in the ventricular chamber would be jeopardized and blood will not be ejected to supply the brain and other parts of the body.

Conducting Tissue of the Heart

Unlike skeletal muscle, cardiac muscle has the capacity to contract on its own in the absence of stimulation by nerves or hormones. This property is referred to as **automaticity,** which is a result of specialized cardiac muscle tissue (autorhythmic cells) in the heart known

💡 ECTOPIC AND ARTIFICIAL PACEMAKERS

At times cells in areas other than the SA node may produce abnormal impulses. Such areas are known as **ectopic pacemakers.** The impulses may be generated occasionally, producing extra beats or it may pace the heart for a short duration of time. Some factors that trigger such ectopic activity are nicotine, caffeine, drugs such as digitalis, and electrolyte imbalance.

When the heartbeat is too slow, too fast, or irregular, **artificial pacemakers** may be recommended. Wires run to the atria, the ventricle, or both regions from a small device, which stimulates the heart at the rate of 70–80/minute. More sophisticated pacemakers modify the stimulus according to the circulatory demands as during exercise. The control device may be implanted into the body or worn outside on a belt.

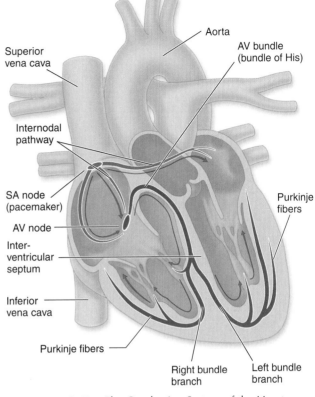

FIGURE 8.10.   The Conducting System of the Heart

as the **conducting system.** The conducting system network initiates and conducts and distributes electrical impulses.

The components of the conducting system are shown in Figure 8.10. It includes the **sinoatrial (SA) node,** located in the wall of the right atrium; the **atrioventricular (AV) node,** located at the junction of the atrium and ventricle; the conducting cells of the **internodal pathway** that interconnect the SA and the AV nodes and convey impulses to the muscles of the atrium; the **atrioventricular (AV) bundle** (bundle of His)**;** the **right** and **left bundle branches** that convey impulses towards the right and left ventricle; and the **Purkinje fibers** that distribute the impulses to the ventricular muscle fibers.

Generation of Rhythmic Impulse

The action potential of conducting tissue is different from that of skeletal muscle or the ventricular muscle described above. The cells in the conducting system are smaller than other muscle fibers of the myocardium and, unlike the others, cannot maintain a stable, resting membrane potential. Every time these cells reach their resting potential after depolarization, there is a slow leak of positive ions into the cell, raising the potential toward threshold and triggering another action potential (see Figure 8.11B). The rate at which action potentials are triggered is fastest in the SA node, about 80–100 times/minute. The other parts of the conducting system also have an unstable resting potential, how-

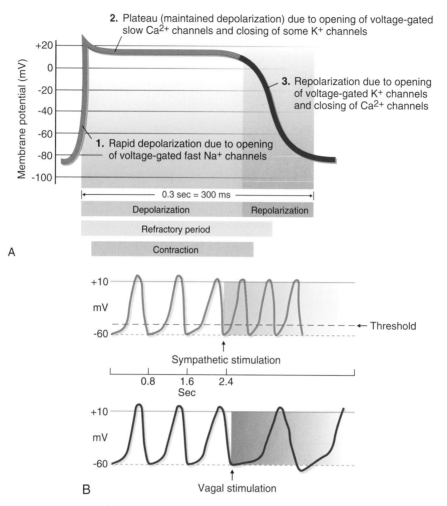

FIGURE **8.11.** Action Potentials in the **A,** Cardiac Muscle; **B,** SA Node and the Effects of Stimulation of Sympathetic Nerves and Parasympathetic Nerves

ever, action potentials are triggered here at a slower rate. For example, the AV node can generate action potentials at the rate of 40–60/minute; the rest of the conducting system generates at an even slower rate. Because the SA node generates action potentials at the fastest rate, the heart rate is normally determined by its pace. Hence, the SA node is known as the **pacemaker.**

Conduction of Impulses

Impulses generated by the pacemaker are conducted rapidly to the AV node along the internodal pathway. At the same time, the impulses are conducted to the atrial muscle, and the two atrium contract as a functional syncytium. The impulses do not travel to the ventricle directly from the atrium as a result of the presence of the nonconducting connective tissue of the fibrous skeleton, which separates the atrium from the ventricle.

At the AV node, the conduction of impulses that have reached it from the SA node is slowed down. This is advantageous, as it gives the atrium enough time to contract and propel the blood into the ventricles. The cells of the AV node can conduct impulses at

a maximal rate of about 230/minute. As each impulse can produce a ventricular contraction, this is the maximal heart rate of an individual.

The connection between the AV node and the AV bundle is the only route through which impulses can pass from the atrium to the ventricle. The AV bundle

---

✚ Heart Rate and Impulse Conduction Terms

Arrhythmia, dysrhythmia—irregular heart rate (abnormality of rhythm)
Bradycardia, brachycardia, bradyrhythmia—slowness of the heartbeat, usually defined as a rate lower than 50 beats/minute.
Fibrillation—contraction of the heart in an irregular and disorganized fashion
Heart block—abnormality in the conduction of electrical impulses from atria to ventricle or through the ventricle
Tachycardia, polycardia, tachyrhythmia, tachysystole—an increase in heart rate usually applied to rates higher than 90 beats/minute.

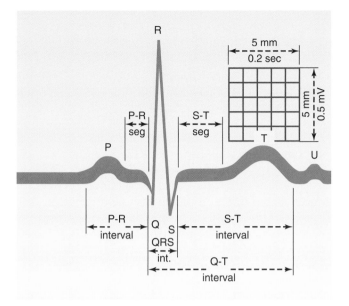

FIGURE 8.12.   Electrocardiogram

splits into right and left bundle branches located in the interventricular septum. From here, impulses travel through the Purkinje fibers that rapidly conduct impulses to all ventricular muscle fibers. Ventricular contraction proceeds from the apex in a wave and spreads toward the base, squeezing the blood toward the base where the large vessels are located.

An Overview of the Electrocardiogram

By placing electrodes on the surface of the chest wall, the electrical changes that occur in the heart can be recorded. The **electrocardiogram (ECG)** (see Figure 8.12) is the recording of these electrical activities. The general direction of conduction of the electrical impulse is from the SA node through the atria to the AV node, then along the AV bundle in the interventricular septum to the apex, and then along the ventricular wall toward the base of the heart (Figure 8.10). When the impulse is conducted, the inside of the myocardial cell becomes positive and the outside becomes negative. If electrodes are placed over the chest wall and the electrical impulse travels toward it, the recording of the electrode shows a positive or upward deflection (of course, the electrode has to be positive). When the impulse moves away from the electrode, it shows a negative deflection. Typically, the electrical activity during each contraction of the heart is recorded as a series of positive and negative waves, with each part of the wave representing impulse conduction along different parts of the heart.

The first, small, positive upward deflection, the **P wave,** represents the depolarization in the atria. The complex of negative and large, positive deflection **QRS complex** represents the depolarization of the ventricle. The repolarization activity of the atria oc-

curs at the same time as the QRS complex. The last, positive upward deflection, the **T wave,** represents the repolarization of the ventricle. The distance between the beginning of the P wave and the QRS complex—the **PR interval**—indicates the time taken for the impulse to travel from the atria to the ventricle.

Because the recording device, such as recording paper, moves at a standard speed, the distance between the different waves indicates the duration taken for the impulse to travel from one region to another. Also, the height of the waves indicates the size of the muscle tissue (i.e., hypertrophied muscle tends to produce a larger wave). By placing the electrodes in different standard parts of the chest wall, arms, and legs, the electrical activity of the heart can be captured in various "viewpoints"—from the side, from above, or from below. Typically, electrodes are placed on the arms and legs and at six chest positions. The instrument used to record the electrical changes is called an **electrocardiograph.**

A lot of information can be obtained by analyzing an ECG. Irregularities in heart rate, size of different chambers, location of pacemaker, presence and location of damaged or dead cardiac tissue, rate of conduction, and conduction defects are just a few conditions that can be detected and diagnosed.

Cardiac Centers, Innervation of the Heart, and Factors Affecting Heart Rate

The rhythmic contraction of the heart, as described, is a result of regular action potentials produced in the pacemaker. But this rhythm can be altered by the action of autonomic nerves that innervate the heart (see Figures 8.11 and 8.13). Postganglionic sympathetic neurons arising from the cervical and upper thoracic

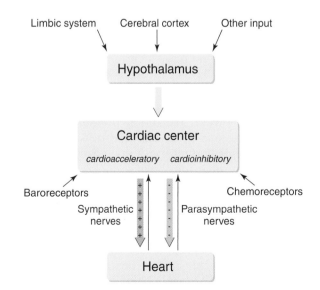

FIGURE 8.13.   A Schematic Representation of the Innervation of the Heart, Cardiac Centers, and its Communications

ventricle. Parasympathetic fibers reach the heart via the vagus nerve (cranial nerve X).

Both the sympathetic and parasympathetic neurons communicate with the **cardiac centers** located in the medulla oblongata. One part of the cardiac center is the **cardioacceleratory center.** Neurons from this center increase the heart rate and force of contraction of the heart via their communication with the sympathetic nerves. When the sympathetic nerves to the heart are stimulated, they increase the rate at which the SA node generates impulses and the heart rate increases.

The **cardioinhibitory center,** another part of the cardiac center, acts via the parasympathetic nerves (vagus nerve), slowing the heart rate and decreasing the force of contraction.

The cardiac centers have many other communications. They have connections with higher centers like the hypothalamus. The hypothalamus, in turn, has communications with various parts of the nervous system. In this way, the activity of the heart can be affected by numerous factors.

In addition to the hypothalamus, the cardiac centers receive input regarding the status of the cardiovascular system—blood pressure, blood volume, stretch of the chamber walls of the heart—through afferent (sensory) autonomic nerves. Some of the important input it receives is from baroreceptors and chemoreceptors. These receptors, located in and near the walls of large blood vessels, detect changes in blood pressure (from baroreceptors), carbon dioxide, hydrogen ion, and oxygen levels in the blood (from chemoreceptors), and the impulses from them reach the cardiac center via the glossopharyngeal nerve (cranial nerve IX) and the vagus nerve (cranial nerve X). The cardiac center, in turn, ensures that adequate blood supply is maintained to vital organs, such as the brain.

Anger, painful stimuli, exercise, inspiration, reduced oxygen levels, adrenaline and noradrenaline in the blood, fever, increase in body temperature, and thyroid hormones all increase the heart rate. In general, stimuli that increase heart rate also increase blood pressure. Due to blood pressure regulatory mechanisms, compensatory changes in heart rate are seen. Heart rate is slowed by increased activity of the baroreceptors—when the blood pressure increases, expiration, fear, and grief, among others.

Another factor that alters SA node pace is the ionic composition of the extracellular fluid. For example, an increase in extracellular potassium increases the heart rate. Calcium and sodium ion levels also have an effect.

Heart rate is also affected by the individual's age, gender, physical fitness, and body temperature. For example, infants have a faster heart rate. Adult females have a slightly higher heart rate than adult males. A physically fit individual has a slower heart rate. A decrease in temperature slows down the heart rate, by reducing metabolism.

Blood Supply to the Heart

Even as the heart pumps blood to the rest of the body, it must supply adequate blood to its own walls as the muscles contract and relax, rhythmically and continuously. The circulation to the heart is known as the **coronary circulation** (see Figures 8.7 and 8.14), which consists of an extensive network of blood vessels.

The **left** and **right coronary arteries** are the first branches off of the aorta, and they originate at the base of the ascending aorta. The right coronary artery follows the coronary sulcus (sulcus, which demarcates the junction of the atria and ventricle) and gives off branches that supply the right atrium, ventricles, parts of the conducting system and descends posteriorly between the two ventricles as the **posterior interventricular branch,** supplying the interventricular septum. The left coronary artery supplies blood to the left ventricle, left atrium, and the interventricular septum. It also follows the coronary sulcus on the left side as the **circumflex artery.** Anteriorly, a large branch descends between the ventricles as the **anterior interventricular branch.**

Both coronary arteries have several communications with each other, known as **anastomoses.** The

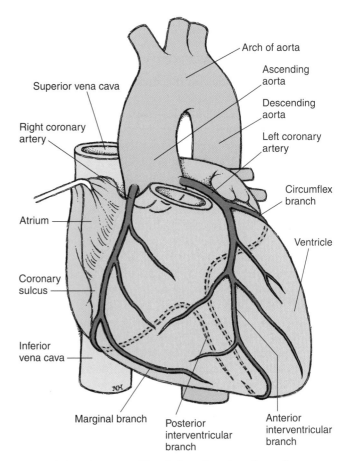

FIGURE 8.14. Coronary Circulation. Anterior view of coronary arteries

Cardiac Cycle

Many cyclical or sequential events occur in the heart between the beginning of one heartbeat and the next. All events that occur associated with one heartbeat are known as the **cardiac cycle** (see Figure 8.15). During the cycle, each heart chamber contracts and relaxes. The period of contraction is known as **systole,** and the period of relaxation is known as **diastole.** At a heart rate of 75 beats/minute, the duration of each cardiac cycle is about 800 milliseconds, with systole lasting for about 270 milliseconds and diastole for about 530 milliseconds. When the heart rate increases, the duration of diastole is shortened more than the systole. This results in the reduction of time available for ventricular filling (occurring when the ventricle relaxes). If the heart rate is unusually fast, there is too little time for the ventricles to fill and little blood is pushed into the large arteries. The person becomes unconscious as a result of reduced blood flow to the brain.

During systole or the contraction phase, the blood inside the chamber is ejected out and, during diastole or the relaxation phase, the chamber gets filled with blood and the cycle continues. The right direction of blood flow is determined by the presence of valves and difference in pressure between the chambers.

arteries divide many times in the walls of the heart to form a network of capillaries. These capillaries eventually form veins, which drain into the **great cardiac vein.** The great cardiac vein begins on the anterior surface of the ventricles along the interventricular sulcus and then travels in the coronary sulcus to reach the posterior aspect of the heart to drain into a larger vein, the **coronary sinus.** The coronary sinus drains into the right atrium.

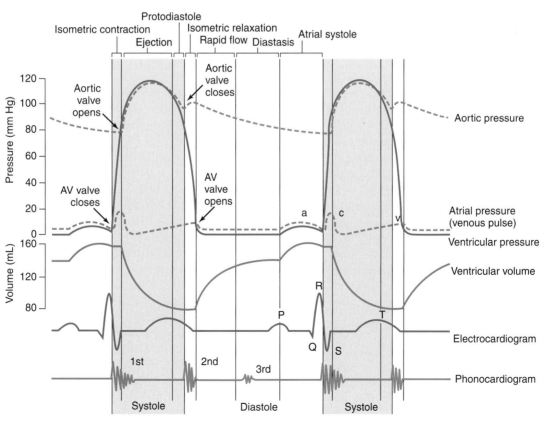

FIGURE 8.15. Cardiac Cycle

For proper flow, the sequence of contraction of the atria and ventricle has to be precise, with the atria contracting just before the ventricles. The presence of the conducting system and the difference in rate of impulse conduction through them ensures that atrial and ventricular muscles contract at different times.

Atrial Diastole and Systole

Blood flows into the atria via the superior and inferior vena cavas during atrial diastole. The atrial diastole lasts for about 700 milliseconds. When the SA node produces an action potential, the atria contract (**atrial systole**). Because the impulse takes time to reach the ventricular muscles, the ventricles are relaxed at this time, and the AV valves are open and blood from the atria enter the ventricle easily.

Ventricular Systole and Diastole

When the impulse reaches the ventricles, they contract (**ventricular systole**). The pressure in the ventricles rises above that of the pulmonary trunk and aorta, and the semilunar valves that were closed during the diastole of the ventricle are pushed open and blood is ejected into the blood vessels. At the same time, the AV valves are pushed close (Figure 8.9). This is primarily responsible for the **first heart sound** or the "lubb" heard when using the stethoscope or placing the ear or hand on the chest wall superficial to the heart.

The muscles begin to relax after about 270 milliseconds (i.e., when the heart rate is 75 beats/minute). When the ventricles relax, the volume increases and the pressure decreases. When the pressure drops below that of the pulmonary trunk and aorta, the semilunar valves (Figure 8.9) close with a snap. This is responsible for the **second heart sound** or the "dubb" sound. Because the pressure is less than that of the atria, the AV valves open and blood flows in.

The first and the second heart sounds give an idea of the duration and activities of the cardiac cycle. The duration between the first and second sound indicates the duration of ventricular systole; the duration between the second and first sound, the duration of ventricular diastole.

✚ Murmurs

At times, when the blood flow is rapid and turbulent or flows through narrowed or abnormal openings between the chambers or if the valves are leaky and fail to close properly, abnormal sounds, referred to as **murmurs,** are heard. The location on the chest wall where the murmur(s) is best heard and when (i.e., at which phase of the cardiac cycle it is heard) helps a clinician identify the abnormality.

Pressure Changes

The blood pressure in the two atria is just a few mm Hg. The pressure in the right ventricle is much less than that of the left and is equal to about 25 mm Hg. This is because the lungs offer little resistance to blood flow. Because the left ventricle has to pump blood to the rest of the body, it encounters more resistance, and the pressure in the left ventricle is as high as 120 mm Hg during systole. The pressure in both the ventricles drops close to 0 mm Hg during the relaxation phase.

The blood pressure in the aorta, while reaching 120 mm Hg during ventricular systole, does not drop to 0 mm Hg during diastole. Instead, the pressure is about 80 mm Hg. This is because the elastic walls of the aorta expand when blood rushes in during systole and recoil back during diastole, increasing the pressure in the lumen. For the same reasons, the pressure in the pulmonary trunk is higher than pressure in the right ventricle during diastole.

The pressure in the blood vessels during ventricular systole is known as the **systolic pressure** and that during diastole is known as the **diastolic pressure.** It is usually expressed as systolic pressure/diastolic pressure and, in this case, the blood pressure in the aorta is 120/80 mm Hg.

Volume Changes

When the ventricle contracts, not all of the blood is ejected into the large blood vessels. There is some blood remaining in the chamber, and this is known as the **end-systolic volume.** The volume of blood ejected during each contraction is known as the **stroke volume,** and it is equal to about 70 mL. When the heart contracts more forcefully, the stroke volume increases and end systolic volume decreases. The volume of blood ejected from the ventricle every minute is known as the **cardiac output.** In a resting supine man, it averages about 5.0 liters/minute (heart rate × stroke volume).

The volume of blood pumped out of the ventricles depends on the volume of blood *returning* to the heart through the veins. This volume is known as **venous return.** Venous return is normally about 5.0 liters/minute (5.3 qt/min) and depends on the cardiac output (volume of blood pumped out), blood volume (volume of blood inside the blood vessels), skeletal muscle activity (blood flow through the veins is facilitated by the contraction and relaxation of the skeletal muscles around it—skeletal muscle pump), and all other factors that affect the rate of blood flow through the vena cava.

The volume of blood remaining in the ventricle at the end of ventricular diastole is known as the **end-diastolic volume.** The end diastolic volume determines, to a large extent, the stroke volume (volume of blood pumped out with each ventricular contraction).

Apex Beat

Because the base of the heart is fixed to the mediastinum and the apex is free, the ventricle moves up and hits the anterior wall of the chest every time the ventricles contract. The location on the chest wall where the ventricle hits it is known as the **apex beat.** Usually, the apex beat can be located in the fifth left intercostal space, a little medial to the midclavicular line. If the heart is enlarged or if the mediastinum has been pushed to the left by fluid in the right lung or pulled to the left by collapse of the left lung, the apex beat is shifted to the left and sometimes may be felt in the left axilla.

Arterial Pulse

The blood forced into the aorta during ventricular systole not only moves the blood forward in the vessel but also sets up a pressure wave that travels along the arteries. The pressure wave expands the walls of the arteries as it travels and this expansion is felt as the **pulse** in arteries located more superficially. Because the pulse correlates with the ventricular systole, the rate of ventricular contraction can be measured by counting the pulses felt. The regularity, rate, and force of ventriclular contraction can be evaluated by taking the pulse. For the various arterial pulsations and their locations on the surface of the body, **see page 484**.

Venous Pulse

Normally, venous pulsation is not seen or felt, as the pressure is too low. Because there is no valve between the superior vena cava and the right atrium, abnormally increased pressure in the atrium may produce venous pulsations that can be seen in the neck along the jugular veins. This is known as the **jugular venous pulse.**

FACTORS AFFECTING CARDIAC OUTPUT

If a person exercises, cell metabolism and oxygen requirement increases. This implies that blood flow to the active tissue has to increase. Increase in blood flow is, in turn, caused by an increase in cardiac output. When the tissue is inactive, oxygen demands decrease, and it would be efficient for the body to decrease cardiac output in such situations. Therefore, it is important for the body to alter the cardiac output according to needs to maintain homeostasis.

Cardiac output can be varied by altering the heart rate and stroke volume (see Table 8.3). Both the heart rate and stroke volume are controlled to a large extent by the autonomic nerves (**see page 370** for regulation of heart rate). The sympathetic nerves speed the heart rate and increase the stroke volume by mak-

Table 8.3	
Effects of Various Conditions on Cardiac Output	
Condition or Factor	
No change	Sleep
	Moderate changes in environmental temperature
Increase	Anxiety and excitement
	Eating
	Exercise
	High environmental temperature
	Pregnancy
	Epinephrine
	Histamine
Decrease	Sitting up or standing from lying position
	Rapid arrhythmia
	Heart disease

ing the myocardial muscles contract more forcefully. Adrenaline and noradrenaline (from the adrenal medulla) in the blood have the same effect as sympathetic stimulation. The parasympathetic innervation of the heart slows down the heart rate. The vagus nerve carries parasympathetic fibers to the heart.

The stroke volume of the heart is affected by (A) the degree of stretch of muscle fibers before it contracts (**preload**), (B) the force of contraction of individual fibers (**contractility**), and (C) the resistance that needs to be overcome to eject the blood out of the ventricles (**afterload**) (e.g., pressure in the aorta).

The initial length of the cardiac muscle fibers also has an effect on the force of contraction. When the ventricles are filled with more blood, the muscle fibers are stretched optimally so that there is maximal overlap of actin and myosin fibers (**see page 185**), increasing the strength of contraction. Therefore, when more venous blood returns to the heart, the force of cardiac muscle contraction is automatically increased. During exercise, for example, there is dilation of blood vessels in the skeletal muscles, with resultant reduction in peripheral resistance and increased flow of blood back to the heart via veins. This relationship between the end diastolic volume and force of contraction during systole is known as the **Frank-Starling law of the heart.**

The force of contraction of individual fibers (contractility) can be increased by various agents that facilitate entry of calcium into the myocardial fibers. Stimulation of sympathetic nerves to the heart, presence of adrenaline, noradrenaline in the blood, and increased calcium levels in the blood are some factors that increase contractility.

Contractility is decreased by parasympathetic stimulation, inhibition of sympathetic activity, increased potassium levels in the blood, acidosis, and presence of drugs that decrease calcium into the myocardial fibers, among others.

The stroke volume is also affected by resistance to blood ejection from the ventricles (afterload). You may recall that when the pressure inside the ventricle exceeds that of the pressure in the arteries (pulmonary trunk/aorta), the semilunar valves are opened and blood is ejected out of the ventricle. Any factor that increases the pressure in the arteries would resist the outflow and, thereby, decrease stroke volume. Increased blood pressure (hypertension) and narrowing of the aorta are a few conditions that increase afterload.

The body has the capacity to increase the cardiac output to many times its resting level. The ratio between a person's maximum cardiac output and the cardiac output at rest is known as the **cardiac reserve.** On average, the heart can increase the output four to five times its resting level. Professional athletes may have a cardiac reserve as high as eight to nine times the resting level. Individuals with cardiac disease may have little cardiac reserve, restricting them from participating in any activity that requires an increase in cardiac output.

Blood Vessels and Circulation

The blood that is pumped out of the ventricles enters the two large blood vessels—the **aorta** and **pulmonary trunk** (Figures 8.7 and 8.8). The blood vessels carry blood from the heart to the tissue and back to the heart. The blood flows through the vessels primarily because of the pumping of the heart. In the case of the blood returning from the body to the heart, the elastic recoil of the artery walls during diastole, compression of veins by skeletal muscles during contraction, and the negative pressure created in the thorax during inspiration help draw blood toward the heart (venous return).

Aneurysm

An **aneurysm** is a bulge in a weakened blood vessel wall. It has serious consequences if it ruptures.

The blood from the right ventricle flows to the lungs via the pulmonary trunk and back to the left atrium via the pulmonary veins and this is known as **pulmonary circulation.** The blood from the left ventricle flows to the rest of the body via the aorta and back to the right atrium via the vena cava and this is known as **systemic circulation.** The systemic circulation is made up of numerous different circuits in parallel (see Figure 8.16), which allows for wide variations in regional blood flow without changing the total systemic flow. For example, blood flow to the gastrointestinal system alone can be increased at mealtime.

STRUCTURE AND FUNCTION OF BLOOD VESSELS

In both the pulmonary and systemic circulation, blood flows through different kinds of blood vessels, each suited to its function (see Figure 8.17 and Table 8.4). The **arteries** conduct blood *away* from the heart toward the tissue. The large, **elastic arteries** divide and redivide into smaller midsized **muscular arteries.** The midsized arteries divide into smaller arteries. The smallest arteries are called **arterioles,** the major function of which is to regulate blood flow to the region. From the arterioles, the blood moves into **capillaries** where exchange between blood and tissue is possible. The capillaries join to form **venules,** and then **veins,** which return blood from capillaries to the heart.

Artery and vein walls contain three layers: **tunica interna** or **tunica intima, tunica media,** and **tunica externa** or **tunica adventitia** (Figure 8.17). Tunica interna is the inner layer that comes in contact with blood. It consists of a smooth layer of simple squamous epithelium known as **endothelium,** with an underlying layer of connective tissue with elastic fibers. The tunica media has sheets of smooth muscle arranged as circular (and longitudinal in large arteries) layers around the lumen; it is the thickest layer in arteries. When the smooth muscle contracts, because of the organization of fibers, the diameter of the lumen is narrowed and blood flow is reduced. On relaxation, the opposite happens. A network of autonomic nerves located in the wall innervates the muscle fibers. The smooth muscle fibers respond to local changes in the environment, nerves, and circulating hormones. The tunica media also contains some elastic fibers that allow the blood vessel to stretch easily when the pressure of blood increases.

The tunica externa is the outermost layer made up of connective tissue and a few elastic fibers. This layer is the thickest in veins and contains smooth

Table 8.4

A Comparison of Artery and Vein Characteristics

Characteristic	Artery	Vein
Direction of blood flow	from heart to tissue	from tissue to heart
Size of wall	thicker	thinner
Sectional view	rounded lumen (due to thick wall)	oval or collapsed lumen (due to thin wall)
Content of smooth muscle and elastic fibers	more	less
Valves	absent	present
Pulsations	felt	not felt

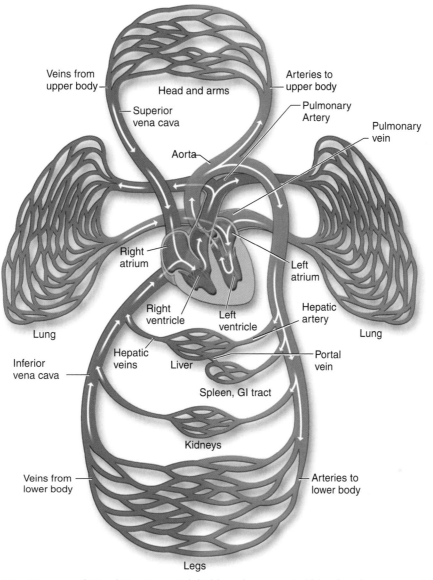

FIGURE **8.16.**   Diagram of Circulation in an Adult (blue, deoxygenated blood; red, oxygenated blood)

muscle and elastic fibers. This layer helps to anchor the vessels in place and stabilizes them as they pass through and around tissue.

The walls of the arteries and veins give them strength to withstand the blood pressure. Because the pressure in veins is much less, the walls are thinner than that of arteries. The presence of muscle fibers allows for the caliber of lumen to change and, thereby, alter blood supply according to the needs of the region perfused. When the artery is narrowed or constricted, it is termed **vasoconstriction.** If the diameter of the lumen is increased by relaxation of smooth muscles, it is termed **vasodilatation.**

The elastic fibers allow the blood vessel to expand during systole and recoil during diastole. The diastolic recoil is important because it keeps the blood flowing, even in the relaxation phase of the heart.

Otherwise, blood flow to the organs would be in spurts. As a result of the thickness of the walls, diffusion cannot occur across arteries and veins and they serve only to conduct blood.

The walls of large blood vessels are too thick to get their nutrients directly from the blood that flows through them. They get their nutrients from tiny blood vessels that perfuse the walls. These vessels are known as **vasa vasorum** (*vessels of vessels*).

The arteries are further classified as **elastic arteries, muscular arteries,** and **arterioles.** The *elastic arteries* or *conducting arteries* have a high density of elastic fibers that help them withstand the pressure changes that occur in the cardiac cycle. They also provide the elastic recoil for maintaining diastolic pressure; therefore, by recoiling, they propel the blood forward when the ventricle is relaxing. These arteries are

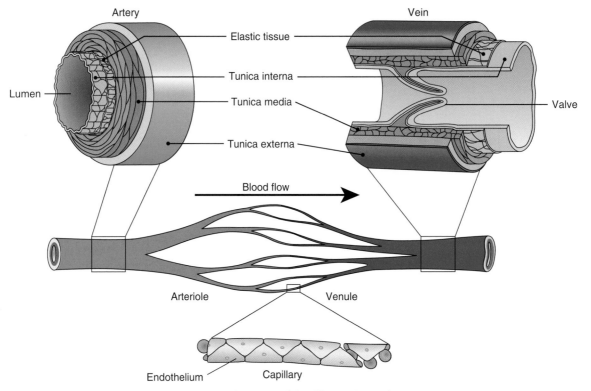

FIGURE **8.17.**   Structure of Capillary, Vein, and Artery

large, with a diameter of up to 2.5 cm (1 in). Because their main function is to conduct blood to the muscular arteries, they are also known as **conducting arteries.** The aorta, pulmonary trunk, and the larger branches, such as the brachiocephalic, common carotid, subclavian, vertebral, and common iliac arteries, are of this type.

The *muscular, midsized* or *distribution arteries* are smaller, with a diameter of about 0.4 cm (.2 in). The tunica media of these arteries have more muscle. As a result of the greater muscle content, these arteries are capable of altering blood flow to the organs they supply by constricting or dilating. Hence, these arteries are known as **distributing arteries.** The arteries

supplying the arm and leg (e.g., brachial artery, radial artery) are of this type.

The *arterioles* are about 30 μm (0.001 in) or less with a thick, muscular tunica media. They, along with the muscular arteries, are responsible for most of the resistance that opposes blood flow in the circulation and are known as **resistance vessels.**

Most tissues receive blood from more than one artery. The branches of the two or more arteries that supply the same tissue communicate with each other. This communication is known as **anastomoses** (singular, **anastomosis**). As a result of the presence of anastomoses, when one of the arteries is obstructed, the blood supply to the tissue is not totally cut off because the other artery(s) compensate. This alternate route of blood flow to the tissue is known as **collateral circulation** to that tissue. Some tissue receives blood from only one artery. These arteries are known as **end**

Arteriosclerosis

In arteriosclerosis, the walls of the arteries thicken and toughen. In one type of **arteriosclerosis,** known as **atherosclerosis,** there is deposition of lipid in the tunica media and injury of the endothelial lining. As a result, the resistance to blood flow is increased and blood pressure increases. Also, the rough endothelial lining encourages platelet adhesion and clot formation. This may narrow the lumen and block blood flow or the clot may become dislodged and block smaller blood vessels (**embolism**). Complications of atherosclerosis include myocardial infarction and stroke, among others.

DON'T PINCH PIMPLES ON THE SIDES OF YOUR NOSE!

Why? The facial vein communicates with the veins inside your skull via the ophthalmic vein (vein draining your eye). There is a potential danger of facial infections, especially near the nose, entering the facial vein and then the skull, causing meningitis.

arteries. When end arteries are obstructed, the tissue loses its blood supply and necrosis (cell death) ensues.

Capillaries

Capillaries are the only vessels that allow exchange of nutrients, wastes, gases, electrolytes etc. across their walls, and they are known as **exchange vessels.** They are as small as the diameter of a red blood cell (RBC) and often the RBCs travel single file as they squeeze through the capillaries. The thinness of wall, extensive surface area, and slow movement of blood through them allows exchange to take place easily and efficiently. Because these are microscopic vessels, the flow of blood through them is known as **microcirculation.**

The capillary (see Figure 8.18) is lined by endothelium attached to a basement membrane. It does not have tunica media or externa. Most capillaries have a complete endothelial lining with small gaps between the cells. These are known as **continuous capillaries.** Continuous capillaries are found in skeletal muscle, smooth muscle, connective tissues, and lungs. Other capillaries have pores in the plasma membrane of the endothelial cells that permit rapid exchange of water and larger solutes **(fenestrated capillaries).** Such capillaries are found in the glomeruli of the kidneys, endocrine glands, and villi of the small intestine. In certain areas, such as the liver, spleen, and bone marrow, the capillaries have large pores between the endothelial cells. They are so large that they even allow plasma protein to pass through. Such capillaries are known as **sinusoidal capillaries** or **sinusoids.** The presence of sinusoidal capillaries in the bone marrow allows the cells manufactured here to get into the blood.

The network of capillaries varies from region to region in accordance to the metabolic activity of the tissue they supply. Tissue such as the kidney, liver, muscles, and nervous tissue have an extensive network as a result of their high metabolic rate. When the activity of the tissue is diminished, the blood flow is restricted to only a few channels of the capillary network. When the tissue is active, the entire network fills with blood.

The structural arrangement of the capillary bed enables rapid changes in blood flow. From the arteriole, a **metarteriole** emerges to supply 10–100 capillaries. Contracting or relaxing the smooth muscle fibers that surround the proximal end of the metarteriole regulates blood flow to these capillaries. The distal end of the metarteriole opens into a venule known as a **thoroughfare channel.** When oxygen requirement is low, blood goes directly from the metarteriole into the thoroughfare channel without going into the capillaries. Each capillary that branches from the metarteriole has a circle of smooth muscle known as the **precapillary sphincter** (see Figure 8.19). Contraction of this sphincter can reduce or cut off blood flow through that capillary. The precapillary sphincter is particularly sensitive to chemicals in the interstitial fluid around it. For example, if oxygen levels drop and waste products accumulate, they relax, increasing the blood flow.

Each capillary network may receive blood from more than one artery. This ensures that even if one artery is blocked, the tissue is not totally deprived of nutrients. Only about 25% of capillaries have blood flowing through them at rest. More capillaries are opened when the metabolic needs of the tissue are increased.

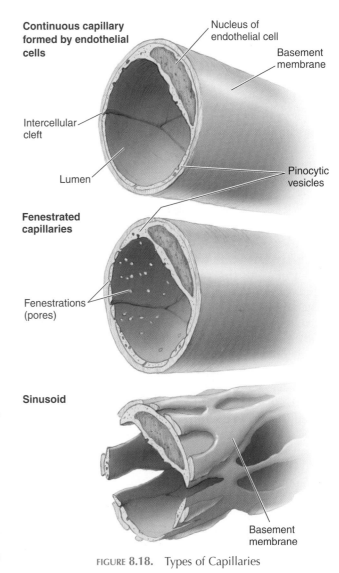

Continuous capillary formed by endothelial cells

Nucleus of endothelial cell

Basement membrane

Intercellular cleft

Lumen

Pinocytic vesicles

Fenestrated capillaries

Fenestrations (pores)

Sinusoid

Basement membrane

FIGURE 8.18.   Types of Capillaries

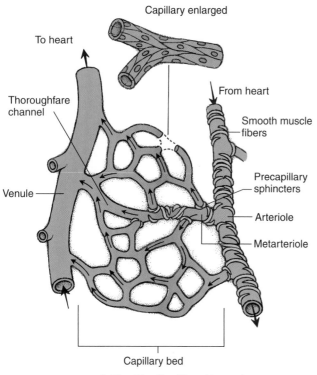

FIGURE 8.19.   The Capillary Network

Exchange Across Capillaries

The primary function of the cardiovascular system is to ensure that blood reaches the capillaries where exchange of nutrients and waste products occur. Remember that exchange can occur only in the capillaries and all other vessels serve to conduct blood to and remove blood from the capillaries. Many physical factors determine the rate of exchange and the direction of movement (**see page 508**). Diffusion, vesicular transport, osmosis, and filtration are the primary factors that affect exchange.

Substances that can move easily across the capillary endothelium (directly through the plasma membrane, through the gaps in or between the endothelium) do so by **diffusion** (**see page 28** for a description of the diffusion process). Oxygen, carbon dioxide, glucose, amino acids, and steroid hormones are examples of substances that move by diffusion. Lipid-soluble substances, such as oxygen, carbon dioxide, and steroidal hormones, diffuse through the plasma membrane. Water-soluble substances, such as glucose and amino acids, pass through gaps in the cells and between the cells. The direction of movement is determined by the concentration gradient. For example, oxygen and glucose that are of a higher concentration inside the capillaries move out while carbon dioxide and other waste products that are of a higher concentration in the cells move into the capillaries. If the gaps between the capillary endothelial cells are large, even plasma proteins move out of the capillaries.

Large, lipid-insoluble substances may be transported by **vesicular transport** (**see page 30**). Here, the plasma membrane of the endothelial cells facing the blood indents to engulf the substance and form a vesicle (endocytosis). The vesicle is transported across the cytoplasm to the other side of the cell where it fuses with the plasma membrane to be extruded into the interstitial compartment (exocytosis).

Movement of Fluid Across the Capillaries

The movement of fluid across the capillaries is determined by the difference between the forces that pull/push the fluid *out of* the capillaries and forces that pull/push the fluid *into* the capillaries. Such forces are a result of the processes **osmosis** and **filtration** (**see pages 29 and 30** for a description of the processes).

The **blood hydrostatic pressure** tends to push the fluid out of the capillaries. This pressure is generated by the pumping action of the heart and is equivalent to the blood pressure in the capillaries. The hydrostatic pressure is comparable to the force that pushes water out of a leak in a garden hose; if the tap is opened further, more water gushes out of the leak. The blood hydrostatic pressure is about 35 mm Hg.

The **interstitial hydrostatic pressure** tends to push the fluid back into the capillaries. This is the pressure of fluid between the cells. Normally, there is little fluid in the tissue spaces as they are removed by the lymphatic vessels. In the body, this pressure is negligible—about 0 mm Hg or negative.

The particles inside the blood that are unable to move out of the capillaries are responsible for the **blood colloid osmotic pressure.** Think of the endothelial wall of the capillaries as the semipermeable membrane that allows water and some solutes to go through but is impermeable to larger particles. The blood colloid osmotic pressure tends to pull the fluid into the capillaries. The plasma proteins are mainly responsible for this force, which is about 26 mm Hg.

The blood colloid osmotic pressure is opposed by the **interstitial fluid osmotic pressure.** This force is a result of the large particles present in the interstitial compartment. The force tends to move the fluid out of the capillaries into the interstitial compartment. There are few particles, such as proteins, present in this compartment as they are removed quickly by the lymphatic capillaries. This force is, therefore, very small, only about 0.1–5 mm Hg. (see Figure 8.20)

The net balance of all of these pressures determines whether fluid leaves or stays inside the capillaries. If the net pressure that pushes fluid out of the capillaries is more than the net pressure that draws fluid in, fluid would move into the interstitial compartment (filtration). If the net pressure that draws fluid into the capillaries is more than the net pressure that pushes the fluid out, fluid would move into the capillaries (reabsorption). The **net filtration pressure** can be calculated using the figures given above.

Net filtration pressure = pressure that pushes fluid out (filtration) – pressure that pulls fluid in (reabsorption) = (blood hydrostatic pressure + interstitial fluid osmotic pressure) − (interstitial hydrostatic pressure + blood colloid osmotic pressure) = (35 mm Hg + 1 mm Hg) − (0 mm Hg + 26 mm Hg) = 10 mm Hg. At the arterial end, the net pressure of 10 mm Hg tends to push the fluid out.

As the blood flows through the capillaries from the arterial to venous end, the blood hydrostatic pressure decreases to about 16 mm Hg. At the venous end, therefore, the net pressure tends to draw the fluid into the capillaries. Net filtration pressure at venous end = (16 mm Hg + 1 mm Hg) − (0 mm Hg + 26 mm Hg) = −9 mm Hg. (i.e., the pressure that pushes fluid out is less than the pressure that pulls fluid in) Hence, fluid moves into the capillary at the venular end.

About 85% of the fluid in the body that moves into the interstitial compartment moves back into the capillaries. The remaining fluid and the proteins that may have escaped into the interstitial compartment are removed by the lymphatic vessels and returned to the circulatory system. Everyday, about 3 liters (3.2 qt) of fluid are returned to the circulatory system by the lymphatic vessels. If excessive fluid accumulates in the interstitial compartment, it is termed **edema.**

DO GIRAFFES DEVELOP EDEMA?

What happens when giraffes lower their heads to drink water? Although these long-legged animals are also affected by gravity, edema does not develop in their legs because they have tight skin and fascia—similar to antigravity suits. They also have an effective muscle pump which helps with venous return.

When giraffes lower their heads, the movement of the jaw muscles helps push the blood back to the heart. Also, valves in the jugular vein prevent backflow.

Venules and Veins

The capillaries empty into small veins known as **venules.** In some areas, there are direct connections between arterioles and venules. This is referred to as **arteriovenous anastomoses** (AV anastomoses) or **shunts.** Such anastomoses allow blood to bypass the capillaries and flow directly into veins. Shunts are in abundance in the skin and are controlled by the sympathetic nervous system. They permit the blood flow to be varied over a wider range —a useful function for temperature regulation.

The venules form thin-walled, midsized veins that join and rejoin to form **large veins.** The branches of veins are referred as **tributaries.** In most regions, the

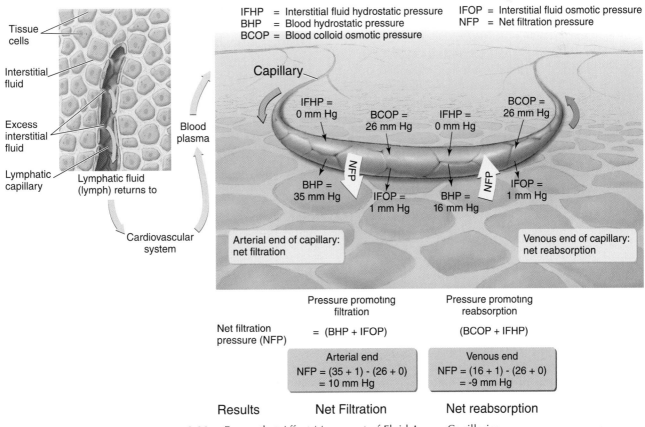

FIGURE **8.20.**   Forces that Affect Movement of Fluid Across Capillaries

veins accompany arteries and lie parallel and close to them. The walls of the veins have three layers; however, they are much thinner than those of arteries. The lumen of the vein is much larger than that of arteries and can, therefore, accommodate more blood than arteries. Hence, the veins may serve as blood reservoirs. Many veins also have valves in them. Venous valves are thin folds of the tunica interna that direct blood toward the heart. Valves help with the venous return by preventing backflow of blood.

In some regions, the vein is very thin, with just a thin endothelial wall and no smooth muscles. The surrounding connective tissue replaces the tunica media and externa. Such veins are known as **venous sinus** or **vascular sinus.** Venous sinus are found in the cranial cavity—between the dura mater. The coronary sinus of the heart (the vein that drains the wall of the heart) is also a vascular sinus.

Venous Return

As blood flows from larger arteries through arterioles and capillaries, the blood pressure drops and is only 10% of that in the arteries when it reaches the venules. The pressure is so low that it cannot even oppose the force of gravity. The volume of blood returning to the heart from the veins—the **venous return**—depends on the pressure difference between the venules to the right ventricle. Although the pressure difference is low, venous return is equal to the amount of blood pumped out of the heart as a result of additional mechanisms.

To help with the venous return, veins have one-way valves. In addition to valves, the pulsation of the arteries lying parallel to them and compression resulting from contracting skeletal muscle (**skeletal muscle pump**) that surrounds them helps to squeeze venous blood towards the heart against the force of gravity.

Respiratory movement also helps to return blood to the heart (**respiratory pump**). During inspiration, pressure decreases in the thoracic cavity and the thoracic volume increases. At the same time, the pressure increases in the abdominal cavity as the diaphragm descends during inspiration. This squeezes

the abdominal veins. The resultant unequal pressure creates a "sucking" effect that pulls blood toward the heart.

Volume in Blood Vessels

The blood volume (approximately 5.0 liters [5.3 qt]) is unevenly distributed among the arteries, veins, and capillaries at any given time. Most of the blood (60%–65%) is contained in the venous system, as the walls are thinner and more distensible. For this reason, the veins are also referred to as **capacitance vessels.** The veins serve as reservoirs of blood (**blood reservoirs**) and, when the blood volume drops as in severe bleeding or dehydration, they constrict and increase the blood volume in the arteries and capillaries. The veins of the abdominal organs, such as the liver and spleen and the veins of the skin, are important blood reservoirs.

At rest, about 5% of the blood volume is present in the capillaries. The systemic arteries hold about 15% of the blood volume. About 8% of the volume is in the heart and 12% in the pulmonary vessels.

MAJOR SYSTEMIC ARTERIES

Figure 8.21 is an overview of the systemic arteries. Only the major arteries relevant to bodyworkers are described. The large artery from the left ventricle is the **aorta.** It is the largest of arteries and begins at the aortic semilunar valve. The **right** and **left coronary arteries** branch off just above the valve. The aorta passes superiorly for a short distance as the **ascending aorta** and curves to form the **arch of the aorta** before it passes inferiorly as the **descending aorta.**

Three major branches leave the arch of the aorta. These are the **brachiocephalic,** the **left common carotid,** and the **left subclavian arteries.** The brachiocephalic artery, after ascending a short distance, forms two branches—the **right subclavian** and the **right common carotid.** The carotids supply the structures in the head and neck, and the subclavian delivers blood to the arms, shoulders, chest wall, back, and to the central nervous system.

Arterial Supply to the Upper Limbs

The subclavian artery is known as the **axillary artery,** after it leaves the thoracic cavity and passes the superior border of the first rib. The axillary artery crosses the axilla and enters the arm, at which point it is referred to as the **brachial artery.** The brachial artery supplies the upper arm. At the antecubital fossa, it divides into the **radial artery** (which follows the radius) and the **ulnar artery** (which follows the

---

✔ Varicose Veins

In some individuals, the valves of the vein may not function properly, allowing backflow and pooling of blood in the veins. Other than the cosmetic problem, these bloated and distorted veins can lead to various complications, such as thrombi (blood clots inside blood vessels), emboli (loose, dislodged clots), and painful ulcers.

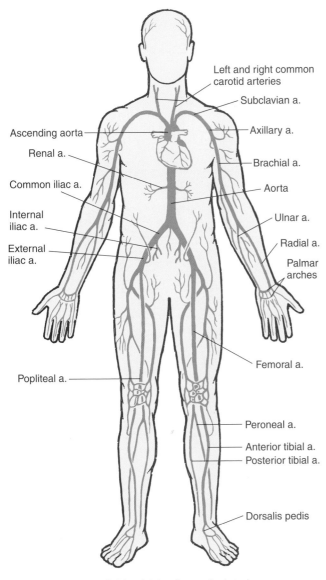

Ascending aorta

Renal a.

Common iliac a.

Internal iliac a.

External iliac a.

Popliteal a.

Left and right common carotid arteries

Subclavian a.

Axillary a.

Brachial a.

Aorta

Ulnar a.

Radial a.

Palmar arches

Femoral a.

Peroneal a.

Anterior tibial a.
Posterior tibial a.

Dorsalis pedis

FIGURE **8.21.**   Major Systemic Arteries

sure). The external carotids supply the neck, esophagus, pharynx, larynx, lower jaw, and face.

Arterial Supply to the Brain

The internal carotids supply blood to the brain. The brain is also supplied by the **vertebral arteries,** which are branches of the subclavian arteries. The brain is extremely sensitive to changes in blood supply. If the circulation to it is interrupted for several seconds, the person can become unconscious. Irreversible brain damage can be produced if the supply is cut off for more than 4 minutes. The internal carotids and the vertebral arteries anastomose and form a circle near the brainstem inside the skull. This is known as the **circle of Willis.** The major branches from the circle are the **anterior, middle,** and **posterior cerebral arteries.** Most often, it is the middle cerebral artery affected in a person with stroke.

Arterial Supply to the Thorax

The arch of aorta becomes the descending aorta or **thoracic aorta** and descends to the left of the vertebra along the posterior thoracic wall. It is located closer to the midline as it reaches the diaphragm. It then passes through the aortic hiatus of the diaphragm and becomes the **abdominal aorta.** As the thoracic aorta descends, it gives off many branches to the viscera (**visceral branches**) and to the thoracic wall (**parietal branches**). The visceral branches supply the bronchi, pericardium, esophagus, and other structures in the mediastinum.

Arterial Supply to the Abdomen and Pelvis

At about level T12, the thoracic aorta pierces the diaphragm and becomes the **abdominal aorta,** which lies posterior to the peritoneal cavity. It divides into two major arteries at level L4—the **right** and **left common iliac arteries.** The abdominal aorta delivers blood to the abdominopelvic organs and most of the major branches are unpaired and arise anteriorly and enter the mesentery. The major arteries are the **celiac artery,** which supplies blood to the stomach (left gastric branch), spleen (splenic branch), and liver (common hepatic artery); the **superior mesenteric artery,** which supplies the pancreas, duodenum, small intestines, and most of the large intestines; and the **inferior mesenteric artery,** which supplies blood to the terminal parts of the colon. Five paired arteries, the **inferior phrenics, suprarenal, renal, gonadal,** and **lumbar arteries,** also arise from the abdominal aorta.

The left and right common iliac arteries carry blood to the pelvis and lower limbs. Each common il-

ulna to the wrist). The radial and ulnar arteries supply the forearm. It is the radial artery that is palpated at the wrist to take the pulse. At the wrist, the arteries anastomose to form two arches—the **deep** and **superficial palmar arches**—from which branches supply the hand, thumb, and fingers.

Arterial Supply to the Head and Face

The left and right common carotid arteries ascend in the tissue of the anterior aspect of the neck. Their pulsations can be palpated on either side of the trachea. Each divides into the **external carotid** and **internal carotid arteries.** A slight bulge in the internal carotid artery just as the common carotid artery branches, known as the **carotid sinus,** indicates the location of the baroreceptors (receptors that detect blood pres-

Superficial Pulses

The pulse of an artery located close to the surface of the body can be felt by using the fingertips and squeezing the artery lightly against a solid mass, such as bone. The pulsations that can be felt are the *temporal, facial, common carotid, brachial, radial, femoral, popliteal,* and *dorsalis pedis arteries.*

Temporal artery: can be felt on the side of the head (often visible in elderly, thin individuals).

Facial artery: crosses the body of the mandible as it enters the face in front of the masseter muscle. It can be felt by grasping the cheek between the thumb and index finger about 2 cm behind the angle of the mouth.

Common carotid artery: can be felt on either side of the trachea in the neck

Brachial artery: can be felt in the anterior aspect of the elbow, just medial to the biceps tendon; it is better felt with the arm extended; the stethoscope is placed over this artery when measuring blood pressure in the arm

Radial artery: can be felt on the lateral aspect of the anterior surface of the wrist, applying light pressure against the lower end of the radius

Femoral artery: can be felt with the hip extended, in the midinguinal point

Popliteal artery: can be felt in the back of the knee in the middle of the popliteal fossa. It is better felt with the person lying prone with the leg extended.

Dorsalis pedis artery: can be felt in the middle of the dorsum of the foot between the tendons of the extensor digitorum longus and extensor hallucis longus tendon

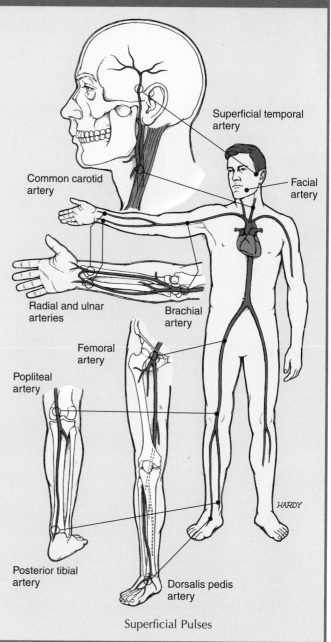

Superficial Pulses

iac artery divides into the **internal** and **external iliac arteries** at the level of the lumbosacral joint. The internal iliac supplies the organs in the pelvic cavity, such as the uterus, urinary bladder, the external genitalia, the internal and external walls of the pelvis, the medial side of thigh, and the vagina. The external iliac arteries supply the lower limbs.

Arterial Supply to the Lower Limbs

The external iliac crosses the surface of the iliopsoas muscle and penetrates the abdominal wall midway between the anterior superior iliac spine and the pu-

bic symphysis and emerges on the anteromedial surface of the thigh where it is called the **femoral artery.** The femoral artery continues inferiorly and is posterior to the femur at the popliteal fossa. Here it is called the **popliteal artery.** It divides here into the **posterior** and **anterior tibial arteries.** The posterior tibial gives rise to the **peroneal artery.** When the anterior tibial reaches the foot, it becomes the **dorsalis pedis artery.** The posterior tibial artery branches as it reaches the foot and forms the **medial** and **lateral plantar arteries.** Anastomoses connect the dorsalis pedis artery with the plantar arteries to form two arches, the **dorsal arch** and the **plantar arch.**

SYSTEMIC VEINS

Drainage From the Brain, Head, and Neck

Figure 8.22 is an overview of the major veins. The superior vena cava receives blood from the tissue and organs of the head, neck, chest, shoulders, and upper limb. Inside the skull, the smaller veins drain into large vessels known as **sinuses.** The venous sinuses converge and ultimately leave the skull as the **internal jugular vein.** The internal jugular vein descends parallel to the common carotid artery in the neck. Posteriorly, the skull is drained by the **vertebral veins** that leave the skull and descend within the foramen in the transverse processes of the cervical vertebrae.

From regions outside the skull and neck, the veins of the head drain into the **external jugular vein,** which lies just beneath the skin, on the anterior surface of the sternocleidomastoid muscle.

Drainage From the Upper Limbs

The upper limb, like the lower limb, has two sets of veins—the **superficial** and the **deep.** In the hand, **digital veins** empty into the **superficial** and **deep palmar veins** that interconnect to form the **palmar venous arches** (similar to the palmar arches of arteries).

The superficial veins empty into the **cephalic vein,** which ascends along the radial side of the forearm, the median **antebrachial vein,** and the **basilic vein,** which ascends on the ulnar side. The basilic vein ascends in the upper arm, medial to the biceps brachii muscle. Anterior to the elbow, the superficial **median cubital vein** passes medially and obliquely from the cephalic to the basilic vein. Usually, blood is collected for examination or donation from the median cubital vein.

The *deep veins* are positioned parallel to the arteries and carry the same names. The **deep palmar veins** drain into the **radial vein** and **ulnar vein.** After crossing the elbow, these veins fuse to form the **brachial vein.** The brachial vein, on entering the axilla, is called the **axillary vein.** The superficial basilic vein joins the brachial vein near the axilla.

The cephalic vein joins the axillary vein on the lateral surface of the first rib to form the **subclavian vein.** The subclavian passes medially and merges with the internal and external jugular veins on each side to form the **brachiocephalic vein.** At the level of the first and second rib, near the heart, the right and left brachiocephalic veins join to form the **superior vena cava.** The superior vena cava is joined by the **azygos vein** inside the thorax. The azygos vein collects blood from the thoracic cavity.

Drainage From the Lower Limbs

The lower limbs and abdomen are drained by the inferior vena cava. In the foot, the capillaries in the sole of each foot form **plantar veins** that join to form the plantar **venous arch.** Similar to the upper limb, there are two sets of veins—**superficial** and **deep.** The deep veins lie parallel to the arteries and are called by the same names as the arteries. The **anterior tibial vein,** the **posterior tibial vein,** and the **peroneal veins** join at the popliteal fossa to form the **popliteal vein.** On reaching the femur, the popliteal vein is referred to as the **femoral vein.** The femoral vein penetrates the abdominal wall and becomes the **external iliac vein.**

The surface anatomy of the *superficial veins* is important, as it is a common site for varicosities. Some of the capillaries of the foot join on the superior surface of the foot to form the **dorsal venous arch.** Two superficial veins are formed from the dorsal venous arch—the **great saphenous vein** and the **small saphenous vein.** The great saphenous vein ascends along the

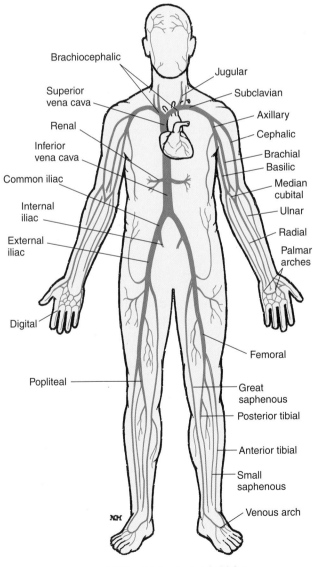

Brachiocephalic

Jugular

Superior
vena cava

Subclavian

Renal

Axillary

Inferior
vena cava

Cephalic

Common iliac

Brachial

Internal
iliac

Basilic

External
iliac

Median
cubital

Ulnar

Radial

Palmar
arches

Digital

Femoral

Popliteal

Great
saphenous

Posterior tibial

Anterior tibial

Small
saphenous

Venous arch

FIGURE **8.22.**   Major Systemic Veins

✓ **Venous Thrombosis**

Formation of thrombus is one complication of varicose veins. Thrombus may form in the superficial or deep vein, and it may be accompanied by inflammation. This condition is known as thrombophlebitis. It usually presents as pain, swelling, and muscle tenderness in and around the area.

A simple test for deep vein thrombus is the Homan's sign, in which the ankle is dorsiflexed with the knee extended. If a thrombus is present, pain is felt in the calf.

---

medial aspect of the leg and thigh and drains into the femoral vein near the inguinal region. The small saphenous vein arises from the dorsal venous arch and ascends along the posterior and lateral aspect of the calf where it drains into the popliteal vein.

Drainage From the Pelvis and Abdomen

In the pelvis, the external iliac vein is joined by the **internal iliac vein** on each side, to form the right and left **common iliac veins.** At the level of L5, the right and left common iliac veins join to form the **inferior vena cava.**

The inferior vena cava lies posterior to the peritoneal cavity, parallel to the aorta. Some of the major veins that join it in the abdomen are the **lumbar veins, gonadal veins** (from the testes/ovaries), **hepatic veins** (from the liver), **renal veins** (from the kidney), **suprarenal veins** (from the adrenal glands), and **phrenic veins** (from the diaphragm).

Portal Circulation

The circulation of blood in the stomach and intestines is unique in that the capillaries formed in the walls of the gut eventually drain into the **hepatic portal vein,** which empties into sinusoidal capillaries in the liver (see Figure 8.23). The **inferior mesenteric, splenic,** and **superior mesenteric veins** are some important tributaries that join to form the hepatic portal vein. This circulation is referred to as the **hepatic portal system.** The blood in the hepatic portal vein contains nutrients absorbed from the gut, which it carries to the liver for storage, metabolic conversion, or excretion. After passing through the liver sinusoids, blood collects into the **hepatic veins** that empty into the inferior vena cava. This unique circulation is important because the liver helps maintain the composition of blood in the systemic circulation, even if the digestive activities vary greatly. Simply put, it does not allow glucose or other nutrients to be dumped into the systemic circulation every time an individual eats!

The liver not only receives deoxygenated blood from the hepatic portal vein, but also oxygenated blood via the **hepatic artery,** a branch of the celiac trunk. This blood, together with blood from the portal vein, drains into the hepatic veins.

Dynamics of Blood Flow

The cardiovascular system faces many challenges. It has to maintain blood flow to all tissue, taking care to continue perfusion of vital organs such as the brain and heart, no matter what the situation. When activity increases in one tissue, blood flow has to increase in this region without compromising flow to the brain and heart. For efficiency, blood flow has to be reduced to inactive tissue. Many of the biophysical principles come into play when this system meets these challenges.

Some of the important biophysical considerations that help us understand the circulation of blood are those that apply to any liquid:

- blood (like any liquid) flows from an area of *high pressure* to one of *low pressure*
- if the *difference in pressure* is high, flow is increased
- blood flow is decreased if the resistance is more (resistance is any force that opposes movement); in the cardiovascular system, it is referred to as the **peripheral resistance.**

BLOOD PRESSURE

Arterial blood pressure must be high enough to overcome peripheral resistance and maintain blood flow through capillaries. The force of contraction of the ventricle raises the pressure to about 120 mm Hg (**systolic pressure**), and the elastic recoil of the arteries maintains the pressure at about 90 mm Hg during ventricular diastole (**diastolic pressure**). This is enough pressure to keep the blood flowing continuously to all parts of the body. However, if there is increased resistance to flow, more pressure is needed.

💡 mm Hg

This unit is used to measure blood pressure and is an abbreviation for millimeters of mercury. For example, if the pressure is 10 mm Hg, it is the pressure required to push a column of mercury to a height of 10 millimeters. Because mercury is heavy, the numbers are small. If water is used instead of mercury, the height of the column will be many feet and the numbers will be large and cumbersome to use. In fact, the first measurement of blood pressure was made in a horse using the height of water as the unit and the tube had to be more than 8 feet long.

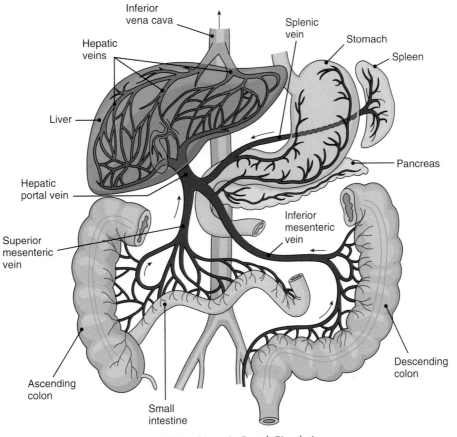

FIGURE **8.23.** Hepatic Portal Circulation

If pressure is high, the work of the heart is increased and, if the pressure is too high, the heart may fail. If the pressure is too low, even if the heart is not taxed, it may not be sufficient to perfuse the brain. Hence, the blood pressure has to be constantly monitored and maintained.

PERIPHERAL RESISTANCE

Peripheral resistance is the resistance offered in the tissue; it has a relationship to blood flow and blood pressure.

$$\text{Flow} = \frac{\text{Pressure}}{\text{Resistance}}$$

If resistance increases, the blood pressure has to be increased to maintain flow.

The major factors that contribute to the peripheral resistance are *friction between the blood and vessel walls,* which largely depends on the *length* of vessels; the *caliber (diameter)* of blood vessels and the *viscosity (consistency)* of blood; and *type of flow* (i.e., whether the flow is turbulent or smooth).

The peripheral resistance increases as the total length of blood vessels increases. As a result, the blood pressure has to be increased to maintain blood flow to the tissue. In individuals who are obese, there is an increase in total blood vessel length to supply the adipose tissue. This may be one cause of hypertension observed in obese individuals.

The peripheral resistance in the body is mainly a result of the alteration in the caliber of blood vessels. Of the blood vessels, the arterioles offer the most resistance. The high content of smooth muscle in the arteriole walls enables adjustment of resistance according to regional needs. Sympathetic stimulation creates contraction of smooth muscle.

Blood viscosity is largely determined by the percentage of the volume of blood occupied by red blood cells. If the red blood cell content increases, viscosity increases, and the heart has to work harder to push the blood forward.

Regulation of the Cardiovascular System

The ultimate objective of the cardiovascular system is to ensure that the tissue blood flow meets the demands for oxygen and nutrients at the right time and

💡 BLOOD PRESSURE MEASUREMENT

The ideal method for measuring blood pressure would be to put a tube connected to a measuring device, directly inside an artery. This, of course, would be cumbersome and an indirect method for measuring blood pressure is used. Because the pressure of blood also pushes against the walls of the artery other than propelling the blood forward, the pressure exerted on the sidewall is measured.

The instrument used to measure blood pressure is a **sphygmomanometer.** In brief, this instrument consists of a rubber bag with two tubes leading from it. The bag is usually covered with cloth, with a removable fastening that secures the bag firmly around the limb. One tube is connected to a device that measures pressure in mm Hg. The other tube is connected to a rubber bulb with a one-way valve that lets air in or out of the rubber bag. The bag is wrapped firmly around the arm (or leg) and air is pumped into the bag. When the air pressure in the bag is above that of the artery, the wall of the artery is fully compressed and no blood passes through. If the air is let out slowly, the pressure in the bag decreases and, at one point when the pressure reaches just below that of the systolic pressure of the artery, some blood squeezes through the compressed artery during systole. As the pressure in the bag is lowered even more, more and more blood passes through the narrowed artery. At a pressure below diastole, the caliber of the artery returns to its original size and blood flows through it as before.

When blood flows through a normal artery, no sound is produced when lightly placing a stethoscope on the body. This is because the flow is streamlined (like water flowing quietly in a stream where there is no obstruction). If the artery is narrowed or compressed, sound is produced as the flow becomes turbulent (like a stream flowing fast or over pebbles). By placing a stethoscope over the brachial artery (or popliteal artery in the leg) when the rubber bag of the sphygmomanometer is being deflated and listening to the sounds produced, blood pressure can be measured. At high pressure, with the artery fully compressed, no sounds are heard. When blood squirts through the artery when the pressure is just below systolic pressure, a sound is heard, and this is the systolic pressure. Sound is heard as long as the artery is compressed and the flow is turbulent. No sounds are heard when blood does not flow or if the flow is streamlined. The pressure at which the sound disappears (or become faint) is taken as the diastolic pressure.

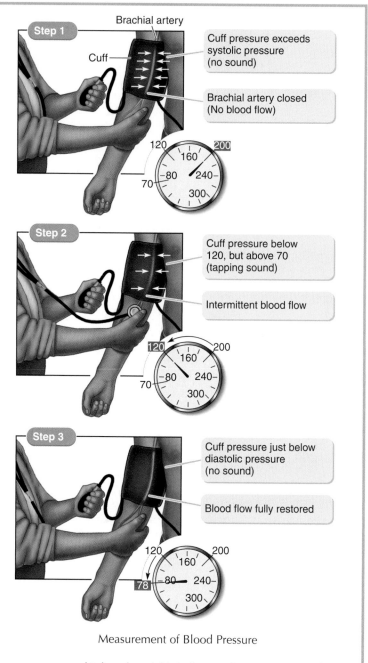

Measurement of Blood Pressure

region, without drastically altering blood flow to vital organs such as the brain. This is achieved by manipulating the cardiac output (output of the heart), peripheral resistance (changing the diameter of resistance vessels), and altering the amount of blood pooled in the veins. Three regulatory mechanisms are involved to achieve the objective: **local mechanisms, neural mechanisms,** and **endocrine mechanisms.** These mechanisms increase blood flow to active tissue and increase and decrease heat loss from the body by redistributing the blood. If blood loss occurs, they maintain blood flow to the heart and brain. If the loss is severe, they maintain blood flow to these vital organs at the expense of other parts of the body.

LOCAL MECHANISMS

The tissues are able to regulate, to some extent, their own blood flow. This capacity is referred to as **autoregulation.** Autoregulation can be compared to the

Hypertension

A person is said to have high blood pressure or hypertension if the pressure is consistently greater than 140/90 mm Hg. Hypertension increases the load on the heart, making the heart work harder. The cardiac muscle hypertrophies, increasing its oxygen needs. As a result, there is an increased risk of developing angina and myocardial infarction. The high pressure also stresses the blood vessels and there is a greater chance of developing arteriosclerosis, aneurysms, rupture of blood vessels, and stroke.

water supply to our houses. A pumping station pumps water to houses in a certain locality. However, individuals in each house are able to regulate the water according to their needs. Similarly, the heart pumps blood to the body, but each organ has the capacity to regulate the blood flow to it according to its needs. For example, the vascular smooth muscles contract and reduce the caliber of the vessel automatically when they are stretched by increased blood flow. When a tissue becomes active, blood flow automatically increases. This is brought about by the accumulation of "vasodilator substances." Changes in pH, decreases in oxygen, and increases in carbon dioxide, temperature, potassium ions, and lactic acid, all outcomes of active metabolism, tend to relax the vascular smooth muscles and automatically increase blood flow. In injured tissue, release of histamine from damaged cells has the same effect.

By autoregulation, blood flow reduces in injured arteries and arterioles. This is because the arterioles constrict strongly, partly as a result of the liberation of the chemical serotonin from platelets and other vasoconstrictor substances by the endothelial cells. When cold, the smooth muscles of vessels in the skin contract and produce vasoconstriction as a result of direct stimulation by cold.

Other than regulating blood flow on a short-term basis, tissue has the capacity to increase or decrease the number and length of blood vessels according to

Massage and Postural Hypotension

It is relatively common for individuals to feel dizzy when suddenly getting up from the massage table. As massage has an effect on the sympathetic system reducing vasomotor tone, sudden posture change can result in pooling of blood in the legs and symptoms of postural hypotension. It is advisable for the therapist to caution clients to get up slowly and sit on the table for sometime, allowing for compensatory mechanisms to adjust the pressure before getting off.

long-term needs. New blood vessels may be formed (**angiogenesis**) or blood vessels that are already present may be remodeled (**vascular remodeling**).

NEURAL MECHANISMS

The innervation of the heart was discussed on **page 471**.

All blood vessels of the body other than capillaries and venules have smooth muscles in the walls, which are innervated by sympathetic nerves. The sympathetic nerves produce vasoconstriction in almost all tissue. However, the sympathetic nerves to the skeletal muscle produce vasodilatation. There is a constant discharge of impulses via the sympathetic nerves, and all blood vessels are in a state of some vasoconstriction, even at rest. This is known as the **vasomotor tone** or **vascular tone.**

The sympathetic nerves are controlled by groups of neurons located in the medulla oblongata known as the **vasomotor area** or **vasomotor center.** The activity of the vasomotor center and, thereby, that of sympathetic nerves, is altered by many factors. Figure 8.24 gives the various factors that stimulate and inhibit the center.

Neurons from the cerebral cortex have an effect on the center via the hypothalamus. These are responsible for the increase in blood pressure and heart rate produced by emotions such as anger or sexual excitement. Inflation of the lungs results in vasodilatation. Oxygen and carbon dioxide levels in the blood have a direct effect on the activity of the center, and input from sensory nerves can affect the center as well. For example, pain sensations increase blood pressure, however, prolonged severe pain may cause vasodilatation and fainting. Another important factor that af-

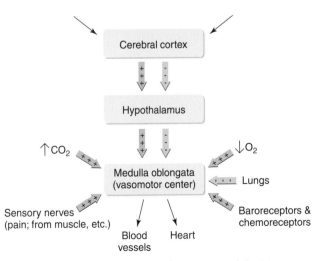

FIGURE **8.24.** Factors That Affect the Activity of the Vasomotor Center. (green arrows, stimulation; and pink arrows, inhibition of the center)

fects the vasomotor center is the input from **barore-ceptors.**

Baroreceptors are stretch receptors found in the walls of the heart and blood vessels. The arterial circulation is monitored by receptors located in the walls of the carotid sinus and aortic arch. The venous pressure is monitored by other receptors present in the right and left atria, vena cava, and pulmonary veins. The arterial baroreceptors and their activity are described below.

Afferent nerves from the carotid sinus and aortic arch baroreceptors reach the vasomotor center via the glossopharyngeal and vagus nerves. When the pressure in the arteries increases, the walls are stretched and these receptors are stimulated. The impulses are carried to the vasomotor center where they have an inhibitory effect. The decrease in the activity of the center results in vasodilatation, fall in blood pressure, and heart rate. The opposite happens when the blood pressure drops in the arteries. This baroreceptor reflex is a powerful mechanism, which regulates the blood pressure from moment to moment.

The chemoreceptors (**see page 564**) under respiratory system) located in the carotid and aortic bodies have an effect on the cardiac center and vasomotor center, in addition to the respiratory center, resulting in vasoconstriction and bradycardia. However, this effect may be overridden by other regulatory mechanisms.

In addition to those previously mentioned, many other reflexes (beyond the scope of this book) affect blood pressure.

ENDOCRINE MECHANISMS

Many hormones in the circulation have an effect on blood pressure, volume, and flow. It is brought about by direct effect on the smooth muscles of blood vessels or on the kidney tubules.

The hormones secreted by the adrenal medulla have a potent vasoconstrictor effect. The adrenal medulla (**see page 403**) is innervated by sympathetic nerves and secrete **adrenaline** and **nonadrenaline** into the circulation when stimulated. Both hormones increase the force and rate of contraction of the heart. While producing vasoconstriction in general, adrenaline causes vasodilatation in skeletal muscles and the heart.

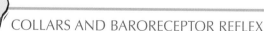

COLLARS AND BARORECEPTOR REFLEX

Tight collars can apply pressure on the neck and press on the carotid sinus. The baroreceptors are stimulated and produce a reflex slowing of the heart, dilatation of blood vessels, and drop in pressure. The reduced blood supply to the brain may make the person feel dizzy or even faint.

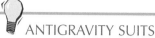

ANTIGRAVITY SUITS

To compensate for the gravitational effects, *G suits* are worn. These are double-walled pressure suits containing water or compressed air that compress the abdomen and legs with a force proportionate to the G force.

Vasopressin or **antidiuretic hormone** secreted by the posterior pituitary gland also has a vasoconstrictor effect. As the names suggest, the hormone also reduces excretion of water in the kidneys, increasing the blood volume and blood pressure.

Another potent vasoconstrictor is **angiotensin II** (**see page 411**). The hormone **aldosterone,** secreted by the adrenal cortex, helps increase blood volume by stimulating the kidneys to reabsorb water and sodium ions from the urine. In this way, both blood volume and blood pressure are maintained.

Atrial natriuretic peptide is another hormone secreted by cardiac muscles in the walls of the right atrium. It is secreted when the walls of the atria are stretched excessively. This hormone *reduces* blood volume and blood pressure by increasing the excretion of water and sodium in the urine, reducing the activity of vasoconstrictor hormones and causing vasodilatation.

In summary, the cardiovascular system is regulated by many mechanisms, some with short-term and others with long-term effects, some producing local and others producing generalized effects, all working toward the goal of meeting the needs of various tissues, without compromising blood flow to the vital organs. The regulatory mechanisms—local, neural, and endocrine mechanisms—work in an integrated manner to maintain homeostasis. The various drugs used for treating hypertension act on one or more of these mechanisms.

COMPENSATORY ADJUSTMENTS

The regulatory mechanism activity can be better appreciated by examining how they come into play during both everyday activities and abnormal conditions.

The compensatory adjustments made by the cardiovascular system to some of the challenges faced by the circulation, normally in everyday life and abnormally in disease, are considered below. The challenges considered are:

- Compensations for gravitational effects
- Exercise
- Shock
- Cardiac Failure.

Compensations for Gravitational Effects

As a result of the effect of gravity when standing, the mean blood pressure in the feet of a normal adult is 180–200 mm Hg and the blood pressure in the head is about 60–75 mm Hg. If the person stands still, about 300–500 mL (0.317–0.53 qt) of blood tends to pool in the veins of the lower limbs and fluid tends to move out of the capillaries into the interstitial fluid as a result of the increased hydrostatic pressure (edema formation).

All this results in a reduction of blood returning to the heart and the stroke volume drops. If there were no compensatory mechanisms, the resultant drop in blood flow to the brain will result in prompt loss of consciousness.

The major compensation is caused by the stimulation of the carotid sinus and aortic arch baroreceptors when there is a slight drop in blood pressure. Stimulation results in immediate increase in heart rate to increase cardiac output and generalized vasoconstriction via the sympathetic nerves. In addition, there is an increase in renin levels, with formation of angiotensin II producing further vasoconstriction. Aldosterone levels also increase, conserving water, increasing blood volume, and maintaining blood pressure.

In the brain, local mechanisms play a part in increasing blood supply and maintaining consciousness. The accumulation of carbon dioxide, lack of oxygen, and changes in pH have a direct effect on blood vessels causing vasodilatation. Also, brain tissue extracts more oxygen from each unit of blood.

Prolonged standing, especially if standing still, produces additional problems because of the fluid moving into the interstitial compartment. As long as the person is moving, the contracting muscles compress the veins and return blood to the heart. If the person stands still, venous return is decreased, and the person faints as a result of reduced brain perfusion. Fainting can be considered as a compensatory mechanism because, when the person falls to the ground, the effect of gravity is removed and venous return is restored.

Some people develop a fall in blood pressure, dizziness, dimness of vision, and even fainting when suddenly standing up. This is called **orthostatic** or **postural hypotension.** When the blood volume is low, as in dehydration, or when the compensatory mechanisms do not function well, as when taking an-

tihypertensives or in those individuals with diabetes, the effects are more significant.

Effects of Acceleration

The effects of gravity on the circulation are multiplied during acceleration or deceleration, whether on an elevator, a fast rides in an amusement park, or on a rocket. Gravity is measured by **G force,** with 1 G equal to the earth's surface. The force is referred to as **positive G** when it is acting from head to foot, and negative G when acting from foot to head. At accelerations equal to about 5 G, as a result of the excessive pooling of blood in the lower limbs and a drop in blood pressure and volume, vision fails in 5 seconds (**blackout**), and unconsciousness follows.

Negative G causes an increase in cardiac output and intense congestion of the head and neck vessels. A severe, throbbing headache and mental confusion (**redout**) result. Tiny blood vessels, especially around the eye, may rupture as a result of high blood pressure and congestion.

Exercise and Training

With exercise, extensive compensatory adjustments are made throughout the body, especially in the cardiovascular and respiratory systems.[1]

Muscle Blood Flow

At rest, muscle blood flow is as low as 2–4 mL/100 g (0.55–1.1 cu inches/lb) per minute. However, even the thought of exercise increases the blood flow via the sympathetic vasodilator fibers. When the muscle contracts, the blood vessels are compressed. If the tension reaches about 70% of maximum, no blood flows through the contracted muscles; however, when the muscle relaxes between contractions, blood flow increases significantly by autoregulation. The accumulation of local metabolites, increase in CO_2 and decrease in O_2 levels, etc., directly affect the smooth muscle of blood vessels to relax and more capillary beds to open. Fluid enters the interstitium faster and lymphatic flow is greatly increased. The increase in temperature and change in pH facilitates the absorption of O_2 from the hemoglobin and transport of CO_2. All of these changes make it possible for the muscle to drastically speed its metabolism.

Changes in Systemic Circulation

The response of the systemic circulation to exercise depends on whether the exercise is **isometric** or **isotonic** (exercise is isometric when the muscle does not decrease in length when the tension increases, e.g., pushing against a wall).

TICKLE YOUR BRAIN. . .

Given your knowledge of the regulatory mechanisms of the cardiovascular system, what do you think will be the effect of zero gravity on the body?

In isometric exercise, the blood flow to the steadily contracting muscle is decreased as the vessels are compressed. The systolic and diastolic pressure increases significantly, and the heart has to work harder. In isotonic exercise, as a result of vasodilatation in the skeletal muscle, the blood pressure does not rise as much.

Cardiac output is increased by increasing both heart rate and stroke volume. The rise is in proportion to the severity of exercise. The cardiac output can sometimes exceed 35 L/minute. In children, the heart rate may be higher than 200 beats/minute during exercise. Venous return is significantly increased, aided by the contracting muscles and the suction effect of rapid and deep inspiration. After stopping the exercise, the circulation returns to normal, and the recovery time depends on the severity of exercise and the fitness of the individual.

Temperature Regulation

Heat generated during exercise is dissipated by dilation of vessels to the skin. Some heat is lost in the expired air as well. Increased production and evaporation of sweat are major sources of heat loss.

Effect of Training on the Cardiovascular System

Training produces changes in the heart and muscle that increases the efficiency of oxygen delivery.[1] The changes produced are related to the initial fitness level, genetic makeup, training frequency, training type, and training duration and intensity. Of the various types of exercises some, such as aerobic exercise that exercises larger muscles, have greater effects on the cardiovascular system. Walking, running, cycling, and swimming are some examples of aerobic exercises.

Individuals who have had long-term aerobic training have larger hearts, greater end-diastolic ventricular volume, larger stroke volume and a lower heart rate, both at rest and during exercise. The larger heart enables them to increase cardiac output much more than individuals who are sedentary. Because of this increase in efficient use of energy, the heart is less taxed and does not have to increase the cardiac output as much as in sedentary individuals for the same intensity of exercise. The changes produced in the heart vary according to the type of exercise. For example, resistance-trained athletes (such as weight lifters) have a thicker ventricular wall compared with endurance athletes. But the endurance athletes tend to have a greater cavity size.

The resting heart rate of a trained athlete may be as low as 40–60 beats/minute. This is a result of the imbalance between sympathetic and parasympathetic stimulation of the heart caused by training.

At the microscopic level, training results in thickening of individual myofibrils and an increase in the number of myofilaments, mitochondria, enzymes, and blood flow per unit area of muscle. The changes produced are reversible and, if training is discontinued, decrease to pretraining levels within weeks.

With aerobic training, the plasma volume increases. This is a result of increased synthesis and production of albumin. The red blood cell mass is also increased with resultant increase in total blood volume.

With endurance training, more mitochondria and enzymes required for metabolism are present in the muscle. The number of capillaries per unit area is higher. The blood flow to the skeletal muscle in question is also increased. The result is better perfusion, with more availability of oxygen and less accumulation of metabolites.

Other changes that occur with regular exercise include a reduction in blood pressure (both systolic and diastolic) and increased ability of the body to dissolve blood clots by facilitating fibrinolytic activity. In addition, regular exercise reduces the incidence of anxiety and depression and increases the overall sense of well-being. The incidence of numerous diseases is reduced in those who exercise regularly. See page 195-200 for more on physical conditioning.

Shock

Shock is a loosely-used term, with a great deal of confusion and controversy. There is a marked difference between the effects produced by electric shock, spinal shock, or shock in the circulatory system.

Shock in the circulatory system refers to conditions that cause profound and widespread reduction in the delivery of oxygen and nutrients to tissue.[2] There are many conditions that result in shock, a result of de-

---

✔ Basic Principles in Treating Shock

The aim in shock treatment should be to correct the cause and help the physiologic compensatory mechanisms. Medical help should be called for promptly; however, the compensatory mechanisms could be helped by:

- taking care not to overheat the body because it produces cutaneous vasodilatation and further reduction in venous return and cardiac output
- eliminating the effect of gravity and pooling of blood in the lower extremities; the person should lie down; raising the foot end by 15–30 cm (.5–1 foot) helps increase venous return
- remembering that although the head-down position is helpful, it also causes the contents of the abdomen to be pushed against the diaphragm, making adequate ventilation difficult.

Table 8.5

Types of Shock and Examples of Conditions

Hypovolemic Shock (decreased blood flow)

Bleeding

Injury

Severe Burns

Surgery

Distributive, Vasogenic, or Low Resistance Shock (marked vasodilation)

Fainting

Anaphylaxis (severe allergic reaction)

Cardiogenic Shock (inadequate cardiac output)

Myocardial infarction

Heart failure

Arrhythmia

Obstructive Shock (obstruction of blood flow)

Large vessel embolism

---

creased blood volume; excessive dilation of blood vessels, with less blood reaching the heart and lungs; malfunctioning of the heart, or obstruction of blood flow in the lungs or heart. Table 8.5 lists the types of circulatory shock, with examples of conditions.

The compensatory mechanisms in hemorrhagic and anaphylactic shock are discussed. The reduction in blood volume by bleeding reduces the venous return and cardiac output, with a resultant drop in blood pressure. This drop is detected by the baroreceptors, and there is a reflex increase in heart rate. There is profound vasoconstriction throughout the body (except in vessels of the brain and heart), and the skin appears pale and feels cool. Contraction of veins and the spleen try to increase the blood volume in the systemic circulation. The increase in breathing helps "suck" blood back to the heart. The increased secretion of vasopressin, renin, aldosterone, adrenaline, and noradrenaline try to bring the blood pressure and volume to normal levels. The thirst center is stimulated and urine production is decreased to increase blood volume by altering water intake and output.

If the vasoconstriction is prolonged, as in severe bleeding, there may be irreversible damage to the kidneys. After moderate bleeding, the plasma volume is restored within 12 to 72 hours by influx of tissue fluid. Erythropoietin levels increase, and the red cells return to normal in 4 to 8 weeks.

If bleeding is severe, the person cannot recover despite the presence of compensatory mechanisms and

is said to be in *irreversible shock*. This is when the blood flow to the brain is so reduced that the cardiac and vasomotor centers stop functioning. Injury to the heart slows and eventually stops the heart.

In anaphylactic shock, which may occur when a person with allergies is reexposed to an allergen, the antigen-antibody reaction releases large quantities of histamine, causing dilation of arterioles and increased permeability of capillaries. Fluid moves out of the circulation, reducing blood volume and pressure. The same compensatory mechanisms as found in hypovolemic shock result.

Cardiac Failure

Cardiac failure is a condition in which the heart is unable to meet the demands made by the body. It invariably happens when the heart is too weak to adequately pump the blood into the circulation. Because edema is one of the manifestations, a relatively common sign observed in various disorders, cardiac failure is considered. Depending on how severe and how fast the failure develops, a person may die, go into shock, or present with congestive cardiac failure.

To understand the signs and symptoms of congestive heart failure, **see Figure 8.16, page 477.** Consider the pulmonary and systemic circulation as roads and imagine a partial roadblock in either the left or the right ventricle. Depending on traffic, the congestion and lineup of vehicles can be as far down as the leg. In cardiac failure, the blood returning to the heart is not pumped out adequately, and the pressure builds up in the vessels leading to the heart.

Now, if the *left ventricle* is failing, pressure builds up in the left atrium, pulmonary veins, capillaries, and pulmonary arteries; in short, the pulmonary circulation. As a result of the increased hydrostatic pressure, fluid moves out of the pulmonary capillaries into the alveoli of the lung with resultant *pulmonary edema*. In this condition, the person has difficulty breathing (**dyspnea**).

Individuals with pulmonary edema feel better when sitting because the fluid tends to accumulate in the lower part of the lung due to gravity.

If the *right ventricle* fails, blood tends to backlog in the right atrium, vena cava, and circulation in various organs. The increased pressure in the right atrium is reflected by the jugular veins because no valve separates the vein from the atrium, and bulging neck veins can be observed. There is backlog in the liver, and it enlarges and presents as pain in the right upper abdomen, deep to the ribs. The buildup of pressure in the veins of the extremities (especially the legs) causes edema, which appears in the most dependent parts. In a supine position, the edema may be observed in the sacral region. If severe, fluid accumulates around the eye, and the face looks puffy. Toward the end of the day, if the person has been upright, the edema may be more in the dorsum of the foot and in the legs.

Because the heart does not pump adequately and tissue perfusion is reduced, the drop in pressure in the aortic arch and carotid artery is detected by the baroreceptors and the sympathetic nervous system is reflexively stimulated. All the regulatory mechanisms discussed come into play. Vasoconstriction and retention of water and sodium as a result of hormonal secretion occurs, worsening matters.

Heart failure treatment is directed at improving contractility of the heart, treating the symptoms, and reducing the load on the heart by eliminating the retained water with diuretics.

Effect of Aging on the Cardiovascular System

HEART

With aging, there is a general increase in collagen fibers in the heart. The size of the heart decreases with age, with some increase in the size of the left ventricle. The exact cause of these changes is difficult to determine because a large number of elderly persons have associated heart disease. The valves begin to thicken as a result of degeneration of collagen fibers and accumulation of lipids and calcium. The contraction force of the heart is decreased, reducing cardiac output and blood flow to organs. With age, blood flow to organs such as the brain and kidney are reduced as a result of changes in cardiac output and in blood vessels supplying the organs. There is a decline in maximum heart rate.

BLOOD VESSELS

The aorta thickens and becomes less elastic. There is an increase in connective tissue, with a reduction in elastic tissue in large arteries. This results in needing greater pressure to push the blood into the stiffened arteries, with a resultant rise in systolic blood pressure. The smooth muscles of the blood vessels respond less well to the sympathetic nerves and cardiovascular responses to exercise and stress, etc., are blunted. The baroreceptors are also less sensitive with age, which is one reason why elderly persons feel dizzy when they suddenly change posture (orthostatic hypotension). The basement membrane around the capillaries thickens, slowing down the exchange rate of nutrients and waste products between cells and blood.

BLOOD

Part of the bone marrow is replaced with connective tissue and fat slowing down the production of blood cells. As a result, red blood cells are reduced in number. There is a tendency for blood to clot as a result of increased platelet activity. Total blood cholesterol tends to increase together with an increase in low-density lipoproteins (LDL) and a decrease in high-density lipoproteins (HDL), making the person more susceptible to such conditions as atherosclerosis.

EFFECT OF REGULAR EXERCISE

Many studies have shown that adequate physical exercise can delay and reduce the cardiovascular changes that result from age.[1] Studies also show that the incidence of heart disease is much less in physically active individuals.[1]

Massage and the Cardiovascular System

Massage has a significant effect on the cardiovascular system.[2-19] Locally, massage produces vasodilatation in the tissue and speeds the removal of toxins that cause aches and pains.[4-8] The produced vasodilatation improves circulation and, thereby, the availability of oxygen and nutrients to the area. This has been shown to enhance recovery after intense exercise or injury.[9] In one study, in contrast to those previously cited, the massage of 10 healthy subjects failed to show any alteration in limb blood flow,[10] indicating a need for additional research.

The increase in superficial blood flow has been explained as a result of direct mechanical stimulation of superficial capillaries and arterioles, release of histamine, and axon reflex—the same physiologic effects of triple response.[11] The increased blood flow in deeper tissues, such as muscles, is a result of alternating squeezing and relaxing of muscles caused by strokes such as effleurage and petrissage.[8] These centripetal strokes squeeze veins and lymphatic vessels and force blood and lymph toward the heart, decreasing the chance for accumulation of waste and stagnation of blood.[7] Other than the strokes, the use of heat before and during massage also produces dilatation of blood vessels as a result of temperature changes.[12]

It has been shown that blood flow not only increases in the local area during massage but also reflexively in other areas.[13] For example, an increased blood flow has been measured in the limb opposite the one being massaged,[13] and massage in the neck and shoulder area has changed blood flow in the finger.[3]

It is interesting to note that, as early as 1945, massage was shown to increase blood flow in the limbs of individuals with flaccid paralysis.[14,15] This finding illustrates the potential benefit massage may have in improving the healing of ulcers, a common problem in these individuals.

It has been observed that there is a decrease in blood viscosity and a drop in hematocrit during massage as a result of hemodilution.[4,15] This may be of benefit to those individuals prone to thrombus formation. Interestingly, a study of surgery patients showed that intermittent compression and massage of the arms reduced the incidence of deep vein thrombosis, possibly by increasing the fibrinolytic activity in blood.[4] However, additional research is needed to provide evidence that massage is of benefit.

The blood levels of myoglobin and other muscle enzymes have also been shown to increase after deep massage.[16] This may confound the results in patients whose blood is being tested for these enzymes for other purposes.

The inhibitory effect of massage on the sympathetic nerves slows the heart rate and force of contraction and, thereby, the work of the heart.[7] This effect, coupled with vasodilation, produces a drop in blood pressure[3,17] and can also be of benefit to those diagnosed with hypertension.[18] In one study, massage produced a decrease in diastolic blood pressure, anxiety, and levels of cortisol (a hormone that is increased during stress).[19] However, more research is needed to document the long-term effects of massage in lowering blood pressure.

All therapists should obtain a thorough history to identify any cardiovascular condition the client may have that requires special precautions or may be contraindicated. For example, history of hypertension and antihypertensive medication should alert the therapist to possibilities of postural hypotension. History of varicose veins, if severe, has to be associated with possibilities of thrombus, emboli, and ulcers. In individuals taking anticoagulants, there may be a tendency to bleed and bruise easily.

Other than taking a good history, the therapist must observe the surface of the skin for changes in color or pigmentation. Presence of unusually dilated veins, jaundice, edema, cyanosis, pallor, bruises, and bleeding under the skin are just a few that can give the therapist an indication of cardiovascular system activity. It is vital for the therapist to gather sufficient information about any cardiovascular disease that a client has and plan a strategy for management before treatment sessions.

The therapist should be aware of the signs, symptoms, and complications of common cardiovascular diseases in the elderly. Many elderly individuals may be on drugs to treat or prevent progress of the dis-

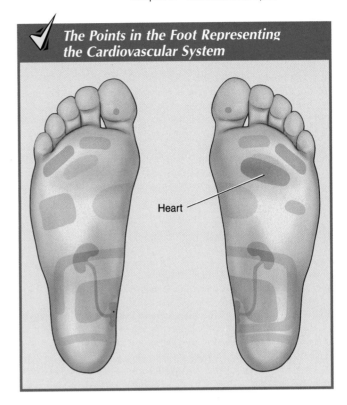

The Points in the Foot Representing the Cardiovascular System

Heart

ease, and the adverse effect of these drugs may have a bearing on therapy.

REFERENCES

1. McArdle WD, Katch FI, Katch VL. Exercise Physiology: Energy, Nutrition, and Human Performance. 5th Ed. Baltimore, Maryland: Lippincott Williams & Wilkins, 2001.
2. Rich GJ (ed). Massage Therapy—The Evidence for Practice. New York: Harcourt Publishers, 2002.
3. Mein EA, Richards DG, McMillin DL, McPartland JM. Physiological regulation through manual therapy. Physical Medicine/Rehabilitation: A state-of-the-art review Phys Med Rehab Clin of N Amer. 2000;14(1):27–42.
4. Knight MTN, Dawson R. Effect of intermittent compression of the arms on deep venous thrombosis in the legs. Lancet 1976;Dec 11, 1265–1267.
5. McCaffery M, Wolff M. Pain relief using cutaneous modalities, positioning, and movement. Hospice J 1992;8(1-2):121–153.
6. Bray R. Massage: Exploring the benefits. Elderly Care 1999 Jul;11(5):15–16.
7. Ernst E, Matrai A, Magyarosy I, et al. Massage cause changes in blood fluidity. Physiotherapy 1987;73:43–45.
8. Hovind, H, Nielsen SL. Effect of massage on blood flow in skeletal muscle. Scan J Rehabil Med 1974;6:74–77.
9. Ylinen J, Cash M. Sports Massage. London: Stanley Paul, 1988.
10. Shoemaker JK, Tidus PM, Mader R. Failure of manual massage to alter limb blood flow: Measures by Doppler ultrasound. Med Sci Sports Exerc 1997;1:610–614.
11. Jacobs M. Massage for the relief of pain: Anatomical and physiological considerations. Phys Ther Rev 1960;40(1):93–98.
12. Thomas S. Massage for common ailments. Stroud, Glos: London: Gaia Books, 1998.
13. Severini V, Venerando A. The physiological effects of massage in the cardiovascular system. Eur Medicophysica 1967;3(165):183.

14. Barr JS, Taslitz N. The influence of back massage on autonomic functions. Phys Ther 1970;50:1679–1691
15. Wakim KG, Martin GM, Terrier JC, et al. The effects of massage on the circulation in normal and paralysed extremities. Arch Phys Med 1949;30(March):135–144.
16. Bork K, Korting GW, Faust G. Serum enzyme levels after whole body massage. Arch Dermatol Forsch 1971;240:342–348.
17. Ashton J. In your hands. Nurs Times 1984;80(19):54.
18. Zang F. An introduction to keeping-fit massage (1). J Trad Chin Med 1993;13(2):120–123.
19. Hernandez-Reif M, Field T, Krasnegor J, Theakston H, Hossain Z, Burman I. High blood pressure and associated symptoms were reduced by massage therapy. J Bodywork Movement Ther 2000;4:31–38.

SUGGESTED READINGS

Ganong W. Review of Medical Physiology. 21st Ed. California: Appleton & Lange Medical, 2003.
Andrade CK, Clifford P. Outcome-Based Massage. Baltimore: Lippincott Williams & Wilkins, 2001.
Arkko PJ, Pakarinen AJ, Kari-Koskinen O. Effects of whole body massage on serum protein, electrolyte and hormone concentrations, enzyme activities and hematological parameters. Int J Sports Med 1983;4:265–267.
Ching M. The use of touch in nursing practice. Aust J Adv Nurs 1993;10(4):4–9.
Corbett M. The use and abuse of massage and exercise. Practitioner 1972;208:136–139.
Redick DS. Should patients with acute myocardial infarctions receive back massage? Focus Crit Care 1986;13(3):42–46.
Nawroth A. Massage—the anthroposophic approach. J Anthroposophic Med 1995;12(2):43–49.
Sabri S, Roberts VC, Cotton LT. Prevention of early deep vein thrombosis by intermittent compression of the leg during surgery. Br Med J 1971;4(394).
Ylinen J, Cash M. Sports Massage. London: Stanley Paul, 1988.

Review Questions

Multiple Choice
Choose the best answer to the following questions:

1. The blood volume in a young adult is
   A. 1.5–3 liters.
   B. 4–6 liters.
   C. 7–8 liters.
   D. 8–10 liters.

2. The normal blood pH range is
   A. 6.8–7.0.
   B. 7.0–7.1.
   C. 7.35–7.45.
   D. 7.55–7.65.

3. All of the following hormones regulate blood pressure EXCEPT
   A. antidiuretic hormone.
   B. angiotensin II.
   C. adrenaline.
   D. thyroxine.

4. Which of the following plasma substances most contributes to blood osmotic pressure?
   A. Water
   B. Plasma proteins
   C. Glucose
   D. Hormones and enzymes

5. Which of the formed elements actively participate in blood clotting?
   A. Platelets
   B. Erythrocytes
   C. Neutrophils
   D. Eosinophils

6. The hormone that increases production of red blood cells is
   A. adrenaline.
   B. erythropoietin.
   C. angiotensin.
   D. atrial natriuretic peptide.

7. A person who is blood group O+ has the following antibodies EXCEPT
   A. B antibodies.
   B. A antibodies.
   C. Rh antibodies.
   D. A and B antibodies

8. Which white blood cells constitute the largest percentage in a healthy individual?
   A. Neutrophils
   B. Basophils
   C. Eosinophils
   D. Lymphocytes

9. Which white blood cells are involved in allergic reactions and parasitic infestations?
   A. Neutrophils
   B. Monocytes
   C. Eosinophils
   D. Lymphocytes

10. Platelets are formed in the
    A. spleen.
    B. tonsils.
    C. bone marrow.
    D. lymph nodes.

11. All of the following are examples of anticoagulants EXCEPT
    A. heparin.
    B. warfarin.
    C. streptokinase.
    D. vitamin K.

12. A person with a high hemoglobin level is said to have
    A. anemia.
    B. hemophilia.
    C. thrombus.
    D. polycythemia.

13. In a healthy adult, the approximate volume of blood pumped out by the heart in 1 minute is
    A. 80 mL.
    B. 250 mL.
    C. 2 L.
    D. 5 L.

14. The blood vessel(s) that carries oxygenated blood from the lungs to the left atrium is the
    A. pulmonary artery.
    B. pulmonary vein.
    C. vena cava.
    D. aorta.

15. The valve that prevents backflow of blood into the right atrium is the
    A. pulmonary valve.
    B. mitral valve.
    C. aortic valve.
    D. tricuspid valve.

16. In the ECG, ventricular depolarization is denoted by the
    A. P wave.
    B. QRS complex.
    C. T wave.
    D. PR interval.

17. The cardiac centers are located in the
    A. spinal cord.
    B. medulla oblongata.
    C. hypothalamus.
    D. cerebral cortex.

18. The first branches of the aorta are the
    A. brachiocephalic arteries.
    B. common carotid arteries.
    C. coronary arteries.
    D. subclavian arteries.

19. In a healthy adult, the blood pressure measured in the left ventricle during ventricular contraction will be about
    A. 120 mm Hg.
    B. 60 mm Hg.
    C. 20 mm Hg.
    D. 0 mm Hg.

20. The pressure wave that expands the walls of the arteries is felt as the
    A. first heart sound.
    B. pulse.
    C. apex beat.
    D. murmur.

21. Cardiac output is increased by all of the following conditions EXCEPT
    A. low body temperature.
    B. exercise.
    C. anxiety.
    D. pregnancy.

22. The vessels responsible for most of the resistance that opposes blood flow in the circulation are the
    A. elastic arteries.
    B. arterioles.
    C. capillaries.
    D. veins.

23. The vessels where exchange of nutrients occur are the
    A. elastic arteries.
    B. arterioles.
    C. capillaries.
    D. veins.

Fill-In
Complete the following:

1. Old red blood cells are destroyed by macrophages in the organs _____ , _____ and bone marrow.

2. The globin part of hemoglobin is converted into _____ and recycled.

3. The heme part is broken into the metal _____ and a pigment _____ . Excess production of this pigment is responsible for the condition _____.

4. The heart is wedged between the two lungs in the _____ of the thorax.

5. The _____ is a serous membrane that surrounds the heart.

6. In cardiac muscle, the _____ help convey the force of contraction and impulses from one cell to another.

7. Cardiac output is equal to _____ × heart rate.

8. The first heart sound is a result of the closure of the _____ valves.

9. Physical conditioning causes a(n) _____ (increase, decrease) in heart rate. The maximal cardiac output is _____ (increased, decreased). The capillary network in the skeletal muscles is _____ (increased, decreased) and the blood pressure may be _____ (increased, decreased).

10. The hormone _____ increases the heart rate and force of contraction.

11. The _____ and _____ are blood vessels that transport blood. Exchange can only take place in _____ .

12. The type of blood vessels with the highest percentage of smooth muscle in their wall and greatest resistance to blood flow are _____ .

13. Three hormones that produce vasoconstriction are _____ , _____ , and _____ .

14. The major veins that drain into the right atrium are the _____ and _____ .

True–False

(Answer the following questions T, for true; or F, for false.)

1. Coagulation is an antigen-antibody process.

2. For clotting to occur, many factors found in the platelets, plasma, or other tissue fluids are required.

3. Type B blood group individuals have antibodies against B antigens in the plasma.

4. A person who is of Rh+ group has the Rh antigen on the red blood cells.

5. Under normal circumstances, the plasma of a person who is Rh- has antibodies against Rh antigen.

6. The conducting system of the heart includes the sinoatrial node, atrioventricular node, and the Purkinje fibers.

7. The ECG is a recording of the muscle contractions of the heart.

8. The pressure in the right ventricle is more than that in the left ventricle.

9. The apex beat is a result of the closure of the atrioventricular valves.

10. Stimulation of the sympathetic nerves causes an increase in force of ventricular contraction.

11. If the heart is removed from the body and coronary circulation is maintained together with the temperature, oxygen, and nutrients required, it is possible for the heart to continue beating.

12. The sympathetic nerves to the heart, if stimulated, slow the heart rate and force of contraction.

13. The apex beat is the sound heard during ventricular contraction.

14. The stroke volume is the volume of blood pumped out of the heart per minute.

15. The pulse is produced by the closure of the aortic and pulmonary artery.

16. Systolic pressure is the pressure measured during ventricular contraction.

Matching

Match the following (write a, b, c, d, e, or f next to descriptions 1–6):

1. ____ A pigment derived from red blood cells
2. ____ Agglutination
3. ____ Coagulation
4. ____ A type of antigen on the surface of red blood cells
5. ____ Another term for platelets
6. ____ Formation of blood clot in the walls of blood vessels

a. thrombosis
b. Rh factor
c. clumping of red blood cells
d. bilirubin
e. a process where fibrinogen gets converted to fibrin
f. thrombocytes

Match the following (write a, b, c, or d next to descriptions 1–4):

1. ____ Valve between aorta and left ventricle
2. ____ Valve between pulmonary trunk and right ventricle
3. ____ Valve between the right atrium and right ventricle
4. ____ Valve between the left atrium and left ventricle

a. mitral valve
b. aortic valve
c. tricuspid valve
d. pulmonary valve

Short-Answer Questions

1. What are the functions of plasma proteins?

2. If a client has jaundice, what are the possible causes of bilirubin increase?

3. How does the neutrophil participate in the immune process?

4. What are the possible reasons for excessive, prolonged bleeding in an individual?

5. Why is it important to monitor an Rh-positive fetus in an Rh-negative mother? What is the role of the immune system in this case?

6. Where is the apex beat located? Locate the apex beat on your colleague with the palm of your hand.

7. What is the approximate location of the heart on the anterior chest wall?

8. As if you were a red blood cell and had just entered the right atrium, trace your route to reach the left atrium.

9. If you, the red cell, now had to return to the right atrium, what route would you take to reach the left atrium in a hurry? If you had all the time in the world and wanted to take the longest route, how would you go? (Of course, the red blood cells have no choice, such as you are being given).

10. If you had varicose veins in the leg and the long saphenous vein was affected, where would you find the enlarged vein? Trace it on the surface of your (or your colleagues') leg.

11. Locate and palpate the following arteries on yourself: common carotid, femoral, brachial, radial, popliteal, and dorsalis pedis.

12. What are the changes produced in the cardiovascular system when a person gets up from lying down? How do these changes occur?

13. What is the effect on the blood pressure when a person does isometric exercises? How is this effect different when isotonic exercises are performed?

14. What are the effects of training on the circulation in skeletal muscle?

Case Studies

1. Mr. Mathison has lived with a diagnosis of hypertension for more than 4 years. Initially, he was advised to exercise and watch his diet. Because his blood pressure continued to be high, his physician prescribed certain drugs. Mr. Mathison had been a client of Mary (the massage therapist) for more than one year.

   One day, Mary had just finished the massage and left the room; Mr. Mathison was dressing. Mary's heart almost stopped when she heard the loud crash and thud of a falling body. She found Mr. Mathison lying on the floor with a small gash on his forehead, caused by the table edge as he fell. Before Mary could react, Mr. Mathison sat up sheepishly and said, "You know, these dizzy spells have been coming on and off ever since I started the drugs. Don't worry, it is definitely not due to your treatment."

   But Mr. Mathison's statement did not dispel the thoughts that circled in Mary's head. "Could massage have precipitated this? What is hypertension anyway? How do drugs reduce high blood pressure? Could I have done anything to prevent this from happening in the clinic?"
   A. What is the normal range of blood pressure?
   B. What is hypertension?
   C. What is meant by orthostatic hypertension?
   D. How is blood pressure regulated in the body?

2. The town where this massage therapist had a clinic consisted largely of elderly people. Almost all of the clients that she saw had some health problem. There was Mr. Mathison, who had startled her the other day by falling unconscious. Mr. Snyder, the 65-year-old farmer, although active all his life experienced a mild heart attack last month. Mrs. Rose, poor lady, had been suffering from varicose veins for more than 8 years.
   A. What cardiovascular changes occur with aging?
   B. What are varicose veins? What vein is commonly affected?
   C. What is edema?
   D. Identify the precautions to be taken when treating an elderly client.

3. Mrs. Carman was the wife of one of the wealthiest businessmen in the town. This was her first visit, and Robert, who had opened the clinic only a month ago, was a little nervous. To Robert's dismay, when Mrs. Carman removed her clothes and wrapped herself in a towel, he saw what looked like bruises all over her back. The first thought that crossed his mind was that Mrs. Carman was a victim of spousal abuse. But on questioning Mrs. Carman, Robert found out that Mrs. Carman bruised easily and that it was a family tendency. What could it be? Was it safe to massage Mrs. Carman? Was Mrs. Carman telling the truth? Should she talk to her family physician? What a dilemma!
   A. What is your advice to Robert?
   B. How does blood clot?
   C. What are the factors that cause excessive bleeding?

4. The folks in the town called Mrs. Bloomsberry "Mrs. Paleberry" behind her back. Mrs. Bloomsberry (what an extraordinary name!) was the palest individual the therapist had ever seen. During every visit, Mrs. Bloomsberry explained that her pallor was a result of pernicious anemia and that she was being treated.
   A. What is the normal red blood cell count?
   B. Where are red blood cells manufactured?
   C. What is anemia?
   D. What are the causes of anemia?
   E. What is pernicious anemia?
   F. How is pernicious anemia responsible for skin color change if it has something to do with blood?
   G. Is massage safe in this case?

5. The first infant massage a massage therapist performed was a nerve-racking experience. The infant's (just a few months old) skin had a yel-

lowish tinge. The therapist knew that indicated jaundice. But jaundice was a symptom of hepatitis, wasn't it? Isn't hepatitis infectious? Are there other causes of jaundice? For a start, what actually is jaundice? The therapist had washed his hands carefully before and after the massage. Perhaps the child did not have hepatitis after all, as there was no history of fever.
A. What would/should a therapist do in this situation?
B. Can you provide answers to the therapist's questions?

6. A colleague had referred a client to Maria. Her colleague knew that this client had been diagnosed as HIV-positive. During discussion sessions in their massage therapy school, Maria had argued vehemently that she would massage a client diagnosed with AIDS with no qualms. Now she was going to put her words into action. Maria was equipped with the knowledge required. For example, she knew what AIDS was, how it spread, and the precautions she needed to take. She also knew what AIDS could do to the immune system. Now she had the task of overcoming her psychological barriers.
A. How does the body defend itself from infections?
B. What should/would you do in Maria's situation?
C. What precautions could be taken by a therapist to prevent spread of infection?

Answers to Review Questions

Multiple Choice

1. b	2. c	3. d	4. b	5. a	6. b
7. c	8. a	9. c	10. c	11. d	12. d
13. d	14. b	15. d	16. b	17. b	18. c
19. a	20. b	21. a	22. b	23. c	

Fill-In

1. spleen, liver
2. amino acid
3. iron, bilirubin, jaundice
4. mediastinum
5. pericardium
6. intercalated disks
7. stroke volume
8. atrioventricular valves
9. decrease in heart rate, increased cardiac output, increased capillary network in skeletal muscles, blood pressure is decreased
10. adrenaline
11. arteries and veins, capillaries
12. arterioles
13. adrenaline, angiotensin II, vasopressin
14. inferior vena cava and superior vena cava

True–False

1. False. Clumping or agglutination is an antigen-antibody process
2. True
3. False. Type B will have antibodies against A antigen
4. True
5. False. Antibodies will be present only if the person has been previously exposed to the Rh antigen.
6. True
7. False. It is the electrical changes that are recorded
8. False. Because blood drains into the right atrium via the veins (with low pressure), and the resistance to outflow through the pulmonary trunk is very low, the pressure in the right ventricle is low
9. False. It is a result of the contact of the apex of the heart against the chest wall when the ventricle contracts
10. True
11. True
12. False. It does the opposite
13. False. It is a result of the contact of the apex of the heart against the chest wall when the ventricle contracts
14. False. The definition is for cardiac output. Stroke volume is the volume of blood pumped out with every ventricular contraction
15. False. The pulse is a pressure wave
16. True

Matching

1. 1–d
   2–c
   3–e
   4–b
   5–f
   6–a
2. 1–b
   2–d
   3–c
   4–a

Short-Answer Questions

1. Plasma proteins maintain the pH of the blood. Certain proteins are antibodies that recognize specific antigens; certain proteins are clotting factors; certain proteins are transport carriers

for hormones, metals, amino acids, fatty acids, enzymes, and drugs. They are important for keeping water inside blood vessels and maintaining blood volume by exerting osmotic force.

2. Abnormal red blood cells in blood; Rapid breakdown of red blood cells by spleen, liver, and bone marrow; liver problems; obstruction of bile duct.

3. Neutrophils seek out bacteria and other foreign tissue, phagocytize, kill, and digest the organisms. The toxic enzymes present in the cytoplasmic granules help kill the organism. The neutrophils can enter tissue spaces by diapedesis and aggregate in areas with infection. They are attracted to infection sites by chemicals secreted by other neutrophils and injured cells.

4. Connective tissue disorders that result in weak blood vessel wall; deficiency of platelets; lack of any factors required for clotting, e.g., lack of factor VIII (hemophilia); abnormal functioning of the fibrinolytic system that breaks up clots; anticoagulant medications.

5. It is important to monitor the Rh-positive fetus in an Rh-negative mother because the mother can develop antibodies against the Rh-positive antigen present in the fetus if she is exposed to the antigen. The antigen-antibody reaction that results can cause clumping and destruction of fetal red blood cells. Anemia, jaundice, low birth weight, and death (erythroblastosis fetalis) are some complications.

6. The apex beat can be located in the fifth left intercostal space, a little medial to the midclavicular line. If the heart is enlarged, the apex beat would be shifted.

7. The right border would extend from the third costal cartilage to the sixth costal cartilage about 1 cm from the right margin of the sternum; the lower border would extend across the xiphisternal junction to the fifth left intercostal space, just medial to the midclavicular line; the left border would extend from the apex beat to the second intercostal space, 1 cm away from the left margin of the sternum; and the upper border would extend along a line joining the upper point of the right and left borders.

8. right atrium—right ventricle—pulmonary trunk—pulmonary arteries (to lungs) —arterioles—capillaries—venules—pulmonary veins—left atrium

9. left atrium—left ventricle—aorta—coronary arteries—arterioles—capillaries—veins—coronary sinus—right atrium; left atrium—left ventricle—aorta—common iliac artery—external iliac artery—femoral artery—to capillaries in toes—venules—femoral vein—external iliac vein—common iliac vein—inferior vena cava—right atrium

10. The great saphenous vein ascends along the medial aspect of the leg and thigh and drains into the femoral vein near the inguinal region.

11. Common carotid—on either side of the trachea in the neck; femoral—in the midinguinal point; brachial—anterior aspect of the elbow, just medial to the biceps tendon; radial—lateral aspect of the anterior surface of the wrist; popliteal—back of the knee in the middle of the popliteal fossa; dorsalis pedis—middle of the dorsum of the foot between the tendons of the extensor digitorum longus and extensor hallucis longus.

12. When a person is lying down, the effect of gravity is removed. On getting up, the effect of gravity blood tends to pool in the leg. The blood pressure drops and blood supply to the brain is reduced. The major compensation is initiated by stimulation of the baroreceptors, with a resultant immediate increase in heart rate, stroke volume, and cardiac output. There is generalized vasoconstriction via the sympathetic nerves. In addition, there is an increase in levels of renin, aldosterone, etc., producing vasoconstriction and increased blood pressure.

13. Both diastolic and systolic pressure increase as contracting muscles compress blood vessels.

14. Training increases the capillary network in the trained muscle. The total blood flow to the trained muscle increases with training.

Case Studies

1. **A.** The normal range is 90–120 mm Hg systolic pressure and 60–90 mm Hg diastolic pressure.

   B. Hypertension is a persistent increase in blood pressure above the normal range.

   C. Orthostatic hypotension is the drop in blood pressure on changing posture.

   D. The blood pressure is regulated by local (autoregulation), neural (innervation of the blood vessels and heart); vasomotor center (baroreceptors); and endocrine mechanisms (hormones, such as adrenaline, noradrenaline; vasopressin; angiotensin II; and atrial natriuretic peptide).

   What Mr. Mathison exhibited is probably orthostatic hypotension. The drugs given for hypertension reduce sympathetic activity or inhibit the hormones that produce vasoconstriction. Because massage reduces sympathetic activity, it could make the situation worse, as Mr. Mathison was on antihypertensives. Mary could have avoided the situation by taking a good history. She would have been aware of his dizzy spells and realized the possible cause. She could have cautioned the client to get up slowly and sit on the table for some time, allowing for compensatory mechanisms to adjust the pressure before standing.

2. **A.** In the heart, there is a general increase in collagen fibers; the size of the heart decreases with some increase in the size of the left ventricle; a large number of elderly persons have associated heart disease; the valves begin to thicken as a result of collagen fiber degeneration and lipid and calcium accumulation; the force of heart contraction is decreased, reducing the cardiac output and blood flow to organs. Blood flow to organs such as the brain and kidney is reduced as a result of cardiac output changes and in blood vessels supplying the organs. The maximum heart rate declines. In the blood vessels, the aorta thickens and becomes less elastic; there is an increase in connective tissue, with a reduction in elastic tissue in large arteries, resulting in greater pressure needed to push the blood into the stiffened arteries and a rise in systolic blood pressure; the smooth muscles of the blood vessels respond less well to the sympathetic nerves, and cardiovascular responses to exercise, stress, etc., are blunted. The baroreceptors are also less sensitive with age, which is a reason why elderly persons may feel dizzy when they suddenly change posture (orthostatic hypotension). The basement membrane around the capillaries thickens, slowing down the exchange rate of nutrients and waste products between cells and blood. Part of the bone marrow is replaced with connective tissue and fat, slowing down blood cells production. As a result, red blood cells are reduced in number. There is a tendency for blood to clot as a result of increased platelet activity. Total blood cholesterol tends to increase together with an increase in low-density lipoproteins (LDL) and a decrease in high-density lipoproteins (HDL), making a person more susceptible to conditions such as atherosclerosis.

B. Varicose veins are abnormally dilated and tortuous veins. The long saphenous vein is commonly affected.

C. Edema is abnormal increase in fluid in the interstitial compartment. It is a complication of varicose veins.

D. Some precautions to be taken when treating an elderly client are: Take a good history to determine if the person has cardiovascular

diseases; observe surface of skin for changes in color or pigmentation (e.g., cyanosis, jaundice, edema, dilated veins, bruises, and bleeding under the skin) Take suitable precautions as the elderly are prone to orthostatic hypotension.

3. **A.** It is important for a massage therapist to learn the details of bleeding tendencies. This will help learn the severity of the problem. It would be advisable for the therapist to talk to the client's physician before proceeding with massage. In severe cases, even mild pressure can cause bleeding under the skin. Robert was right to think about spousal abuse as it could cause bruising.

B. The fundamental reaction in the clotting process is the conversion of fibrinogen to fibrin. For this conversion, many clotting factors, such as calcium and prothrombin, are required. Vitamin K is also required. Platelets are important in the clotting process.

C. See answer to Short-Answer question no. 4. for factors that cause excessive bleeding.

4. **A.** The normal red blood cell count is approximately 5 million cells/cubic millimeter of blood.

B. The formation site of red blood cells varies from age to age. In the fetus, the cells are formed in the liver and spleen. In children, the cells are formed in the marrow cavities of all bones. By age 20, the blood cells are manufactured in the upper end of the humerus and femur and in flat bones such as the sternum, pelvis, and vertebra.

C. Anemia is a condition in which there is a reduction of red blood cells and/or hemoglobin content.

D. There are many causes of anemia. Conditions that result in an increased destruction rate of red blood cells and a decreased production rate and blood loss all cause anemia.

E. Pernicious anemia is a condition in which there is a reduction of intrinsic factor, a factor (secreted by the stomach and required for absorption of vitamin B_{12}). Vitamin B_{12} is needed for the manufacture of red cells.

F. Oxygenated hemoglobin is responsible for the red color of blood. The skin appears pale if there is reduced amount of hemoglobin in the blood.

G. It is safe to massage this individual. Severe anemia can lead to cardiac failure and the therapist should ensure that such complications do not exist in the client.

5. **A.** and **B.** Jaundice is a result of increased levels of bilirubin. Jaundice could be a result of in-

creased destruction of red blood cells, liver problems, or obstruction to the bile duct. Hepatitis refers to inflammation of the liver. The most common cause of hepatitis is viral hepatitis, an infectious condition. Mild jaundice in an infant could be a result of the immature liver unable to cope with the red blood cells destruction that occurs as fetal hemoglobin is replaced by adult hemoglobin. Jaundice in an infant could also be a result of Rh incompatibility or congenital deformities of the liver or bile duct. It is important for the therapist to get clearance from a pediatrician, especially if the jaundice is severe.

6. **A.** The body possesses natural barriers (**see page 520**) that prevent easy entry of microorganisms. The white blood cells provide the body with powerful defenses against infection. AIDS affects the functioning of the lymphocytes.

   B. It is important for Maria to learn if the client has any AIDS complications, such as super-infections or tumors. She has to decide if she is comfortable treating this client because psychological barriers can have a bearing on the therapy. Immunity is suppressed in AIDS. Maria should ensure that she does not have infections when she treats the client.

   C. There are many precautions that can be taken by a therapist to prevent spread of infection: washing hands before and after treating any client; ensuring that no contact is made with bodily secretions; cleaning the table with disinfectants; laundering linen appropriately; clearing policies for treating clients with different infections.

Coloring Exercise

The internal structures of the heart (anterior view). Color the chambers and blood vessels that contain oxygenated blood red. Color the chambers and blood vessels that contain deoxygenated blood blue. Identify the structure indicated by the label lines. Color all valves green.

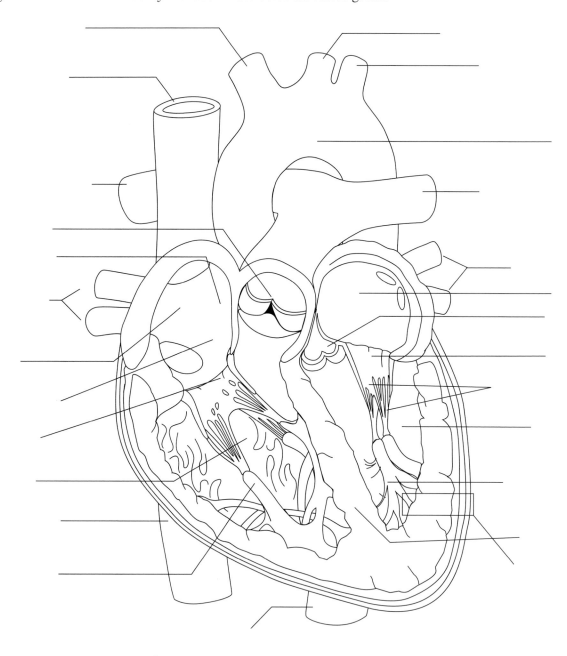

Cardiac cycle. On the diagram, shade the column that identifies ventricular systole pink, atrial systole blue, ventricular diastole purple. On the ECG tracing, label the different waves and name the activity that occurs during the period (e.g., ventricular depolarization, ventricular repolarization, atrial depolarization). The label lines indicate the opening/closing of the various valves. Write the name of the valve beside the label and whether it opens/closes at that time.

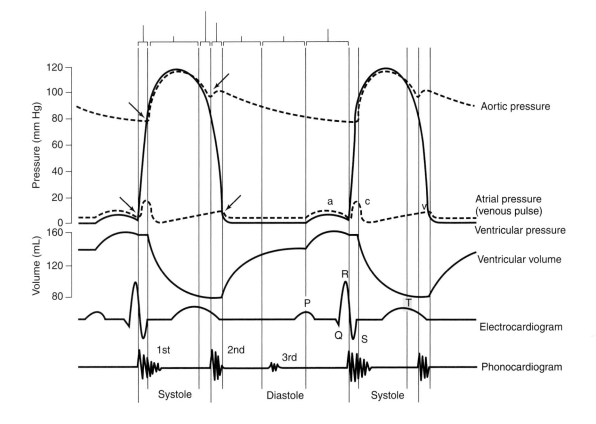

Forces that affect movement of fluid across capillaries. In the diagram, draw arrows indicating the direction of movement of fluid for each of the labeled forces in the arterial and venous end of the capillaries. Color the arterial end of capillary red and its venous end blue.

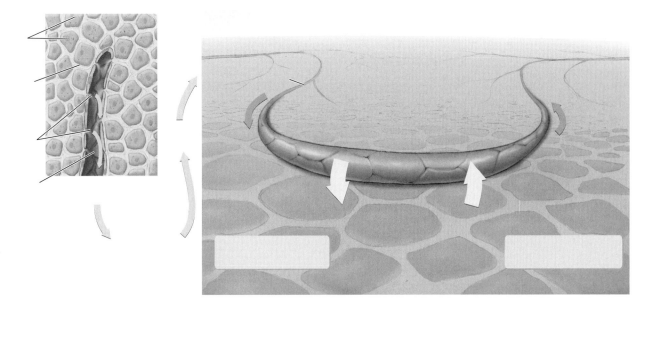

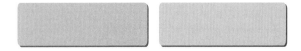

Major systemic arteries. Label the major arteries indicated by leader lines.

Major systemic veins. Label the major veins indicated by leader lines.

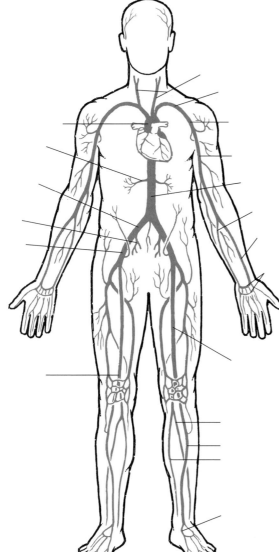

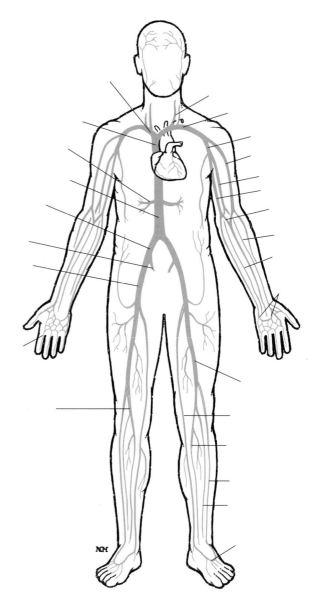

CHAPTER 9

Lymphatic System

Objectives

Lymphatic System

On completion of this chapter, the reader should be able to:

- Identify the fluid compartments of the body and the volume of fluid in each compartment.
- Describe the role of different factors that affect the movement of fluid between the fluid compartments.
- Define edema.
- Describe the formation and flow of lymph.
- Describe the factors that affect the rate of lymph production and removal.
- Identify the structures that belong to the lymphatic system.
- List the functions of the lymphatic system.
- Describe the direction of lymph movement in different parts of the body.
- Describe the structure of a lymph node.
- Identify the major groups of lymph nodes and the regions they drain.
- Describe the effects of massage on the lymphatic system.
- Describe the specific techniques that are effective in reducing edema.

Immunity

- Define immunity.
- Differentiate between specific and nonspecific immunity.
- Differentiate between active and passive immunity.
- Define innate, humoral, and cellular immunity.
- Describe the role of lymphocytes in immunity.
- Identify the locations where lymphocytes are manufactured.
- Define antigen and antibody.
- Describe how antibodies work.
- Explain the basis of immunization.
- List the diseases against which immunization is available.
- Explain how the disease AIDS affects immunity.
- Define the term autoimmune disease.
- List examples of autoimmune diseases.
- Define allergy.
- Explain the mechanism of allergy.
- Define anaphylaxis and describe how it occurs.
- Describe the changes that occur in the lymphatic system and immunity with aging.
- Describe the effects of massage on immunity.

(continued)

- List the general causes of disease.
- Describe the different routes through which infection can spread.
- Describe the strategies that the therapist can use to prevent self-infection and infection of others in the clinic.

*W*ater, *waste products, and nutrients in the body are constantly exchanged between the cells and the fluid around them. Some of this fluid flows in and out of blood vessels and the rest is found around the cells. The lymphatic system helps remove larger particles and drain the excess fluid that accumulates around the cells back into the circulatory system. At the same time, defense cells located in the lymphatic system screen the fluid and defend the body by removing foreign agents.*

In this chapter, the fluid compartments of the body, factors that maintain fluid volume in each compartment, and the physiologic basis of edema are considered. The components of the lymphatic system, its role in the maintenance of immunity, and the mechanism of immunity are also addressed.

Body Fluid Compartments

Did you know that an adult body contains approximately 40 liters (84.5 pt) of water? Visualize the volume of 40 1-liter milk containers in the dairy section of your grocery store. About 25 liters (52.8 pt) of this fluid is found inside the cells—**intracellular fluid** (see Figure 9.1). The remaining 15 liters (31.7 pt) is

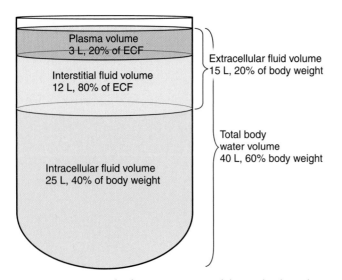

FIGURE 9.1. Major Fluid Compartments of the Body (the values are approximate for a 70 Kg man)

found outside the cells—**extracellular fluid.** Of the extracellular fluid, about 12 liters (25.4 pt) are located between the cells (**interstitial fluid)** and 3 liters (6.3 pt) are located inside blood vessels as **plasma** or **intravascular fluid** (remember that the blood volume of about 5 liters (10.6 pt) is made up of this fluid, together with the blood cells).

The fluid in the blood and the interstitial region is continuously being mixed as it diffuses in and out of the blood capillaries. Therefore, the waste products of the cells, which have diffused out into the space between the cells (**interstitial space**), enter the blood and are transported to the excretory organs, while the nutrients required by the cells enter the interstitial space from the blood by diffusion.

Despite the rapid mixing of extracellular fluid, the volume of fluid in the plasma and the interstitial region remains constant. The various physical forces that cause movement through the pores in the capillaries maintain this constancy.

PHYSICAL FORCES THAT CAUSE MOVEMENT OF FLUID BETWEEN COMPARTMENTS

One force that tends to push fluid out of the capillaries is **capillary hydrostatic pressure** (see Figure 8.20). In the body, this pressure is equal to about 17 mm Hg. If you can imagine a nick in your garden hose, 17 mm Hg is equivalent to the pressure that forces the water out through the nick. If you increase the flow of water through the garden hose by opening the tap, more water will leak out of the nick. Similarly, any factor that causes an increase in the pressure inside capillaries will increase the volume of water moving out of the capillaries. For example, if there is more blood flowing through the capillaries as a result of artery dilatation, or if more pressure builds in the capillaries because blood flow into the vein is impeded, more fluids will move out of the capillaries.

Another force that affects fluid movement between the fluid compartments is **interstitial colloid osmotic pressure,** caused by the proteins in the interstitial fluid. These proteins draw water from the capillaries toward the interstitial compartment by osmosis, causing a pressure equal to about 5 mm Hg (If necessary, review the section on membrane transport mechanisms **in Chapter 1, page 28** that discusses osmosis, diffusion,

> ***Pitting Edema***
>
> This term describes severe edema in which "pits" are formed when pressure is applied to the skin with the fingertips.

etc.). If more protein leaks into the interstitial compartment from the capillaries or from the cells, more water is drawn from the capillaries by osmosis. This situation occurs when an area of the body is inflamed. During inflammation, the capillaries dilate and protein leaks out of the capillaries, drawing water along with them. This is one mechanism that produces swelling.

The interstitial compartment has a *negative* **hydrostatic pressure** equal to −6 mm Hg, about the same as the suction force around your garden hose. This force, if exerting its effect alone, will tend to suck the fluid out of the capillaries. However, if this force is positive, the fluid tends to move from the interstitial compartment to the inside of capillaries.

The plasma protein inside the capillaries is another force that plays a part in fluid movement. These proteins, similar to the interstitial fluid protein, draw fluid into the compartment in which they are located; in this case, the plasma. This force is called **plasma colloid osmotic pressure** and is approximately 26 mm Hg. In conditions such as severe malnutrition in which plasma protein is decreased, less fluid is drawn into the blood vessels and more moves into the interstitial compartment, producing swelling. This swelling, caused by fluid accumulation in the interstitial compartment, is known as **edema.** The movement of fluid out of the capillaries also depends on the **permeability of capillaries.**

Normally, the excess fluid and protein that accumulates in the interstitial fluid compartment is removed by the **lymphatic system.** The activity of the lymphatic system determines the volume of fluid present. Edema results if lymph drainage from a region is reduced.

Therefore, there are various forces acting in different directions simultaneously, and the direction in which the fluid moves into or out of the capillaries depends on which net force predominates.

Can you now determine which of the above forces draws fluid out of the capillaries and which draws fluid into the capillaries?

EDEMA

When the net force pushing fluid out of the capillaries predominates, fluid tends to accumulate in the interstitial fluid compartment. Edema caused by low output of the lymphatic system, with resultant high levels of protein in the interstitial fluid is called **lymphedema.** The physiologic factors that result in edema are listed in Table 9.1. Try to think of conditions that may present with edema as a result of one or more of these physiologic causes.

The Lymphatic System

In general, the fluid moving out of the capillaries exceeds that entering it from the interstitial fluid compartment. Also, large protein particles tend to accumulate in this compartment. These proteins may be particles that have leaked from the blood into the in-

> ***Terms Associated With Edema***
>
> **Anasarca**—generalized edema
> **Angioneurotic edema,** or **angioedema**—localized edema of subcutaneous or mucosal regions, usually a result of allergic reactions to food or drugs
> **Ascites**—excessive fluid in the peritoneal cavity
> **Cardiac edema**—edema resulting from congestive cardiac failure
> **Cerebral edema**—swelling of the brain tissue
> **Dependent edema**—edema that occurs only in those regions exposed to the effect of gravity (e.g., edema of the lower limb on prolonged standing and edema in the sacral region in the supine position)
> **Effusion**—excessive fluid in a cavity (e.g., in the joint capsule, pleural cavity [pleural effusion], pericardial cavity [pericardial effusion])
> **Hydrocele**—collection of fluid in a saclike cavity (e.g., serous fluid collection in the cavity around the testis)
> **Myxedema**—nonpitting edema associated with hypothyroidism. The presence of increased mucins (proteoglycans) in the edema fluid is responsible for the nonpitting nature.
> **Nonpitting,** or **brawny edema**—swelling of subcutaneous tissue that cannot be indented easily by compression
> **Pitting edema**—edema that produces indentations when pressure is applied for a short duration
> **Pulmonary edema**—fluid in the lungs, usually resulting from obstruction to pulmonary venous outflow (e.g., left heart failure)
> **Swelling**—an abnormal enlargement of a part of the body; one cause of swelling is edema.

Table 9.1

Causes of Increased Interstitial Fluid Volume—Edema

Increased filtration (capillary hydrostatic) pressure

  Dilation of arterioles

  Constriction of veins

  Increased venous pressure (heart failure, leaky heart valves, obstruction to veins, increase in extracellular fluid volume, effect of gravity)

Changes in osmotic pressure

  Decreased plasma protein levels

  Accumulation of osmotically active particles in the interstitial space

  Increased capillary permeability

  Histamine and related substances

Inadequate lymphatic drainage

---

terstitial fluid, cell waste products, or remains of dead tissue. Being large, these proteins cannot be easily removed by the capillaries, however, another mechanism—the **lymphatic system**—is in place to remove excessive fluid and proteins.

FUNCTIONS OF THE LYMPHATIC SYSTEM

The function of the lymphatic system is to return excess fluid and protein from the interstitial fluid compartment back into the blood circulation (see Figure 9.2). If the protein is not returned to the blood, the plasma colloid osmotic pressure will drop, and it will not be possible for fluid to stay inside the circulatory system.

Defense is another important function of this system. Lymphoid tissue is responsible for the production, maintenance, and distribution of **lymphocytes,**

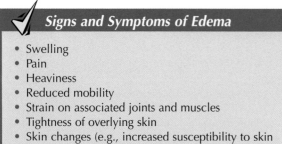

Signs and Symptoms of Edema

- Swelling
- Pain
- Heaviness
- Reduced mobility
- Strain on associated joints and muscles
- Tightness of overlying skin
- Skin changes (e.g., increased susceptibility to skin breakdown, infection, and injury; delayed wound healing; lower skin temperature as a result of reduced blood flow in the area
- Sensory disturbances of the hand and foot
- Psychological disturbances owing to alterations in body image, sexuality, and social acceptance

a class of white blood cells that participates in defense. The white blood cells in the lymphatic system remove foreign agents that have entered the interstitial region.

In the intestine, lymphatics help carry fat and large particles to the liver. In the kidney, adequate lymphatic flow is required for concentrating the urine.

COMPONENTS OF THE LYMPHATIC SYSTEM

The lymphatic system is an anatomical system consisting of **lymph vessels, lymph,** specialized cells called lymphocytes (described in the section on Immunity), **lymphoid organs,** and collections of **lymphoid tissue** in different parts of the body.

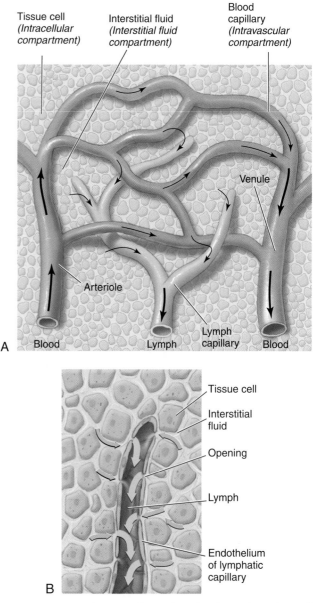

FIGURE **9.2.**   **A,** Formation of Lymph and Relationship of Lymph Capillaries to Tissue Cells and Interstitial Fluid Compartment. **B,** Lymph capillary.

Lymph Vessels

The lymphatic system is similar to the cardiovascular system because it, too, has vessels, often called **lymphatics.** Lymphatics are present in almost all the regions of the body; however, they are absent from the central nervous system and such regions as the cornea, lens, cartilage, and epithelium that lack a blood supply.

The smallest vessels—the **lymphatic capillaries**—arise as blind-ended tubes in the interstitial spaces (Figure 9.2). These capillaries have thinner walls, and they are larger than blood capillaries. The lymph capillaries are highly permeable and allow large particles to easily enter the vessel. The endothelial cells lining the capillaries have gaps that allow the particles to enter. In addition, the cells overlap with each other, with the overlap acting as one-way valves. **Anchoring filaments**—proteins attached to the endothelial cells—also help adjust the width of the gaps. When there is more fluid inside the lymph capillaries, the width of the gap becomes smaller, allowing less fluid in and preventing backflow of fluid. When there is more fluid in the interstitial compartment, the anchoring filaments are pulled and the gap widens, allowing more fluid to enter the capillaries.

The lymph capillaries in the intestines (**lacteals**) are located in the center of the villi. The lymph in the lacteal carries a high fat content, giving the lymph a creamy, white appearance. Lymph flowing through the lacteals is referred to as **chyle.**

From the periphery, the networks of capillaries join and rejoin others to form larger **lymphatic vessels** (see Figure 9.3). The lymphatic vessels resemble veins, with an endothelium, smooth wall muscles, and adventitia. The inner lining of these large vessels is thrown into folds to form valves. Lymph vessels have numerous valves located every few millimeters, giving the vessels a beaded appearance. At various intervals, the lymph vessels open into lymphatic tissue called **lymph nodes.** Lymphatic vessels from the lymph nodes join others and progressively become larger until they communicate with two collecting vessels, the **thoracic duct** or **left lymphatic duct,** the largest of these vessels, and the **right lymphatic duct.** The lower end of the thoracic duct is enlarged and is known as the **cisterna chyli.**

The thoracic duct and the right lymphatic duct are located in the thoracic cavity. The thoracic duct is about 38–45 cm (15–17.7 in) long and runs parallel to the vertebral column. The right lymphatic duct is much shorter, about 1.5 cm (0.6 in) long. Both ducts open into the blood vessels in the neck (on the left and right side, respectively) at the junction of the subclavian and internal jugular vein. Thus, lymph is emptied into the blood circulation.

The thoracic duct collects lymph from the left side of the body and from the right side of the body inferior to the diaphragm. The right lymphatic duct collects lymph from the right side of the body superior to the diaphragm (i.e., the right side of the head and neck, the right upper limb, the right side of the thorax, the right lung, the right side of the heart), and part of the liver.

Lymph and Lymph Flow

The lymph or lymph fluid, a clear, pale yellow fluid, is the overflow fluid from the tissue spaces with the same composition as the interstitial fluid. It carries large proteins and waste from different parts of the body.

Although lymph vessels, unlike blood vessels, do not have extensive smooth muscle around them, these smooth muscles play a pivotal role in the movement of lymph. The smooth muscles possess intrinsic contractile properties: i.e. they contract rhythmically and in phases. This property known as the intrinsic lymph pump helps lymph flow. The activity of the lymphatic smooth muscles is altered by physical stimuli (e.g. interstitial fluid pressure; lymph pressure), chemical stimuli (e.g. circulating hormones; local secretions from endothelium of lymph capillaries and immune cells). The one-way valves in lymph vessels also help direct the fluid. Lymph is also propelled to a large extent by the passive and active movements of skeletal muscles. In addition, the pulsation of arteries lying close to the lymph vessels helps propel the lymph. Another important mechanism that draws the lymph upward is the respiratory movements. When a person inspires, the pressure drops in the thorax and increases in the abdomen. This difference in pressure is sufficient to "suck" the lymph into the thorax and the venous system. Changes in posture, passive compression, and massage can also aid lymph flow. The smooth wall muscles of the lymphatic vessels also help move lymph by contracting when distended. The rate of flow increases with physical activity. It has been estimated that about 2–4 liters of lymphatic fluid and the equivalent of 25% to 50% of the total circulating plasma protein is returned to the circulation every day.

Lymph Nodes

As lymph flows toward the blood circulation, at various points it passes through lymph nodes (see Figure 9.4). Lymph nodes are small organs of about 1–2 cm (0.4–0.8 in) that filter large particles and remove foreign substances before lymph empties into the veins. They may be oval, round, elongated, or bean-shaped. Lymph nodes are also centers for proliferation of the lymphocytes. They are usually found in the subcutaneous tissue (superficial nodes) or muscle fascia and body cavities (deep nodes). Lymph nodes are numerous; there are more than 600 lymph nodes in the body.

Lymph nodes are often found in clusters, especially in the axilla, groin, the side of the neck, thorax, and abdomen. The lymph nodes are located along the lymph vessels that lead from the tissue to the larger

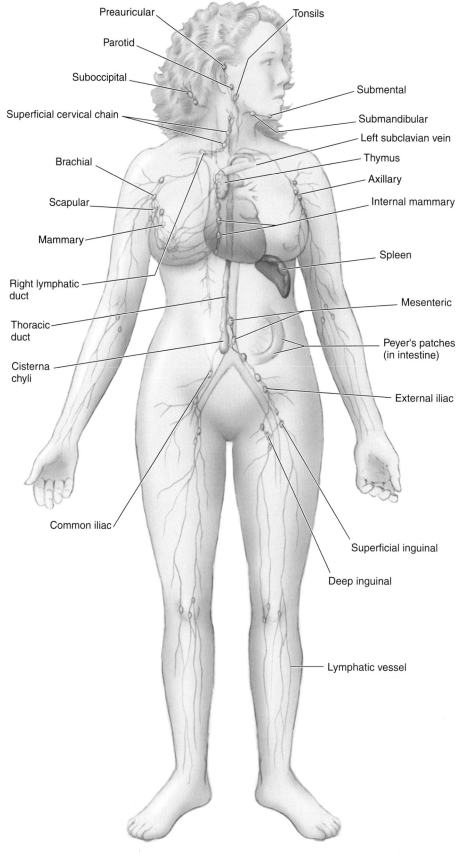

FIGURE 9.3.   Lymphatic Drainage and Location of Major Lymph Nodes

ducts. Each lymph node processes lymph from a specific, adjacent anatomic site.

A lymph node is surrounded by a connective tissue **capsule.** The connective tissue of the capsule extends into the lymph node as **trabeculae,** dividing it into smaller compartments. The trabeculae and the meshwork of connective tissue inside the lymph node provide the framework for the lymph node and also help slow the flow of lymph as it passes through. The lymph node contains numerous lymphocytes and **macrophages,** types of white blood cells involved in the defense of the body (**see page 459**), arranged in clusters called **germinal centers.**

Tiny lymph vessels, called **afferent vessels,** bring the lymph *into* the lymph node. In the lymph node, the lymph flows through irregular channels (**sinuses**) that contain the white blood cells. Sinuses are present under the capsule (subcapsular sinuses), between the

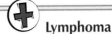

Lymphoma

Lymphoma is a malignant disorder of the lymphatic structures that presents as painless, progressive enlargement of a single or group of lymph nodes. Cancerous cells may spread to other areas of the body.

connective tissue (trabecular sinuses), and in the center of the lymph node (medullary sinuses). An **efferent vessel** takes lymph *away* from the node after it is screened by the cells located inside the node. These vessels emerge from the side of the lymph node through a small indentation known as the **hilus.**

If confronted by a foreign organism, white blood cells destroy the organism. At the same time, their multiplication is triggered. Certain lymphocytes produce **antibodies,** proteins manufactured to destroy the specific organism (**antigen**). Antibody production causes lymph nodes that drain an infected area to become enlarged and painful during the infection, a condition called **lymphadenitis.** Sometimes, the lymph vessels are also inflamed and appear as thin, red streaks around the infected region, a condition called **lymphangitis.**

In addition to lymph vessels and lymph nodes, the lymphatic system includes the lymphoid organs; the **thymus, spleen,** and lymphoid tissue found in the **tonsils, appendix,** and **intestine.**

The Thymus

The thymus (see Figure 9.5) is a flat, long structure with two lobes located in the mediastinum, inferior to the thyroid gland in the neck, posterior to the sternum. If you were able to pull your sternum forward and peek behind it, you would find it there! The thymus is surrounded by a connective tissue capsule. Similar to other lymphoid tissue, the thymus contains lymphocytes, macrophages, and reticular epithelial cells.

The thymus is fully developed at birth, and it continues to grow until puberty. After puberty, it slowly decreases in size. The thymus is important in the development of the immune system. The lymphocytes processed in the thymus are called the **T lymphocytes.** In the absence of the thymus, immunity is significantly lowered. The thymus is considered an endocrine organ because it secretes the hormone thymosin (**see page 411**).

The Spleen

The spleen (Figures 9.3 and 9.6) is an oval organ that is about as size of a clenched fist. It is located on the upper left quadrant of the abdomen, deep to ribs 9, 10, and 11, inferior to the diaphragm in contact with the stomach, splenic flexure of the colon, and the left kid-

Lymphotomes and Watersheds

Foldi and Kubic divided the body into different lymphatic drainage areas. In the skin, these drainage areas are called "lymphotomes." The line between any two adjoining areas is called a watershed. Foldi and Kubic claim that collateral lymphatics connect adjoining "lymphotomes" across watersheds. Massaging the lymph across the watershed may provide an alternate route for lymph to drain from a blocked lymphotome. (Redrawn from Tappan FM, Benjamin PJ. Tappan's Handbook of Healing Massage Techniques, 3rd Ed p 227. Copyright 1998. Adopted with permission from Prentice-Hall, Inc, Upper Saddle River, NJ)

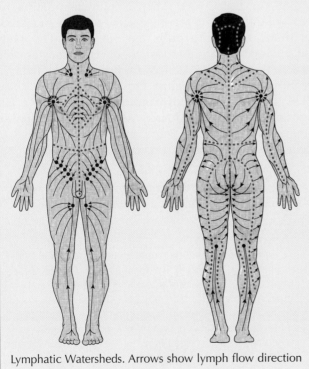

Lymphatic Watersheds. Arrows show lymph flow direction

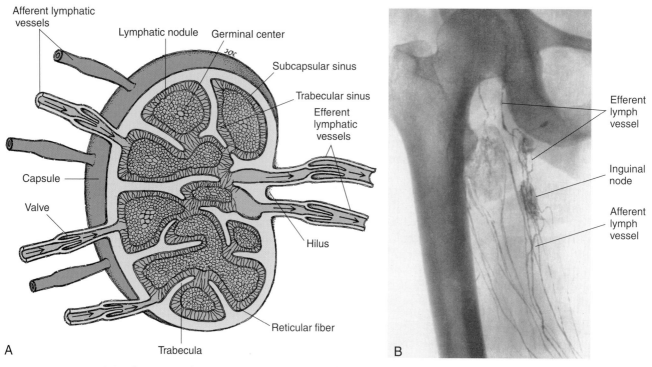

FIGURE 9.4. Some Lymphatic Structures. **A,** Section through a lymph node. **B,** inguinal lymphogram, showing the afferent lymph vessels, efferent lymph vessels, and inguinal nodes. Reproduced with permission from Authors: Battezzati M, Donini I. The Lymphatic System, 2nd Ed. John Wiley & Sons, Chichester West Sussex 1972.

ney. It is the largest mass of lymphoid tissue in the body. The spleen is covered by a connective tissue capsule from which trabeculae extend to the interior, providing the framework. Microscopic examination reveals that the spleen is composed of two, distinct kinds of tissue, the **white pulp** and **red pulp.** The white pulp contains an abundance of lymphocytes and macrophages, which destroy foreign tissue and manufacture antibodies against the foreign tissue. These cells surround branches from the splenic artery. The red pulp consists of dilated veins called **venous sinuses,** which are filled and surrounded by cords of cells, consisting of red blood cells, macrophages, lym-

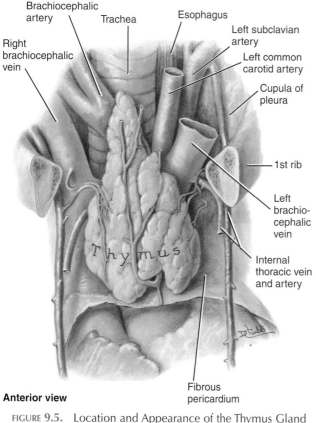

Anterior view

FIGURE 9.5. Location and Appearance of the Thymus Gland

Splenomegaly

An abnormally enlarged spleen is referred to as **splenomegaly.** Normally, the spleen is beneath the left ribs and cannot be felt by palpating the abdomen. An enlarged spleen can be felt in the left upper quadrant of the abdomen as a firm, uniform mass that moves with respiration. An enlarged spleen may be a sign of an infectious condition such as typhoid fever and malaria or anemia that results from rapid destruction of red blood cells. Splenomegaly is also seen in many other conditions, including leukemia and lymphoma.

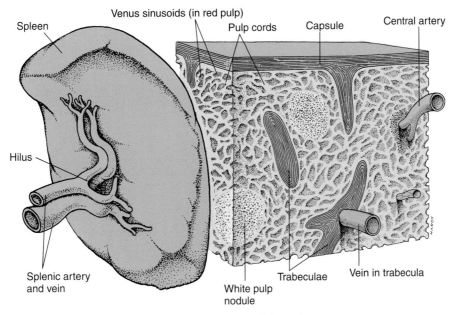

FIGURE **9.6.** Structure of the Spleen

phocytes, plasma cells, and other white blood cells. Tributaries of the splenic vein are closely associated with the red pulp. Within the red pulp, platelets are stored and injured and/or old red blood cells and platelets are destroyed. Before birth, the spleen also manufactures red blood cells.

The spleen is richly supplied with blood vessels; at any given time, it holds about 350 mL (11.8 oz) of blood. This volume of blood can be quickly sent back into the circulation when there is severe bleeding; therefore, the spleen serves as a blood reservoir. Unfortunately, as a result of its vascularity, profuse bleeding can occur into the peritoneal cavity if the spleen is damaged as a result of trauma to the abdomen. In such situations, the spleen is removed **(splenectomy)** to prevent the person from bleeding to death. Other structures, such as the bone marrow and liver, take over the functions of the spleen.

The Tonsils

The tonsils (see Figure 10.2) are collections of lymphoid tissue (lymphocytes and macrophages) located under the mucous membrane in the mouth and the back of the throat. They help protect against foreign agents that may enter the body through the nasal and oral cavities. The tissues located on either side of the throat are known as the **palatine tonsils.** Those located in the throat near the posterior opening of the nasal cavity are the **pharyngeal tonsils, or adenoids.** The paired collections of lymphoid tissue at the base of the tongue are known as **lingual tonsils.**

Intestinal Lymphoid Tissue

Lymphoid tissue located in the submucosa of the intestines and in the appendix defends the body against foreign agents that may enter the system through the gut. In the gut, the lymphoid tissues are scattered in patches. In the intestine, these patches are known as **Peyer's patches.**

DRAINAGE ROUTE OF LYMPH

Knowledge of the direction and route of lymph drainage is important for many reasons (see Figure 9.3 and box - Lymphotomes and Watersheds page 513). Massage therapists can apply the massage strokes along the direction of lymph drainage and speed lymph movement. Surgeons can plan the extent of surgery or radiation in persons with cancer because cancer cells can be carried by lymph to the nodes draining the area. When treating some types of cancer, the lymph nodes draining the area are removed or irradiated together with the cancerous tissue.

Upper Limbs

Lymphatic vessels in the arm (see Figure 9.7) consist of superficial and deep groups, which anastomose.

✚ Tonsillitis

Tonsillitis is an inflammation of the tonsil. Removal of the tonsils, or tonsillectomy, is performed in cases of chronic inflammation.

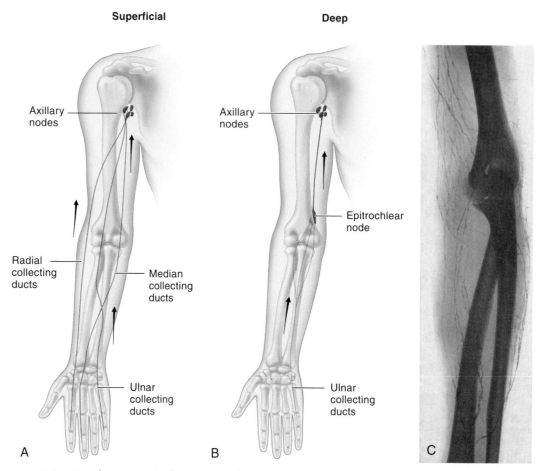

Superficial

Deep

Axillary nodes

Axillary nodes

Epitrochlear node

Radial collecting ducts

Median collecting ducts

Ulnar collecting ducts

Ulnar collecting ducts

A

B

C

FIGURE 9.7. Lymph Drainage in the Upper Limbs. **A,** Supra fascial collecting ducts. **B,** Superficial ulnar collecting ducts of the forearm and deep collecting ducts of the arm. **C,** Lymphogram of the left arm (antero-posterior) view, showing the middle lymphatic group of the forearm. The radiopaque material was injected into a dorsal lymphatic vessel of the hand. Reproduced with permission from Battezzati M, Donini I. The Lymphatic System. 2nd Ed. John Wiley & Sons, Chichester West Sussex 1972.

The superficial vessels are present in the subcutaneous tissue, while the deep vessels drain the muscle, periosteum, and bone. Each finger has one to two collecting ducts that join in the dorsum of the hand to form five or six larger trunks, joined with collecting ducts from the palm. In the forearm, three groups of drainage vessels are present—the ulnar group, the radial group, and the median group. The deep group of vessels travels along the deep arteries.

In the arm, the lymph from the ulnar and deep groups of vessels are screened by nodes located in the elbow (**epitrochlear nodes**) and then by nodes in the axilla (**axillary nodes**). The radial and middle groups join to ultimately drain into the axillary nodes.

From the axillary node on the left extremity, lymph flows to the neck region where it joins the thoracic duct. Lymph from the right extremity flows in the same direction as the left, except that it drains into the smaller, right lymphatic duct. Both ducts empty into the junction of the subclavian and internal jugular veins (Figure 9.3).

Head and Neck

The lymph from the right side of the chest, face, and scalp also flows toward the right axilla and into the right lymphatic duct. The lymph from the left side of face and scalp flows into the thoracic duct. Both sides are screened by numerous lymph nodes located in the neck (**cervical nodes**). Lymph from the nose, lips, and teeth drains through the **submental** and **submaxillary nodes** located in the floor of the mouth before it reaches the cervical nodes. **Preauricular lymph nodes,** located in front of the ear, drain the superficial tissue and skin on the lateral side of the head and face (Figure 9.3).

Lower Limbs

There are two groups of collecting ducts in the leg, the superficial group and the deep group (see Figure 9.8). The superficial vessels arise in the subcutaneous tissue, and the deep arise from the muscles, periosteum, and bone. The two systems are connected by anastomotic channels supplied with valves that allow lymph to flow from deep to superficial. There are also collateral connections between the different groups.

In the superficial group, one to two collecting ducts arise from each toe and join on the dorsum of the foot, forming five to six larger trunks on the anterior aspect. These are joined by certain vessels arising in the plantar surface. In the anterior aspect of the leg, there are three major superficial groups of vessels: the medial, lateral, and median groups. The three groups converge on the medial aspect of the knee to course with the great saphenous vein and reach nodes in the inguinal region.

On the posterior aspect, two groups of collecting ducts, the retromalleolar (medial and lateral), are formed. These vessels drain lymph from the plantar surface and heel of the foot. They run upward and medially to join the collecting ducts in the thigh. Some of the lateral vessels join the deep vessels and follow the small saphenous vein to reach the **popliteal nodes,** located in the posterior aspect of the knee.

All superficial groups of vessels ultimately join in the lower third of the medial aspect of the thigh to travel with the great saphenous vein and drain into nodes located in the upper part of the thigh, the **inguinal nodes** (Figures 9.3 and 9.4B).

The deep vessels follow the deep vessels on the leg, to reach the popliteal nodes and eventually drain into the inguinal nodes. From here, the vessels carry the lymph into the abdomen and empty into the lower end of the thoracic duct.

Breasts

The lymph drainage from the breast is important in cases of breast cancer. Eighty-five percent of the lymph flows into the respective axillary nodes. The remaining lymph drains into nodes located posterior to the sternum and lymph vessels located in the pectoralis muscle. Certain vessels drain into nodes situated in the supraclavicular region (Figure 9.3 and box - Lymphotomes and Watersheds page 513).

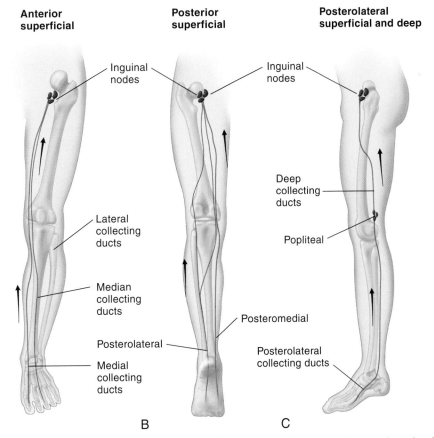

FIGURE **9.8.** Lymph Drainage in the Lower Limbs. **A,** The three anterior groups of supra fascial collecting ducts. **B,** The posterior groups of supra fascial collecting ducts. **C,** The posterolateral supra fascial collecting ducts of the leg and deep lymphatics of the thigh. Reproduced with permission from Battezzati M, Donini I. The Lymphatic System. 2nd Ed. John Wiley & Sons, Chichester West Sussex 1972.

✚ Elephantiasis

Also known as filariasis, this disorder is caused by threadlike filarial worms that are injected into the bloodstream by mosquitoes. The worms block lymphatic flow in different areas and swelling occurs due to accumulation of fluid. If the legs are affected they can become as large as an elephant's, hence the name!

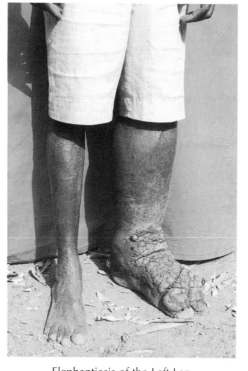

Elephantiasis of the Left Leg

Massage and the Lymphatic System

Massage has positive effects on lymph drainage. It is believed that the effects of massage are equal to the circulatory effects produced by the contraction of muscles.[1] Appropriate strokes and drainage techniques can help with the movement of lymph and reduce edema.[1,2] Passive exercise often used in conjunction with massage also encourages lymph drainage. Massage over lymph nodes can speed lymph drainage and hasten the resolution of swelling resulting from adhesions. Massage has been shown to be particularly effective in relieving postsurgical swelling and pain and for enhancing the rate and quality of healing.[3]

The removal of edema fluid reduces the incidence of fibrosis in the location. In addition, pain can be relieved by removing those chemicals and waste products dissolved in the fluid that stimulate pain receptors.

 Breast Cancer and Edema

In some breast cancer cases, the cancerous growth, as well as a wide area of tissue and lymph nodes draining the breast, is removed (mastectomy). Such procedures can interfere with normal draining of lymph from the upper limb. This may result in edema of the limb on the side of the growth. However, lymph drainage may be restored by the reestablishment of new lymphatic vessels, which grow back into the area.

MASSAGE AND LYMPHEDEMA

Some studies[4,5] have proven the positive effects of **complex physical therapy** (CPT) in those with lymphedema. CPT, or complex physical drainage (CPD) or complex decongestive physiotherapy (CDP), is a treatment consisting of massage, compression bandaging, an active exercise program, and skin care. The treatment is given for 1 to 2 hours/day for a few weeks, followed by use of support hosiery. It is designed to improve lymphatic drainage and remove stagnant proteins from the tissues. CPT has been found to be effective in patients with lymphedema following cancer surgery in which lymph nodes have been removed.

Prior to massaging the affected area, it is important for the therapist to obtain detailed information about the onset; duration; cause; previous treatments, such as physiotherapy, radiotherapy, chemotherapy, surgery, and medications; skin infections; and loss of function. All of these factors can affect treatment protocol. The therapist needs to assess the hardness of the edema, the condition of the skin and nails, and restriction of active and passive movements. Periodic measurements of the circumference of the limb may give an idea of the progress made with the treatment. The therapist should be open to modifying the treatment plan, according to objective and subjective improvements seen in the patient. Alteration of treatment may include changing the direction or sequence of the massage strokes.

The massage technique used for lymphedema is called **manual lymph drainage**.[6] The techniques help clear edema by facilitating lymph flow through the col-

✓ Types of Lymphedema

Lymphedema may be classified as primary (idiopathic) or secondary, depending on its etiology. Primary edema may be congenital or a result of unknown causes. Secondary lymphedema may be a result of obstruction or trauma to the lymphatic system (e.g., surgical removal of lymph nodes, radiotherapy, or infection).

Lymphostasis, Lymphedema, and Compensation

Lymphostasis, or stagnation of lymph, results when normal lymph flow is impeded. It may be caused by congenital malformation of the lymph vessels; mechanical obstruction, such as extrinsic or intrinsic compression; traumatic or surgical injuries; radiation; or inflammation of lymphatic vessels and nodes. Removal of lymph nodes and radiotherapy in the treatment of cancer, infection (e.g., filariasis), and trauma are common causes of lymphostasis.

Lymphedema is the accumulation of lymph that results from lymphostasis. Protein and fluid tend to accumulate in the interstitial fluid compartment (**lymphedema**). With time, the protein precipitates, triggering proliferation of fibroblasts and formation and accumulation of elastic and collagen fibers with resultant thickening of connective tissue and hardening and enlargement of the structure. Lymph vessels caught in the fibrous tissue perpetuate the situation.

When the lymphatic vessels dilate, the valves become incompetent and lymph flows backward. The pressure in the lymphatic capillaries pushes lymph from the vessels into the interstitial compartment and, at times, into the blood capillaries. Lymph also flows through collateral anastomotic channels that exist between various groups of collecting ducts. They may also drain backward through collaterals that exist between lymphatic trunks of other regions. For example, if the axillary nodes are removed, lymph may drain backward through collaterals to the deltoid group of collecting ducts that drain directly into the supraclavicular lymph nodes. Regeneration of lymph vessels can also occur to compensate for lymphostasis. For example, when a lymph node is excised, a dense network of capillary vessels is formed to connect the afferent and efferent vessels.

laterals and collecting ducts. Superficial effleurage and superficial lymph drainage techniques are used to remove fluid and assist drainage, and kneading with the finger tips or hand is used to soften areas of hardened edema. Superficial effleurage refers to gliding strokes with pressure that deforms the subcutaneous tissue down to the investing layer of the deep fascia. Superficial lymph drainage technique refers to very gentle stretches of the skin, superficial fascia, and the lymphatic vessels in the direction of lymphatic flow, followed by gentle release of the stretch.

Initially, the proximal area of drainage is massaged to facilitate flow from distal areas. For example, with edema in the upper limbs, neck, anterior and posterior trunk, and axilla are massaged first. Following massage of the proximal area, the affected area is massaged in sections. For example, the upper extremity is divided into four sections—the deltoid, upper arm, forearm, and hand. The deltoid region is massaged first, moving the edema fluid into the proximal area. Then the upper arm is massaged, moving the edema fluid into the deltoid region. Next, the edema fluid is massaged from the forearm to the upper arm. The edema from the hand is subsequently massaged to the proximal area. This sequence of strokes is repeated many times everyday.

Following massage, the area is bandaged, using low-stretch bandages to increase tissue pressure, support the connective tissue, and maintain the reduction obtained from the massage. Active exercise programs specifically designed to clear proximal areas prior to distal areas further help drain lymph.

At times, a pneumatic pump (mercury compression pump)[7] may be used to assist drainage. Here, the affected limb is placed in a cylindrical metal tank and pressure is applied around the limb through a rubber sleeve. Drugs that help remove excess plasma protein may be administered in addition to other forms of lymphedema treatment. Support hosiery, in the form of stockings, sleeves, or gloves, are also available in various sizes, lengths, styles, and compression ratings to keep edema under control.

PNEUMATIC MASSAGE THERAPY

Pneumatic massage therapy refers to the use of pneumatic devices to reduce edema. Here, a sleeve with multiple cuffs is applied over the edematous limb and compressed air is sent into the sleeve. By systematically inflating and deflating the various cuffs, pressure is applied to the subcutaneous tissue in a wavelike pattern, facilitating lymph drainage.

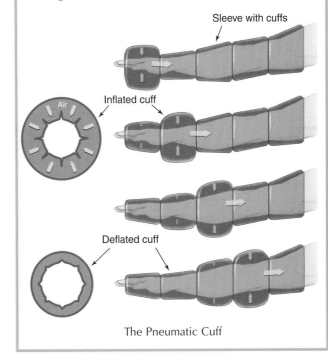

The Pneumatic Cuff

- Increase in the formation and return of lymph through contraction of the lymphatic vessels as a result of mechanical stress
- Direct lymph movement initiated by the direction of the stroke and compression of tissue by manipulation
- Reduced pain by counterirritant analgesia
- Psychological effects, such as reduction of anxiety and relaxation.

Lymphedema is a disabling condition and CPT, by removing edema from the limbs, relieves pain and discomfort and improves the well-being of the patient. It is possible to maintain and improve the benefits produced by CPT because the connective tissue that has proliferated is eventually reabsorbed and overstretched skin regains its elasticity, while new collateral vessels improve lymphatic drainage.

MASSAGE AND LOCALIZED SWELLING

Edema may be localized, as in bursitis, joint effusion, and trauma. If the swelling is a result of acute inflammation, rest, ice or application of cold for 10 to 15 minutes, compression, and elevation (RICE) should be used. Techniques, such as connective tissue massage,[1] may be used if the edema is chronic and associated with fibrosis.

CANCER AND MASSAGE

In individuals with cancer, many issues need to be addressed. Some forms of cancer tend to spread via the lymphatics, and deep massage may speed the spread. This topic is controversial; it is advisable to seek medical advice before massaging an individual with cancer.

It is possible that massage therapists may encounter one or more painless, abnormally enlarged lymph nodes, often unnoticed by the client, during a massage session. Such swellings need to be investi-

✓ **Contraindications to Lymph Drainage Techniques**

- Acute inflammation as a result of infection
- Untreated cancer with metastasis
- Allergic reactions
- Recent thrombosis
- Cardiac failure.

gated by a medical professional to rule out cancer or other disorders.

In many conditions, the spleen may be enlarged and palpable through the abdominal wall. If enlarged, the spleen can rupture if excessive pressure is applied to the left upper quadrant of the abdomen. Therapists should be cautious when treating clients with conditions that may cause splenomegaly (e.g. hemolytic anemia, malaria, cirrhosis).

Immunity

Rapid progress has been made in the field of immunology. This section gives only a brief overview sufficient to help the massage therapist understand the relevant clinical conditions related to immunity.

Immunity is the ability of the body to resist infection and disease by activation of specific defense mechanisms. The human body has many different defense mechanisms. Some of them are **nonspecific;** they do not differentiate one type of threat from another. Others are **specific,** developing defenses specifically against one particular type of threat. Both types of defense need to be functioning to provide adequate defense to the body (see Figure 9.9).

NONSPECIFIC IMMUNITY

Nonspecific defenses are present from birth, and they include physical barriers, phagocytic cells, immunologic surveillance, liberation of a variety of chemicals, inflammation, and fever.

Physical Barriers

Physical barriers prevent or make it difficult for foreign organisms to enter the body. For example, the skin is multilayered, and the epithelial cells are interlocked or held together by tight junctions that make it difficult for organisms to enter the body. The presence of keratin in the epidermis provides resistance against bacterial enzymes, acids, and alkalis. Also, the skin's accessory structures provide additional protection. The hair protects against mechanical abrasion. Secretions from sebaceous glands contain chemicals (lysozymes) that have antibiotic properties. Even if microorganisms penetrate the epidermis, they are confined to one area by the fascia.

Entry of organisms through the mucous membranes of the respiratory, gastrointestinal, urinary, and reproductive tracts is also effectively prevented. The respiratory tract is lined by mucus-secreting cells. The microorganisms that enter tend to settle on

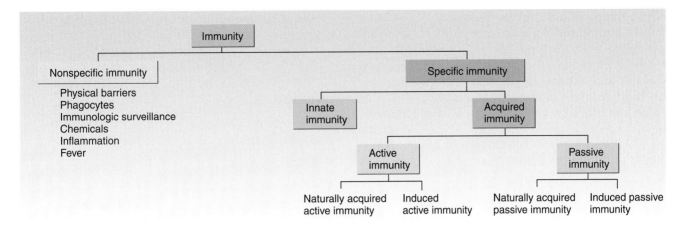

FIGURE **9.9.** Types of Immunity

the mucus. Cilia—hairlike projections on the surface of respiratory cells—help move the mucus toward the mouth, and it is then swallowed. Reflexes, such as coughing and sneezing, also help as defense mechanisms in the respiratory tract. Nasal hair filters and traps microorganisms in the nasal passages.

In the digestive tract, saliva has antimicrobial properties. The highly acidic environment and the protein-digesting enzymes in the stomach kill pathogens. Defecation and vomiting also help expel microbes from the body. The genitourinary tract is frequently flushed with urine, which is a deterrent for growth of microorganisms, and the pH of the vagina is not conducive to microbial growth. Other secretions, such as tears, sweat, and nasal secretions, contain lysozyme, an enzyme capable of breaking down the cell walls of bacteria. The secretions also help to wash away microorganisms.

Phagocytes

Phagocytes are white blood cells (see **page 459**) that patrol the tissue. If they encounter foreign or dead organisms, phagocytes engulf them into their cytoplasm and digest them. Phagocytes are attracted to the site of infection by chemicals, such as microbial products, components of white blood cells, damaged tissue cells, and activated complement proteins, in a process known as **chemotaxis.** The phagocytes then adhere to the plasma membrane of the organism a process called **adherence.** The cell membrane then extends around the microorganism to engulf it (**ingestion),** after which lysosomes containing digestive enzymes fuse with the vacuole containing the organism. The organism is then killed and digested, and the residue (**residual body**) is extruded from the cell by exocytosis. **Neutrophils** and **eosinophils** are the smallest phagocytic cells; often referred to as the **microphages.** They serve as the "first line" of defense.

The larger **macrophages** are modified monocytes of the circulation that have wandered into the tissues. Almost all tissue harbors macrophages and this diffuse collection of phagocytic cells is known as the **reticuloendothelial system. Wandering** or **free macrophages** are attracted to sites of injury or infection by chemicals liberated in the affected tissue **(chemotaxis).** They then squeeze out from the blood between the endothelium of capillaries in a process called **emigration,** or **diapedesis. Fixed macrophages** are modified monocytes that remain in the same location.

The fate of microorganisms engulfed by phagocytic cells varies. Some organisms are engulfed and destroyed by lysosomal enzymes. Other microorganisms, such as those in tuberculosis, may not be destroyed inside the cell unless other cells assist the macrophage. At times, the macrophages secrete toxins into the interstitial fluid in the vicinity of the organism in order to destroy them. Fixed macrophages rely on the fluid movement around them to phagocytize the organisms.

Immunologic Surveillance

Another form of nonspecific immunity is immunologic surveillance. Cells known as **natural killer**

➕ **Leukemia**

Leukemia is a cancerous multiplication of white blood cells in the bone marrow and lymph tissue. A key sign of leukemia is an abnormally large number of white blood cells in the blood. Unfortunately, these cells are immature and abnormal and do not improve the immune status.

(NK) **cells** constantly survey the tissue of the body. These lymphocytes recognize any antigen that is foreign to the body. At times, the body's own cells may become abnormal. These cells, too, are recognized by NK cells and destroyed. NK cells are different from other lymphocytes in that they recognize *all* cells that look different. These cells are important in destroying cancer cells and cells infected by viruses, among others. NK cells are present in the blood, spleen, lymph nodes, and red bone marrow.

Chemicals

Chemicals liberated by different cells are important in immunity. There are many different types of chemicals, some of which are described below.

Cytokines

Cytokines are small proteins that inhibit or facilitate normal cell function, such as cell growth and differentiation. For example, certain cytokines (chemotactic agents) attract phagocytes to the area, some cause fever by affecting the hypothalamus, and others stimulate proliferation of white blood cells. Cytokines are secreted by cells such as lymphocytes, macrophages, fibroblasts, and endothelial cells. Interleukin, tumor necrosis factor, lymphotoxins, perforin, macrophage migration-inhibiting factor, and interferons are examples of cytokines.

Interferons are small proteins released by activated lymphocytes, macrophages, and tissue cells infected by viruses. Interferons bind to surface receptors on normal cells and trigger the cell to release antiviral proteins in the cytoplasm. These proteins prevent the virus from multiplying inside the cells. Interferons also help to activate macrophages and NK cells. Certain types of interferons reduce inflammation in an injured area.

Complement System

The complement system is similar to the clotting system. It includes a number of inactive enzymes in the blood plasma, one of which, when activated, triggers a sequence of events that activate the other enzymes of the system. There are 11 enzymes belonging to this system, labeled from C1–C9 (C1 has 3 subtypes). When C1 is activated, it sequentially activates the other enzymes. The activated enzymes trigger the necessary defense mechanisms. For example, one consequence of complement activation is inserting pore-forming molecules into the cell membranes of foreign cells that literally punch holes through the membrane. Another is stimulating granulocytes, mast cells, and platelets to release histamine. Histamine dilates the blood vessels (redness) and allows fluid to leak out (swelling). Some

of the activated complements and enzymes attract leukocytes to the site. By "sticking" to the surface of the organisms, the enzymes alert the leukocytes to the "enemy."

Histamine

Histamine is a chemical liberated by a variety of tissue cells, including mast cells, basophils (a type of white blood cell), and platelets. Histamine causes vasodilatation (which brings more blood to the area of injury or infection), increases vascular permeability (which allows fluid to enter the injured area and dilute the toxins released; it also allows white blood cells to migrate to the area easily), and increases glandular secretion. Other actions include contraction of smooth bronchi muscles in the respiratory tract and attraction of eosinophils.

Kinins

Kinins are derived from plasma protein and have effects similar to those of histamine: increase in vascular permeability, vasodilatation, attraction of white blood cells to the area, and stimulation of pain receptors.

Prostaglandins

Prostaglandins are lipids that are secreted by almost all cells. These chemicals have varied actions, such as smooth muscle relaxation, vasodilatation, and stimulation of pain receptors.

Leukotrienes

Similar to prostaglandins, leukotrienes are also lipids and have similar actions. Mast cells and basophils primarily secrete leukotrienes.

Pyrogens

Pyrogens are chemicals released by white blood cells (and other cells) that cause an increase in body temperature (fever). An example of a pyrogen is interleukin-1, a type of cytokine.

Inflammation

Inflammation is discussed on **page 69.**

Fever

A person has "fever" if his body temperature is maintained above 37.2°C (99°F). Pyrogens reach the hypothalamus—the temperature-regulating area of the brain—and reset the "thermostat" to a higher temperature. This increase in temperature tends to inhibit some viruses and bacteria and also speeds the body's metabolism and, thereby, the activity of defense cells.

SPECIFIC IMMUNITY

Specific immunity is an immune response directed against a specific agent. Agents, such as bacteria, viruses, toxins, foreign tissue, and parasites that are recognized by the body as foreign and stimulate immune responses, are called **antigens.** Antigens may be the whole microorganism or a part of it, such as flagella, capsule, cell wall, toxins, pollen, the white of an egg, incompatible red blood cells, foreign cells, or tissue. Chemically, antigens are usually proteins, but nucleic acids, lipoproteins, glycoproteins, and large polysaccharides may all act as antigens.

Lymphocytes play a key role in the development of specific immunity. Immunity against specific threats may be either **innate** or **acquired.**

Innate Immunity

Innate immunity is genetically determined. For example, certain viruses and bacteria that affect lower animals, do not affect humans. This type of immunity is present even if the individual has not been previously exposed to the threat. However, in diseases such as AIDS (see **page 527**), in which all aspects of specific defense are depressed, unusual microorganisms may affect the individual.

Acquired Immunity

Acquired immunity is not present at birth. This type of immunity is obtained later. Acquired immunity may be obtained **actively** or **passively.**

Active immunity is produced when an individual is exposed to a foreign organism. Active immunity is long-lasting and can protect the individual from the disease for a long time, even a lifetime. A person may be naturally exposed to the organism, as when a person has chickenpox (**naturally acquired active immunity**), or he or she may be deliberately exposed to a modified or harmless organism, as in certain types of immunizations (**induced active immunity**). Immunizations stimulate the individual's immune system to develop specific defenses against harmful organisms (such as polio). If the individual comes in contact with the pathogen in the future, the defense mechanism is ready.

Passive immunity is not a result of active stimulation of an individual's immune system. Antibodies against specific organisms manufactured by the mother are transferred to the developing fetus in the womb. Antibodies are also secreted in breast milk and this, too, helps protect the infant. In emergency situations, as in epidemics, antibodies (produced by another person) against specific organisms may be injected into susceptible individuals to prevent them from getting infected. Many elderly people and those at higher risk are injected this way against specific organisms. For example, antibodies may be given for hepatitis B, tetanus, and anthrax. However, this type of defense is only temporary and lasts for only a short time (see **page 526**).

LYMPHOCYTES

Lymphocytes (see Figure 9.10) are key constituents of the immune system. This white blood cell group recognizes foreign agents and produces "ammunition" to destroy them. They not only *recognize* but also *remember* the agents that they have encountered and react more rapidly and with greater force if they are encountered again. If the other white blood cells are considered foot soldiers, lymphocytes can be compared with the Federal Bureau of Investigation (FBI), with their collection of criminal profiles. As there are specialists in the FBI, the lymphocytes, too, are also specialized into different subtypes (see Figure 9.11). These subtypes have specific functions; however, they integrate closely and defend the body together.

Formation and Processing of Lymphocytes

In the fetus, lymphocytes develop in the bone marrow. Some lymphocytes migrate to the thymus and are transformed into those cells responsible for one immunity arm, **cell-mediated immunity.** The lymphocytes that are processed in the **T**hymus, are called **T lymphocytes.** Other lymphocytes, the **B lymphocytes,** are responsible for **humoral immunity.** These lymphocytes are named for the organ in birds, the bursa of Fabricius, where they were first discovered. In man, with no tissue equivalent to the bursa of Fabricius, such processing is thought to occur in the liver, bone marrow, or spleen. After processing, the T and B lymphocytes migrate to the lymph nodes and bone marrow.

ANTIBODY FACTORIES

Today, it is possible to produce large quantities of the same antibody by special techniques. A single lymphocyte can be fused to a tumor cell (which then multiplies) to form a "factory" that produces the antibody that the lymphocyte originally produced, only in large quantities. The antibodies produced in this way are known as monoclonal antibodies, and they can be used to treat various diseases.

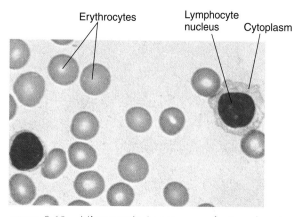

FIGURE **9.10.**   Microscopic Appearance of a Lymphocyte

Humoral Immunity, Cell-Mediated Immunity, and Role of Lymphocytes

One way that lymphocytes participate in immune reactions is by antibody production (see below) that reacts to antigens that are foreign to the body. This type of immunity is called **humoral immunity,** or the **antibody-mediated immune response.** Humoral immunity is primarily effective against antigens present in the body fluids.

Another immune reaction involves direct contact between the foreign agent and immune cells. This reaction is known as **cell-mediated immunity.** Exam-ples of cell-mediated immune reactions are allergy (see **page 529**) and transplant rejection. Cell-mediated immunity is particularly effective against pathogens located within cells (e.g., fungi, viruses, and parasites), cancer cells, and tissues that are foreign to the body (e.g., transplanted organs and tissues).

Humoral Immunity

When viruses, bacteria, or other foreign agents enter the body, they are ingested by macrophages. The macrophages then display the antigen on the surface of the cell membrane. The antigens presented are recognized as foreign by specific T and B lymphocytes. On recognition, the lymphocytes differentiate and proliferate. In the humoral immune response, B lymphocytes differentiate into **memory cells** and **plasma cells.**

Memory cells store data about a particular antigen for future use. Plasma cells produce specific **antibodies (or immunoglobulins)** against this protein. Immunoglobulins are glycoproteins that circulate in the blood. Each Y- or T-shaped molecule is composed

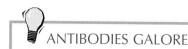

ANTIBODIES GALORE

It has been calculated that the body is capable of producing 10^8–10^{10} different antibodies.

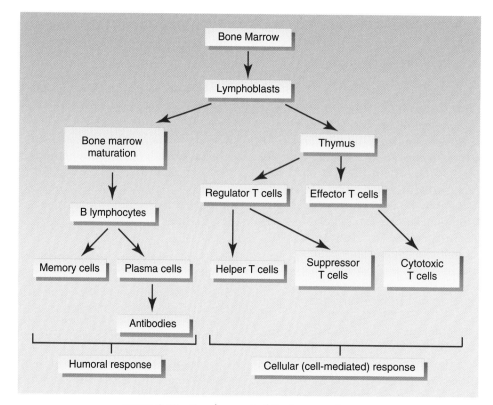

FIGURE **9.11.**   Development of the Immune System

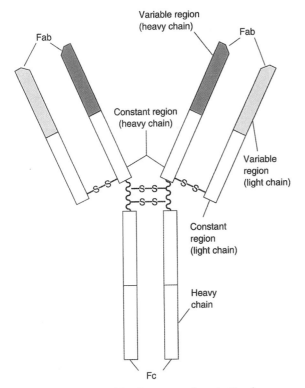

FIGURE **9.12.**   The Structure of an Antibody

of four polypeptide chains (two heavy and two light chains), with a carbohydrate chain attached to each heavy chain. Each chain has a variable region that matches the specific antigen (see Figure 9.12) and a constant region. The structure of the constant regions of the antibody is common to all other antibodies of the same class.

There are five antibody classes; IgG, IgA, IgM, IgD, and IgE. The classes of antibodies differ from each other in their constant regions. This difference confers slightly different properties and biological roles to each class. An apt analogy for these five classes is to compare them to different types of weapons used to attack an enemy. Special weapons are used for ground-to-ground combat, others for surface-to-air combat, and others are used under water! For example, IgA is secreted in tears, saliva, and intestinal secretions and protects the body from invasion by specific organisms. IgA antibodies are secreted in breast milk. Maternal IgG antibodies cross the placenta before birth and provide resistance to the fetus. IgE antibody, if bound to specific antigens, prompts mast cells and basophils to release histamine.

Antibodies are manufactured to be specific for a particular antigen. They can be compared to a key that fits a specific lock. For example, if a person has been exposed to the chickenpox virus, plasma cells manufacture antibodies specific to the chickenpox virus. Memory cells are also formed against the virus. If the person is exposed a second time to the same virus, the memory cells are stimulated and large quantities of antibodies are produced against the chickenpox virus.

How Do Antibodies Work?

Antibodies work in different ways. Some antibodies *neutralize* the antigens when they combine and prevent them from exerting their effects. Others may *lyse the cell* on which the antigen is present. In addition, when antibodies are bound to antigens on the surface of bacteria, they *attract other white blood cells,* such as macrophages and neutrophils, to engulf them. Antibodies may also result in the release of histamine and other *chemicals* from cells. Also, some of these defense mechanisms are partly caused by *stimulation of the complement system.*

Recognition of Self and Nonself

Although each cell in the body has antigens (substances capable of provoking antibody formation) on its cell membrane, lymphocytes are able to distinguish "self" from "nonself." In every individual, certain genes code for the production of unique glycoproteins. These glycoproteins are present on the surface of every cell in the body, identifying it as self. These glycoproteins, known as **major histocompatibility complex** (MHC), can be compared to an identification badge given to members of a particular association. Therefore, in general, antibodies are not developed against cells belonging to self. Even if it does, the body protects itself from attacks by its own defense cells in many ways. For example, T cells that develop against self are killed in the thymus early in life. Also, B cells that are exposed to high concentrations of antigens become less responsive. Since B cells are exposed to a high concentration of self antigens, they do not react against them. Rarely, cells of self are recognized as foreign by the body's own lymphocytes. The resultant immunologic reaction is responsible for the signs and symptoms of **autoimmune diseases.**

Basis of Skin Tests

Skin tests determine if a person has been exposed to certain antigens. A small quantity of a specific antigen is injected just under the skin, usually on the forearm. If the person has been exposed and the immune mechanisms are normal, the region becomes red and inflamed within 2 to 4 days, indicating that the person has developed antibodies against the antigen. However, further investigation is needed to determine if the person is presently infected because the antibodies may have been developed much earlier. One common skin test is the *tuberculin skin test* (to test for exposure to the tuberculosis bacilli).

Primary and Secondary Responses on Exposure to Antigens

The initial response of the body on the first exposure to antigens is known as the **primary response.** After exposure to the antigen, it normally takes about two weeks for antibody levels to peak. During this time, B cells are converted to plasma cells that secrete antibodies specific for the antigen. The antibody levels do not remain elevated for long after the first exposure. If the individual is exposed to the antigen a second time, the presence of memory cells stimulates rapid production of antibodies. In the **secondary response,** antibody levels quickly reach peak levels (see Figure 9.13). The levels are much higher than those of the primary response and remain elevated for a longer time. Secondary responses can occur even if many years have elapsed after the first exposure to the antigen.

T Cells and Cell-Mediated Immunity

T cells are activated when exposed to an antigen on the surface of foreign agents or when cells such as macrophages present the foreign antigen on their cell membrane after ingesting the foreign agent. Similar to B cells, there are different subtypes of T cells, each with specific functions. The **cytotoxic/ effector/killer T cells** attack and destroy cells that carry the antigens that initially activated them. One mechanisms they use for the attack is to punch holes in the cell membrane of the foreign cell. They may also provoke a reaction inside the foreign cell that results in death.

Helper or **inducer T cells** recognize foreign antigens and infected cells and help activate the B cells to produce antibodies (Figure 9.11). They also partici-

Stress and Immunity

One effect of stress is an increase in the levels of glucocorticoids (steroids). Glucocorticoids depress the inflammatory response by inhibiting mast cells and making capillaries less permeable, which are all part of a normal defense reaction. They reduce the number and activity of phagocytic cells in tissue. The activity of lymphocytes is also significantly reduced in stress. This reduction in immunity makes an individual more susceptible to infections.

pate in cell-mediated immunity in which the cytotoxic T cells and natural killer cells recognize virus infected cells and foreign antigens. Helper T cells also induce the macrophages and monocytes to fight infection. Another type of T cell, the **suppressor T cell,** suppresses the immune reaction by inhibiting both B and T cells. **Memory T cells** remember the antigenic properties and respond quickly and vigorously if the same antigen is reintroduced into the body.

The T cells are responsible for transplanted organ and tissue rejection. When tissue from another individual is transplanted into the body, the T cells recognize the antigens on the transplanted cells as foreign and produce an immune reaction that kills the foreign tissue—rejects it. This reaction is observed even when the tissue is from a close relative, unless the tissue is from an identical twin.

IMMUNIZATION

The process of immunization or vaccination capitalizes on the functions of lymphocytes. It relies on the primary and secondary responses of active immunity and passive immunity.

Passive Immunization

An individual can be immunized in emergencies by injecting large quantities of antibodies (produced outside) against the specific disease. For example, in a cholera epidemic, a large population may need to be immunized quickly before the disease spreads. In this case, direct injection of antibodies provides a temporary form of immunity. Rh-negative mothers carrying Rh-positive fetuses are routinely given antibodies against Rh antigens soon after delivery. These antibodies destroy Rh antigens that may have leaked into the mother's circulation from the fetus. If antibodies do develop, they can attack the next Rh-positive fetus and jeopardize its life. These are both examples of passive immunization, in which the individual's immune system is not stimulated to produce his or her own antibodies.

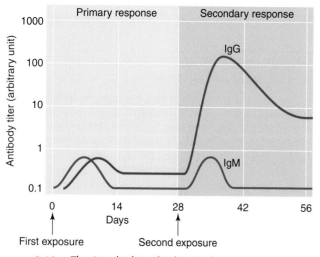

FIGURE 9.13. The Level of Antibodies in the Primary and Secondary Responses to a Specific Antigen

Active Immunization

In active immunization, by being exposed to the specific antigen, the individual produces his or her own antibodies. The antigen may be in the form of small quantities of pathogens that are similar to but not as lethal as the one producing disease. Or, the antigen could be in the form of killed pathogens. Such vaccines have been developed against many diseases. Vaccines against diseases such as diphtheria, polio, tetanus, whooping cough, and measles are routinely given to children. Many of these vaccines are given more than once to stimulate a secondary, long-lasting response to the antigen.

Rarely, some forms of immunization procedures produce adverse effects. Methods are available to identify those children prone to develop these rare adverse effects; parents must make an informed choice about immunization in these cases.

If a large population of individuals who have not been immunized against a particular infection exists in one area, the entire population becomes vulnerable to that infection. In these situations, an epidemic of that particular disease has the potential to infect the entire population. To a large extent, the possibility of such a situation has been minimized as, those who have been immunized are shielding individuals who have not been immunized from contracting these deadly diseases.

ABNORMALITIES OF THE IMMUNE SYSTEM

Immunodeficiency States

AIDS

The Virus

Acquired immune deficiency syndrome (AIDS) develops after infection by the **human immunodeficiency virus** (HIV). There are three subtypes of this

---

VACCINES FOR ACTIVE IMMUNIZATION

Vaccines for active immunization of normal civilian adults in the United States

Vaccines	Schedule and Target Group
Combined diphtheria and tetanus toxoids	Every 10 years; all adults
Inactivated influenza vaccine for current year	All adults from age 65
Live measles vaccine	One dose. All adults without history of previous infection or immunization.
Live mumps vaccine	One dose. All adults without history of previous infection or immunization
Live rubella vaccine	One dose. All females

Adapted from: National Immunization program. Available at http://www.cdc.gov/nip/recs/adult-schedule.pdf

---

virus: HIV-1, HIV-2, and HIV-3. Because most individuals infected with HIV-1 virus eventually develop AIDS (unlike those infected by the other subtypes), this subtype is considered the most significant.

HIV and the Immune System

HIV belongs to a class of viruses called retrovirus. Retroviruses carry their genetic information as RNA rather than DNA. The virus has a protein coat that surrounds the RNA strand and reverse transcriptase enzyme (the enzyme that helps RNA to be converted to DNA inside the host cell). A bilipid layer coat encloses the virus. Proteins embedded in the coat help the virus enter the host cell (see Figure 9.14). The virus is fragile and does not live for long outside the body. Once inside the body, the virus targets helper T cells and macrophages.

In certain cells, the infection enters a latent phase in which the cell serves as a reservoir from which the virus can be released for a period of many years. In other cells, such as helper T cells, the virus may behave differently. After it enters the cell, it sheds its protein coat and, with the help of reverse transcriptase, alters the genetic material within host cell nucleus. Soon, the cell begins to manufacture viral proteins, which then affect more and more cells. The infected cells are ultimately killed, reducing the number of helper T cells in the body. Because helper T cells coordinate both cell-mediated and humoral immunity, the infected individual becomes immunodeficient. Suppressor T cells are not affected, which helps to further depress the immune response. As a result, the body is vulnerable to many types of infections.

Microorganisms that ordinarily do not affect humans (**opportunistic infections**) tend to infect the affected individual with lethal consequences. The

---

Strategies for Suppressing Immune Reactions

In certain situations, immune reactions are deliberately suppressed (e.g., to prevent rejection of transplants). Certain drugs that kill T cells by destroying all rapidly dividing cells may be used; however, these drugs increase an individual's risk for infection and cancer. Alternately, certain drugs, such as cyclosporin that specifically kill T lymphocytes without affecting B lymphocytes and steroids that suppress T-cell formation, may be given. Recently, antibodies have been developed to selectively destroy lymphocytes. However, all of these drugs have adverse effects, some of them severe.

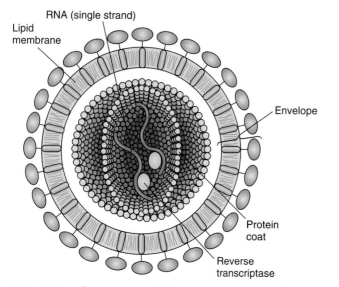

RNA (single strand)

Lipid
membrane

Envelope

Protein
coat

Reverse
transcriptase

FIGURE **9.14.**   The Structure of the Human Immunodeficiency Virus

surveillance activity of the immune system is also depressed and abnormal (cancerous) cells normally recognized and destroyed by the immune system survive, increasing the risk of cancer.

Spread of the Virus

HIV is spread from one individual to another through intimate contact. Although all body secretions, including tears, saliva, and breast milk, of the infected individual contain the virus, the major route of spread is via semen, vaginal secretions, and transfusion of contaminated blood and from an infected mother to the fetus. It has also been shown that the risk of viral transmission of the virus is higher with male-to-male contact as compared with female-to-male. There is a higher rate of transmission by anal intercourse because the delicate lining of the anal canal is easily damaged. Presence of ulcers or wounds in the genitals increases the risk further.

Other than contracting HIV through transmission of contaminated blood (this is rare as donors are now carefully screened for AIDS before taking blood), needle sharing by drug users increases the risk. In the United States, approximately 2,000 babies are born infected with HIV each year. This is a result of the transmission of the virus across the placenta from in-

fected mothers. The virus is not transmitted by insect bites or by casual contact, such as hugging and sharing of household items.

Course of the Disease

Initially, a few weeks after exposure to HIV, the infected individual may experience flulike symptoms, with lymph node enlargement. At this time, antibodies against the virus begin to form. Available tests can detect the presence of these antibodies in the blood within 2 to 6 months of exposure. The course of the disease is variable and further symptoms may not appear for 5 to 10 years. However, the virus continues to multiply in the lymphoid tissue, depleting the T cells, and depressing the immunity. The Centers for Disease Control and Prevention in Atlanta, Georgia, has classified HIV disease based on the T cell count. The symptoms do not usually appear until the number of specific T cells is low. Those individuals with very low counts are categorized as having late-stage HIV disease and include all patients with AIDS.

Early symptoms of AIDS are initially mild, including lymph node enlargement, weight loss, and diarrhea. Soon, the person develops life-threatening infections. Infections as a result of unusual microorganisms are observed. As a result of immunologic surveillance depression, the risk of cancer is high. A normally rare cancer, known as Kaposi's sarcoma, is common. Kaposi's sarcoma is characterized by purple/brown/blue growths that appear on the hands, feet, and trunk. The lesions are caused by abnormal multiplication of endothelial cells of blood vessels. In people with AIDS, the lesions tend to quickly spread to different areas of the body. Infection of the nervous system by HIV, eventually produces dementia. The average life expectancy after diagnosis is 2 years.

Prevention

The best defense is to avoid exposure to HIV. Sexual contact with infected individuals should be avoided because all forms of sexual contact increase the risk of viral transmission. Condoms are recommended when a partner's sexual history is not known. The only condoms to be used are those made of materials, such as latex, that block the passage of the virus.

HIV is destroyed when exposed to heat (57.2°C [135°F] for 10 minutes) or disinfectants, such as hydrogen peroxide, household bleach, and even standard dishwashing and clothes washing liquids.

Treatment

Unfortunately, there is no cure for AIDS. Rapid progress is being made in developing a vaccine that may provide HIV immunity. The survival rate of AIDS patients is increasing as a result of the development of drugs that slow the progress of the disease and improved antibiotic therapies against secondary infections. During treatment, the psychosocial issues involved with the disease are important.

Cancer

One treatment option for cancer patients is to give drugs that target the rapidly multiplying cells. These drugs, in addition to attacking cancer cells, destroy mother cells that manufacture lymphocytes and, thus, reduce immunity. Radiation therapy, another cancer treatment option, also has similar serious adverse effects.

Organ transplants

The immune system in individuals who have received transplants (e.g., skin, kidney, bone marrow) is deliberately suppressed by drugs to prevent immune cells from attacking the foreign tissue. These drugs make these individuals more prone to infection.

Autoimmune Disorders

Autoimmune disorders result when the immune system mistakenly targets normal body cells and tissues. Normally, self-proteins that have antigenic properties are ignored. Even if the antigens are targeted by some defense cells, they are quickly destroyed by natural killer cells.

In autoimmune disorders, however, the immune system malfunctions and antibodies known as **autoantibodies** develop against the antigens present in

specific self-tissue (see Probable Autoimmune Diseases for typical examples of autoimmune disorders).

Allergy

It is important for massage therapists and other health professionals to obtain a detailed history of allergy to avoid serious consequences in the clinic.

Allergies are considered an inappropriate, excessive, or abnormal response to antigens. The antigens in allergic reactions are often referred to as **allergens.** Allergens may be inhaled, ingested, injected, or introduced by direct skin contact. In an allergic reaction, the inflammatory response produced by antigen-antibody complexes may be extensive, and some normal cells in the region may also be destroyed along with infected or injured cells. The sensitization of a specific individual to an allergen is dependent on the individual's genetic makeup, the physical and chemical properties of the allergen, how the person is exposed, and the quantity of the allergen.

According to the type of reaction and the immune mechanisms involved, allergies are classified into four categories:

- **Immediate hypersensitivity, IgE mediated disorder,** or **type I allergy** (more common)
- **cytotoxic reactions, antibody-mediated disorder,** or **type II allergy**
- **immune complex disorders; complement-mediated disorder,** or **type III allergy**
- **delayed hypersensitivity, T-cell-mediated hypersensitivity reactions,** or **type IV allergy.**

Immediate Hypersensitivity, IgE-Mediated Disorder, or Type I Allergy

In immediate hypersensitivity or type I allergy, antibodies begin to develop against the allergen when a person is first exposed to it. Because the primary response to the antigen is slow, the reaction may be mild. The antibodies (IgE type) developed in this encounter get bound to the cell membrane of basophils and mast cells throughout the body. The change that occurs after the first exposure to the allergen is known as **sensitization.** The tendency of certain individuals to produce large quantities of these antibodies may be a result of their genetic makeup, which is why certain allergies are common in family members.

After sensitization, if the individual is exposed to the allergen again, the bound antibodies trigger the basophils and mast cells to liberate their secretions, such as prostaglandins, heparin, and histamine, into the surrounding tissue. These secretions are responsible for the dramatic symptoms observed in allergic individuals such as vasodilatation, increased vascular permeability, bronchi constriction, pain receptors stimula-

Probable Autoimmune Diseases (not all-inclusive)

- Rheumatoid arthritis
- Scleroderma
- Systemic lupus erythematosus
- Insulin-dependent diabetes mellitus (type I)
- Myasthenia gravis
- Ulcerative colitis.

tion, and itching. Increased secretion, observed as watery eyes, nasal discharge (rhinitis), and sneezing, also occurs. The basophils, macrophages, and other white cells attracted to the area are, in turn, stimulated to liberate their own chemicals, which further extends and multiplies the initial effects.

The extent of the response varies from individual to individual and from one location to another. If the individual's skin is exposed to the allergen, the reaction may be restricted to the local area. Type I hypersensitivity that is localized, such as hay fever or allergic rhinitis, dermatitis, or eczema; food allergies; or gastroenteritis are referred to as **atopic disorders.** Atopic disorders are a type of genetically determined hypersensitivity, and individuals with this type of allergy are usually allergic to more than one environmental allergen. Typical allergens causing allergic rhinitis and allergic asthma are pollen from grasses, weeds, and trees, dust mites, animal dander, feathers, and fungal spores. Allergens that cause contact dermatitis in previously sensitized individuals include cosmetics, hair dyes, metals, drugs/creams applied to the skin, and latex (e.g., latex gloves). Almost any food can produce allergies. Shellfish, legumes, cow's milk and egg whites are common food allergens.

Symptoms develop dramatically when the allergen has entered the circulation, leading sometimes to death. This kind of a dramatic reaction is known as **anaphylaxis.** Deaths that result from transfusion of incompatible blood and penicillin injections are anaphylactic reactions. Here, the allergen enters the circulation and is quickly carried to mast cells throughout the body. The vasodilatation that results and the movement of fluid out of the dilated capillaries can lead to a sudden drop in blood pressure and **anaphylactic shock.** Welts or hives may develop on the skin surface. The constriction of bronchi that accompanies anaphylaxis can lead to breathing difficulties. If this condition is not treated immediately, the individual may collapse within minutes and die.

Cytotoxic Reactions, Antibody-Mediated Disorder, or Type II Allergy

Examples of cytotoxic reactions or type II allergy are reactions produced in the fetus as a result of Rh incompatibility and certain drug reactions. The reaction results in cell lysis, leading to reduction in red blood cells (anemia), white blood cells, and platelets.

Immune Complex Disorders; Complement-Mediated Disorder, or Type III Allergy

In immune complex disorders or type III allergy, antigen-antibody complexes are deposited in the blood vessel walls or in the kidneys. The complexes activate complement proteins and result in local inflammatory reactions. Examples of type III allergic reactions are glomerulonephritis and the vasculitis (inflammation in blood vessels) that occurs in systemic lupus erythematosus.

Delayed Hypersensitivity, T Cell-Mediated Hypersensitivity Reactions, or Type IV Allergy

Delayed hypersensitivity or type IV allergies result in delayed reactions and are mediated by cells, not antibodies. T cells that have been exposed to an antigen are stimulated by a second exposure. The T cells attach to the antigen and usually produce a localized inflammation 24 to 72 hours after exposure. A typical example of type IV allergic reactions is the reaction that occurs around transplanted tissue and the reaction to skin tests, such as tuberculin tests, performed in individuals suspected of having tuberculosis.

The type IV reaction in an individual who has received a transplant is caused by the presence of the MHC antigens on the cell surface of the transplanted tissue. These antigens invoke an immune reaction (host versus graft disease). Conversely, the MHC antigen of the host tissue provokes an immune reaction in the graft tissue (graft versus host disease).

Allergy Treatment

Certain allergy symptoms can be treated with antihistamines. Other forms of treatment include administration of corticosteroids to reduce inflammation; epinephrine or adrenaline to increase blood pressure and dilate the bronchi, and use of supportive equipment to monitor and regulate the vital signs.

The Lymphatic System, Immunity, and Aging

As an individual ages, the resistance to all types of infection is decreased. This may, in part, be due to altered lifestyle such as reduced exercise and diet. Malignancies are more common in the elderly. The immune response to vaccines is also diminished. The incidence of autoimmune diseases increases, which may be a result of the overall decrease in immune function. Natural killer cell activity decreases, leading to the proliferation of abnormal cells such as cancer cells. The number of T lymphocytes diminishes with age. Both T and B lymphocytes become less responsive to antigens; atrophy of the thymus with resultant decrease in hormone secretion may play a part in this decreased response. B cell function is decreased and the quantity of antibodies produced when the body is challenged with antigens is reduced.

Basic Concepts of Health and Disease

Health is defined by the World Health Organization as "a state of complete physical, mental, or social well-being and not merely the absence of disease or infirmity." Health is an ideal state that all of us strive for and may, perhaps, achieve. Most people consider health and disease as two opposite points of a spectrum and usually place themselves close to the midpoint of this spectrum.

The term **disease** literally means "absence of ease." One way of viewing disease is to consider it as a disruption in the mechanisms of the body that maintain homeostasis. The causes of disease are varied and different fields of medicine explore different aspects of disease. **Pathology** is the study of the nature of diseases and the changes that diseases produce in the body's structure and function.

COMMON TERMS

Standard terms are used by health professionals in relation to diseases. The problems described by the patient are **symptoms; signs** are evidence of disease that can be observed by the health professional. For example, the complaint of pain in a region is a symptom; swelling felt in the area is a sign. The cause of the disease is referred to as its **etiology.** When the actual cause has been identified and named, the disease or condition is said to be **diagnosed,** or that a **diagnosis** has been made. The predicted outcome of the disease is termed the **prognosis.** The prognosis of a disease can be good or bad, depending on the history of individuals who have had the disease earlier. Many individuals are predisposed to diseases as a result of factors such as age, sex, race, environment, or genetic makeup. Such factors are called **risk factors** or **predisposing factors** for disease.

GENERAL CAUSES OF DISEASE

Human disease results from the action of various injurious agents on cells and tissue, causing biochemical or structural damage. Disease may be caused by:

- Impaired energy production (e.g., reduced nutrition or reduced availability of oxygen to tissues)
- Impaired immune responses
- Genetic abnormalities inherited from a parent or acquired by radiation, viruses, drugs, or chemicals
- Metabolic toxic agents such as alcohol, drugs, and heavy metals

- Physical agents (e.g., mechanical trauma, heat and cold, radiation injury)
- Chemical agents such as industrial and agricultural chemicals and toxic waste
- Infectious agents
- Abnormal development and growth.

INFECTION AND INFECTION PREVENTION

Among the various causes of disease, infectious agents gain importance in the clinic, as they can be transmitted from person to person.

Infectious agents can be grouped into the following categories. Arranged in order of structural complexity, they include prions, viruses, rickettsiae, chlamydiae, bacteria, fungi, algae, protozoa, metazoa, and Insecta.

Prions are proteins that do not have genetic material. However, they are infectious and capable of duplication. Some diseases associated with prions are Creutzfeld-Jakob disease, kuru, scrapie and, in animals, mad cow disease (bovine spongiform encephalopathy)

Viruses are the smallest of these agents. They contain DNA or RNA strands enclosed in a protein coat and require a living cell for replication and survival. On entering a host cell, the virus directs the nucleus of the cell to function differently and enable viral replication. New viral particles are formed in the host cell and these particles are liberated into the extracellular fluid to infect more cells.

Rickettsiae, chlamydiae, and **bacteria** are simple cells that are small (about 1 micron), with the DNA material enclosed in a cell membrane. They lack a nuclear membrane. These organisms need specific environments for survival. The rickettsiae and chlamydiae, similar to viruses, mainly depend on host cells for survival. Some bacteria are aerobic organisms that require oxygen for energy; others are anaerobic organisms that can survive without oxygen.

Algae, protozoa, and **fungi** are microorganisms that have membrane-bound organelles and a nucleus. Algae are organisms that produce oxygen as a product of photosynthesis. Protozoa are unicellular organisms that may contain flagella. They have a more complex life cycle. Fungi are microorganisms that grow as a mass of branching, interlacing filaments and include molds. Yeasts, which are also forms of fungi, do not have a branched appearance.

Metazoa and **Insecta** are multicellular parasites that affect humans. Metazoa include worms and flukes, and Insecta includes ticks, fleas, and *Sarcoptes scabiei* (which causes scabies) that transmit or cause disease.

The ability of the infectious agent to cause disease is called **pathogenicity.** Organisms that readily cause disease are said to be **virulent.** Organisms that cause disease only when the immunity in a host is low are called **opportunistic pathogens.** Knowledge of the characteristics of the various organisms helps humans construct strategies to keep infections at bay.

PATHWAYS OF INFECTION

The various routes by which organisms gain entrance to the body are protected by defense mechanisms. If these mechanisms are breached in some way, infection can occur. Once inside the body, the infection may spread directly via the bloodstream or lymphatics. One method of containing and preventing infections is to protect these pathways and maintain the barriers. Think of the various ways by which this protection can be achieved as the different pathways of infection are addressed.

Skin

Keratinized epithelium, sweat, and sebum are some protective barriers present in skin. When the continuity of skin is breached by laceration, burns, or reduced blood supply, the barrier is no longer effective, and the risk of infection increases.

Infection may be acquired through the skin *by direct physical contact* (e.g., herpes simplex, ringworm, impetigo), by *infection when the skin is disrupted* (e.g., tetanus), or *by injection into the skin by vectors* carrying infectious agents (e.g., malarial parasites injected by mosquitoes). Infections may also be acquired by *injection by humans,* such as transfusion of infected blood and blood products and contaminated needles. Certain infections are spread by *direct penetration of the skin by the infectious agent* (e.g., hookworm larvae).

Infection may also be transmitted *by indirect contact* with infected body fluids via towels, shared utensils, or bedding.

Respiratory Tract

Entry of pathogens through the respiratory tract is prevented by the presence of mucus and cilia that move the mucus toward the mouth. Defense cells, antibody secretions, and lymphoid tissue (tonsils) in the mouth and pharynx also protect the respiratory tract. Depression of the cough reflex by drugs; interference with ciliary transport, as in alcoholism, cold, and loss of ciliated cells as a result of smoking; and bronchial obstruction as a result of various causes can all contribute to the weakening of the barrier and an increased risk of infection. Inhalation of droplets carrying infectious agents is the usual mechanism of transmission.

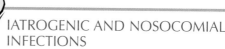

IATROGENIC AND NOSOCOMIAL INFECTIONS

Iatrogenic infection—an infection caused by diagnostic or therapeutic interventions, such as the insertion of a urethral or intravenous catheter.

Nosocomial infection—an infection occurring in a patient that was neither present nor incubating at the time of hospital admission.

Gastrointestinal Tract

This tract is protected by lysosomes, antibodies present in various secretions and the pH of secretions that are not conducive to growth and multiplication of microorganisms. The mucosal lining and the growth of natural intestinal flora in the colon also serve as a protective barrier. Entry of infectious agents through the gastrointestinal tract is via infected food and drink, including fecal contamination.

Genitourinary Tract

This tract is normally sterile. But risk of infection is increased by obstruction of urinary flow, catheterization, and alteration in normal flora by prolonged use of broad-spectrum antibiotics and others. Entry of infection through this tract is more common in women because of the shortness of the urethra.

Immunity and Massage

Taking a history of the immune status of every client is recommended. A detailed allergic history should also be taken to avoid the occurrence of an asthmatic attack or anaphylaxis. Certain chemicals in the massage oils or traces of detergents in linen or even certain essential oils may result in itching and rashes in allergic individuals. Therefore, proper pre-

✓ *Massage and Immunity*

By relieving stress, massage may boost the various functions of the immune system. The number of natural killer cells and their activity increase with massage, suggesting that massage may strengthen the immune system. A significant improvement in immune function has been shown in HIV-positive men after massage. This finding implies that massage can be used as an adjuvant therapy in those with immune-related disorders.

cautions should be taken when treating people with known allergy.

It is important for therapists to address the immune status of the client coming to the clinic. Individuals on dialysis, those undergoing chemotherapy or radiation therapy for cancer, those with AIDS, and the elderly are some examples of clients whose immune system may be depressed. Usually, a person with depressed immunity complains of recurrent infections, unexplained weight loss, and persistent fatigue. These clients should not receive treatment even when the therapist has a mild infection. Conversely, it is possible for immunocompromised individuals harboring infections such as tuberculosis to infect massage therapists. Suitable precautions must be taken.

When a client has a disease, one primary questions that must be addressed is, "Is this disease infectious?" If it is infectious, the therapist should have enough information about the condition to decide if massage is indicated or contraindicated. The therapist should be well informed about infectious diseases to recognize them and avoid further harm to the client, the therapist, and to other clients visiting the clinic. Clients with communicable infections should not be treated when the infection is active.

Therapists can use many simple strategies to prevent infection. All health professionals should consider immunization against diseases for which vaccines are available as a result of the working environment and frequent contact with those who are ill. Care of hands such as keeping fingernails short and frequent hand washing can be helpful disease prevention. Clean, well-ventilated clinics, with proper washing of linen and use of disinfectants can definitely control spread of disease. One of the most important strategies, however, is good, well-balanced nutrition; a healthy, active lifestyle; and a positive outlook in life.

REFERENCES

1. Andrade CK, Clifford P. Outcome-Based Massage. Baltimore: Lippincott Williams & Wilkins, 2001.
2. Foldi M. Anatomical and physiological basis for physical therapy of lymphodema. Experientia 1978;33(suppl):15–18.
3. Salvo SG. Massage Therapy. Principles & Practice. Philadelphia: W.B. Saunders, 1999.
4. Mason M. The treatment of lymphoedema by complex physical therapy. Aust J Physiotherapy 1993;39(1):41–45.
5. Pflug JJ. Intermittent compression in the management of swollen legs in general practice. Practitioner 1975;215:69–76.
6. Lerner R. What's new in lymphedema therapy in America? Int J Angiology 1998;7:191–196.
7. Airaksinen O, Kolari PJ, Pekanmaki K. Intermittent pneumatic compression therapy. Crit Rev Phys Rehabil Med 1992;3(3): 219–237.

SUGGESTED READINGS

Battezzati M. The Lymphatic System. Revised Ed. New York: John Wiley & Sons, 1972.
Jackson A. Massage therapy enhances the immune system. Nurs Times 1996;92(51):50.
Kenney RA. Physiology of Aging: A Synopsis. 2 Ed. Chicago: Year Book Medical, 1989.
Kinser C, Colby LA. Therapeutic Exercise: Foundations and Techniques. 2nd Ed. Philadelphia: F.A. Davis, 1990.
Kirshbaum M. Using massage in the relief of lymphoedema. Prof Nurse 1996;11(4):230–232.
Kuchera ML, Kuchera WA. Osteopathic Considerations in Systemic Dysfunction. Kirksville, MO: KCOM Press, 1991.
Pflug JJ. Intermittent compression; a new principle in treatment of wounds. Lancet 1974; ii (355):356.
Scull CW. Massage–Physiological basis. Arch Phys Med 1945;26: 159–167.
Starling EH. The influence of mechanical factors on lymph production. J Physiol 1894;16:224.
Wakim KG. Physiologic effects of massage. In: Licht S, ed. Massage, Manipulation and Traction. Huntington, NY: Robert E. Keirger, 1976:38–42.
Whinfield AL. The effect of massage on the swollen leg. J Brit Podiatr Med 1995;50(4):47–49.

Review Questions

Multiple Choice

1. The function of the lymphatic system includes all of the following EXCEPT
   A. draining interstitial fluid.
   B. transporting dietary lipids.
   C. protecting against foreign agents.
   D. producing red and white blood cells.

2. Humoral immunity primarily affects
   A. pathogens located intracellularly.
   B. cancer cells.
   C. pathogens located extracellularly.
   D. transplanted tissue.

3. Peyer's patches are found in the
   A. distal ileum.
   B. stomach.
   C. lymph nodes.
   D. tonsils.

4. The functions of the lymph nodes include all of the following EXCEPT
   A. Producing lymphocytes.
   B. Storing protein.
   C. Filtering lymph.
   D. Screening lymph for foreign agents.

5. The axillary lymph nodes drain lymph from all of the following regions EXCEPT the
   A. forearms.
   B. abdomen.
   C. hands.
   D. breasts.

6. The functions of the spleen include all of the following EXCEPT
   A. producing bile.
   B. destroying red blood cells.
   C. serving as a blood reservoir.
   D. forming bilirubin.

7. On comparing the primary and secondary immune responses, the secondary immune response
   A. occurs less rapidly than the primary response.
   B. produces a lower level of antibodies.
   C. is shorter.
   D. may be elicited years after the first antigen exposure.

8. Examples of nonspecific immunity include all of the following EXCEPT
   A. antibody production.
   B. fever.
   C. physical barriers.
   D. immunologic surveillance.

Fill-In

1. The two major body fluid compartments are the
   _____ and _____ compartments. The _____ compartment consists of the interstitial and vascular compartments.

2. Edema is a condition in which there is excessive fluid in the _____ fluid compartment.

3. The forces that result in movement of fluid *into* the capillaries include the intravascular osmotic pressure and _____. An increase in the hydrostatic pressure inside the capillaries will result in fluid movement _____ (into/out of) the capillaries.

4. The components of the lymphatic system include lymph vessels, _____, and
   _____.

5. _____ is the lymph node group located in the upper part of the thigh.

6. _____ are modified monocytes of the circulation that have wandered into the tissue.

7. The principal factors that help return lymph from tissue to the blood vessels in the neck are
   _____, _____,
   _____, and _____.

True–False
(Answer the following questions T, for true; or F, for false):

1. Infection can be acquired though direct physical contact with an infected person, injection into the skin by insects, and direct penetration of the skin by the infectious agent.

2. Opportunistic pathogens are organisms that affect a healthy individual if given the slightest opportunity.

3. Interstitial colloid osmotic pressure is generated by protein and other particles located in the interstitial compartment.

4. Lymphocytes are manufactured in the bone marrow.

5. The thoracic duct drains lymph from the right upper limb.

6. The spleen is located in the right upper quadrant of the abdomen.

7. Histamine causes local vasoconstriction.

8. Passive immunity is when a modified antigen is injected to provoke an immune reaction.

9. AIDS can be transmitted by sharing household items, such as clothes, with the infected individual.

10. Allergy is an inappropriate, excessive, or abnormal response to antigens.

11. Lymphatic vessels have one-way valves.

12. Lymph vessels communicate directly with adjacent blood vessels.

13. Each lymph capillary originates as a blind-ended tube.

14. The clinical characteristics of acute inflammation include pain, redness, swelling, and heat.

15. Antibodies are highly specific proteins also known as immunoglobulins.

Matching–A

1. _____ Cells capable of producing antibodies
2. _____ A substance secreted by mast cells that produces vasodilatation
3. _____ Antigens that help lymphocytes recognize cells belonging to self
4. _____ White blood cells that are capable of engulfing microorganisms

a. antibodies
b. antigens
c. histamine
d. complement system
e. cytokines
f. major histocompatibility complex
g. phagocytes
h. T cells

5. _____ Includes a number of inactive enzymes present in blood plasma
6. _____ Lymphocytes that are processed by the thymus
7. _____ Cells that recognize other cells that are foreign and destroys them
8. _____ Small proteins that can inhibit or facilitate normal cell functions such as cell growth and differentiation
9. _____ Glycoproteins that circulate in the blood as part of the globulin fraction; also known as immunoglobulins
10. _____ Substances recognized by the body as foreign that stimulate immune responses

i. plasma cells
j. natural killer cells

Matching–B
Match the immunity type to each clinical scenario.
1. _____ Mr. Jones has been given an injection of antibodies against a specific disease that is prevalent in the country he intends to visit.
2. _____ Three-month-old Kate is immune to some diseases because of the antibodies transmitted to her through breast milk.
3. _____ Polio drops have been administered to one-year-old John as part of the immunization schedule.
4. _____ Sara did not get chickenpox when her friend Jack did because she had chickenpox when she was nine.
5. _____ The entire company workforce is immunized against tetanus.

   a. artificially acquired active immunity
   b. artificially acquired passive immunity
   c. naturally acquired active immunity
   d. naturally acquired passive immunity

Short-Answer Questions
1. In what direction should massage strokes be applied to help drain lymph from the following areas:
   a. Lower limb
   b. Upper limb
   c. Face and scalp
2. What are lymph nodes?
3. Identify the location of at least 4 major lymph node groups in your body.

4. What is meant by
   a. passive immunity?
   b. active immunity?
   c. acquired immunity?
   d. innate immunity?
5. What is an antigen?
6. What is an antibody?
7. A massage therapist has inadvertently treated a person with tuberculosis. The therapist consults the physician, who advises a skin test. What is the basis of skin tests?
8. It is advisable for massage therapists to be immunized against some diseases. What is the basis for immunization?
9. List some diseases for which vaccines are available.
10. List three causes of disease.
11. How does manual lymphatic drainage help with lymph movement?

Case Studies
1. Mrs. Albright comes in for a relaxation massage. She had just returned the day before from a trip to Mexico. As she lies on the table, the therapist notices that Mrs. Albright's feet are swollen. "Definitely edematous," he tells himself. On questioning Mrs. Albright, he learns that the swelling had developed during the long flight. "At the rate at which the number of seats are being increased in each plane, we will soon be expected to sit cross-legged or sit on the floor to occupy less space," Mrs. Albright laughs.
   A. What is the cause of Mrs. Albright's swelling? Explain in terms of forces that affect fluid movement in and out of the interstitial compartment.
   B. Is massage of the feet indicated or contraindicated in this condition?
   C. Can massage help? If so, what are the massage techniques that you would use?
   D. What other questions would you ask Mrs. Albright if you were the therapist?

2. Mrs. Raman is a newer client at the clinic. She has come in at the insistence of her friend, Mrs. Albright. This lady is shy and always wears ankle-length dresses, no matter how hot the weather is. When the therapist gives the first massage, she discovers why Mrs. Raman is hesitant to expose her legs. Mrs. Raman's left leg looks like an elephant's leg: rough and huge, with large and distorted toes that have only enough toenail to indicate the presence of toes. The right leg is dainty and beautiful. Mrs. Raman reveals to the therapist that she contracted filariasis eight years ago, and her leg has been in this condition since then.

A. What kind of disease is filariasis? Is it infectious?

B. What causes the swelling in Mrs. Raman's case? Explain in terms of forces that affect fluid movement in and out of the interstitial compartment.

C. If the therapist chose to massage the leg, would she be infected?

3. Forty-year-old Kathleen had major breast cancer surgery one month ago. Her right breast was removed, together with extensive right axilla tissue. She has noticed that, following surgery, her right arm becomes swollen toward the end of the day. Kathleen has been told to keep her arm elevated above heart level as often as possible. Kathleen also notices that massage helps relieve the aching, heaviness, and pain she experiences in her arm by day's end.

A. Why did Kathleen's right limb swell?

B. What caused the heaviness and pain?

C. How is this swelling related to surgery?

D. What causes Kathleen's swelling? Explain in terms of forces that affect fluid movement in and out of the interstitial compartment.

E. How does massage help?

F. What other treatment may help reduce the Kathleen's swelling?

4. Mr. Joseph is a chronic alcoholic. He quit drinking six months ago, after joining Alcoholic Anonymous. Alcoholism, however, has taken its toll. Mr. Joseph has the biggest potbelly the therapist has seen. Mr. Joseph's enlarged abdomen is not a result of a thick layer of fat, but a result of fluid collected in the peritoneal cavity. His face is puffy and his legs are mildly swollen. The therapist knows that Mr. Joseph has been diagnosed with liver disease.

A. In this case, how is the edema related to the liver problem? Explain in terms of forces that affect fluid movement in and out of the interstitial compartment.

B. Can massage help reduce Mr. Joseph's edema?

5. Mr. Labat is a client who had a heart attack last year. He seemed well every time he came in for a massage and is a cheerful man, with a smile for every one. The therapist looks forward to Mr. Labat's appointments because he always tells interesting stories. On this occasion, the therapist notices that Mr. Labat's legs are swollen. She also notes some edema around his lower back. Mr. Labat states that he has been having pain on his left shoulder for the past week, along with mild swelling in his legs every night. He is going to see his physician the next week.

A. Given Mr. Labat's medical history, what could be the reason for his left shoulder pain?

B. What could be the cause of Mr. Labat's swelling? Explain in terms of forces that affect fluid movement in and out of the interstitial compartment.

C. Should the therapist treat all edema the same way?

6. Mrs. Cartier, one of the therapist's regular clients in the six years after opening her practice, was recently diagnosed with AIDS.

The therapist noticed that Mrs. Cartier had lost a lot of weight since her last pregnancy, which she attributed to complications during labor. Mrs. Cartier had lost large quantities of blood during labor 10 months ago and had been given many blood transfusions soon after. Following the pregnancy, Mrs. Cartier always felt ill, and her physician had ordered tests. Two months ago, Mrs. Cartier had been informed that she had AIDS—possibly contracted through contaminated blood received during blood transfusions. The therapist has read and heard a lot about AIDS, but never before had a client with AIDS.

A. What issues does a therapist have to deal with?

B. If you were the therapist, would you continue to treat Mrs. Cartier? If not, why? If yes, what precautions must you take?

C. What background knowledge about AIDS will you require to treat this client?

6. The therapist attended a 2-day workshop on aromatherapy, and she is excited about all the new products she has splurged on. She bought many kinds of little bottles with exotic names, each capable of producing a totally different aroma. She decided that she would try some on Gina, her first client of the day.

After about 10 minutes of the massage session, Gina complains of an itching sensation all over her body. "Do you think something from the sheets is causing the itch?" Gina inquires.

"No, I don't think so." The therapist replies. "But I can change the sheets if you like." When Gina lies down on the fresh sheets, to her dismay, the therapist notices that Gina's back and legs, which had just been massaged, were beginning to turn an angry red, with localized areas of swelling.

A. What is happening to Gina?

B. How could the therapist have avoided this situation?

C. How should she deal with the present situation?

D. What could be the cause of Gina's swelling ? Explain in terms of forces that affect fluid movement in and out of the interstitial compartment.

8. The young physician, newly appointed in the rural area where the therapist worked, is enthusiastic and sincere. He cares about the community and wants to concentrate more on preventive medicine. The therapist learns through the grapevine that the physician is going to recommend that all women—especially those of reproductive age—are immunized against German measles. The therapist has not been immunized. Some of her clients expressed concern because they heard that immunization can produce adverse effects.
   A. What is immunization?
   B. How does it work?
   C. Against which diseases can an individual be immunized?
   D. Should therapists be immunized against specific diseases?
   E. What are the potential adverse effects of immunization?

Answers to Review Questions

Multiple Choice

1. D. The lymphatic tissue manufactures lymphocytes, a type of white blood cell. Red blood cells are not manufactured in the lymphatic system.
2. C
3. A
4. B
5. B
6. A. Bile is produced by the liver. Bilirubin, a breakdown product of red blood cells, is a component of bile.
7. D
8. A

Fill–In

1. intracellular, extracellular, extracellular
2. interstitial
3. interstitial hydrostatic pressure, out of
4. lymph, lymph organs, lymphocytes
5. Inguinal
6. Macrophages
7. presence of one-way valves, passive and active movement of skeletal muscles, pulsation of adjacent arteries, respiratory movements

True–False

1. True
2. False. These organisms do not normally infect healthy individuals. They can be pathogenic in immunodeficient individuals.
3. True
4. True
5. False. The lymph flows into the right lymphatic duct from the right upper limb.
6. False. The spleen is located in the left upper quadrant. The liver is located in the right.
7. False. The primary effect of histamine is to relax the smooth muscle of blood vessels and make the capillaries more permeable.
8. False. The description is that of active immunity. In passive immunity, the immune system is not challenged.
9. False
10. True
11. True
12. False, Only the thoracic duct and the right lymphatic duct communicate directly with the vein.
13. True
14. True
15. True

Matching–A

1. i   2. c   3. f   4. g
5. d   6. h   7. j   8. e
9. a   10. b

Matching–B

1. b   2. d   3. a   4. c   5. a

Short-Answer Questions

1. a. Toward the thigh. The proximal region should be worked on first before proceeding to distal areas.
   b. Toward the axilla. The proximal region should be worked on first before proceeding to distal areas.
   c. Toward the neck.
2. Lymph nodes are small organs, surrounded by a capsule. They filter large particles and remove foreign substances before the lymph drains into the veins. They are also centers of proliferation of immune cells.
3. Major groups of lymph nodes include the axillary, cervical, abdominal, thoracic, and inguinal lymph nodes.
4. a. Passive immunity results from infusion of already formed antibodies into an individual. It does not stimulate the immune system.

b. Active immunity is produced when an individual is normally or artificially exposed to the foreign agent.

c. Acquired immunity is not present from birth, but obtained later.

d. Innate immunity is genetically determined.

5. An antigen is a foreign agent that provokes an immune response.

6. An antibody or immunoglobulin is a protein produced by the plasma cells that is specific to an antigen.

7. In a skin test, a small amount of altered antigen is subcutaneously introduced. If the person has been previously exposed to the antigen, inflammation is produced in the area of injection. The presence of inflammation and the timing of its appearance determine whether a person has been previously exposed to this particular antigen.

8. The basis of immunization is the reaction of the body when exposed to altered antigens.

9. Some examples are measles, mumps, rubella, tetanus, hepatitis, and influenzae.

10. Causes include impaired immune responses; genetic abnormalities; impaired energy production; metabolic toxic, physical, chemical, and infectious agents; and abnormal development and growth.

11. In manual lymphatic drainage, mechanical compression moves lymph toward the heart.

Case Studies

1. A, The swelling is a result of the pressure put on the veins in the back of legs as one sits. Lymph flow relies on muscle movement. When seated on the plane, it was unlikely that Mrs. Albright could move freely. The effects of gravity also play a part in reducing venous return. As a result, plasma hydrostatic pressure increases, resulting in edema.

   B, She can be massaged, provided that she is not at risk for venous thrombosis.

   C, Massage, especially manual lymphatic drainage, would be helpful.

   D, The therapist should rule out all other causes of edema by taking careful history.

1. A, Filariasis is a parasitic infection transmitted by the bite of an infected mosquito.

   B, The swelling is a result of inefficient lymphatic drainage. The filarial worm lodges in the lymph nodes, producing an inflammatory reaction. This reaction, in turn, affects drainage in the local area. The accumulation of fluid, together with the protein in the interstitial compartment, is responsible for the signs and symptoms of infection. The protein increases the interstitial colloid osmotic pressure, drawing more fluid into the interstitial compartment.

   C, The therapist will not become infected because the parasite is transmitted by the bite of a mosquito.

3. A, Kathleen's right upper limb swells because of improper lymph drainage resulting from axillary lymph node removal.

   B, The pain and heaviness is a result of fluid accumulation, toxins, and waste products from the tissue in the region.

   C, and D, The cause of edema is the same as in case study two—inadequate lymph drainage.

   E, Massage would help by manually removing lymph from the area and facilitating drainage. The other positive effects of massage, such as reduction of stress and sedation, would be beneficial.

   F, Elevation of the limb, use of intermittent pneumatic devices, and use of elastic stockings are some other forms of treatment. Surgery is another option for severe cases.

4. A, The liver manufactures plasma protein. Plasma protein contributes extensively to the colloid osmotic pressure in plasma that draws fluid into the capillaries. In liver disease, plasma protein levels drop, increasing the movement of fluid into the interstitial compartment.

   B, Massage may not be beneficial in reducing Mr. Joseph's edema.

5. A, Mr. Labat may be exhibiting signs of heart failure. Typically, pain originating from the heart is referred to the left side of the chest, left shoulder, and down the arm.

   B, The swelling may also be a sign of cardiac failure. When the heart is unable to push the blood out of the ventricles, blood tends to dam up in the proximal areas. For example, if the right heart fails, blood accumulates in the veins, resulting in liver enlargement and fluid accumulation in the lower limbs.

   C, It is important for therapists to determine the cause of edema before treating a client. In Mr. Labat's case, massage may help get fluid back into the veins and overload the heart, making the condition worse.

6. A, Many issues need to be dealt with in this case: How comfortable is the therapist with treating people with AIDS? What is the therapist's attitude toward people with AIDS? How knowledgeable is the therapist about AIDS and its transmission? What are the signs and symptoms? What is the course of

the disease? Based on all issues, it is up to the therapist to decide whether she can provide quality treatment to the client.

B, Some precautions that must be taken include the avoidance of direct contact with bodily secretions. The therapist should use protective barriers if necessary. Contact with clients should be avoided if the therapist has open cuts, wounds, ulcers, or dermatitis with open lesions. If the therapist is inadvertently exposed to the client's blood or body fluids, the area should be scrubbed with 10% povidone iodine and washed with water for 10 minutes or more, and the therapist should report to a medical service as soon as possible.

C, The therapist should be knowledgeable about the disease course; the mode of transmission of HIV; the signs, symptoms and complications of AIDS; and treatment and adverse effects.

7. A, Gina is probably having an allergic reaction. It is important to obtain a thorough medical history before massaging a client. Extra precaution needs to be taken with those with history of any form of allergy.

B, The therapist should have tested the client for an allergic reaction to this new product by applying a minute amount to a small area of skin before using it over the entire body.

C, The product should be removed and the skin quickly washed. If the reaction is mild, antihistamines may be helpful. If the reaction is extensive, medical help should be sought. If the client goes into shock, medical help should be called immediately.

D, During an allergic reaction, antigens attach to sensitized mast cells, causing release of hista-

mine and other chemical mediators that increase capillary permeability. Blood vessels dilate, increasing blood flow and capillary hydrostatic pressure (pushes fluid into the interstitial compartment). Plasma protein moves into the interstitial compartment through the permeable capillaries (increases interstitial osmotic pressure, drawing out fluid).

8. A, Immunization or vaccination is the process of developing immunity against a specific foreign agent.

B, It can be performed in two ways. In some cases, antibodies produced outside the body against a specific agent are injected to provide temporary immunity. In most vaccines, small quantities of a foreign agent are modified to nullify its virulence. The agent is injected into the body to prompt the manufacture of antibodies.

C, There are a wide range of diseases against which immunization is available, including measles, mumps, rubella, polio, whooping cough, tetanus, meningitis, and typhoid.

D, Because therapists come in contact with many clients, it may be wise to be immunized against infectious diseases (for which immunization is available) that are prevalent in the country in which they work. All therapists should receive the recommended tetanus boosters.

E, Usually, vaccine adverse effects are minor and localized to the site of injection. Redness, pain, and mild fever are some common adverse effects. Adverse effects vary with the type of immunization. It is important to research an individual vaccine's adverse effects before vaccination.

Coloring Exercise

On the diagram, identify the structures indicated by label lines. Shade the area of the body supplied by the right lymphatic duct using your favorite color. Color all lymph nodes blue.

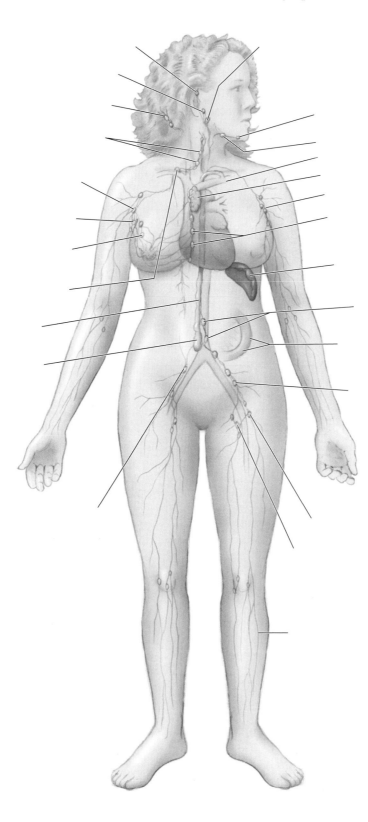

CHAPTER 10

Respiratory System

Objectives **On completion of this chapter, the reader should be able to:**

- List the functions of the respiratory system.
- Explain how the body is protected from debris and pathogens entering through the respiratory tract.
- Identify the components of the respiratory tract and describe the function(s) of each component.
- Identify the factors that affect the caliber (diameter/size) of the bronchi and bronchioles.
- Define the various lung volumes and capacities.
- Describe the origin, insertion, and actions of the muscles involved in respiratory movement.
- Describe the physiological processes involved in the exchange of gases in external and internal respiration.
- Explain how Boyle's law, Henry's law and Dalton's law apply to the exchange and transport of gases in the body.
- Describe the pulmonary circulation.
- Explain how oxygen is transported in the blood.
- Explain how carbon dioxide is transported in the blood.
- Identify the factors that affect the transport of oxygen by hemoglobin.
- Describe the oxygen-hemoglobin dissociation curve and the effect of various factors such as pH, CO_2 levels, and hydrogen ions.
- Describe respiration control and regulation.
- Identify the factors that affect the rate and depth of respiration.
- Describe the effects of exercise on the respiratory system.
- Describe the effects of aging on the respiratory system.
- Describe the effects of smoking on the respiratory system.
- Describe the effects of massage on the respiratory system.
- Explain the role of postural drainage before and during massage.
- Identify the special techniques used in association with postural drainage.

E*very living cell in the body requires energy to maintain and perform its functions. Most cells use oxygen for metabolizing nutrients to produce this energy. In the process, carbon dioxide is produced. The body needs to constantly replenish the used oxygen and eliminate the carbon dioxide. The cardiovascular system circulates the blood, providing the required oxygen and removing the carbon dioxide from the tissues. Simulta-neously, it transports the blood to the respiratory system, which replenishes the oxygen and removes the carbon dioxide by diffusion of gases between air and blood.*

For diffusion to occur easily, the structure in question has to be thin and delicate, with a wide surface area. It should also be protected because such a structure becomes vulnerable to attack by pathogens. In ad-

dition, exposure of a wide surface area to air can lead to excessive loss of water by evaporation. The architecture of the human respiratory system deals with all these issues as it carries out its function.

This chapter describes the structures of the respiratory system and the physiologic processes involved in carrying out its important functions.

Functions of the Respiratory System

The primary function of the respiratory system is to *provide* the required *oxygen* and *remove carbon dioxide* from the body. By the removal of carbon dioxide, this system helps *maintain the pH of the blood* at 7.4. Another important respiratory system function is to help with the *production of sound* (e.g., speaking, singing).

The upper part of the respiratory system houses the sensory receptors for *smell,* which are stimulated by chemicals present in the air the body breathes. The respiratory system helps eliminate *some water and heat* as air is breathed in and out. The movement of the respiratory muscles and the resultant changes in volume and pressure inside the thoracic cavity *help increase venous return and lymphatic drainage.* In addition to these functions, certain cells in the respiratory system help *activate angiotensin I,* a hormone involved in regulating blood pressure and volume (see page 411).

The Anatomy of the Respiratory System

The respiratory system is made up of passages that conduct air from the environment into the body and respiratory surfaces that are involved in gas exchange. The respiratory system is classically divided into the **upper** and **lower respiratory tracts.** The upper respiratory tract includes the **nose, nasal cavity, paranasal sinus,** and the **pharynx** (throat). The lower respiratory tract (larynx and below) includes all structures below the pharynx and includes the **larynx** (voice box), **trachea** (wind pipe), **bronchi, bronchioles,** and the **alveoli** of the lungs (see Figure 10.1). Functionally, the respiratory system can be classified as the conducting part and the respiratory part. The conducting part includes those structures that are only involved in conducting the air from the atmosphere to the lungs. All structures from the nose to the last part of the bronchioles belong to this category. The respiratory part includes the structures where gas exchange takes place and includes the last part of the bronchioles and distal structures.

UPPER RESPIRATORY TRACT

The Nose and Nasal Cavity

The air that reaches the lungs enters the body through the **nose.** The external part of the nose is made up of bone, hyaline cartilage, muscle, adipose tissue, and skin and is lined internally by mucous membrane. The superior part of the nose is bony; made up of the frontal, nasal, and maxillary bones. The inferior part is cartilaginous and more flexible. The openings on the inferior aspect of the nose are known as the **nostrils,** or **external nares.** The nostrils open internally into a wider area known as the **nasal cavity** (see Figure 10.2). The nasal cavity is divided into the right and the left regions by the **nasal septum.** The anterior and inferior portion of the nasal septum is made of hyaline cartilage (feel it); the superior part is made up of bone. Inferiorly, the nasal cavity is separated from the oral cavity by the maxillary and palatine bones; this is the **hard palate,** the hard portion of the roof of the mouth. From the posterior part of the hard palate, a fleshy partition—the **soft palate**—separates the pharynx into the **nasopharynx** and **oropharynx.**

The first portion of the nasal cavity widens into the **vestibule,** which is the part seen when looking up the nostrils. This region is covered with coarse hair that extends across the nostrils and helps prevent larger particles, such as sand and sawdust, from entering the nasal cavity.

The nasal cavity is divided into smaller chambers by three, irregular, shelflike projections from the lateral wall of the nose known as the **superior, middle,** and **inferior conchae.** The air passes through the passages—the **superior, middle,** and **inferior meatus**—that are present between the conchae. The meandering, turbulent pathway for air created by the conchae helps churn the air that has entered and enables large particles to stick to the mucus lining, slowing entry and providing sufficient time for the air to be altered to the body temperature and become saturated with water. In addition, the eddy produced carries air to the superior region of the nasal cavity

DEVIATED SEPTUM

The nasal septum may be located more to the left or to the right in certain individuals, which may be responsible for the frequent nasal block and congestion these individuals experience. In certain individuals, a deviated septum may cause them to snore.

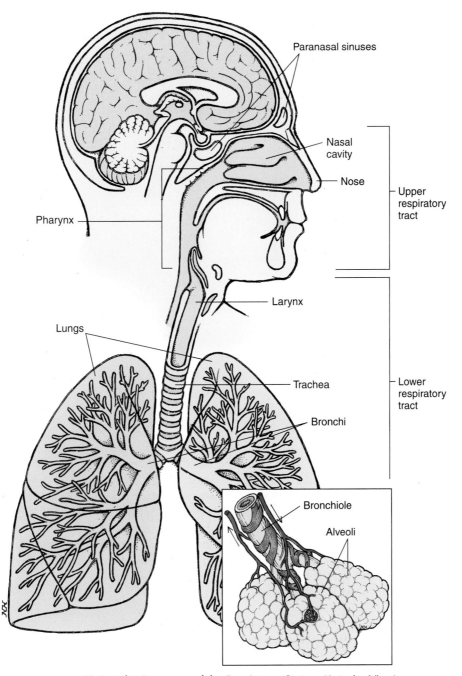

FIGURE **10.1.**   The Structures of the Respiratory System (Anterior View)

where the smell receptors (**olfactory receptors**) are located. The posterior part of the nasal cavity opens into the pharynx through the **internal nares.**

Other than the external and internal nares, the nasal cavity has many other openings. The **nasolacrimal duct**—the tear duct that opens into the nose from the conjunctiva of the eye. This is the reason why the nose becomes "leaky" when a person cries. The tears that enter the nose keep the cavity moist. The openings of the **paranasal sinus** are located in the nose.

The Nasal Epithelium

The nasal epithelium, or mucosa, is suited to clean the air that enters the nasal cavity and to bring it to body temperature and humidity. As mentioned, coarse hair prevents large particles from entering. The epithelium is a **stratified squamous type** that can withstand abrasion and friction. Then the epithelium changes to **pseudostratified ciliated columnar epithelium.** The cilia, tiny hairlike projections on the cell membrane, move rhythmically in one direction.

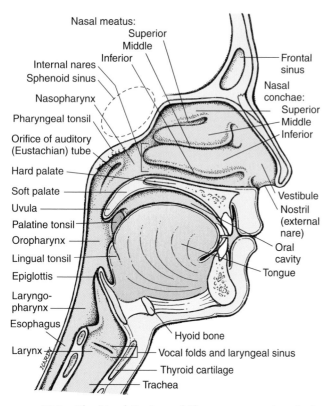

FIGURE **10.2.** The Nasal Cavity and Pharynx as seen in a Sagittal Section of the Head with Nasal Septum Removed

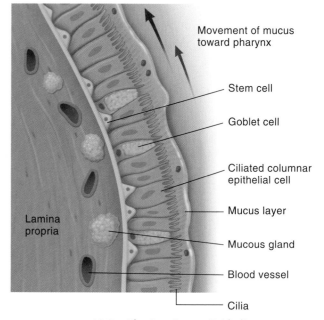

FIGURE **10.3.** The Respiratory Epithelium

Interspersed among the ciliated columnar cells are **goblet cells,** which secrete a sticky mucus (see Figure 10.3). The cilia of the epithelium help move the mucus, together with any adhering dust and pathogens, toward the back of the nose. The movement of the cilia and mucus, similar to the movement of a conveyor belt, is sometimes referred to as the mucous escalator. From the back of the nose, the mucus enters the pharynx and is eventually swallowed.

The connective tissue lining the epithelium (**lamina propria**) contains many **mucous glands,** which secrete mucus into the nasal cavity, and a large network of blood vessels. These vessels help bring warm blood close to the surface. This mechanism helps warm and humidify the cool, dry air that enters. This process is important because the body can lose a lot of heat and moisture via the breathed air. Animals,

such as dogs, use this mechanism for cooling the body by panting.

The Olfactory Mucosa

The superior part of the nasal cavity has specialized tissue that contains the nerve endings of the first cranial nerve—the olfactory nerve. These nerve endings, receptors for the sense of smell, are located along the superior nasal conchae, the superior portion of the nasal septum, and the inferior part of the cribriform plate (see Figure 10.4). The receptors are stimulated by chemicals in the air that dissolve in the mucous

Bleeding Nose
The extensive network of blood vessels in the nose is responsible for the nosebleeds that commonly occur. Nosebleeds, also known as **epistaxis,** are more common in individuals who have allergies, bleeding disorders, hypertension, or upper respiratory tract infections.

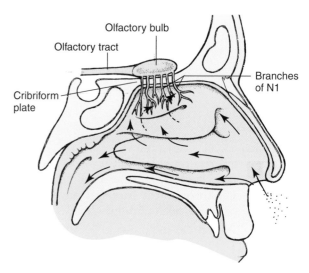

FIGURE **10.4.** The Location of the Olfactory Nerves. The location of the olfactory nerve on the left side of the nasal cavity with the septum removed.

secretion. The olfactory nerves penetrate the tiny openings in the cribriform plate and carry the sense of smell to the brain. To get a better sense of a smell, we sniff forcefully to draw air in and reach the portion of the nasal cavity that houses the olfactory epithelium (also see **page 356**).

Paranasal Sinus

The paranasal sinus (see Figure 10.5), or air cells of the nose, are cavities present in the lateral and superior walls of the nasal cavity. The **sphenoid sinus**—located posteriorly and superiorly—is closely related to the pituitary gland; therefore, the pituitary gland is often approached for surgery through the nasal cavity and the sphenoid sinus. The paired **maxillary sinus** are located in the maxillary bones. The maxillary sinus have a greater tendency to become inflamed (sinusitis) because the sinus opening to the nasal cavity is located closer to the roof of the sinus (rather than the floor), making drainage more difficult. There are many **ethmoid sinus** located in the ethmoid bone in the superior and posterior part of the nasal cavity. The **frontal sinus** are located deep to the medial part of the eyebrows. All of these sinus are air-filled cavities that communicate with the nasal cavity, and they are lined by the same epithelium as the rest of the nasal cavity.

The sinus help humidify and heat the air that enters the body. In addition, they lighten the weight of

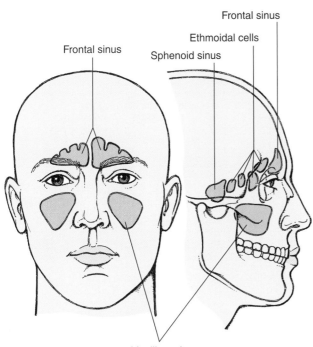

FIGURE **10.5.** Sectional Anatomy of the Skull, Showing the Paranasal Sinus Location

> ### 💡 EUSTACHIAN TUBE AND HEARING
>
> The opening and closure of the eustachian tubes are responsible for the sudden change in hearing (popping in the ears) that occurs when swimming under water or ascending to high altitudes.
>
> When a person has a cold or sore throat, the inflammation and edema in the pharynx can result in closure of the eustachian tube opening and may affect hearing. With time, the air in the tube may get absorbed into the blood vessels, producing a partial vacuum in the region and severe ear pain. The latter is more common in babies because the opening is small. In babies, because the short eustachian tube makes it easier for infections in the throat to spread to the ear, middle ear infection often accompanies upper respiratory tract infection.

the head. The resonance produced as a result of their presence gives the voice its specific characteristics.

The Pharynx

The region that extends between the posterior part of the nasal cavity—the internal nares and the larynx—is known as the **pharynx** (Figure 10.2). Both the respiratory and digestive systems share part of this region. The superior wall of the pharynx is in close contact with the axial skeleton; the lateral walls are muscular. The pharynx is divided into three parts: the **nasopharynx,** the **oropharynx,** and the **laryngopharynx** (Figures 10.1 and 10.2).

Nasopharynx

The nasopharynx region extends between the internal nares and the soft palate and lies superior to the oral cavity. Some lymphoid tissue—the **pharyngeal tonsils** or the **adenoids**—are located in the posterior wall.

The **Eustachian tubes,** or **auditory tubes,** which connect the middle ear to the pharynx, open into the nasopharynx. The opening opens and closes, equalizing the air pressure in the middle ear to that of the atmosphere. This is needed for proper conduction of sound during hearing.

Oropharynx

The oropharynx is the region of the pharynx that is common for the passage of food and air. This region lies between the soft palate and the base of tongue. The epithelium lining the oropharnyx changes from the delicate, pseudostratified ciliated columnar of the nasopharynx to the rugged, stratified squamous epithelium because there is scope for abrasion and friction from food. The posterior part of the tongue contains some lymphoid tissue—the **lingual tonsils.** The

Laryngitis

Infection of the larynx (laryngitis) is often accompanied by hoarseness of the voice as a result of vocal cord inflammation. Acute, severe swelling in the larynx, especially in children, can be dangerous because it can block off the glottis and obstruct air passage.

palatine tonsils are located to the side. Thus, the tonsils prevent passage of pathogens beyond this point.

Laryngopharynx, or Hypopharynx

The inferior most region of the pharynx is the laryngopharynx. The larynx is located anterior to the laryngopharynx.

LOWER RESPIRATORY TRACT

The Larynx

The larynx, or voice box (see Figure 10.6), is the region that connects the pharynx to the trachea (windpipe). It can be felt just below the jaw in the upper, anterior part of the neck. The larynx is largely carti-

lage, with ligaments and muscles attached. The **epiglottis, thyroid cartilage,** and **cricoid cartilage** are the larger cartilages. The epiglottis, located internally close to the base of the tongue, is shaped like a shoehorn. With each swallow, it moves posteriorly to close the narrow opening of the larynx (the **glottis**) to prevent entry of food into the larynx.

The thyroid cartilage is shaped like a shield and is commonly known as the Adam's apple. It forms the anterior and lateral wall of the larynx. Superiorly, ligaments attach the thyroid cartilage to the hyoid bone. Inferiorly, ligaments attach it to the cricoid cartilage. The cricoid cartilage is ring-shaped and is, in turn, inferiorly attached to the cartilage of the trachea (Figure 10.6).

Vocal Cords

Other smaller cartilages—**arytenoids, cuneiform,** and **corniculate,** elastic ligaments, and tiny muscles are located in the larynx. Two elastic ligaments, known as the **true vocal cords,** extend between the thyroid cartilage and arytenoid cartilage and go across the glottis. These ligaments are stretched and relaxed by laryngeal muscles that move the cartilage. The air that passes through the opening vibrates the vocal cords and produces sound. The size of the glot-

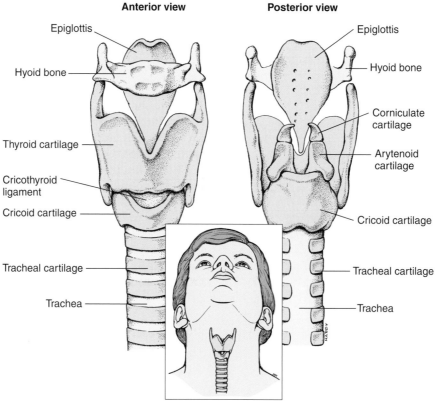

FIGURE **10.6.**   The Larynx

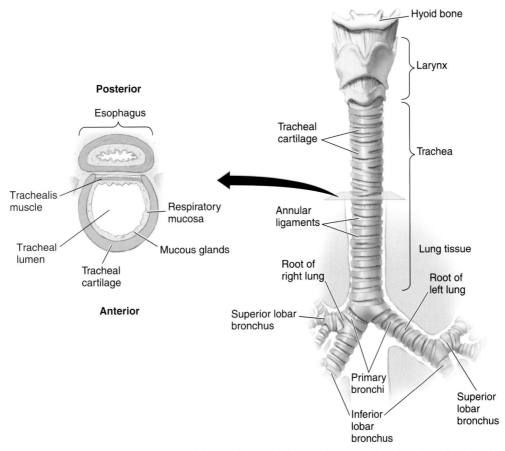

FIGURE **10.7.** Transverse Section of the Trachea and the Esophagus and trachea (anterior views)

tis and the length and tension of the vocal cords determine the pitch of the sound produced. In males at puberty, the larynx enlarges in size and the vocal cords thicken and lengthen, making the voice deeper and lower pitched. Just superior to the true vocal cords are folds of mucosa known as the **false vocal cords,** or **ventricular folds.** The mucosa inferior to the vocal cords is lined with pseudostratified ciliated columnar epithelium.

The sound production in the larynx is known as **phonation.** However, for words to be formed, this sound must be modified by **articulation.** Articulation requires voluntary muscle movement of the lips, cheeks, and tongue, etc. The pharynx, mouth, nasal cavity, and sinus act as resonating chambers.

Cough Reflex

The larynx contains sensitive nerves that trigger the cough reflex if large particles inadvertently enter this region. The cough reflex results in deep inspiration, followed by contraction of the expiratory muscles, with the glottis closed and the vocal cords tightened. This results in increased lung pressure. Suddenly, the glottis is opened, allowing a forceful blast of air to come through, dislodging the irritant from the laryngeal region into the pharynx and beyond.

The Trachea

The trachea (Figures 10.1 and 10.7) is a tube about 11 cm (4.3 in) long and 2.5 cm (1 in) wide. It extends from the cricoid cartilage to the T5 vertebra, where it branches in two—the **right** and **left primary bronchi.** It is kept patent by 16–20 C-shaped cartilage (the opening of the C faces posteriorly), attached to each other by ligaments. The posterior part of the trachea is closed off by a smooth muscle, the **trachealis** muscle. The cartilage prevents the trachea from collapsing every time there is a pressure change produced between the inside of the trachea and the atmosphere (in the neck region) as one breathes. The

---

INTUBATION

In certain situations, a tube is passed via the pharynx and through the glottis to open the respiratory passage. This procedure is known as intubation.

softer, posterior aspect of the trachea allows for expansion of the esophagus as food passes.

The Bronchi and Bronchioles

The trachea branches into the right and left **primary bronchi** at the level of the second costal cartilage at the sternal angle (superior border of the fifth thoracic vertebra) in the mediastinum. Both bronchi have cartilage similar to the trachea, with the right bronchus wider and more in line with the trachea. Therefore, foreign particles that enter the trachea (a rare occurrence) tend to lodge in this bronchus. The bronchi enter the lungs at the **hilus,** the medial region of the lung, through which blood vessels, nerves, lymphatics, and bronchi enter.

The primary bronchi divide repeatedly to form smaller bronchi and **bronchioles.** The bronchi located outside the lungs are known as **extrapulmonary bronchi** and the remainder, **intrapulmonary bronchi.** The primary bronchi divide into three on the right and two on the left known as **lobar,** or **secondary bronchi.** Each bronchus moves air in and out of the respective **lobes** of the lungs (see below). The lobar bronchi become smaller and branch again to form the **tertiary,** or **segmental bronchi.** The tertiary bronchi branch further to form tiny, **terminal bronchioles,** which are about 0.3–0.5 mm (0.01–0.02 in) wide. The terminal bronchioles are continuous with the **respiratory bronchiole,** which are the thinnest and most delicate of bronchioles.

The lung tissue supplied by each tertiary bronchi is called a **bronchopulmonary segment.** There are ten bronchopulmonary segments in each lung, each made of many lobules. Each lobule (see Figure 10.8) is wrapped in elastic connective tissue and has an arteriole, venule, lymphatic vessel, and a branch from the terminal bronchiole. If there are tumors or abscesses in any bronchopulmonary segment, the segment can be surgically removed without affecting the surrounding lung tissue. Knowledge of the direction of bronchi supplying the segments helps therapists facilitate drainage of secretions from specific segments by changing the posture of the patient.

All structures from the nasal cavity to the terminal bronchiole serve only as conducting passages for the air that enters. Exchange of gases between the air

and the blood only takes place in the region of the respiratory bronchioles and beyond.

Bronchial Smooth Muscle and Its Control

Bronchi walls lose cartilage as they branch and become smaller. Instead, the walls have more smooth muscle. Contraction and relaxation of these smooth muscles alter the caliber of the bronchi and bronchioles regulating the volume of air entering different regions of the lungs. The smooth muscles of the bronchi and bronchioles are innervated by the autonomic system. The sympathetic nerves relax the smooth muscles and increase the caliber of the passages, making it easier for air to enter the lungs; the parasympathetic nerves have the opposite action. In addition to nerves, chemicals such as leukotrienes and substance P, secreted locally by white blood cells and other cells, and CO_2 levels have an effect on bronchial smooth muscles. This is why asthma tends to worsen during, or soon after, respiratory infections in which white blood cell activity is increased. Also, allergen exposure and resultant inflammation can trigger an asthmatic attack.

The Alveoli

The respiratory bronchioles are connected to larger spaces, called **alveolar ducts,** into which open smaller chambers known as the **alveoli** (Figure 10.8). The alveoli (singular, alveolus) are lined by a single layer of squamous cells. The alveoli walls contain elastic fibers that help reduce the volume of the alveoli when air is breathed out. The alveoli give the lungs a spongy appearance. The alveoli increase the surface area for exchange of gases; each lung contains about 150 million alveoli. The total surface area made available for gas exchange by the alveoli is approximately 150 m² (179 yd²). The alveoli are surrounded by an extensive network of capillaries. Thus, the air that enters the alveoli is separated from the blood by only the thin, single layer of endothelium of the capillaries, a basement membrane, and the thin wall of the alveoli—a distance of about 0.1μm. These layers that separate air from blood are known as the **respiratory membrane.**

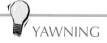

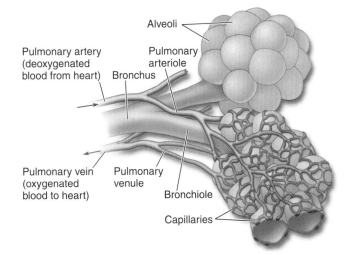

FIGURE **10.8.**   A Portion of a Lobule of the Lung

Labels (left to right / top to bottom): Alveoli; Pulmonary arteriole; Pulmonary arteriole; Bronchus; Pulmonary artery (deoxygenated blood from heart); Pulmonary vein (oxygenated blood to heart); Pulmonary venule; Bronchiole; Capillaries

Alveoli Defense and Lubrication

Many macrophages patrol the alveoli and eliminate pathogens that have escaped other defense mechanisms of the respiratory system.

The thin, moist lining of the spherical alveoli tends to collapse and stick together because of surface tension. (Surface tension is the force produced by the attraction of water molecules to each other. When water surrounds gas, the attraction between the water molecules rather than between air and water, produces a force that is directed inward. It is surface tension that causes a drop of water to attain a spherical shape.) Specialized cells, known as **type II cells, septal cells,** or **surfactant cells,** produce an oily secretion (**surfactant**), which lubricates and reduces the surface tension of the liquid coating the alveoli. Surfactant is a detergentlike mixture of phospholipids and lipoprotein. If not present in sufficient amounts, it will be difficult for air to enter the alveoli, similar to the difficulty faced when two, wet, glass surfaces, placed one over the other, are pried apart. In the absence of surfactant, the alveoli tend to collapse during expiration.

THE PULMONARY CIRCULATION

The blood reaching the alveoli is that of the pulmonary circulation (see **page 463**). Blood that has circulated through the body, with most of the oxygen removed, enters the right atrium via the superior and inferior vena cava and proceeds to the right ventricle. Contraction of the right ventricle pumps this blood into the pulmonary trunk. The pulmonary trunk divides into right and left pulmonary arteries, which take the blood to the right and left lungs, respectively. As in all organs, the arteries divide to form arterioles and capillaries. It is this network of capillaries that surround the alveoli and participate in gas exchange. The capillaries join and rejoin to form venules and veins. Ultimately, four pulmonary veins (**Figure 8.7**) transport the oxygenated blood into the left atrium, where they enter the left ventricle and then are pumped into the aorta and distributed to the rest of the body. Bronchial arteries—branches from the aorta—bring oxygenated blood to the bronchi and other lung tissue. Most blood from the bronchial arteries returns to the heart via the pulmonary veins. Some reach the heart through veins that ultimately reach the heart via the superior vena cava.

The blood vessels in the lungs, unlike those in other tissue, constrict when there is less oxygen in the surrounding region. This is advantageous because it helps direct blood to better-ventilated parts of the lung.

THE LUNGS

The paired lungs are organs comprised of bronchi, bronchioles, alveoli, connective tissue, blood vessels, lymphatics, and nerves (see Figure 10.9). The right and left lungs are situated on either side of the **mediastinum** (the part of the thoracic cavity that lies between the lungs). The lung is somewhat conical, with the apex projecting just above the first rib. The base of the lung is related to the superior surface of the diaphragm, which separates the thorax from the abdomen. The lungs take the same contour as the inner wall of the thorax, and the lung surface in contact with the thoracic wall is known as the **costal surface.** Medially, the **mediastinal surface** of the lung is in contact with the structures of the mediastinum.

The lungs are separated into **lobes** by deep fissures. The *right* lung has three lobes (the **superior, middle,** and **inferior**); the *left* lung has only two lobes (the **superior** and **inferior**). A deep, **oblique fissure** separates the superior and the inferior lobe. In the right, a **horizontal fissure** separates the superior and the middle lobes. The right lung appears larger than the left lung; in the left, a lot of space is taken by the heart and great blood vessels. The right lung is shorter, however, because the diaphragm is higher in the right as a result of the presence of the liver inferiorly.

THE PLEURA

The **pleura** is a membrane that surrounds the lungs. Similar to the pericardial membrane and pericardial

---

⊕ Pleuritis and Pleural Effusion

At times, the pleura become inflamed and fluid tends to collect in the pleural cavity, restricting the movement of the lungs. The inflammation is referred to as pleuritis, or pleurisy, and the fluid collection as pleural effusion.

cavity, the pleura is a double membrane with a cavity in between (Figure 10.9). The layer in close contact with the lungs is the **visceral pleura.** The other layer lines the thoracic cavity, diaphragm, and the mediastinum (other than the hilus) and is known as the **parietal pleura.** A good analogy of the pleural cavity anatomy is to think of the lung as a fist being pushed into a balloon partly filled with air. The layer of the balloon close to the fist would be the equivalent to the visceral pleura; the other layer, the parietal pleura. The space between the layers, the **pleural cavity,** is filled with some fluid (**pleural fluid**) rather than air as in the balloon. The pleural fluid provides lubrication and minimizes friction when the lungs move during breathing.

Mechanics of Respiration

To fully understand the mechanics of respiration, the learner is encouraged to review the structure of the thoracic cavity (the ribs, the costal cartilage, sternum, clavicle, thoracic vertebrae, and related articulations described on **page 109.**)

Respiration refers to the movement of air in and out of the lungs and the exchange of gases. It includes two processes—**external** and **internal respiration.** External respiration refers to all processes involved in the absorption of oxygen and the removal of carbon dioxide from the air spaces in the lung and pulmonary capillaries. Internal respiration refers to the absorption of oxygen by cells and the removal of carbon dioxide from them by the blood in the capillaries. **Cellular respiration** refers to the process of use of oxygen and production of carbon dioxide for ATP production by cells.

EXTERNAL RESPIRATION

For external respiration, the air must be physically moved from the atmosphere into the lungs. This involves increasing and decreasing the size of the thoracic cavity by movement of the chest wall and action of the respiratory muscles. This process is known as **pulmonary ventilation,** or **breathing.** The process of drawing air *into* the lungs is termed **inspiration** or **inhalation,** and the process of moving the air *out of* the lungs is referred to as **expiration** or **exhalation.**

WORK OF BREATHING
Lung disease can affect the total amount of energy required for ventilation. In some cases, up to 30% of the total energy of the body may be used just to bring the air into the lungs.

The rate at which air flows is not only influenced by the pressure differences between the atmosphere and the thoracic cavity but also by the surface tension in the alveoli, the compliance of the lungs (the ease with which the lungs expand), and the resistance offered by the airways.

Pressure Changes During Pulmonary Ventilation

Knowledge of basic physics will help you understand how air is moved in and out of the thoracic cavity. According to **Boyle's law,** the pressure inside a closed chamber is inversely related to the volume. Simply, if the volume in a closed container is reduced, the pressure of gas in the container increases. For example, if volume is reduced by half, the pressure would double. If volume is doubled, the pressure would be half of what it was originally. This is the principle behind movement of air in and out of the thoracic cavity.

The parietal pleura lines the inner wall of the thoracic cavity and the visceral pleura lines the outside of the lungs. The pleural fluid keeps the two membranes in close contact by surface tension. Also, the pressure in the pleural cavity, which is less than that of the atmosphere, a partial vacuum, keeps the two layers opposed. When the thoracic cavity increases in volume by the action of muscles and movement of the thoracic cage, it draws the pleura and, therefore, the lungs with it. This results in a drop in pressure inside the lungs (Remember, when the volume increases, the pressure decreases). Because the nasal cavity communicates with the outside atmosphere, air flows into the lungs to equalize the pressure—inspiration.

Conversely, if the thoracic volume decreases, pressure inside the lungs increases (a decrease in volume increases the pressure), and the air flows out of the lungs through the nose to equalize the pressure with that of the atmosphere—expiration. Normal expiration is passive, and the change in thoracic volume is caused by the relaxation of the inspiratory muscles and the elastic recoil of the chest wall and the lungs that were stretched during inspiration.

The difference in the oxygen and carbon dioxide levels in the air and blood causes the gases to move by diffusion from the region of higher concentration to that of lower concentration across the alveoli. Thus, carbon dioxide diffuses from the blood to the air and oxygen from air to the blood. Respiration takes place using these physical principles.

Surface Tension and Pulmonary Ventilation

The luminal surface of the alveoli has a layer of fluid. Because water molecules have a greater attraction between each other than with gas molecules, an inward directed force is created. This inward force—surface

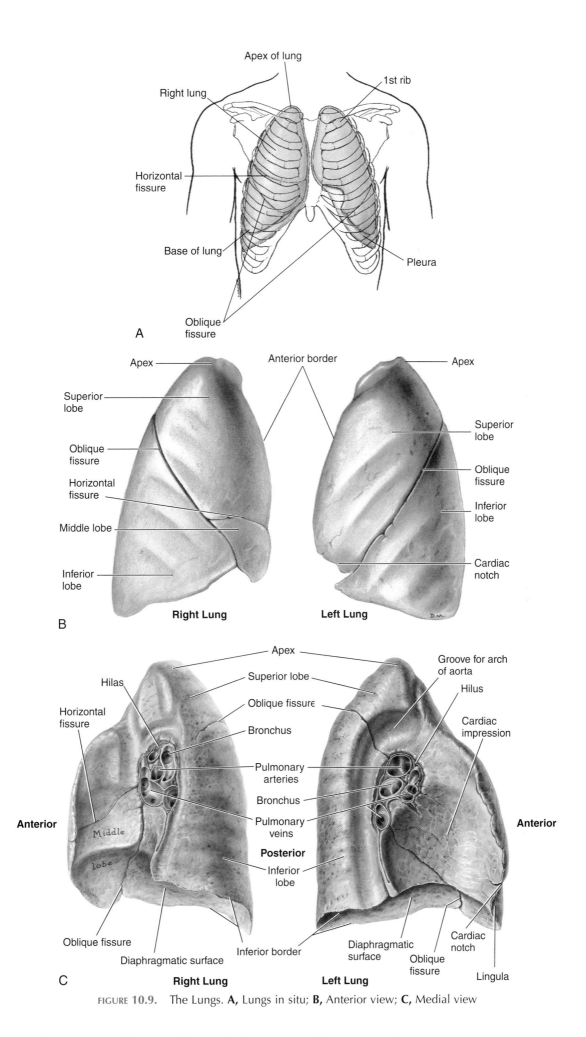

Apex of lung

Right lung

1st rib

Horizontal fissure

Base of lung

Pleura

Oblique fissure

A

Apex

Anterior border

Apex

Superior lobe

Oblique fissure

Horizontal fissure

Middle lobe

Inferior lobe

Superior lobe

Oblique fissure

Inferior lobe

Cardiac notch

B

Right Lung

Left Lung

D.M.

Apex

Groove for arch of aorta

Hilas

Superior lobe

Hilus

Horizontal fissure

Oblique fissure

Bronchus

Cardiac impression

Pulmonary arteries

Bronchus

Anterior

Middle

lobe

Pulmonary veins

Anterior

Posterior

Oblique fissure

Inferior lobe

Cardiac notch

Diaphragmatic surface

Inferior border

Diaphragmatic surface

Oblique fissure

Lingula

C

Right Lung

Left Lung

FIGURE 10.9. The Lungs. **A,** Lungs in situ; **B,** Anterior view; **C,** Medial view

tension—tries to draw the alveoli into the smallest possible diameter. Therefore, the alveoli tend to collapse during expiration. During inspiration, this force opposes entry of air into the alveoli. Surfactant, secreted by the type II cells, reduces the surface tension and the resistance offered during inspiration.

Lung Compliance

Compliance is the change in volume for a unit change in pressure, and it reflects the ability of the lungs to stretch. If more air volume can be brought into the lung with smaller pressure differences between the lung and the exterior, the lung is considered more compliant. For example, lack of surfactant will make the lungs less compliant and make it harder to breathe in. Normal lungs have high compliance because they have elastic tissue that stretch easily. Also, the presence of surfactant reduces surface tension. Respiratory conditions that result in scar tissue formation and reduction of elastic fibers, fluid in the lungs, paralysis of respiratory muscles, or reduced surfactant, lower compliance, increasing the work of breathing. In emphysema, the lungs become more compliant than normal. This, too, is not desirable because there would be a tendency for air to remain in the lungs even after expiration.

Airway Resistance

The resistance to air flow is largely determined by the caliber of the bronchi. By contracting and relaxing the smooth muscle of the bronchi (see page **371** for factors affecting the bronchi caliber), the resistance to airflow can be modified. When the sympathetic nerves are stimulated, the muscle wall relaxes, increasing the diameter of the bronchi and reducing resistance. In conditions such as asthma or obstructive pulmonary disease, the airway resistance is increased, making it harder to breathe. Normally, the airways increase in width during inspiration and reduce during expiration.

Presence of mucus and edema in the airways can also affect resistance. In **cystic fibrosis,** as a result of the presence of a defective gene that carries instructions for a transmembrane protein responsible for the active transport of chloride ions, the transport of salts and water is inefficient. Thick and viscous secretions result, with mucous plug formation, inflammation, predisposition to infection, and an increase in airway resistance.

RESPIRATION MUSCLES

Inspiratory Muscles

Inspiration is an active process where the muscles of respiration (Figure 10.10 and Table 10.1) contract to increase the thoracic volume. The major muscle of in-

Breathing Exercises

Breathing exercises may be used in acute or chronic lung diseases, postsurgically, in those with severe chest deformities that affect respiratory function, and others. Exercises improve ventilation; increase the effectiveness of the cough mechanism; prevent improper ventilation (atelectasis) and perfusion of the lungs; improve the strength, endurance and coordination of the respiratory muscles; promote relaxation; and correct inefficient or abnormal breathing patterns. In addition, respiratory exercises (e.g., yoga breathing [pranayma]) have been used to ease anxiety and reduce stress, etc.

Deep breathing exercise, diaphragmatic breathing exercise, inspiratory resistance training (in which the patient inhales through a handheld resistive training device), incentive respiratory spirometry (in which a visual or auditory feedback is provided through a spirometer), segmental breathing (in which the patient is taught to expand a localized area of his or her lung), glossopharyngeal breathing (in which the tongue and pharynx are consciously used to force air into the lungs), pursed-lip breathing (in which the lips are pursed to create back pressure during expiration) are some breathing exercises used.

Other exercises to mobilize the chest may be used with breathing exercises to treat those with respiratory conditions.

spiration is the diaphragm. The diaphragm is a dome-shaped, skeletal muscle, projecting into the thoracic cavity (see Figure 4.26). Its origin is along the walls of the thorax and insertion is into a centrally placed tendon. The diaphragm is innervated by the phrenic nerve that arises from cervical segments 3, 4, and 5. When the diaphragm contracts, the central tendon is pulled downward into the abdominal cavity, increasing the diameter of the thoracic cavity in the superior-inferior direction. The diaphragm is responsible for 75% of air movement into the lungs.

The external intercostal muscles that originate in the upper rib, with insertion in the lower rib, with the fibers running anteriorly and inferiorly, help elevate the ribs. They are innervated by nerves arising from thoracic segments 1 to 12. The ribs articulate with the vertebrae and sternum in a way that the antero-posterior and transverse diameters are increased when they are lifted up by this muscle (see Figure 3.38). The activity of the external intercostals is responsible for bringing approximately 25% of the volume of air into the lungs.

In addition to the diaphragm and external intercostals, other accessory muscles assist inspiration, including the sternocleidomastoid, scalenes, serratus anterior, pectoralis minor, pectoralis major, and upper trapezius. The sternocleidomastoid muscles help elevate the sternum, and the scalene muscles elevate the

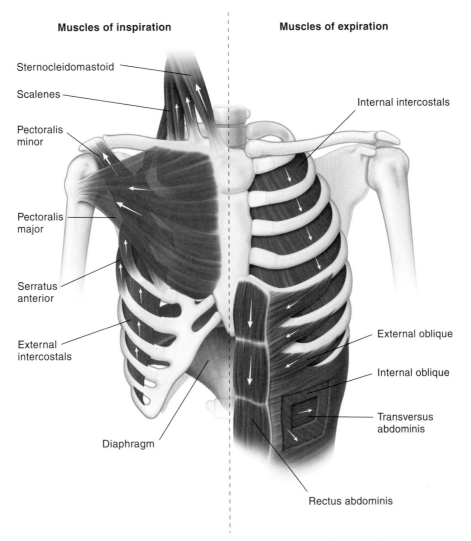

Muscles of inspiration

- Sternocleidomastoid
- Scalenes
- Pectoralis minor
- Pectoralis major
- Serratus anterior
- External intercostals
- Diaphragm

Muscles of expiration

- Internal intercostals
- External oblique
- Internal oblique
- Transversus abdominis
- Rectus abdominis

FIGURE **10.10.**   Muscles of Respiration. Arrows indicate the direction of movement.

upper few ribs, increasing the anteroposterior diameter. Muscles, such as the serratus anterior, pectoralis major and minor, act as muscles of inspiration by elevating the ribs or pulling the ribs toward the arms by reverse muscle action (i.e., the insertion is fixed while the origin moves) when the upper limb is fixed in position. The accessory muscles come into play when respiration is forced, as in individuals with asthma.

HICCUP

Hiccup is a result of involuntary, sudden contraction of the diaphragm. When this occurs, usually at the beginning of inspiration, the glottis suddenly closes, producing the characteristic sound. Prolonged hiccup may be caused by irritation of the phrenic nerve or sensory nerves in the stomach. Sometimes, this can be caused by irritation of certain areas in the brain.

Expiratory Muscles

During normal respiration, the expiration process is passive and caused by the relaxation of the inspiratory muscles described above. In forced respiration, expiration becomes active and is assisted by the internal intercostals and transversus thoracis, which help depress the ribs (Figure 10.10 and Table 10.1). The abdominal muscles, which include the external obliques, internal obliques, transversus abdominis, and the rectus abdominis, help compress the abdomen and force the diaphragm upward.

Other Muscles

The abductor muscles in the larynx contract early in inspiration, pulling the vocal cords apart. The adductor muscles contract reflexively and close the glottis during swallowing or gagging, to prevent food from entering the larynx.

Table 10.1

The Origin, Insertion, Innervation, and Action of Respiration Muscles

Muscles of Inspiration

Muscle	Origin	Insertion	Innervation	Action
Diaphragm	Xiphoid process; cartilage of ribs 4–10; body of lumbar vertebrae	Central tendinous sheet	C3,4, and 5	Increase volume of thoracic cavity; decrease volume of abdominopelvic cavity
External intercostals	Inferior border of each rib	Superior border of lower rib	T1–T12	Raises/elevates ribs, increasing the volume of the thoracic cavity-inspiratory muscle
Sternocleidomastoid	Superior margin of sternum and medial aspect of clavicle	Mastoid process	Cranial nerve XI and C2, C3	Together, they flex the neck; individually, they turn the head to the opposite side
Scalene muscles	Transverse process of cervical vertebrae	Superior surface of first two ribs	Posterior rami of C3–C8	Flexes neck; elevates ribs
Pectoralis major	Body of sternum; cartilage of 2–6 ribs; medial aspect of clavicle	Greater tubercle of humerus	Medial and lateral pectoral nerves (C5–T1)	Flexes; adducts; medially rotates humerus; elevates ribs if humerus held stationary
Pectoralis minor	Anterior aspect of ribs 3–5	Coracoid process of scapula	Medial pectoral nerve (C8 and T1)	Protracts; depresses; laterally rotates scapula; elevates ribs if scapula held stationary
Trapezius	Has a long origin from the occipital bone, ligamentum nuchae; spinal processes of thoracic vertebrae	V-shaped insertion from the lateral 1.3 of clavicle, acromion and spine of scapula	Accessory (cranial nerve XI), third and fourth cervical	Depends on contracting fibers: elevation; depression; adduction; rotation of scapula; elevation of clavicle; extension of head and neck
Serratus anterior	Anterior and superior aspect of ribs 1–9	Anterior aspect of the medial border of scapula	Long thoracic nerve (C5–C7)	Protracts (pulls forward); abducts; medially rotates the scapula; elevates ribs if scapula held stationary

Muscles of Expiration

Muscle	Origin	Insertion	Innervation	Action
Internal intercostals	Superior border of each rib	Inferior border of rib above origin	Intercostal nerves	Depresses ribs, increasing the volume of the thoracic cavity
Rectus abdominus	Superior surface of pubis	Xiphoid; inferior surface of cartilage of ribs 5–7	Anterior rami of intercostal nerves (T7–T12)	Flexes spine; depresses ribs
External oblique	Lower eight ribs	Linea alba and iliac crest	Anterior rami of intercostal nerves (T7–T12)	Flexes spine; depresses ribs
Transversus abdominus	Cartilage of lower ribs; lumbodorsal fascia	Linea alba and pubis Iliac crest	Anterior rami of intercostal nerves (T7–T12)	Compresses abdomen
Internal oblique	Lumbodorsal fascia; iliac crest	Lower ribs; xiphoid; linea alba	Anterior rami of intercostal nerves (T8–T12)	Flexes/bends spine; depresses ribs

Thorax Landmarks and Surface Markings of the Diaphragm

Slide your finger from the suprasternal notch to a transverse ridge where the manubrium meets the body of the sternum at the sternal angle. The second costal cartilage is at the level of the sternal angle. This is where the trachea bifurcates into the right and the left bronchi.

The nipple is over the fourth intercostal space or fifth rib, about 10 cm (3.9 in) from the midline in men and most women. (In older women, the location varies, according to the size and pendulousness of the breast). The right dome of the diaphragm rises to just below the right nipple. The left dome rises to 2.3 cm (0.8–1.2 in) a level just inferior to the left nipple. In the midline, the central tendon is at the level of the xiphisternal junction. During vigorous inspiration, the diaphragm can descend as much as 5–10 cm (2–4 in).

BREATHING PATTERNS, RESPIRATORY VOLUMES, AND CAPACITIES

Breathing Patterns

The number of breaths taken every minute is known as the **respiratory rate;** a normal adult has a respiratory rate of about 12–18 breaths per minute. Children breathe about 18–20 breaths per minute. **Eupnea** is the term for normal, quiet breathing. A pattern of breathing in which the breathing is shallow, with the chest moving outward, is known as **costal breathing.** This movement is a result of the contraction and relaxation of the intercostals muscles that move the ribs. In **diaphragmatic breathing,** the diaphragm moves up and down, pushing the abdominal contents outwards.

Abnormal Breathing Pattern Terms

Apnea—cessation of breathing in the expiratory phase
Cheyne-Stokes breathing—cycles of gradually increasing tidal volumes, followed by cycles of gradually decreasing tidal volumes, followed by apnea
Dyspnea—difficulty breathing
Hyperpnea, or **hyperventilation**—an increase in rate and/or depth of breathing
Orthopnea—difficulty breathing when supine
Tachypnea—rapid, shallow breathing

Respiratory Volumes and Capacities

The respiratory rate and the volume of air moving in and out of the lungs can be easily recorded using the **spirometer,** or **respirometer.** The recording obtained is the **spirogram** (see Figure 10.11). An upward deflection is produced in the recording when a person breathes in through the mouthpiece of the spirometer. Expiration is recorded as a downward deflection. The height of deflection reflects the volume breathed; the horizontal axis reflects time.

At rest, breathing quietly, an adult takes in about 500 mL (30.5 in³) of air. This is known as **tidal volume** (see Table 10.2). Thus, the volume of air breathed in and out every minute during quiet respiration is equal to respiratory rate × tidal volume and is about 6.0 liters (1.6 gal) per minute. This volume is known as the **respiratory minute volume.**

The total volume of air that can be accommodated in the respiratory system is known as the **total lung capacity.** This volume averages about 6 liters (1.6 gal) in men and 4.2 liters (1.1 gal) in women. Of the total lung capacity, the volume of air that a person can breathe in after a normal expiration is much more than the tidal volume. This volume, known as the **inspiratory capacity,** includes the **inspiratory reserve volume** and **tidal volume** (the approximate values in men and women are given in Table 10.2 and Figure 10.11A). The volume of air that a person can breathe out after a normal expiration is known as the **expiratory reserve volume.** Even when a person breathes out as forcefully as possible, there is some air remaining in the lungs. This volume of air is known as the **residual volume.** The residual volume and the expiratory reserve volume together make up the **functional residual capacity. Vital capacity** is the volume of air that a person can maximally breathe out after a maximal inspiration. Sometimes, the volume of air a person can forcefully breathe out in the first second is measured. This volume is known as the **forced expiratory volume in one second** (FEV₁), or **timed vital capacity.** Normally, more than 80% of the total volume expired is expelled in the first second. FEV₁ is reduced in conditions where obstruction to the airway is present. FEV₁ is a useful measurement for monitoring the day-to-day response to drugs, dosage required, and the progress of obstructive diseases in individuals. A small device known as the

Table 10.2

Volumes/Capacities in Men and Women

Volumes and Capacities	Men (mL)	Women (mL)
Residual volume	1,200	1,100
Expiratory reserve volume	1,000	700
Tidal volume	500	500
Inspiratory reserve volume	3,300	1,900
Vital capacity	4,800	3,100

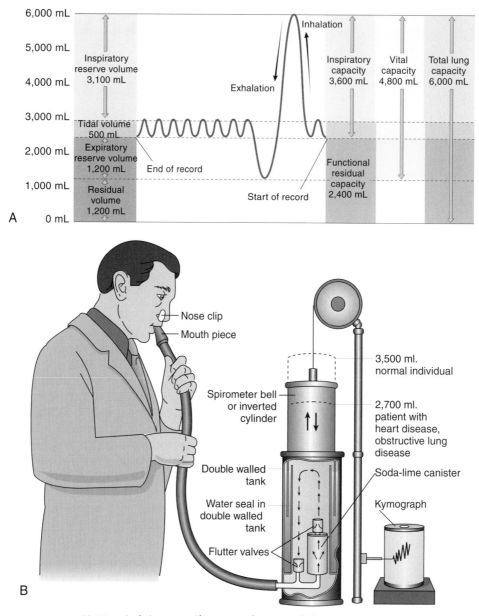

FIGURE **10.11.** **A,** Spirogram, Showing Volumes and Capacities; **B,** Spirometer

peak flow meter is often given to patients to track of their forced expiratory volume. To monitor gas exchange, blood samples may be analyzed to determine the concentration of dissolved gases.

The volumes and capacities, as seen in Table 10.2 differ between men and women. Some volumes also vary with the age and height of the individual. People living in high altitudes and those who have led an active lifestyle since childhood tend to have larger vital capacities.

No matter how large the vital capacity of individuals, what is important is the volume of air that actually reaches the exchange surface—the alveoli. This air, known as **alveolar ventilation,** is equal to 4.2 liters (1.1 gal) per minute. Because the air that occu-

pies the space in the conducting passages (nasal cavity to the terminal bronchiole) are not involved in gas exchange, this volume of air is referred to as **dead space** air. More specifically, this volume of air is known as **anatomical dead space** because this wasted air is a result of the anatomic structure; it occupies about 150 mL (9.2 in³).

Other than the anatomical dead space, some air taken into the lungs may be wasted if the alveoli that they enter do not have a blood supply. Here, although air reaches the exchange surface, there is no blood circulation for gas exchange to take place. The volume of such wasted air is known as **physiological dead space.** In normal individuals, this dead space is low. However, in individuals with such conditions as fibrosis of the lungs, the dead space is large and gas exchange is inadequate.

Gas Exchange

Gas movement between the alveoli and blood is by passive diffusion. The rate of gas exchange can be explained using simple physical laws. **Dalton's law** states that each gas in a mixture of gases exerts its own pressure, behaving as if it is the only gas present. The pressure exerted by the gas is known as **partial pressure** (of that gas e.g. PO_2-partial pressure of oxygen). The addition of the partial pressure of all the gases in the mixture will be equal to the total pressure exerted by the mixture of gases. In atmospheric air, the total pressure exerted at sea level is equal to 760 millimeters of Mercury (mm Hg) or 14.7 pounds per square inch (psi). This pressure can be obtained by the addition of the partial pressure of nitrogen (78.6%), oxygen (20.9%), carbon dioxide (0.04%), water vapor (0.4%) and other gases (0.06%) in the atmosphere. The partial pressure of the gas can be easily determined by multiplying the percentage of the gas in the atmosphere by total atmospheric pressure. Atmospheric air has 20.9% oxygen. Then the partial pressure of oxygen in a region where the atmospheric pressure is equal to 760 mm Hg is: $760 \times 0.209 = 158.8$ mm Hg ($14.7 \times 0.209 = 3.07$ psi). At high altitudes, where the atmospheric pressure is lower, the partial pressure of oxygen would drop even though the percentage of oxygen is the same, directly affecting the rate of gas exchange. For example, if the atmospheric pressure is 740 mm Hg (14.31 psi), then the partial pressure of oxygen would be: $740 \times 0.209 = 154.66$ mm Hg ($14.31 \times 0.209 = 2.99$ psi). That is why, before getting acclimatized, you feel out of breath when you ascend to high altitudes.

Gases move across a permeable membrane from an area of higher partial pressure to an area of lower partial pressure. The rate at which each gas moves

Chronic Obstructive Pulmonary Disease

In a person with chronic asthma or chronic obstructive pulmonary disease, the functional residual capacity is significantly increased (i.e., an abnormally large volume of air remains in the lungs after the person expires). In addition, the forced expiratory volume is decreased as a result of narrowing of the bronchi and difficulty in expiration. As a result, such an individual tends to have an enlarged, barrel-shaped chest, with an increased anteroposterior and transverse diameter.

Hypoxia

Hypoxia is a condition in which there is oxygen deficiency at the tissue level; it has 4 types. **Hypoxic hypoxia** is when PO_2 is reduced in the blood (example: high altitude); **anemic hypoxia** is when the arterial PO_2 is normal but the amount of hemoglobin available to carry oxygen is deficient; **stagnant,** or **ischemic hypoxia,** is when PO_2 and hemoglobin are normal, but the blood flowing to the tissue is inadequate. **Histotoxic hypoxia** is when the tissue cells cannot make use of their oxygen supply (cyanide poisoning).

from a mixture of gases is determined by the difference in its partial pressure. The partial pressure of other gases in the mixture is not a factor. For example, the movement of oxygen in the lungs from the alveoli to the blood is determined by the difference in partial pressure of oxygen in the alveoli and the blood, not by the partial pressure of carbon dioxide or other gases.

Other than partial pressure, the quantity of gas moving across the membrane and dissolving in blood would be determined by how soluble the gas is in plasma. **Henry's law** describes the behavior of gas. Henry's law states that the quantity of gas that will dissolve in a liquid is proportional to the partial pressure of the gas and its solubility coefficient (the volume of gas that dissolves in one unit volume of a liquid at a particular temperature). Carbon dioxide in the body has a higher solubility coefficient (24 times more) than oxygen. Therefore, more carbon dioxide is carried dissolved in plasma. Henry's law explains why we have little nitrogen dissolved in plasma. Although the air has a high partial pressure of nitrogen (79%), little dissolves in plasma because of the low solubility coefficient of nitrogen.

Figure 10.12 is an overview of the difference in the partial pressure of oxygen and carbon dioxide in the alveoli, pulmonary artery and vein and in the systemic artery, vein, and the interstitial fluid.

In addition to the partial pressure and solubility coefficient of carbon dioxide and oxygen, the rate of exchange would be affected by the thickness of the respiratory membrane and the surface area available for exchange. For example, when there is pulmonary edema, fluid in the respiratory membrane increases the distance through which diffusion must take place, with consequent reduction in rate of gas exchange. If a lobe of the lung is collapsed, the surface area for exchange is reduced and less oxygen diffuses.

As the deoxygenated blood in the pulmonary artery passes around the alveoli, exchange of gases occurs quickly, with oxygen moving into the blood from the alveolar air and carbon dioxide from the

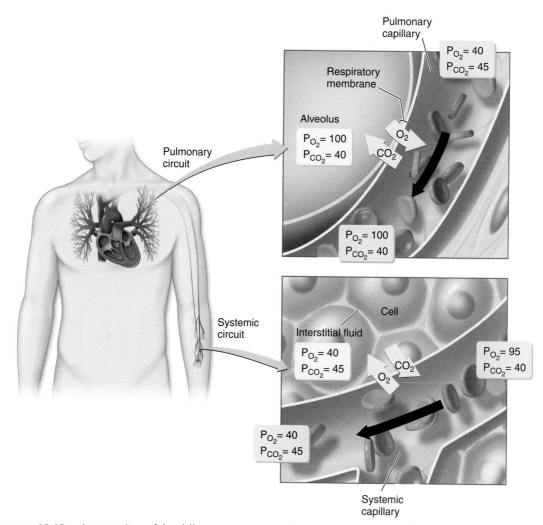

FIGURE **10.12.**   An overview of the difference in the partial pressure of oxygen and carbon dioxide in the alveoli, pulmonary artery and vein, systemic artery, and interstitial fluid (unit = mm Hg)

blood into the air. Although the red blood cells in the blood stay in the capillaries for less than a second (in an exercising individual, about 0.3 seconds), the time is sufficient for exchange to occur.

OXYGEN TOXICITY

Although oxygen is necessary for normal function, prolonged administration of 100% oxygen can be toxic. The situation worsens when it is administered under pressure. Toxicity is a result of the production of the superoxide anion (O_2^-), which is a free radical, and hydrogen peroxide (H_2O_2). If 80% to 100% oxygen is administered for 8 hours or more, irritation of the respiratory passages produces nasal congestion, sore throat, and coughing.

Exposure to oxygen at increased pressures (hyperbaric oxygen) increases the concentration of oxygen dissolved in the plasma. Therefore, it is used during some surgeries for congenital heart disease and for treating gas gangrene, carbon monoxide poisoning, and cyanide poisoning, etc.

TRANSPORT OF GASES

As already mentioned, the solubility coefficient of oxygen is low. Given the difference in partial pressure of oxygen and its solubility coefficient, only about 0.3 mL (0.02 in³) of oxygen can be transported dissolved in 100 mL (0.106 qt) of plasma. This is grossly insufficient for the tissue. With carbon dioxide, much more is produced in the tissue than can be carried dissolved in plasma. Hence, a more efficient mechanism is needed to transport the gases. Hemoglobin, present in red blood cells, with its great affinity for oxygen, enables blood to carry a larger quantity of the gases.

Transport of Oxygen

The primary function of a red blood cell is to transport oxygen and carbon dioxide, and its structure is modified to suit this function. As red blood cells mature, all cellular components not directly related to function are lost. For example, mature red cells do

Abnormal Hemoglobin

The affinity of hemoglobin to oxygen can be altered by changes in the structure of the globular protein chains. Such conditions are usually inherited. **Thalassemia** is a condition in which there is an inability to produce adequate protein chains, resulting in slow red blood cell production and a debilitating anemia and development and growth of the individual can be affected.

Another example of abnormal hemoglobin formation is **sickle cell anemia,** in which defective beta chains are formed. The hemoglobin appears normal when the oxygen levels are high; however, when the levels drop, the structure of the hemoglobin changes and the red blood cells become sickle-shaped and more fragile, with a shorter life span.

not have a nucleus. Ninety-five percent of intracellular protein in these cells is hemoglobin. The cell is small, about 7.4 µm in diameter, and shaped like a biconcave disk, with a narrow central part. This structure helps the cell squeeze through the tiny capillaries without rupturing (see Figure 10.13).

Unique Properties of Hemoglobin

The hemoglobin molecule is made up of four globular protein chains, two **alpha** and two **beta chains** (Fig-

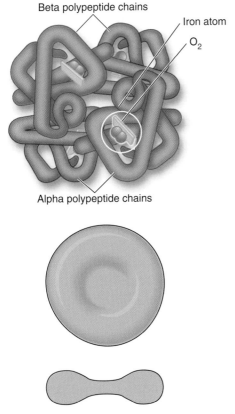

FIGURE 10.13. Biconcave Structure of Red Blood Cell and Hemoglobin Molecule

ure 10.13). Each chain contains a pigment complex known as **heme,** which has an attached **iron** ion. The iron component of the hemoglobin molecule combines with oxygen to form **oxyhemoglobin.** The linkage of iron to oxygen is weak and can be easily broken in accordance with the oxygen concentration in the surrounding tissue. Each hemoglobin molecule is capable of combining with four molecules of oxygen. There are approximately 280 million hemoglobin molecules in each red blood cell and about 98.5% of the oxygen carried in the blood is bound to hemoglobin.

$$Hb + O_2 \leftrightarrow HbO_2$$
Reduced hemoglobin + Oxygen $\leftrightarrow$ Oxyhemoglobin

The amount of oxygen bound to hemoglobin depends on the oxygen level of its surroundings. If the oxygen level is low, hemoglobin releases the oxygen and carbon dioxide binds to the globin chains. In the capillaries of the lungs, where oxygen levels in the alveolar air are high, carbon dioxide is released and oxygen binds to the hemoglobin. The activity of cells can be maintained only if the hemoglobin levels are within normal range.

Factors Affecting the Binding Property of Hemoglobin

The affinity of hemoglobin for oxygen is unique (see Figure 10.14, which shows the affinity of hemoglobin for oxygen at different partial pressures of oxygen). The affinity varies with the partial pressure of oxygen around it, changes in temperature, and pH. As the partial pressure of oxygen increases around hemoglobin, more oxygen is attached to hemoglobin (i.e., all four sites for oxygen in the heme component of hemoglobin molecule are occupied). When all four sites are attached to oxygen, the hemoglobin is considered fully saturated with oxygen. If two sites are occupied, hemoglobin is considered partially saturated; in this case, 50% saturated. In the alveoli, the partial pressure of oxygen is high and hemoglobin is almost fully saturated. Note that the hemoglobin is more than 90% saturated even when the partial pressure is as low as 60 mm Hg (1.16 psi). This is advantageous because hemoglobin can combine with large quantities of oxygen even when the partial pressure drops as low as 60 mm Hg (as in high altitudes or with some respiratory disorders).

When the partial pressure of oxygen drops below 40 mm Hg (0.77 psi), the hemoglobin becomes less

NORMAL HEMOGLOBIN CONTENT

The hemoglobin content of blood is measured in grams per 100 mL; 14–18 g/dL of hemoglobin are found in the blood of males and about 12–16 g/dL in females.

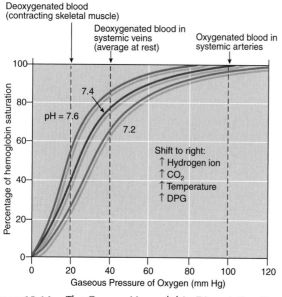

FIGURE 10.14.   The Oxygen-Hemoglobin Dissociation Curve

and less saturated when the partial pressure drops even a little. This characteristic is good because the partial pressure around tissue cells is less than 40 mm Hg. When oxygenated blood reaches the tissue cells, because of this characteristic, oxygen is rapidly and easily detached from hemoglobin. In active tissue, the partial pressure drops even more and even more oxygen is unloaded from hemoglobin.

When the pH drops (i.e., becomes more acidic or the temperature increases slightly), the oxygen-hemoglobin dissociation curve is shifted to the right (Figure 10.14). Also, the accumulation of compound 2,3 diphosphoglycerate (2,3 DPG), which is formed plentifully during metabolism in the red blood cells, facilitates dissociation of oxygen from hemoglobin. This implies that when 2,3 DPG levels are high, hemoglobin gives up oxygen easily at a higher partial pressure of oxygen. In active tissue, the temperature increases slightly because of the increase in metabolism. The liberation of carbon dioxide and production of lactic acid make the environment more acidic. All of these factors—change in temperature, drop in pH, and accumulation of 2,3 DPG—alter the characteristic of hemoglobin, making it unload more oxygen even at a higher partial pressure of oxygen. In this way, the tissues increase oxygen availability according to their activity.

High Altitude and Hemoglobin Levels

At high altitudes, the partial pressure of oxygen in the atmosphere is low, lowering the availability of oxygen in the air. The body adapts to the low levels by increasing red blood cells and hemoglobin content. This way, even if the hemoglobin molecules do not get saturated with oxygen, there are more in number

to combine with oxygen. The increase in hemoglobin content and red blood cells is initiated by the hormone **erythropoietin** (see page **455**), whose levels increase when oxygen levels drop.

Transport of Carbon Dioxide

Carbon dioxide, a byproduct of aerobic metabolism, is transported in the blood in three ways that are reversible (see Figure 10.15). Because it is about 20 times more soluble in blood than oxygen, about 7% of carbon dioxide dissolves in plasma. Twenty-three percent combine with hemoglobin to form **carbaminohemoglobin.** The remaining 70% are converted to carbonic acid in the presence of the enzyme carbonic anhydrase found inside red blood cells. The carbonic acid dissociates easily and rapidly into hydrogen ions and bicarbonate ions.

$$CO_2 + H_2O \leftrightarrow H_2CO_3 \leftrightarrow H^+ + HCO_3^-$$
carbon dioxide + water ↔ carbonic acid ↔
hydrogen ion + bicarbonate ion

Most hydrogen ions formed in this reaction bind to hemoglobin molecules. Thus, hemoglobin molecules serve as buffers, preventing these ions from altering the pH of blood. The bicarbonate ions move out of the red blood cells into the plasma in exchange for chloride ions, which move into the cells from the plasma (**chloride shift**). Because deoxygenated hemoglobin forms carbamino compounds more easily and has a greater affinity for hydrogen ions than oxygenated hemoglobin, transport of carbon dioxide is facilitated in venous blood.

Regulation of Respiration

Having learned that the muscles involved in respiration are skeletal muscles, one might wonder how we are able to breathe rhythmically and regularly on a continuous basis. At the same time, it is fascinating to consider the many ways the rate and depth of respiration is altered in everyday activity.

TRAINING IN HIGH ALTITUDES

Athletes train in high altitudes to give them the added edge of having more hemoglobin to bring oxygen to the tissues; however, they need to start training sufficiently early—a least a few weeks before competition because it takes some time for red blood cells and hemoglobin to be manufactured. However, the resultant high hemoglobin content and red blood cells make the blood viscous, increasing the workload of the heart with a potential for cardiac failure.

Pulmonary capillary   Systemic capillary

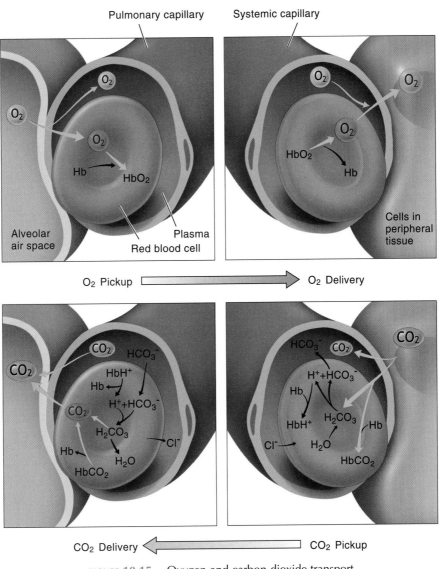

O_2 Pickup ⟹ O_2 Delivery

CO_2 Delivery ⟸ CO_2 Pickup

FIGURE 10.15. Oxygen and carbon dioxide transport

Carbon Monoxide Poisoning

Carbon monoxide is an odorless gas found in cigarette smoke, automobile exhaust, and oil lamps, etc. Unfortunately, hemoglobin has a high affinity for this gas (240 times that for oxygen), even if levels are low. In addition, the bond formed with hemoglobin is strong. Therefore, exposure to carbon monoxide results in the formation of **carboxyhemoglobin.** Once formed, carboxyhemoglobin becomes unavailable to transport oxygen to the tissue. Because the oxygen dissolved in plasma is not altered in carbon monoxide poisoning, respiration is not significantly affected in these situations because the chemoreceptors are stimulated only by the changes in the *dissolved* oxygen content of plasma.

Carbon monoxide poisoning is deadly because the gas is odorless and not easily detected. Also, because it does not increase respiration, the person can slowly be poisoned without knowing it.

The carbon monoxide, nicotine, tar, and other carcinogens in cigarette smoke are responsible for many of the health hazards of smoking, whether actively or passively.

A person with suspected carbon monoxide poisoning is treated with pure oxygen at high partial pressure with a hope that this would displace the carbon monoxide and increase the level of dissolved plasma oxygen.

ONDINE'S CURSE

Ondine's curse is a rare condition in which the voluntary control of respiration is intact and the involuntary component is disrupted. The name is derived from a German legend:

Ondine, a water nymph, had an unfaithful, mortal lover. To punish the lover, the king of the water nymphs cast a curse on him, taking away all the lover's automatic functions. The lover could only stay alive by remaining awake and remembering to breathe. Finally, from exhaustion, the lover fell asleep and died by forgetting to breathe!

Think of musicians who play a wind instrument or the control singers have over the force of respiration. We can hold the breath for a short period, as in diving, but are forced to breathe involuntarily after some time. Breathing stops every time food is swallowed. The thought of an impending competition, makes us breathe faster. Without conscious effort, respiratory rate and depth alter, according to the oxygen requirements of the body. We breathe more heavily when we exercise, and our breathing is matched to the rate at which we use oxygen. All of these alterations are caused by complex regulatory mechanisms of respiration.

AUTOREGULATION IN TISSUE

Tissue can alter oxygen delivery. In active tissue, the increase in temperature, drop in pH, and increase in the concentration gradient of oxygen between the interstitial fluid and blood promote the unloading of oxygen from hemoglobin. In addition, the smooth muscle of the arterioles supplying the tissue are relaxed by an increase in hydrogen ions, change in potassium levels, and increase in carbon dioxide levels (all of which occur in rapidly metabolizing tissue). In this way, more blood is diverted to the tissue that needs oxygen.

AUTOREGULATION IN LUNGS

In the lungs, pulmonary blood flow is increased toward those alveoli where partial pressure of oxygen is higher (i.e., toward well-ventilated alveoli). In this way, gas exchange is increased by avoiding collapsed alveoli. Note that this reaction is opposite that which occurs in the systemic capillaries. Also, the smooth muscle of the bronchi and bronchioles are sensitive to the partial pressure of carbon dioxide in the lungs and relax when carbon dioxide levels are high. This improves ventilation as the caliber of the bronchi increase in those areas of the lungs that are well perfused by deoxygenated blood with a high carbon dioxide content. In addition to this type of local control of perfusion and ventilation, the brain controls the rate and depth of respiration.

RESPIRATORY CONTROL SYSTEM OF THE BRAIN

In brief, spontaneous respiration is produced by rhythmic discharge of impulses from the respiratory area of the brain (see Figure 10.16) via motor nerves to the respiratory muscles. Breathing will stop if the connection from the brain to the motor nerves is severed. However, the rhythmic discharge of impulses from the brain can be altered by many factors such as changing levels of oxygen, carbon dioxide, and hydrogen ions (pH) of the blood. This explains the increase in respiration when active. Also, the nervous connections of the respiratory area with other regions of the brain and with other parts of the body affect the rate of discharge of impulses. This explains how respiration can be altered voluntarily as in singing, involuntarily before and during exercise, and in many other situations.

Respiration is controlled by two separate neural mechanisms. One voluntary and one involuntary. Nerves from the cerebral cortex communicate with the motor neurons that directly innervate the diaphragm and the other respiratory muscles. This is responsible for the voluntary component. Other areas of the brain—classically referred to as the **respiratory centers**—located in the medulla and pons are responsible for the involuntary or automatic component. They, too, communicate with the motor neurons supplying the respiratory muscles. The final out-

A Few Clinical Terms

Asphyxia—occlusion of the airway
Cyanosis—bluish discoloration of the tissue resulting from high levels of deoxygenated hemoglobin
Epistaxis—Loss of blood from the nose
Hypercapnia—increased partial pressure of carbon dioxide in arteries
Hypocapnia—decreased partial pressure of carbon dioxide in arteries
Hypoxia—oxygen deficiency at the tissue level
Rales—hissing, whistling, scraping, or rattling sounds produced in the respiratory tract; occurs when airways are narrowed
Rhonchi—coarse rattling or popping sounds, indicating airway congestion
Stridor—a loud, high-pitched sound; generally indicates obstruction at the level of the larynx
Wheezing—a whistling sound produced during respiration as a result of bronchospasm

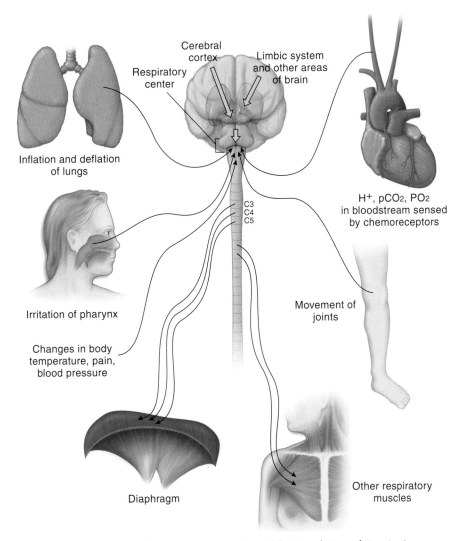

Cerebral cortex

Respiratory center

Limbic system and other areas of brain

Inflation and deflation of lungs

Irritation of pharynx

Changes in body temperature, pain, blood pressure

C3
C4
C5

H+, pCO2, PO2 in bloodstream sensed by chemoreceptors

Movement of joints

Diaphragm

Other respiratory muscles

FIGURE **10.16.**   A Schematic Representation of the Regulation of Respiration

come or action depends on whether the motor nerves are inhibited or stimulated.

Respiratory Centers

Three areas in the brainstem participate in the regulation of respiration. These centers are actually a network of neurons, with their cell bodies located in the medulla and pons.

The medulla has the **respiratory rhythmic center.** This center has two groups of neurons. One group is situated dorsally—the **dorsal respiratory group**—and contains neurons that control the motor neurons that supply the diaphragm and the external intercostal muscles. During quiet respiration, these neurons are active for about 2 seconds, stimulating the muscles and resulting in inspiration. Then they become inactive for about 3 seconds when the muscles relax and expiration occurs passively.

Sleep Apnea

In certain individuals, breathing cessation for short periods during sleep (sleep apnea) may produce such symptoms as early morning headache and fatigue. **Sleep-apnea syndrome** may occur at any age. One cause of sleep apnea is believed to be the failure of the genioglossus muscle (that pulls the tongue forward) to contract during inspiration. As a result, the tongue falls backward, obstructing the airways.

Sudden Infant Death Syndrome (SIDS), in which apparently healthy infants between the ages of 1 week and 12 months are found dead, often in their cribs, is thought to be a result of hypoxia and may be a form of sleep apnea. The incidence of SIDS has decreased significantly as a result of the public campaign by pediatricians, recommending that infants be placed on their backs during sleep rather than in the side or prone positions and encouraging parents to place babies to sleep on firm mattresses.

Another group of neurons in the medulla, situated ventrally, the **ventral respiratory group,** is active during forced respiration. They communicate with the motor neurons that innervate the accessory respiratory muscles and stimulate the accessory muscles during inspiration and expiration. The neurons involved in inspiration and expiration are reciprocally innervated (i.e., when the inspiratory neurons are active, the expiratory neurons are inhibited simultaneously).

The pons has collections of neurons known as the **pneumotaxic center** and **apneustic center.** Both adjust the output of the respiratory rhythmic centers of the medulla. They adjust the rate and depth of respiration in response to stimuli received from other parts of the brain and the rest of the body. For example, the pneumotaxic center reduces the duration of inspiration and facilitates the onset of expiration. The primary effect of this center is to stop inspiration before the lungs are over inflated. When this center is active, the respiratory rate is increased. The apneustic center has the opposite effect, increasing the duration of inspiration and inhibiting expiration.

CHEMICAL CONTROL OF RESPIRATION

The level of oxygen, carbon dioxide and hydrogen ions can alter respiration. This alteration is a result of special receptors that monitor the levels of these substances. These special sensors (**chemoreceptors**) are located near the aorta, carotid artery (**peripheral chemoreceptors**), and the medulla near the respiratory center (**central chemoreceptors**).

The chemoreceptors near the large blood vessels are known as **aortic bodies** and **carotid bodies.** The chemoreceptors are small structures, about 2 mg (0.03 g) in weight and a few millimeters wide, located near the arch of the aorta and the bifurcation of the carotid arteries, respectively. The cells of these bodies are surrounded by large, fenestrated (with many gaps) capillaries. The blood flow through these bodies is considered the highest at 2,000 mL per 100 g of tissue compared with that of the brain at 54 mL per 100 g and that of the kidney with 420 mL per 100 g. The cells are closely associated with sensory nerve fibers that travel from the bodies to the brain via the glossopharyngeal and vagus nerves.

The cells in the chemoreceptors are sensitive to the levels of dissolved oxygen in the plasma, increasing levels of carbon dioxide, and increase in hydrogen ions. When oxygen levels drop or carbon dioxide and hydrogen ion levels increase, the receptors are stimulated and take impulses to the respiratory center, which responds by increasing the rate and depth of respiration.

In addition to these bodies, there are special cells located close to the respiratory center, in the medulla, which are stimulated by higher carbon dioxide and hydrogen ion levels and lowered oxygen levels in the cerebrospinal fluid.

OTHER MECHANISMS THAT CONTROL RESPIRATION

Other than chemoreceptors, respiration is affected by stimulation of receptors in the airways and lungs. Impulses generated by these receptors are carried by the vagus nerve to the respiratory centers. These receptors respond to stretch and, when the lungs are over inflated, inhibit inspiration. This is considered a protective reflex that prevents overinflation of the lungs and is referred to as the **inflation reflex (Hering-Breuer reflex).**

Nerves from the hypothalamus and limbic system communicate with the respiratory centers, altering breathing when in pain or when emotional. For example, sudden severe pain can cause respiration to temporarily cease. Prolonged somatic pain can bring about an increase in respiratory rate.

Research shows that even active and passive movements of joints stimulate respiration. Proprioceptors that monitor movement of joints and muscle stimulate the respiratory center even before changes in pH and oxygen and carbon dioxide levels are produced. Changes in blood pressure and state of the heart can affect respiration as well. A sudden rise in blood pressure decreases the rate of respiration through the influence of baroreceptors on the respiratory center. Receptors from the mouth and pharynx also have an effect and are responsible for alterations when vomiting, gagging, and swallowing.

During sleep, the control of respiration is less rigorous and sensitivity to changing levels of carbon dioxide is reduced; hence, brief periods of apnea may be observed.

In summary, the regulation of respiration is a complex process in which the activity of respiratory centers that generate rhythmic impulses to the respira-

---

ARTIFICIAL RESPIRATION

In conditions such as drowning and carbon monoxide poisoning, artificial respiration may prove lifesaving. In **mouth-to-mouth breathing,** a volume equal to about twice the tidal volume is blown into the victim's mouth 12 times a minute, with the victim supine and neck extended. Expiration is passive as a result of the elastic recoil of the lungs.

To treat chronic respiratory insufficiency, mechanical respirators may be used. Negative pressure, by means of a motor, is applied to the chest at regular intervals, moving the chest wall in a manner similar to normal breathing. Intermittent positive pressure breathing machines produce periodic increases in intrapulmonary pressure by air "pulses" being administered through a face mask.

tory muscles is altered by many stimuli—some stimulatory and some inhibitory—arising from other parts of the brain and outside the nervous system.

Effect of Exercise on the Respiratory System

Many cardiovascular and respiratory mechanisms come into play to meet the oxygen needs of active tissue and to remove the extra carbon dioxide and heat produced during exercise.

Even before the start of exercise, respiratory rate and depth are altered as a result of the psychic stimuli on the respiratory center. Soon after the onset of exercise, there is an abrupt increase in ventilation, probably a result of afferent stimuli from proprioceptors. When exercise is continued, there is a gradual increase in ventilation, presumably a result of changes in arterial pH, Pco_2 and Po_2.

The amount of oxygen entering the pulmonary capillaries is increased by many mechanisms. During exercise, the volume of blood in the pulmonary circulation is increased from 5 L/minute (1.3 gal/min) at rest to as high as 20–35 liters/minute (5.3–9.2 gal). The gas exchange surface area is increased as more pulmonary capillaries open up and are better perfused. In addition, the pressure gradient between alveoli air and blood is increased, speeding the rate of diffusion. This is because more oxygen is used by active tissue and the deoxygenated blood carried to the lungs has a lower partial pressure of oxygen. At the tissue level, the increase in carbon dioxide production, temperature increase, and lactic acid production all contribute to rapid unloading of oxygen from hemoglobin to the tissues.

If exercise is prolonged and strenuous, the respiratory and cardiovascular changes are not sufficient to keep up with oxygen use. As a result, energy is derived by anaerobic means, with accumulation of lactic acid (**oxygen debt**). After cessation of exercise, respiration reduces abruptly as a result of reduced neural stimulus. Respiration slows down further as arterial pH and Pco_2 return to normal. However, the respiration does not reach basal levels until the O_2 debt is repaid, which may take as long as 90 minutes.

Effect of Cold on the Respiratory System

The effect of cold varies with the type and duration of application. When cold application is in the form of a douche (a douche is an application of water by an apparatus that drives or throws water upon the surface

Effects of Smoking on the Respiratory System

It is well known that smoking is hazardous to the respiratory system not only affecting the smoker, but also those exposed to secondhand smoke. The irritants in smoke can increase mucous secretion with resultant obstruction to air flow. Smoke also has a direct effect on the ciliary action of the lining of the airways. This, in turn, reduces the clearing of mucus and debris from the area. The mucus eventually dries and plugs the smaller bronchi. One function of mucus is to remove the adhered microorganisms. With the mucous stagnation in chronic smokers, there is a greater risk of respiratory infections. Repeated infection, inflammation, and healing can have a detrimental effect on the elasticity of the bronchi and lungs, leading to irreversible chronic respiratory diseases. The nicotine in the smoke constricts terminal bronchiole, reducing pulmonary ventilation. The carbon monoxide in smoke binds to hemoglobin, reducing oxygen carrying capacity.

Smoking predisposes individuals to many lung diseases, such as cancer, chronic obstructive pulmonary disease, bronchitis, bronchiectasis, and emphysema. Other health hazards of smoking include cataracts; hearing loss; tooth decay; osteoporosis; heart disease; clotting tendency of blood; stomach ulcers; miscarriages; low-birth-weight infants; sudden infant death syndrome; deformed sperm; Buerger's disease; and a greater risk of cancer of the mouth, salivary gland, pharynx, stomach, esophagus, kidney, bladder, penis, pancreas, colon, anus, and breast.

It is important for therapists to join hands with other health professionals to educate the public and encourage colleagues and clients to stop smoking.

of the body or any part of it), the effect is to produce short, gasping respiratory movements. This effect is more pronounced if the douche is applied to the chest or upper part of the body. In asthmatics, a cold douche to the chest tends to produce a paroxysm of asthmatic breathing because of reflex vasoconstriction of pulmonary vessels and resultant reduction in surface area for gas exchange. If cold application is in the form of a cold bath, following the initial increase, there is a slowing of the respiratory rate, with an increase in depth of respiration.

Effect of Aging on the Respiratory System

Change that occurs in the muscles and skeleton with aging can decrease lung function. The elderly client may have kyphosis/scoliosis that decreases respiratory movement. Osteoporosis of the ribs and vertebrae and calcification of the cartilage may contribute to stiffness of the chest wall. The respiratory muscles (diaphragm, intercostals, etc.) weaken, reducing the efficiency of breathing.

With age, elastic tissue in the lungs alter, with a reduction in the lung's elastic recoil. This compensates for the stiffness of the chest wall, making it easier for the lungs to expand. The alveoli become larger with age, reducing the surface area for exchange. The capillaries in the alveoli also decrease. In general, the work of breathing increases, and the elderly tend to rely on the movement of the diaphragm more than chest wall movement. As a result, small changes in intra-abdominal pressure, such as a heavy meal or change in body position, tend to compromise breathing.

All of the above anatomical changes have significant effects on lung function. More air remains in the lung after expiration; forced expiratory volume and vital capacity decrease. The small airways tend to collapse during shallow breathing, reiterating the importance of deep breathing exercises in older individuals.

Changes also occur in the respiratory centers, with the response to reduced oxygen and increased carbon dioxide levels blunted. The cough reflex is impaired, with reduced force, volume, and air flow rate expelled during a cough. Cilia in the mucosa decrease with age, reducing the lung's capacity to clear mucus and foreign agents that have settled on the mucus. The activity of the macrophages that wander in the lungs is also decreased, together with a reduction in antibodies secreted in the lungs. All this makes the elderly more prone to respiratory diseases.

The changes that occur with aging are worsened when associated with smoking, obesity, and immobility. As with effects of aging on all other body systems, here too, there is wide variation between individuals.

Respiratory System and Massage

Massage can have many positive effects on the respiratory system. A relaxation massage can slow the respiratory rate through its inhibitory effect on the sympathetic system. It can be beneficial to clients with breathing difficulty, especially if fatigued respiratory muscles are targeted. People with breathing difficulty often tend to alter their posture to reduce the effort of breathing. Massage, by relaxing these muscles, can have a profound effect on relieving the aches and pains originating from these muscles, and it has the potential to increase vital capacity and lung function by relaxing tight respiratory muscles and stretching fascia.

The client's position may need to be altered according to the respiratory problem. Clients with breathing difficulty or requiring sinus drainage may be more comfortable in **Fowler's position** in which the head end is raised 30 to 90 degrees, with the hips and knees slightly flexed. In conditions in which respiratory secretions are excessive, changing the pa-

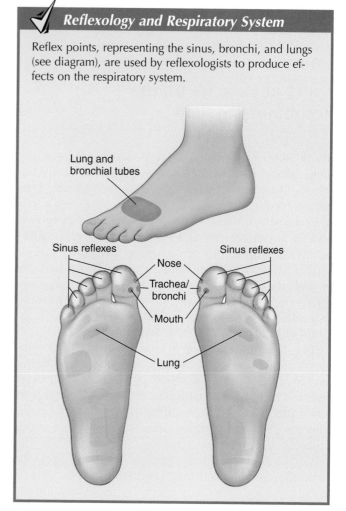

Reflexology and Respiratory System

Reflex points, representing the sinus, bronchi, and lungs (see diagram), are used by reflexologists to produce effects on the respiratory system.

Lung and bronchial tubes

Sinus reflexes   Sinus reflexes

Nose

Trachea/bronchi

Mouth

Lung

tient's posture before and during massage may be beneficial. The **Trendelenburg position,** in which the symphysis pubis forms the highest point of the trunk and the long axis of the trunk forms an angle of about 45 degrees with the horizontal, may be used to drain secretions from basal regions. However, such a position may be uncomfortable for those with breathing difficulties because the abdominal organs are pushed against the diaphragm.

Postural drainage (bronchial drainage)[1,2] clears the airways of secretions by placing the client in different positions, allowing gravity to assist with mucous drainage. The positions are based on the direction of the bronchi supplying different bronchopulmonary segments and lobes. The goal of postural drainage is to prevent accumulation of secretions and to remove secretions that have already been accumulated. Postural drainage is particularly beneficial in those with chronic obstructive pulmonary diseases, such as asthma, chronic bronchitis, emphysema, bronchiectasis, and cystic fibrosis. Figure 10.17 indicates the various positions the client may be placed to drain different parts of the lungs. If the client can tolerate it, the position can be maintained for 5 to 10 minutes. Special percussion techniques, such as cupping tapotement (cupped-hand percussion), vibration, shaking, and rib-springing may be used during postural drainage to further mobilize secretions. A study of clients with cystic fibrosis showed that massage was effective in reducing symptoms.[3]

In cupping tapotement,[1] the palmar surface of the hand is cupped, and the cupped hands are alternately used to strike the client's chest wall in a rhythmic fashion. A hollow sound of suction is produced as a vacuum is created when the palm of the hand is lifted from the surface of the skin. This is the stroke of choice for loosening phlegm and mucus in the airways. Cupping should not be applied over bony prominences, over breast tissue in women, and over site of a fracture. It is contraindicated in patients with angina, bleeding tendencies, and cardiac problems.

Vibration is a technique used in conjunction with percussion to mobilize microsecretions. Vibration is applied during expiration; it is performed by placing both hands on the chest wall and gently compressing and rapidly vibrating the chest wall by isometrically contracting the muscles of the upper extremities.

Shaking is a slower form of vibration applied with wide movement of the therapist's hand. Rib-springing is a more vigorous form of vibration in which greater pressure is applied to the chest wall. A springing action

is applied to the chest wall during expiration. A sputum cup should be available for discarding secretions. Secretions should be carefully disposed of, without contaminating the environment. Clients may not expel secretions mobilized by postural drainage and other techniques until 30 to 60 minutes after treatment.

Postural drainage may be used early in the morning to drain secretions accumulated from the night before. It may also be done prior to sleeping to clear the airways before rest. Treatment frequency will depend on the pathology of the patient's condition. At times, postural drainage and percussion techniques may be used as often as every two to four hours.

Breathing humidified, warm air prior to treatment may help dislodge mucus plugs more easily. Many types of equipment exist for humidification and nebulization.[4] In this process, water vapor is added to the gas. Humidification and nebulization are effective in liquefying thick and inspissated secretions.

At times, essential oils, diffused into the air, may produce effects on the body as they are inhaled.[5] The oil may be dispersed with an atomized diffuser; through heat, using a candle; with scented candles; or with a room spray. The effect of the oil on the body depends on the time of day or season or on the client's mood or past experiences related to the smell. Oils, such as lavender and chamomile, are used for their calming ef-

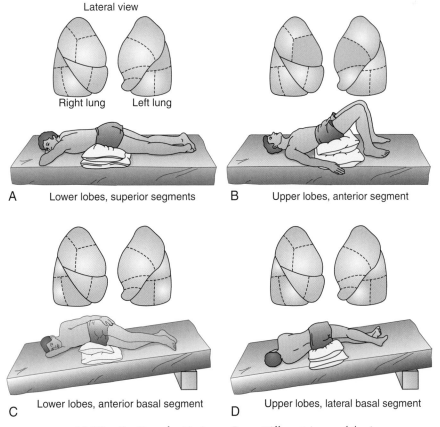

FIGURE **10.17.** Positions for Drainage From Different Areas of the Lungs

Aromatherapy for Respiratory Conditions

Steam Inhalation

Steam inhalation is an effective treatment for conditions such as laryngitis and bronchitis and for soothing dry coughs. Two to three drops of sandalwood and/or frankincense or benzoin may be added to a bowl of steaming, hot water and inhaled for 5 to 10 minutes. Congestion may be relieved by using two to three drops of peppermint and/or eucalyptus oil instead. Hot baths, to which the recommended oil has been added, or use of vaporizers with the recommended oil can have effects similar to steam inhalation. Alternately, a few drops of one of these oils may be added to a handkerchief for inhalation throughout the day.

Gargling

Regular gargling with warm water mixed with four to five drops of tea tree, Spanish sage, clary sage, or thyme may be used to relieve sore throat.

Chest Rub

Four to five drops each of ginger or thyme and lavender or hyssop in 5 tsp/25 mL of carrier oil may be beneficial if applied to the chest and upper back of individuals with upper and lower respiratory tract disorders.

Important Signs and Symptoms of Respiratory Disease

Some important signs and symptoms of respiratory disease include cough, sputum, hemoptysis, breathlessness (dyspnea), wheeze, and chest pain.

Cough is triggered when the irritant receptors located in the mucous membrane of the respiratory tract are stimulated. In healthy individuals, approximately 100 mL (0.106 qt) of mucus is produced each day. This mucus is carried upward by cilia and swallowed.

When there is excessive mucous production, irritant receptors are stimulated and sputum is coughed up. Depending on the respiratory condition, sputum may be clear, white, mucoid, yellow (purulent), rusty, or blood-tinged. When blood is coughed up, it is termed hemoptysis.

Breathlessness or dyspnea is an unpleasant awareness of breathing. Wheeze indicates narrowing of the bronchial tree.

The characteristics of pain from the respiratory structures vary according to where it arises. Diseases within the lung are usually painless because lung tissue does not contain pain receptors. Pain originating in the pleura presents as sharp, well-localized pain that worsens on breathing. Pain from the central part of the diaphragm is referred to the shoulder, and pain from the lateral part is referred to the lower lateral chest wall and upper abdomen. When mediastinal structures are involved, pain is felt in the central part of the chest. Pain from the ribs and muscles are usually localized over the area affected.

fect. Sage, rosemary, pine, and mints are used as stimulants. Many other essential oils are used in specific conditions such as hypertension, insomnia, and depression. Essential oils should be used with extreme caution with individuals with a history of allergies, emphysema, asthma, and other respiratory disorders.

It is important for therapists to ensure that clients with active respiratory infections are not treated in the clinic because respiratory infections invariably spread via airborne particles.[6] Conversely, a therapist with a respiratory infection should not treat clients.

Massage has a positive effect on those with asthma. In a study on children with asthma, the peak expiratory flow rate and other pulmonary functions improved and anxiety and levels of stress hormones were reduced with massage.[7] Before treating clients with history of asthma, the therapist should ensure that the client has the relevant drugs available to prevent undue suffering if an asthmatic attack should ensue during treatment. It should also be ensured that any allergens and other triggers that can precipitate an attack are removed from the vicinity.

REFERENCES

1. Salvo SG. Massage Therapy. Principles & Practice. Philadelphia: W.B. Saunders, 1999.
2. Wade JF. Respiratory Nursing Care. 2nd Ed. St. Louis: C.V. Mosby, 1977.
3. Hernandez-Reif M, Field T, Krasnegor J, Martinez E. Cystic fibrosis symptoms are reduced with massage therapy intervention. J Pediatr Psychol 1999;24,183–189.
4. Miller, Frank B. Encyclopedia Dictionary of Medicine, Nursing & Allied Health. 6 Ed. W.B. Saunders, 1997.
5. Lawless J. The Complete Illustrated Guide to Aromatherapy. Shaftesbury: Element Books, 1997.
6. Premkumar K. Pathology A to Z. A Handbook for Massage Therapists. 2nd Ed. Calgary: VanPub books, 1999.
7. Field T, Henteleff T, Hernandez-Reif M, et al. Children with asthma have improved pulmonary functions after massage therapy. J Pediatr 1998:132,854–858.

SUGGESTED READING

Kinser C, Colby LA. Therapeutic Exercise: Foundations and Techniques. 2nd Ed. Philadelphia: F.A. Davis, 1990.

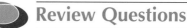

Review Questions

Multiple Choice
Choose the best answer to the following questions:

1. The upper respiratory tract includes all of the following EXCEPT the
   A. trachea.
   B. pharynx.
   C. nasal cavity.
   D. nose.

2. The effects of age on the respiratory system include all of the following EXCEPT
   A. The bones and cartilage of the thoracic cavity lose their flexibility.
   B. The ciliary action of the lining of the respiratory tract increases.
   C. The lung tissue loses its elasticity.
   D. The alveoli become larger, reducing surface area for exchange.

3. The affinity of hemoglobin for oxygen is affected by changes in all of the following EXCEPT
   A. hydrogen ion levels in plasma.
   B. carbon dioxide levels in plasma.
   C. temperature.
   D. calcium ion levels in plasma.

4. Chronic smoking can produce
   A. an increase in ciliary action.
   B. a decrease in mucous secretion.
   C. an increase in oxygen binding capacity of hemoglobin.
   D. a decrease in surface area for exchange.

5. When a person exercises, all of the following happen EXCEPT
   A. the respiratory rate increases even at the thought of exercise.
   B. the movement of the joints affects the respiratory rate.
   C. the increase in pH increases respiratory depth and rate.
   D. the increased production carbon dioxide increases the rate and depth of respiration.

6. Air entering the body is filtered, warmed, and humidified by the
   A. upper respiratory tract.
   B. lungs.
   C. lower respiratory tract.
   D. all of the above.

7. The function of the nasal conchae is
   A. to divide the nasal cavity into a right side and a left side.
   B. to provide surface for exchange of gas.
   C. to create a turbulence in the air to trap small particles.
   D. to provide an opening to the outside of the body.

8. The actual sites of gas exchange within the lungs are the
   A. bronchioles.
   B. pleural spaces.
   C. bronchi.
   D. alveoli.

9. The partial pressure of oxygen in the pulmonary arterial blood is
   A. more than that in the aorta.
   B. the same as that in the right atrium.
   C. the same as that in the left atrium.
   D. more than that in the coronary artery.

10. The partial pressure of carbon dioxide in the aorta is
    A. less than that in the renal artery.
    B. more than that in the pulmonary artery.
    C. the same as that in the right ventricle.
    D. the same as that in the pulmonary vein.

11. Each of the following muscles can elevate the ribs EXCEPT the
    A. scalenes.
    B. external oblique.
    C. external intercostals.
    D. serratus anterior.

Fill–In
Complete the following:

1. Cathleen is breathing at the rate of 12/minute. Her tidal volume is 450 mL. Her minute ventilation is _____ . If the dead space air is 150 mL, her alveolar ventilation per minute is _____ .

2. The volume of air taken in with each inspiration during normal breathing is called _____ .

3. The volume of air remaining in the lungs at the end of forced expiration is called _____ .

4. The volume of air breathed out completely after maximal inspiration is called _____ .

5. The amount of vital capacity that can be forced out in one second is known as _____ .

6. Carbon dioxide is transported in the blood as _____ , _____ , and _____ .

7. The main chemical changes in the blood that stimulate respiration are an increase in _____ , an increase in _____ , and a decrease in _____ levels.

8. The respiratory centers are located in the _____ and the _____ .

9. The volume of air present in the conducting part of the respiratory system is known as _____ .

True–False

(Answer the following questions T, for true; or F, for false):

1. During quiet breathing, there is more muscular work involved when breathing in than when breathing out.

2. As blood passes through the lungs, the CO_2 released into the alveoli is mainly carried as bicarbonate ions.

3. After oxygenation in the lungs, the blood returns to the heart via the pulmonary arteries.

4. The trachea is located anterior to the esophagus.

5. Increase in stimulation of sympathetic nerves to the smooth muscle of the bronchiole will result in bronchoconstriction.

6. As the volume of the thoracic cavity increases, the pressure inside it increases.

7. Nitrogen gas contributes most to the atmospheric pressure.

8. If the atmospheric pressure is 735 mm Hg and the oxygen in the atmosphere is 21%, the partial pressure of oxygen in the atmosphere is 160 mm Hg.

9. Factors that affect the rate at which a gas diffuses across a membrane include the difference in concentration of the gas on the two sides of the membrane, the solubility coefficient of the gas, and the surface area of the membrane.

10. When the hemoglobin carries all the oxygen it can hold, it is considered to be fully saturated.

11. Carbon monoxide has a greater affinity for hemoglobin than oxygen.

12. Of the total amount of air that enters the lungs with each breath, about 50% actually enters the alveoli.

Matching

Match the following structures with the location where they are found. Write a, b, c, d, e, or f next to structures 1–8:

1. _____ adenoids
2. _____ orifice for the auditory tube
3. _____ opening for the frontal sinus
4. _____ cells secreting surfactant
5. _____ bronchioles
6. _____ thyroid cartilage

    a. nasal cavity
    b. nasopharynx
    c. oropharynx
    d. laryngopharynx
    e. larynx
    f. lungs

7. _____ olfactory epithelium
8. _____ alveoli

Short-Answer Questions

1. What are the functions of the nasal cavity?
2. Where is the olfactory mucosa located?
3. Name the various paranasal sinus. Where do the sinus open?
4. What is the function of the paranasal sinus?
5. What prevents food from entering the larynx?
6. What defense mechanisms protect the respiratory system from entry of debris and pathogens?
7. How are the smooth muscles of the bronchi and bronchioles controlled?
8. Trace the path taken by blood to flow from the right ventricle to the left ventricle.
9. Which are the inspiratory and expiratory muscles of respiration?
10. How does inspiration occur?
11. How is oxygen transported in the blood?
12. How does the body meet the oxygen needs of active tissues?
13. What are the possible effects of massage on the respiratory system?

Case Studies

1. Mrs. Hall strongly believed that massage helped her asthmatic condition. She had been suffering from asthma for more than seven years. Mrs. Hall was a frail woman and rather short in stature. Every time Mrs. Hall entered the clinic, the therapist noticed the shape of her chest. It was barrel-shaped, with the ribs flaring out. Mrs. Hall preferred to have seated massage. On some days, the therapist could feel vibrations when she placed her hand over the back of Mrs. Hall's chest. If the therapist's head was close to the chest, she could even hear squeaking sounds. This would happen on the days when Mrs. Hall complained of her asthma "acting up." On those days, the therapist used percussive techniques to help drain secretions.

   A. What is asthma?
   B. Is it infectious?
   C. What are the physiologic processes altered in asthma?
   D. What could be the cause of the sounds in Mrs. Hall's chest?
   E. Why does Mrs. Hall feel more comfortable having a seated massage?
   F. What factors control the caliber of the bronchi?
   G. What muscles are involved in inspiration and expiration?

H. Which muscles should a therapist focus on in clients with respiratory problems?

I. What techniques can a therapist use to drain secretions?

2. It was Monday and Janice, a massage therapist, awakened with a cold. Her eyes were watery and there was a constant "leak" from her nose. Sneezing and coughing, she made her breakfast, unable to even smell the egg when it burned. Janice knew that this was just a cold, everybody seemed to have it. She hoped that it would not spread to her sinus, as it often did whenever she had a cold. She did not feel too ill and wondered if she should go to the clinic—she had at least five clients booked for massage that day.

A. What are sinuses?

B. How many sinuses are there?

C. Where are they located?

D. What is the function of sinus?

E. Why did Janice have difficulty sensing the smell of the burned egg?

F. What is a common cold?

G. Which part of the respiratory tract does it affect?

H. What do you think Janice should do? Should she go to the clinic?

3. John, a teenager, was stabbed through the chest wall when he tried to stop a fight between two of his classmates. The knife pierced the fifth left intercostal space in the lateral part of the chest wall to the lungs. He was diagnosed to have pneumothorax.

A. Name the layers, from superficial to deep, that the knife would have passed through.

B. What is pneumothorax?

Answers to Review Questions

Multiple Choice

1. A. The parts of the respiratory tract located above the larynx form the upper respiratory tract.

2. B. The ciliary action is reduced, not increased, with age.

3. D. Calcium levels do not affect the affinity of hemoglobin for oxygen. An increase in hydrogen levels, carbon dioxide levels, and temperature shift the oxygen-hemoglobin dissociation curve to the right, facilitating the unloading of oxygen from hemoglobin at a higher partial pressure of oxygen.

4. D. With chronic smoking, the alveoli get damaged and the surface area for exchange decreases. Such a change is typical of emphysema.

5. C. The pH drops (i.e., becomes more acidic, with more production of hydrogen ions)

6. A

7. C

8. D. Exchange of gas takes place only in the respiratory bronchioles and alveoli.

9. B. The blood in the pulmonary artery is carrying deoxygenated blood from the tissue. Therefore, it will have less oxygen than the aorta, left atrium, or coronary artery. Because no change takes place when the blood goes from the right atrium to the right ventricle and pulmonary trunk, the partial pressure of oxygen in the pulmonary artery will be the same as that in the right atrium.

10. D. The partial pressure of carbon dioxide will be the same in all arteries (except the pulmonary arteries). Because the blood reaching the aorta is coming from the lungs after exchange of carbon dioxide takes place, the partial pressure of carbon dioxide in the pulmonary veins and aorta will be the same.

11. B. The external obliques help with expiration and pull the ribs downward.

Fill-In

1. respiratory rate × tidal volume (i.e., 12 × 450 = 5,400 mL); respiratory rate × (tidal volume − dead space air) = alveolar ventilation per minute (i.e., 12 × (450 - 150)) = 3,600 mL

2. tidal volume

3. residual volume

4. vital capacity

5. forced expiratory volume in one second

6. bicarbonate, dissolved in plasma and carbamino-hemoglobin

7. hydrogen ion, carbon dioxide, oxygen level (decrease)

8. pons, medulla oblongata

9. dead space air

True–False

1. True. During quiet breathing expiration is passive

2. True

3. False. It is the pulmonary veins that take blood to the heart from the lungs

4. True

5. False. The sympathetics produce bronchodilatation

6. False. The pressure drops as the volume increases

7. True

8. False. 735 × 0.21 = 154.35 mm Hg

9. True

10. True

11. True

12. False. All the air except that in the dead space enter the alveoli. Normal tidal volume is about 500 mL, and the dead space air is equal to approximately 150 mL. The alveolar ventilation is 500 - 150/500 = 70%.

Matching

1. b
2. b
3. a
4. f
5. f
6. e
7. a
8. f

Short-Answer Questions

1. Humidify and warm the air. The hair and cilia help remove debris. It has the olfactory epithelium that helps an individual smell.
2. The olfactory mucosa is located along the superior nasal conchae, the superior portion of the nasal septum, and the inferior part of the cribriform plate.
3. Sphenoid, ethmoid, maxillary, and frontal sinus. They open into the nasal cavity.
4. The function of the paranasal sinus is to humidify and warm the air, contribute toward the resonance of voice, and help lighten the weight of the head.
5. The epiglottis moves posteriorly to cover the larynx when an individual swallows.
6. The hair in the nose, the movement of cilia helps move the mucus towards the throat; the presence of macrophages in the lungs protect the respiratory system from entry of debris and pathogens.
7. The smooth muscles of the bronchi and bronchioles are controlled by autonomic nerves and chemicals such as leukotrienes and substance P secreted locally by white blood cells and other cells have an effect on the bronchial smooth muscles.
8. Right ventricle → pulmonary trunk → pulmonary arteries → arterioles → capillaries → venules → pulmonary veins → left atrium → left ventricle
9. Inspiratory muscles—diaphragm, external intercostals (quiet respiration); accessory muscles—scalenes, sternocleidomastoid, serratus anterior, pectoralis major and minor; expiratory muscles—relaxation of inspiratory muscles (quiet breathing); forced expiration—internal intercostals, abdominal muscles
10. Inspiration occurs by active contraction of the inspiratory muscles. The diaphragm contracts and moves downward, increasing the superoinferior diameter; the external intercostals pull the ribs up, increasing the anteroposterior and transverse diameter. When the thorax volume increases, the pressure drops and air moves into the lungs through the nose.
11. A small volume of oxygen is transported dissolved in the plasma. The rest combines with hemoglobin.
12. The oxygen needs of active tissue are met by increasing the blood flow to the lungs and to the tissue. Cardiac output increases by an increase in stroke volume and heart rate. In addition, the blood vessels to the active tissue dilate. The surface area for exchange in the lungs increases by opening capillaries. The affinity for oxygen is altered by the increase in temperature, drop in pH, and increase in carbon dioxide. Because such changes occur in the environment around the active tissue, the hemoglobin gives up oxygen more readily to the tissue.
13. Massage can produce generalized relaxation of muscles. The respiratory rate is reduced by massage. Percussive techniques and postural drainage are particularly effective in draining secretions. Massaging fatigued respiratory muscles can be beneficial.

Case Studies

1. **A.** Asthma is a condition in which there is a reversible, hypersensitivity of the bronchioles to a variety of stimuli, with narrowing and inflammation of the bronchi and difficulty in breathing.
   B. It is not infectious.
   C. See answer to A.
   D. The sounds produced in the chest are a result of the passage of air through narrowed bronchi and bronchioles. The presence of excessive mucous secretion also contributes to the sound.
   E. When Mrs. Hall is sitting, there is less resistance to the excursion of the diaphragm. Gravity reduces the amount of fluid that can accumulate in the lung tissue.
   F., G., and H. See the answers to Short-Answer Questions 7 and 9.
   H. The therapist can use postural drainage and techniques such as cupping tapotement, vibration, and shaking.
2. **A.** Sinuses are cavities present in the lateral and superior walls of the nasal cavity that open into the nasal cavity.
   B., and C. There are two maxillary, two (or one) frontal, two (or one) sphenoid sinus, and nu-

merous ethmoid sinus. As suggested by their names, they are located in the respective bones.

D. See answers to Short-Answer Question 4.

E. Janice had difficulty sensing smell because congestion in the nose reduces the amount of air reaching the superior part of the nasal cavity where the olfactory epithelium is located.

F. Common cold is an acute inflammation of the upper respiratory tract as a result of viral infection.

G. Upper respiratory tract.

H. Janice should stay away from the clinic until she has recovered from her cold because it is possible for her to spread infection.

3. **A.** Skin—epidermis, dermis, subcutaneous tissue, superficial fascia, adipose tissue, deep fascia, serratus anterior (as the wound is in the lateral part of the chest), external intercostal, internal intercostal, parietal pleura, pleural cavity, visceral pleura, and into the lungs.

B. Pneumothorax is a condition in which there is accumulation of air in the pleural space.

Coloring Exercise

Label the structures in the given diagrams, and color the structures, using the color code.
1. Identify the structures associated with the nose, nasal cavity, pharynx, and larynx. Color all bones yellow; the nasal cavity, pharynx, and larynx, blue; the esophagus, green; and the sinus, red.

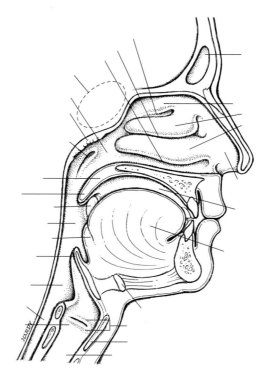

2. Color and identify the muscles of respiration. Draw arrows on the muscles to indicate the direction of movement. Write Inspiratory/Expiratory muscles on the correct side of the dotted line.

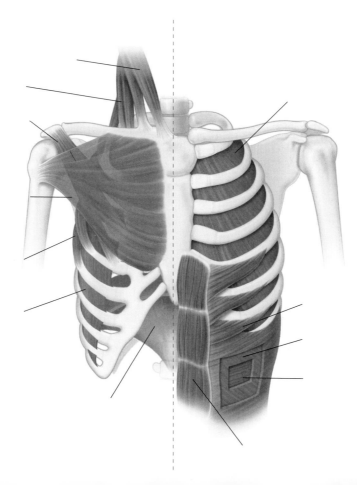

CHAPTER 11

Digestive System

Objectives On completion of this chapter, the reader should be able to:

- List the functions of the digestive system.
- Describe the general structure of the digestive tract walls.
- Describe the structure and location of the peritoneum.
- Describe the process by which movement of food occurs in the gut.
- Describe the regulation of food intake.
- Identify the digestive tract organs and describe their function(s).
- Describe the digestion and absorption of carbohydrates, lipids, and proteins.
- Name the location(s) where water, electrolytes, and vitamins are absorbed.
- Describe the process of defecation.
- Describe the metabolism of carbohydrates, lipids, and proteins.
- List the nutritional requirements of the body.
- Define metabolic rate.
- Describe age-related changes in the digestive tract.
- Identify the possible effects of massage on the gastrointestinal system.

From birth to death, the body is constantly undergoing change. From conception to puberty, anabolism overtakes catabolism. In adulthood, although physical growth is not observed in terms of height, anabolism and catabolism continuously occur. For metabolism to continue, nutrients must be supplied to the body on a constant basis. The gastrointestinal system enables the body to take in nutrients in a variety of forms and convert them into a form acceptable for absorption.

This chapter gives a general overview of the structure and function of the gastrointestinal tract.

Functions of Gastrointestinal System

The gastrointestinal system is the portal through which all nutrients, such as carbohydrates, fats, proteins, vitamins, minerals, and water, required by the body enter. Before the nutrients enter the body, they need to be processed in many ways. Food must be broken down into smaller particles. Once broken into smaller pieces, the different components of food must be reduced to a chemical form that can be absorbed by the epithelium of the gut. The remaining waste material must then be eliminated from the body. For this to occur, many specific processes are involved.

The food must be ingested—taken in via the mouth. This involves conscious choice; areas in the brain regulate the quantity and type of food that is ingested. Once ingested, the food is mechanically processed. This includes breaking the food into smaller pieces and changing the consistency to allow it to be easily swallowed. The mechanically processed food is then ready for digestion. Digestion refers to breaking the food down into small organic pieces using enzymes, assuring that the food particles are small enough to be absorbed by the epithelium covering the gut. Many enzymes manufactured in various parts of the digestive system help with that process.

The enzymes, together with water, acids, electrolytes, and salts, are secreted into the gut to help with digestion. The digested food is then absorbed by the epithelium lining the gut and passed into the circulation and the lymphatics. This material, some of which is processed in the liver, enters the general circulation and is transported to the various tissue of the body, according to their needs. The remaining food—the waste matter—is excreted from the body by a process called defecation. Specialized innervation of the gut helps move the food from the mouth to the anus.

Exposed to the external environment, the digestive system has its own mechanism for protecting the body from bacteria or toxic materials entering the body.

Components of the Gastrointestinal System

The **digestive tract, gastrointestinal** (GI) **tract,** or **alimentary tract** (see Figure 11.1) is a long tube, about 9 meters (29.5 ft) long in the cadaver. The tract begins at the **oral cavity,** continues through the **pharynx** and **esophagus** to reach the **stomach.** The stomach opens into the **small intestine,** where most absorption occurs. From the small intestine, the food moves into the

GASTROENTEROLOGY

Gastroenterology is the medical specialty that deals with the structure, function, diagnosis, and treatment of gastrointestinal tract disorders.

large intestine and, finally, to the rectum (also part of the large intestine) and anus. The **teeth, tongue, salivary glands, liver, gallbladder,** and **pancreas** are considered **accessory digestive organs.** The teeth help to break down the food, and the tongue helps taste, chew, and swallow. The other organs do not come in direct contact with the food; however, they help digest the food chemically by the enzymes they secrete and convey to the lumen by ducts.

Wall of the Digestive Tract

The wall of the digestive tract (see Figure 11.2) has four layers—deep to superficial (i.e., from the lumen to the outer surface of the gut)—the **mucosa, submucosa, muscularis,** and **serosa.**

MUCOSA

The layer surrounding the lumen is the mucosa. The mucosa consists of single layer of **epithelium,** a supportive connective tissue layer (**lamina propria**), and a thin, muscle layer (**muscularis mucosae**). The type of lining epithelium varies from region to region according to function. In areas where this is a likelihood of excessive friction and injury, the epithelium is nonkeratinized, stratified squamous (flat, pavement-like). This type of epithelium is found in the mouth, pharynx, esophagus, and the anus. In areas where absorption or secretion must occur, the epithelium is a simple, columnar type. Most of the gut has this type of epithelium. Scattered between the columnar epithelial cells are exocrine cells (**goblet cells**) that secrete mucus into the lumen and endocrine cells (**enteroendocrine cells**) that secrete hormones into the blood. To increase efficiency, the epithelium is thrown into folds called **villi** in regions where absorption takes place. The folds also allow for expansion when a large meal is ingested. The individual epithelial cells also have folds on the surface facing the lumen known as **microvilli.** The presence of microvilli increases the surface area by 20% and helps improve absorption of nutrients. The epithelium proliferates rapidly and is replaced every 5 to 7 days.

The lamina propria consists of connective tissue. In some areas, this connective tissue contains glands, which open into the lumen and secrete the enzymes and fluids required for digestion. The lamina propria also has nerve endings, blood vessels, and lymphoid tissue. The lymphoid tissue, consisting of lymphocytes and macrophages, protects the GI tract from entry of microorganisms. Some smooth muscle—the muscularis mucosae—is also seen in the lamina propria. Muscle contraction causes the mucosa to be

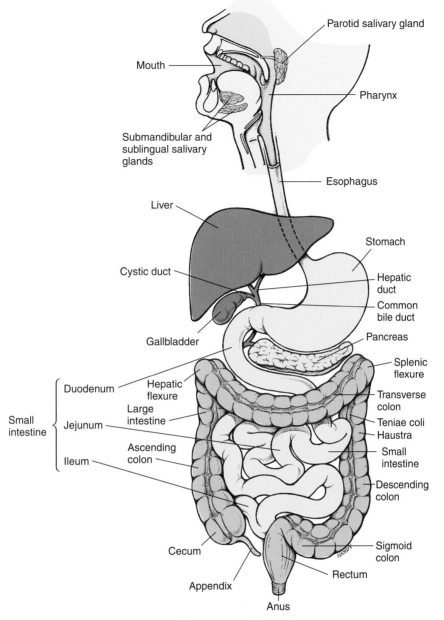

FIGURE **11.1.**   The Digestive System

thrown into folds that increase surface area for secretion and absorption and ensure that the contents of the GI tract come in better contact with the absorptive surface.

Glands not located in the digestive tract also secrete enzymes and fluids. These secretions are expelled into the lumen by ducts that carry the secretion from the glands.

SUBMUCOSA

Outside the lamina propria and its muscles, lies the submucosa. This, too, is a connective tissue layer containing large nerves and blood vessels. The nerves

form a network known as the **submucous plexus,** comprised of both parasympathetic and sympathetic fibers. The parasympathetic fibers stimulate muscle tone and activity and increase glandular secretions. The sympathetic fibers relax the muscles and reduce secretions. However, the circular muscles controlling the openings—the sphincter muscles—are stimulated by the sympathetics.

MUSCULARIS

Just external to the submucosa is another layer of muscles, the **muscularis externa.** The muscularis externa consists of inner circular and outer longitu-

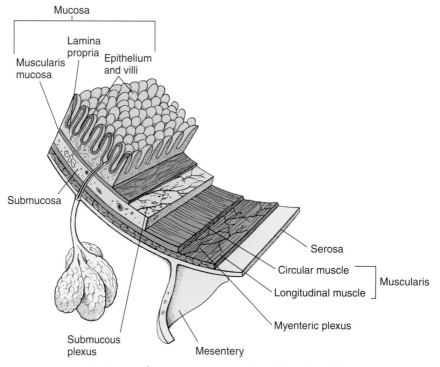

Mucosa

Lamina propria

Muscularis mucosa

Epithelium and villi

Submucosa

Submucous plexus

Mesentery

Serosa

Circular muscle

Longitudinal muscle

Muscularis

Myenteric plexus

FIGURE 11.2.   The Various Layers in the Wall of the GI Tract

dinal smooth muscle. Sandwiched between the circular and longitudinal muscle layers is another network of autonomic (sympathetic and parasympathetic) fibers, the **myenteric plexus.**

The mouth, pharynx, and superior and middle part of the esophagus have skeletal muscle that helps to voluntarily control swallowing. The anus also has skeletal muscle that helps voluntarily control defecation.

SEROSA

Outside the muscularis externa is a connective tissue layer, the **serosa.** In those parts of the gut in the abdomen, the serosa is the smooth membrane known as the peritoneum. In the oral cavity, pharynx, esophagus, rectum, and anus, the serosa is the connective tissue that attaches the part to the surrounding region.

Peritoneum

The peritoneum (see Figure 11.3) is the serous membrane that lines the abdominal cavity. It has a smooth inner lining (simple squamous epithelium) supported by connective tissue. This membrane secretes the **peritoneal fluid,** a clear fluid that lubricates the inside of the abdominal cavity packed with various organs. The peritoneum secretes and absorbs about 7 liters (7.4 qt) of fluid every day.

The best way to describe the way the peritoneum covers the abdominal organs is by analogy. If you tried to push your hand into a partially filled balloon, your fist would be closely covered by one layer of balloon and separated from the other layer by air. This is similar to how the peritoneum covers the organs. The layer close to the organ (your fist) is the **visceral peritoneum,** and the layer away from the organ (the outer layer) is the **parietal peritoneum.** The parietal peritoneum lines the inside of the abdominal cavity. The cavity between the two layers of peritoneum containing serous fluid is the **peritoneal cavity.**

MESENTERY AND OMENTUM

To visualize how the intestine is held in place, imagine that, instead of your fist, you held a pencil side-

Edema in the Abdomen

In people with severe edema, fluid may leak into the peritoneal cavity. This is known as **ascites.** Ascites may be seen in those with generalized edema (e.g., chronic liver disease, kidney failure).

The abdomen can be checked for ascites by placing a hand flat on one side of the abdomen and tapping on the other side. If fluid accumulation is large, the palm of the hand can feel the ripple created by the tap.

ways (i.e., the length of the pencil) and pushed into the partially filled balloon. When the pencil is pushed halfway into the balloon and the inner layer of the balloon covers the pencil, two layers are formed before it continues as the outer layer. Alternately, if you covered a pencil on a table with a piece of tissue paper and then lifted the pencil off the table with two fingers (the pencil still covered with tissue paper), you will find that the tissue paper falls as two layers to the sides of the pencil after covering the pencil. This is how most of the small intestines are covered by peritoneum (the tissue is equivalent to the peritoneum and the pencil to the intestine).

The two layers of peritoneum are close to each other after they cover the intestine and before they continue as the parietal peritoneum lining the abdominal wall. The two layers together form a sheet known as the **mesentery** (Figures 11.3 and 11.4). In this way, the small intestines are positioned in the abdomen and attached to the abdominal wall. The mesentery also prevents the lengthy small intestine from getting entangled. Blood vessels and nerves access the intestine by passing between the two layers of the mesentery.

In addition to the mesentery that holds the small intestine in place, another sheet of modified mesentery falls like an apron from the stomach superiorly, over the anterior aspect of the abdominal cavity. This is

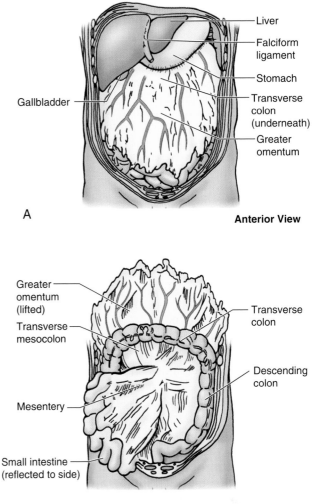

A   **Anterior View**

FIGURE **11.4.**   Peritoneum. **A,** Omentum; **B,** Mesentery

known as the **greater omentum** (Figures 11.3 and 11.4). The omentum contains a lot of adipose tissue and helps pad and protect the abdominal organs and prevents rapid heat loss from the anterior aspect of the abdomen.

Structures located posterior to the peritoneum (i.e., in the posterior abdominal wall covered anteriorly by parietal peritoneum) are said to be **retroperitoneal.** Retroperitoneal organs include the kidneys, adrenal glands, and pancreas.

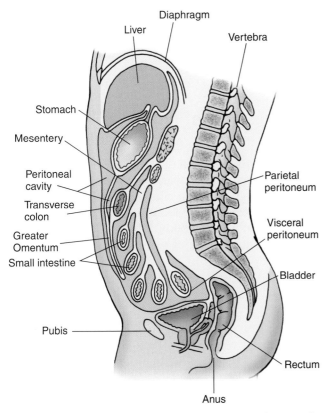

FIGURE **11.3.**   Abdominal Cavity—Sagittal Section (Showing the Peritoneum and Peritoneal Cavity)

Basis of Peritoneal Dialysis

In people with kidney failure and on peritoneal dialysis, the dialysis fluid is injected into the peritoneal cavity. It is left there for some time to allow nutrients to become absorbed and toxins to diffuse out from the blood into the cavity. The fluid is then withdrawn. In this procedure, the peritoneum is used as the membrane across which diffusion occurs.

Movement in the Digestive Tract

The rhythmic contraction of smooth muscle in the wall of the gut helps to propel, mix, and churn the food. The contraction of the smooth muscle is initiated by "pacesetter" cells. The pacesetters are smooth muscle cells in the proximal part of the gut that spontaneously generate impulses and action potential. These impulses travel down the gut via the smooth muscle, as well as the network of autonomic nerves in the wall, creating waves of muscular contraction. The wave of muscular contraction that travels along the length of the digestive tract is known as **peristalsis.** In most areas of the small intestine, other than peristalsis, the circular muscles contract to churn and mix the food material, not necessarily to propel it forward. This movement is known as **segmentation.**

Factors Controlling Digestive Function

The activities of the digestive system are controlled by nerves, hormones, and local mechanisms. Sensory nerves present in the walls of the gut can be stimulated by food material in the lumen and by stretching of the walls. By their communication with the nerve that supplies the smooth muscles, contraction of smooth muscle and secretion of glands in the local area can be affected. In addition, communication of these sensory nerves with the central nervous system can alter activities in various remote parts of the gut.

The gastrointestinal tract is an endocrine factory in itself. Eighteen or more secreted hormones have been identified, with more hormones being identified continually. The hormones secreted in the gastrointestinal tract are transported by the blood and have their effect on other regions of the gut. For example, **gastrin,** a hormone secreted by cells in the stomach, stimulates gastric motility and secretion. Similarly, hormones (e.g., **secretin, cholecystokinin**) from the upper part of the intestine cause an increase in the secretion from the pancreas and relaxation of the sphincter between the small and large intestines.

In addition to hormones, chemicals released locally regulate the activities of the cells. For example, histamine released by cells in the stomach stimulates the adjacent acid-secreting cells. Local mechanisms are important when small areas of the gut must be regulated.

Although the gut appears autonomous, with its own nerve supply, hormones, and local mechanisms, its activities can be modified by other factors. The central nervous system (i.e., the brain and the spinal cord), hormones secreted by other endocrine glands and even changes in the electrolyte content of the blood can modify its activities. That is how stress can cause changes in bowel habits. Individuals with hyperthyroidism tend to have diarrhea, and individuals with hypothyroid, constipation. Many drugs taken for other ailments can also affect the normal functioning of the gut.

An Overview of Nutrition

Nutrition is the function of living plants and animals in which food material is metabolized to build tissue and liberate energy. The first chapter explained the chemical level of regulation and outlined the various chemical components of the body. It follows that the food ingested should consist of all of these components in

Table 11.1

Mean Height, Weight, and Recommended Energy Intake

Age (yr)	Weight (kg) Male	Female	Height (cm) Male	Female	Energy Needs (kcal) (doing light work) Male	Female
11–14	45	46	157	157	2,700	2,200
15–18	66	55	176	163	2,800	2,100
19–22	70	55	177	163	2,900	2,100
23–50	70	55	178	163	2,700	2,000
51–75	70	55	178	163	2,400	1,800
>76	70	55	178	163	2,050	1,600
Pregnancy						+300
Lactation						+500

sufficient amounts to meet the needs of the body at a specific time. Understandably, the needs increase at the time of growth—birth to adolescence and during pregnancy and lactation in women. It also varies according to a person's age, height, weight, and physical activity.

Today, a person's diet, regardless of nutritional needs, varies with affluence, the productivity of the farmers, the availability and accessibility of food, and the food industry. There is confusion among the public because of the numerous books, articles, and advertisements available related to diet. It is important for all individuals to maintain a balanced nutrition because there is evidence that the diet is linked to specific diseases (e.g., a high cholesterol diet is linked to a higher risk of heart disease). See Table 11.1 for the recommended energy intake by individuals of various age groups and physiologic conditions.

Functions of Important Nutrients

PROTEINS/AMINO ACIDS

Proteins are the constituents of structures such as muscle, enzymes, antibodies, some hormones, neurotransmitters, and nucleic acids. They also help transport other substances in the blood. Proteins are required for the body performing many vital functions. Each gram of protein contributes 4 kcal of energy. An average adult woman needs about 40–45 g (1.4–1.6 oz) and an average adult man about 50–60 g (1.8–2.1 oz) of protein per day. A high protein content can be found in such food as eggs, meat, poultry, fish, milk, and cheese. Animal proteins such as this are considered good because they contain all 10 essential amino acids that can be obtained by the body only through diet. Not all plant proteins have all essential amino acids; those on strict vegetarian diets must consume a variety of plant proteins.

CARBOHYDRATES

Carbohydrates, the main source of energy, is stored as glycogen in liver and muscle. It is also a major source of dietary fiber. One gram of carbohydrate provides 4 kcal of energy. Rich sources of carbohydrates are whole grains and grain products, vegetables, and fruits. Consumption of both insoluble and soluble carbohydrates is needed. The insoluble forms (dietary fibers) add bulk to the food and help with bowel movements. An average diet should contain 30–35 g (1.1–1.2 oz) of fiber.

FAT

Fat is needed for the manufacture of cell membranes and steroid hormones. Some fatty acids are required for manufacturing substances such as prostaglandin and other chemical mediators. Another source of energy, each gram provides 9 kcal of energy.

VITAMINS

Vitamins are organic substances present in minute amounts in natural foodstuff that are needed for normal metabolism. Depending on their chemical characteristics, they are classified as **fat-soluble vitamins** and **water-soluble vitamins.**

Vitamins A, D, E, and K are fat-soluble vitamins. Being lipid-soluble, these vitamins are absorbed from the diet, along with the fat content, through the digestive tract. Vitamin D can be manufactured by the skin when exposed to sunlight. The intestinal bacteria manufacture a small amount of vitamin K. Fat-soluble vitamins diffuse across the cell membranes easily and, normally, the body has a large reserve of these vitamins.

Water-soluble vitamins—B_1 (thiamine), B_2 (riboflavin), niacin (nicotinic acid), B_5 (pantothenic acid), B_6 (pyridoxine), folacin (folic acid), B_{12} (cobalamin), biotin, and C (ascorbic acid)—are obtained from the diet and absorbed through the digestive tract. Although most water-soluble vitamins are easily absorbed from the gut, vitamin B_{12} must be bound to intrinsic factor (see **page 587**) secreted by the gastric mucosa before absorption can occur.

Other than the diet, the body obtains water-soluble vitamins from the intestinal bacteria that are capable of manufacturing five of nine water-soluble vitamins. Excess amounts of vitamins are rapidly excreted in the urine. The body does not contain a large reserve of these vitamins, and an individual can show symptoms of vitamin deficiency within a few days to a few weeks.

The function, source, daily requirement, and effect of deficiency and excess of vitamins are given in Table 11.2.

OTHER NUTRIENTS

In addition, the body requires small amounts of such nutrients as calcium, phosphorus, iron, copper, iodine, zinc, fluoride, magnesium, and manganese to function normally (see Table 11.3).

Regulation of Food Intake

Even if it appears otherwise, food intake is generally regulated with great precision. The weight of a normal human is relatively constant over a long period. Studies show that if animals are starved for some time and then permitted to eat as they wish, they only increase their food intake until they regain their lost weight.[1] Similarly, if an animal is force-fed to make it obese and then is allowed to eat freely, the food intake is diminished until the excessive weight gained is lost. The area of the brain known as the **hypothalamus** is responsible for regulating the appetite.

The hypothalamus has two areas—the **feeding center** and the **satiety center.** Stimulation of the feeding center increases food intake, and stimulation of the satiety center reduces food intake. The interaction of both centers regulates how much an individual eats. It has been shown that the cells in the satiety center become less active if the glucose level in the blood reaching the center is low. This, in turn, makes the feeding center more active and more food is taken in. Some other signaling molecules in the blood that affect the hypothalamus and decrease appetite are the hormones glucagon, epinephrine, and leptin (hormone from fat cells). Certain signaling molecules, such as growth hormone, glucocorticoids, insulin, and progesterone, produce an increase in appetite. Many of the drugs given in weight reduction programs reduce the appetite by affecting the food centers in the hypothalamus.

In addition to the hypothalamus, other areas in the brain determine what is eaten. Researchers have shown that lesions in certain areas of the temporal lobe of the brain can make it difficult for an individual to distinguish between edible and inedible and to have a tendency to orally explore all kinds of objects.[1]

Regulation of food intake is a complex process. Other areas of the body other than the brain also have an effect on food intake. Food in the gut can inhibit food intake. It is believed that the amount of fat in the body sends feedback to the brain in some manner that controls the appetite. It is also well known that contractions of the empty stomach—hunger pangs—stimulate appetite. Another major factor for food intake in humans is the culture, environment, and past experiences relative to the taste, sight, and smell of food. Research is underway to explain the actual cause of eating disorders.

Blood Supply to the Digestive Tract

Please refer to **page 483** (arterial supply to the abdomen and pelvis) and **page 486** (portal circulation).

The Structure and Function of Individual Organs of the Digestive System

The digestive tract can be thought of as a very long tube, beginning in the mouth and ending in the anus. The tube is modified in different areas to fulfill spe-

Table 11.2

The Vitamins

Vitamin	Function	Source	Daily Requirement	Effect of Deficiency	Effect of Excess
A	Required for visual pigment, maintains epithelium	Green leafy vegetables	1 mg	Night blindness, retarded growth, deterioration of epithelium	Peeling of skin, liver damage, nausea, loss of appetite
D	Required for normal growth, calcium metabolism	Synthesized in skin; milk, cheese	–	Rickets, bony deformities	Calcium deposits in tissue
E	Prevents breakdown of vitamin A and fatty acids	Vegetables, meat, milk	12 mg	Anemia	–
K	Required for manufacture of clotting factors	Vegetables, manufactured by intestinal bacteria	0.7–0.14 mg	Bleeding tendencies	Liver dysfunction, jaundice
B$_1$ (thiamine)	Coenzyme	Milk, meat, bread	1.9 mg	Beriberi (muscle weakness; nervous and cardiovascular problems)	hypotension
B$_2$ (riboflavine)	Coenzyme; energy formation	Milk, meat	1.5 mg	Epithelial and mucosal deterioration	Itching, tingling sensations
Niacin (nicotinic acid)	Energy formation	Meat, bread, potatoes	14.6 mg	Pellagra (CNS, GI, epithelial and mucosal degeneration)	Itching; burning; vasodilation and death with large doses
B$_5$ (pantothenic acid)	Energy formation	Milk, meat	4.7 mg	Growth retardation; CNS abnormalities	–
B$_6$ (pyridoxine)	Coenzyme	meat	1.42 mg	Growth retardation; anemia; epithelial changes, convulsions	CNS alterations
Folacin (folic acid)	Coenzyme	Vegetables; cereal, bread 0.1 mg	0.1 mg	Growth retardation; anemia; GI disorders; deficiency during pregnancy; CNS abnormalities	–
B$_{12}$ (cobalamin)	Coenzyme	Milk, meat	4.5 μg	Pernicious anemia	polycythemia
Biotin	Coenzyme	Eggs, meat, vegetables	0.1–0.2 mg	Fatigue; muscle pain	–
C (ascorbic acid)	Coenzyme	Citrus fruit	60 mg	Scurvy (epithelial and mucosal deterioration)	Kidney stones

cific functions. Numerous accessory organs in and close to this tube help fulfill these functions. Figure 11.1 illustrates the principal organs of the digestive system. In this section, the digestive system will be described according to the path of food from the mouth to the anus.

THE MOUTH AND ASSOCIATED STRUCTURES

The mouth (see Figure 11.5) opens into the **oral cavity,** or **buccal cavity.** Anatomically, the mouth extends from inside the lips to the **fauces,** a constric-tion or narrowed area that can be seen in the back of the mouth. Beyond this, is the **pharynx.** The roof of the mouth is formed by the **palate.** The anterior two-thirds, the **hard palate,** is hard, containing bone. The posterior one-third, the **soft palate,** has muscle and no bone and is, therefore, soft. The conical downward projection from the soft palate is known as the **uvula.** The soft palate and the uvula project backward from the hard palate and separate the pharynx into the **oropharynx** and **nasopharynx.** They prevent food from entering the nose during swallowing by closing the opening between the nasopharynx and oropharynx.

Table 11.3

The Minerals: Functions and Daily Requirements

Mineral	Importance
Sodium	Major cation in body fluids; needed for cell membrane function
Potassium	Major cation inside cells; needed for cell membrane function
Chloride	Major anion of body fluids
Calcium	Needed for normal muscle contraction, neuron function, bone structure, and blood coagulation
Phosphorus	Bone matrix; part of high-energy compounds (e.g., ATP)
Magnesium	Required for normal cell membrane function; cofactor of enzymes
Iron	Part of hemoglobin; myoglobin
Zinc	Cofactor of enzymes
Copper	Cofactor for hemoglobin synthesis
Manganese	Cofactor of some enzymes

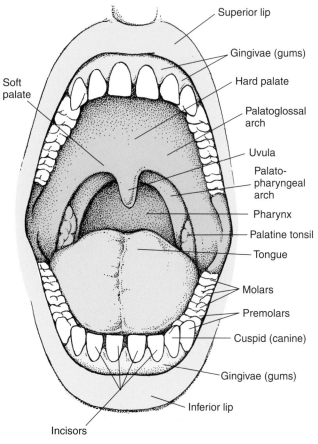

FIGURE **11.5.**   Structures of the Mouth

The fauces, or the posterior region of the mouth, has two mucosal arches on each side. Going from the palate toward the tongue is the **palatoglossal arch,** and behind it, going toward the pharynx, is the **palatopharyngeal arch.** When a person gags, the muscles in the two arches contract and narrow the opening between the mouth and the pharynx, a protective mechanism that prevents unwanted objects from entering the digestive tract.

Between the two arches in the side, lie the **palatine tonsils.** The tonsils are part of the lymphoid system, and they help filter bacteria and toxins that may enter through the mucosa (inner lining) of the mouth.

The Teeth

The teeth (see Figures 11.5 and 11.6) are important for breaking the food into small pieces. This process is known as **mastication** (see **page 203** for the muscles of mastication). The teeth arise from **alveoli,** small sockets in the mandibular and maxillary bones. The tooth is surrounded at the base by the **gums,** or **gingivae.** The bulk of each tooth is a bone-like material called **dentin,** which covers a cavity at the center of the tooth called the **pulp cavity.** Blood vessels and nerves pass through a canal **(root canal)** at the base (root) of the tooth to enter the pulp cavity. Collagen fibers **(periodontal ligament),** from the root of the tooth to the bone, hold the tooth in place. The ligament is reinforced to the bone by **cementum.** The **crown** of the tooth is the portion visible above the gums. The dentin

of the crown is covered by a layer of **enamel,** which is a crystalline form of calcium phosphate.

The teeth are modified according to function; four types have been identified. The blade-like **incisors,** found in the center of the mouth, cut, clip, and nip. The **cuspids,** or **canines**—conical, with a sharp ridge and pointed tip—slash and tear. The **bicuspids,** or **premolars,** with flattened crowns and prominent ridges, help crush, mash, and grind food. The posteriorly located **molars,** larger versions of the bicuspids, crush and grind. In an adult, there are 3 pairs of molars, 2 pairs of bicuspids, 1 pair of cuspids, and 2 pairs of incisors in each jaw.

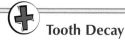

Tooth Decay

Tooth decay results from the action of bacteria in the mouth that secretes a sticky substance that traps food and forms a deposit called plaque. The plaque slowly hardens to form tartar or dental calculus. The tartar protects the bacteria from being destroyed by the saliva. Acids secreted by the bacteria erode the tooth and the result is dental caries.

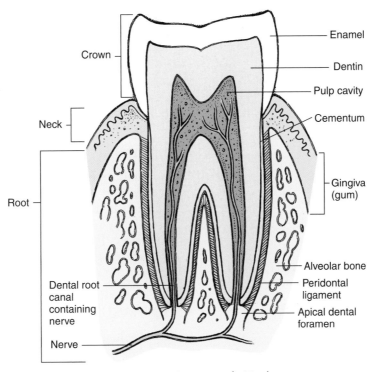

Crown

Neck

Root

Dental root
canal
containing
nerve

Nerve

Enamel

Dentin

Pulp cavity

Cementum

Gingiva
(gum)

Alveolar bone

Peridontal
ligament

Apical dental
foramen

FIGURE **11.6.**   Structure of a Tooth

The **cheeks,** or lateral walls of the oral cavity, are comprised of the buccinator muscles and pads of fat. Anteriorly, the cheek is continuous with the **lip,** or **labia.** The space between the teeth and the cheeks is the **vestibule.**

The Tongue

The tongue is muscular and has its own functions. It positions the food on the teeth, initiates swallowing, has taste buds that help taste food, and plays a key role in speech. The muscles of the tongue are controlled by the hypoglossal nerve (cranial nerve XII). Sensations such as touch, pain, and pressure are carried to the brain by the trigeminal nerve (cranial nerve V). The special sensation of taste is carried by the facial nerve, the glossopharyngeal nerve, and the vagus nerve. The facial nerve carries sensations from the anterior two-thirds of the tongue, and the glossopharyngeal carries it from the posterior one-third. The vagus nerve carries taste sensations from other areas of the mouth, such as the palate and pharynx.

The surface of the tongue appears fuzzy and has minute projections called **papillae.** Most of the taste buds—the sensory organs of taste—are located on the papillae. The taste buds have connections with nerve-endings that carry the sensation of taste to the brain. In humans, there are five basic tastes: sweet, sour, bitter, salt and umami. Bitter substances are best tasted on the back of the tongue; sour along the edges; sweet at the tip; and salt on the dorsum, anteriorly. Taste is sensed when the substances dissolved in the oral fluids come in contact with the taste buds.

SALIVARY GLANDS AND SALIVA

Adjacent to the mouth are many **salivary glands** (see Figure 11.7), which secrete about 1,500 mL (1.59 qt) of saliva per day. Saliva contains two enzymes that begin digestion of fat and carbohydrates (see **page 594**). Mucins (glycoproteins) in the saliva lubricate the food and protect the mucosa of the mouth. Some

FLAVOR OF FOOD

The flavor of food is determined not only by the taste buds, but also by an element of pain stimulation (e.g., hot sauces), smell, consistency, and temperature.

Many diseases can cause diminished taste sensitivity and certain drugs can cause temporary loss of taste sensation.

SWEETENING AGENTS

Saccharin and aspartame are used as sweetening agents when calorie intake must be reduced because they produce satisfactory sweetening in amounts that are just a fraction of the amount of sucrose (sugar) needed.

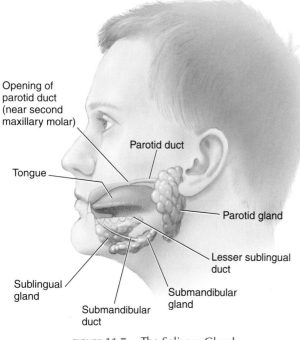

Opening of
parotid duct
(near second
maxillary molar)

Tongue

Parotid duct

Parotid gland

Lesser sublingual
duct

Sublingual
gland

Submandibular
gland

Submandibular
duct

FIGURE 11.7.   The Salivary Glands

immunoglobulins or antibodies are also present in the saliva as the first line of defense against bacteria and viruses. Other proteins that bind toxins, protect enamel (outer coating of teeth), and attack the walls of the bacteria are also present in the saliva.

Saliva performs many important functions. Saliva makes swallowing easier, keeps the mouth moist, helps with speech by facilitating lip and tongue movement, keeps the mouth and teeth clean, and serves as a solvent for the molecules that stimulate taste sensations. Antibacterial properties are provided to the saliva by antibodies and other proteins.

Salivary secretion is increased by stimulation of the autonomic nerves. Food in the mouth and lower end of the esophagus can increase secretion. It is well known that sight, smell, and even the thought of food can increase salivary production.

There are three pairs of salivary glands. The **parotid glands** are large and lie beneath the skin, covering the lateral and posterior aspect of the

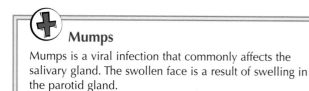

Mumps

Mumps is a viral infection that commonly affects the salivary gland. The swollen face is a result of swelling in the parotid gland.

mandible (i.e., anterior to the ears). A duct from the parotid gland empties the saliva into the vestibule near the upper molar teeth. The **sublingual glands** are located in the floor of the mouth. Many ducts from this gland open under the tongue. The **submandibular glands** are medial to the mandible on its inner surface, in the floor of the mouth.

PHARYNX

The pharynx (see page 545) is the common pathway for food and air and is connected to the nose, throat, and mouth. The pharynx extends from the posterior part of the nose to the entrance of the larynx and esophagus. It is divided into three regions—the **nasopharynx,** the **oropharynx,** and the **laryngopharynx** (**see Figure 10.2**).

ESOPHAGUS

The esophagus (Figure 11.1) is a long tube that transports food from the mouth to the stomach. It is about 25 cm (10 in) long and 2 cm (0.8 in) wide. It is located behind the trachea and travels downward in the posterior part of the thoracic cavity. Before it enters the abdomen, where the stomach is located, it passes through an opening in the diaphragm.

At the proximal end, closer to the pharynx, and at the distal end, closer to the stomach, circular muscles prevent entry of air and backflow of material from the stomach, respectively. The slight narrowing at the lower end of the esophagus is the **lower esophageal sphincter.** If this sphincter does not close properly after the food has entered the stomach, the stomach contents can regurgitate into the lower end of the esophagus. This condition is known as **gastro-esophageal reflux disease.** Because the contents of the stomach are acidic, the walls of the esophagus can become irritated and produce a burning sensation in the epigastric region, referred to as **heartburn.**

Swallowing

After mastication, food material is swallowed. The process of swallowing is known as **deglutition.** Deglutition is only voluntary at the start. Once the food material or bolus reaches the back of the mouth and touches the palatal arches, an involuntary reflex is triggered. The soft palate moves up, closing off the nasopharynx (you don't breath when you swallow!), the larynx moves upward (have you noticed the thyroid cartilage–Adam's apple, bob up and down?), and the epiglottis moves back to close off the larynx and prevent food from entering the respiratory tract. The tongue moves up to the palate. In this way, all exits other than the esophagus are closed. As the food reaches the esophagus, a wave of **peristalsis** (the wave-like movement of the walls of the gut) occurs. In less than 9 seconds, the food is propelled into the stomach. Reverse peristalsis takes place when vomiting occurs.

STOMACH

The stomach is a sac-like, J-shaped expansion of the gut that stores the ingested food and propels the partially digested food into the intestines in smaller quantities. By churning movements, it further breaks down the food particles. The walls of the stomach have an abundance of smooth muscle that run circularly, obliquely, and longitudinally. Contraction of this muscle helps churn the food.

Enzymes (pepsin and gastric lipase) and acid (hydrochloric acid) secreted by the glands in the walls of the stomach help break chemical bonds and partially digest the food. The acid kills many ingested bacteria and provides the right pH for pepsin to start protein digestion. Mucus, made up of glycoproteins and secreted by mucous glands, protects the stomach wall from getting digested. The glands also produce a compound known as the **intrinsic factor.** Intrinsic factor is required for absorption of vitamin B_{12} in the small intestine. A total volume of about 2,500 mL (2.6 qt) of gastric juice is secreted per day.

The stomach is divided into specific regions (see Figure 11.8). The **cardia** is the proximal region, close to the esophagus. The **fundus** is the portion of the stomach that is superior to the junction with the esophagus. The **body** is the area from the fundus to the curve of the J. The **pylorus** is the area of the curve of the J; it narrows into the **pyloric canal** before it opens into the first part of the intestine, the duodenum.

Circular muscles—the **pyloric sphincter**—guard the opening and regulate the amount of food material that enters the duodenum. The consistency of food is changed by the end of the processing by the stomach; watery and acidic, it is known as **chyme.**

The activity of the stomach, similar to the rest of the gut, is controlled by the central nervous system, local nervous reflexes, and gastrointestinal hormones. The gastric secretion increases with the sight, smell, taste, and even thought of food. Other emotions, such as anger, can increase secretions. Fear, anxiety, and stress can reduce the activity. Impulses from the brain reach the gut via the vagus nerve (cranial nerve X). When food arrives in the stomach, secretions are increased by the distension of the stom-

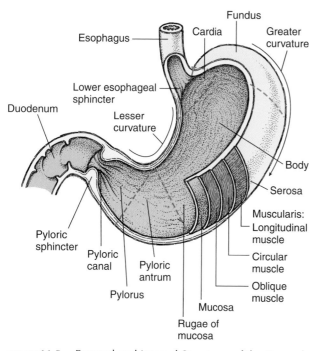

FIGURE 11.8.   External and Internal Structures of the Stomach

ach, presence of undigested material, and pH changes. Food in the intestine has a feedback effect on the rate at which chyme is expelled into the intestine from the stomach. Details of the control mechanisms are beyond the scope of this book but, in short, nerves, local hormones, and local effects superimposed by the central nervous system and hormones secreted elsewhere control the activity.

Digestion of proteins begins in the stomach. The digestion of carbohydrates and lipids that began in the mouth continues in the stomach until the pH drops (becomes acidic). The lining of the stomach is not conducive to food absorption. Few substances such as ethyl alcohol, some water, ions, short-chain fatty acids, and certain drugs (e.g., aspirin) are absorbed here. The major part of digestion and absorption occurs in the small intestine.

SMALL INTESTINE

The small intestine is a long tube approximately 3 m (9.8 ft) long and less than 2.5 cm (1 in) wide. A major part of the abdominal cavity is, therefore, occupied by the small intestine, with the liver occupying the upper right quadrant of the abdomen and the stomach, the epigastric region. About 90% of absorption occurs in the small intestine.

The intestine is divided into three parts: the **duodenum,** the **jejunum,** and the **ileum.** The duodenum is the first part of the small intestine, leading off from the stomach. It is C-shaped, with the pancreas nes-

tled in the curve of the C. The liver is located superior and lateral to the duodenum. Bile secretions from the liver, after being temporarily stored in the gallbladder, flow into the duodenum.

The duodenum, unlike the rest of the small intestine, does not float freely in the abdominal cavity suspended by the mesentery. Instead, the duodenum is in close contact with the posterior part of the abdomen at levels of L1 and L4 and is considered retroperitoneal (behind the peritoneum).

The jejunum, which is continuous with the duodenum, is 1 m (3.3 ft) long. Most digestion occurs here. The ileum, the third region, is the longest at 2 m (6.6 ft). At its distal end, it has circular smooth muscles—the **ileocecal valve.** This area of circular smooth muscle regulates the amount of chyme that enters the cecum, the first part of the large intestine.

The walls of the small intestine have numerous intestinal glands that continue the digestion of food and numerous glands that secrete hormones. About 1.8 liters (1.9 qt) of watery fluid is secreted in the intestines. An abundance of mucus, secreted by the submucous glands, protects the walls of the gut from digestion by enzymes. Because sympathetic stimulation decreases secretion, the duodenum becomes more vulnerable to destruction by chyme and development of ulcers. This is one association between stress and peptic ulcers.

THE PANCREAS

The pancreas (see Figure 11.9) is a gland that lies posterior to the stomach and to the left of the C-shaped curve of the duodenum. The end that lies inside the curve of the C is larger and is known as the **head.** It tapers toward the other end, which extends up to the spleen. This end is the **tail** of the pancreas, with the **body** in between.

The pancreas has two functions—exocrine and endocrine. The exocrine function manufactures enzymes that help with the digestion of proteins, fats,

PROTECTION OF GASTRIC MUCOSA

Gastric secretion is so concentrated that it can cause tissue damage. Fortunately, the healthy gastric mucosa is protected by mucus secretion that forms a 1–3 mm thick layer over the mucosa. The mucosal cells also secrete bicarbonate that, together with the mucus and the tight junction between the cells, protects the stomach lining from becoming irritated and digested.

Substances such as ethanol, vinegar, bile salts, aspirin, and nonsteroidal anti-inflammatory drugs disrupt the barrier and produce gastric irritation.

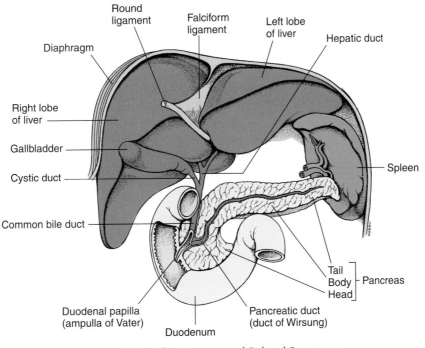

FIGURE **11.9.** The Pancreas and Related Structures

and carbohydrates. The secretions are drained from the gland to the duodenum by the **pancreatic duct.** Before the duct opens into the lumen, it meets with the **common bile duct** that drains bile from the liver and gallbladder. Pancreatic secretion is alkaline; about 1.5 liters (1.6 qt) of pancreatic juice is secreted every day.

The endocrine portion of the pancreas consists of cells known as the **pancreatic islets,** or **islets of Langerhans.** One important hormone secreted by these cells into the blood is insulin, which regulates blood glucose levels.

Pancreatitis

In pancreatitis, the pancreas becomes inflamed and the enzymes spill over into the surrounding tissue, digesting and damaging them. If the islets of Langerhans are destroyed, glucose regulation will be affected and diabetes mellitus results.

THE LIVER

The liver (Figure 11. 9) is the largest organ in the abdomen. It is reddish brown and has a firm consistency. The liver is located in the right upper quadrant of the abdomen, occupying the right hypochondriac, epigastric, and umbilical regions and part of the left hypochondriac. It lies directly below the diaphragm.

The liver is covered by a tough connective tissue capsule over which is the peritoneum.

Unique Blood Supply to the Liver

The liver receives one third of its blood supply via the hepatic artery (see **Figures 8.21 and 8.23**), whose blood is derived from the aorta. The remaining two thirds comes from the hepatic portal vein, which drains blood from the esophagus, stomach, spleen, small intestine, and most of the large intestine. In this way, nutrients absorbed from the gut are processed by the liver before they enter the general

Hepatitis

Hepatitis is a condition that produces inflammation in the liver and inadequate functioning of the hepatocytes. It is most often a result of a viral infection.

There are many different strains of hepatitis virus, such as Hepatitis A, B, C, and E. The incubation period and mode of transmission varies from strain to strain. Hepatitis A, also known as infectious hepatitis, is highly contagious and is transmitted by fecal-oral contamination. Hepatitis B, also known as serum hepatitis, is transmitted through infected blood, serum, or plasma. Serum hepatitis is more serious, often leading to cirrhosis, cancer of the liver, and carrier state.

Surface Marking of the Liver

The most lateral part of the liver lies about midway between the anterior and posterior midline of the thorax beneath the ribs 7–11. Its upper border extends just below the right nipple and goes across the midline of the body to just below the left nipple. The lower border extends from this left end to the 11th rib laterally. The lower margin of the normal-sized liver is not felt in the abdomen. If the liver is enlarged, it is felt in the abdomen below the ribs, as a firm mass that moves with respiration. As a result of its close contact with the diaphragm, the liver is pushed down while inhaling.

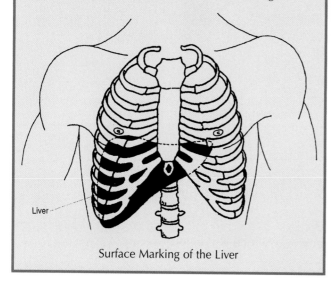

Liver

Surface Marking of the Liver

circulation. After processing in the liver, the blood enters the inferior vena cava via the hepatic vein.

An Overview of the Microscopic Structure of the Liver

The liver is made up of specialized cells called **hepatocytes.** These cells are arranged in single file similar to the spokes of a wheel (see Figure 11.10). At the center of the wheel is the **central vein,** which joins other central veins to form the **hepatic vein.** In the periphery of the wheel, are the blood vessels and ducts for bile. The blood vessels, branches of the **hepatic artery** (containing oxygenated blood from the aorta) and the **hepatic portal vein** (containing blood from the gut, rich in nutrients), open into **sinusoids** (large blood vessels) between the line of hepatocytes. The sinusoids run parallel to the hepatocytes and open into the central vein.

Other cells, **Kupffer cells,** are located in the walls of the sinusoids. Kupffer cells are actually macrophages (white blood cells), which destroy microorganisms that may have entered the blood through the gut.

Tiny channels that carry bile are found between the hepatocytes, along the spokes of the wheel. These channels open into the **bile ductules** located in the periphery of the wheel. The bile ductules ultimately form the **common hepatic duct** that leaves the liver to join the duct from the gallbladder (**cystic duct**).

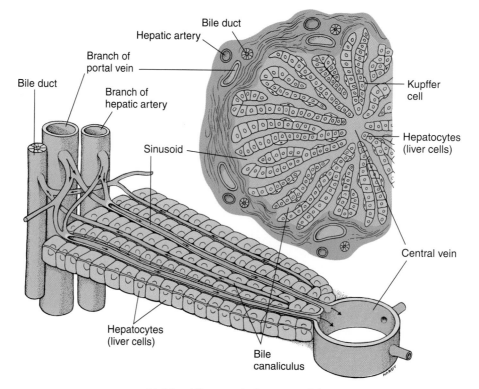

Bile duct

Hepatic artery

Branch of portal vein

Bile duct

Branch of hepatic artery

Sinusoid

Kupffer cell

Hepatocytes (liver cells)

Central vein

Hepatocytes (liver cells)

Bile canaliculus

FIGURE **11.10.**   Microscopic Structure of the Liver

Jaundice

Jaundice, a term given to the yellow coloration of the skin and mucus membrane, is a result of the body's inability to cope with bilirubin, the breakdown product of hemoglobin. When bilirubin levels increase in the blood, it diffuses into the interstitial fluid and produces a yellow tinge to the skin and mucous membrane. Because jaundice is a result of an increase in bilirubin, all people with jaundice are not infectious. Any condition that increases bilirubin levels produces jaundice. For example, if there is a rapid breakdown of red blood cells, faster than the rate at which the liver can cope, jaundice can be observed. When the liver is premature, as in preterm babies, or damaged (hepatitis) or if the bile duct leading to the duodenum is obstructed, jaundice can occur.

The cystic duct and common hepatic duct join to form the **common bile duct,** which opens into the duodenum.

From this description, it can be understood that the liver has an efficient architecture to fulfill its many functions.

Functions of the Liver

Physiology textbooks state that the liver has more than 200 different functions. The most important functions are discussed here. The liver is arranged in such a way that it can screen the blood going into the systemic circulation and adjust the levels of various substances in the blood.

Effect on carbohydrates: The liver helps maintain the blood glucose level. It stores glucose obtained from the gut as glycogen, if the blood level of glucose is too high. If the glucose level drops, the glycogen is converted to glucose to return the blood glucose level to normal. Lipids and proteins are also used to manufacture glucose.

Effect on lipids: Similar to carbohydrates, the liver adjusts lipid levels in blood by mobilizing or storing lipids.

Effect on proteins: Amino acids absorbed from the gut may be stored in the liver for conversion into lipids, carbohydrates, or proteins. When needed, they are broken down. Ammonia is formed when amino acids are broken down. The liver converts the ammonia into urea, which is later excreted by the kidneys.

The liver manufactures most of the plasma proteins such as albumin, proteins required for the clotting process, and proteins used as transport vehicles in the blood. The liver also removes antibodies from the blood.

Removal of waste products: The liver detoxifies toxins and drugs. Many drugs are rapidly converted to ineffective forms by the liver. That is why certain drugs must be given in larger quantities and in frequent doses. Conversely, dosage must be reduced in liver failure.

Removal of pathogens: The Kupffer cells, which are fixed macrophages, remove pathogens and old and damaged blood cells. The breakdown product of hemoglobin (from red blood cells)—bilirubin—is removed from the blood and secreted into the bile for disposal.

Removal of circulating hormones: The liver is important role for removing hormones that circulate in the blood, such as epinephrine, norepinephrine, thyroid hormones, corticosteroids, and sex hormones.

Formation of vitamin D: One important function of the liver is to convert a precursor of vitamin D that is manufactured in the skin or absorbed in the gut into an intermediary product that can be acted upon by the kidney. The kidney is the organ that finally forms vitamin D—one of the hormones that regulates calcium levels in the blood (see **page 60**).

Storage of vitamins: The liver stores many vitamins, especially vitamin B_{12} and the fat-soluble vitamins, A, D, E, and K.

Mineral storage: An important mineral stored by the liver is iron.

Bile synthesis: The liver manufactures bile, the secretion vital for fat digestion and absorption. Bile is a yellow liquid that is mostly water. The most important component of bile is **bile salts.**

Because fat in the diet is not water-soluble, it coalesces to form large drops of fat in the gut. This makes it difficult for the enzymes secreted by the pancreas to act on the fat located deep inside the drop. The bile salts break the large drops into smaller ones, making it easier for the enzymes to act. In addition, the bile salts facilitate the action of the enzymes and help with the absorption of lipids through the mucosa into the body. Most bile salts that enter the gut via the bile duct are reabsorbed into the circulation and recycled by the liver.

Other than bile salts, bile also contains the **bile pigment** bilirubin, which is a breakdown product of hemoglobin.

GALLBLADDER

The gallbladder (Figure 11.9) is a pear-shaped organ in close contact with the inferior surface of the liver.

BILE SALTS AND BILE PIGMENTS

Note that bile pigments and bile salts are different entities. Bile pigments are waste products that give the characteristic color to feces.

Gallstones

For various reasons, the bile in the gallbladder can become so concentrated that it forms crystals—gallstones, or cholelithiasis. If the stones are small, they are not a problem; if big, they may block the duct and produce severe pain.

The gallbladder may be removed if there is chronic inflammation. Removal of the gallbladder does not greatly affect digestion because bile formed in the liver can reach the gut. The bile, however, will be more dilute and its entry into the gut not so well regulated. Individuals who have had cholecystectomy (removal of the gallbladder) may have to avoid food particularly high in fat content.

The cystic duct of the gallbladder joins with the common hepatic duct to form the common bile duct. The function of the gallbladder is to store and concentrate bile that is secreted by the liver. The capacity of a normal gallbladder is about 40–70 mL (1.4–2.4 oz). Because the opening (sphincter) of the common bile duct is closed other than at meal times, the bile that is secreted by the liver is stored in the gallbladder. When stored, some water from the bile is absorbed by the walls of the gallbladder, concentrating it. Contraction of the smooth muscles of the gallbladder and opening of the sphincter is largely caused by **cholecystokinin,** a hormone secreted by cells in the duodenum.

ABSORPTION IN THE SMALL INTESTINE

The absorption is addressed in detail according to food type following the description of the rest of the digestive tract. The small intestine is fully suited for its absorptive function in that its length, presence of villi, and microvilli greatly increase the surface area. Also, the movement of the food material through it is quite slow—about 5 hours for food to pass from the duodenum to the end of the small intestine. In addition, the blood supply and lymphatic supply are extensive.

THE LARGE INTESTINE

The large intestine is much wider than the small intestine. The large intestine (Figure 11.1) is about 6.5 cm (2.6 in) wide and 1.5 m (5 ft) long. The end of the ileum, guarded by the **ileocecal valve** (or sphincter), opens into the large intestine, which begins in the right lower quadrant of the abdomen. The large intestine consists of three regions: the **cecum,** the **colon,** and the **rectum.** The rectum opens into the exterior via the **anus.** The main functions of the large intestine are to absorb water, sodium, and minerals from the chyme and make it more compact; absorb vitamins manufactured by the present bacteria; and, finally, to store fecal matter until it can be expelled from the body. The large intestine removes about 90% of the water in the chyme, reducing the 1–2 liters (1.1–2.1 qt) of chyme to 200–250 mL (about 0.2 qt) of feces passed per day.

The first part of the intestine—the cecum—has a small wormlike projection from the posteromedial side, the **vermiform appendix.** The appendix is about 7.5–15 cm (3–6 in) long, with a variable size and shape. It contains a large amount of lymphoid tissue. In humans, it does not have an important function. Occasionally, the appendix becomes inflamed and produces the typical symptoms of appendicitis.

The colon can be subdivided into four parts—the **ascending colon,** the **transverse colon,** the **descending colon,** and the **sigmoid colon**—all named according to their anatomy. The ascending colon ascends from the right lower quadrant toward the liver in the posterior and lateral aspect of the abdominal cavity. Here, it makes a sharp bend, the **hepatic flexure,** to continue transversely as the transverse colon just inferior to the stomach. To the left, it reaches the spleen before it bends inferiorly to continue as the descending colon. This bend is known as the **splenic flexure.** At the iliac fossa, the descending colon curves inward and descends further as the sigmoid colon, the S-shaped segment of the large intestine. The sigmoid colon lies posterior to the urinary bladder and becomes the **rectum.**

The rectum forms the last 15 cm (6 in) of the digestive tract. When feces enters the rectum, there is an urge to defecate. The **anus** is the last few centimeters of the digestive tract. This region has circular smooth muscles that form the **internal anal sphincter.** Under voluntary control, the circular skeletal muscles located here form the **external anal sphincter.**

The walls of the large intestine have cells that produce large amounts of mucus. No enzymes are released and no digestion occurs here. The longitudinally arranged smooth muscles in the walls of the colon form three bands called **teniae coli.** Because these longitudinal bands are shorter than the length

THE COLON AS A ROUTE FOR ABSORPTION

Because the absorptive capacity of the colon is great, it is a practical route for administration of drugs, especially in children. Anesthetics, steroids, and painkillers are all rapidly absorbed by this route.

Constipation

Constipation is defined as a condition in which there is infrequent or incomplete bowel movements. Many healthy individuals have bowel movements only once in 3 days, and others may defecate once, or even 3 times a day. The only symptoms caused by constipation are mild abdominal discomfort, abdominal distention, and a slight loss of appetite. The symptoms are not a result of absorption of "toxic substances" as many believe. It has been shown that the symptoms are relieved promptly when the rectum is evacuated and caused when it is filled, even with inert substances.

Other symptoms attributed to constipation are invariably because of anxiety or other causes. However, constipation that persists, especially in those individuals who have noticed a change in bowel habits of recent onset, should be examined by a physician.

of the colon, the wall of the colon forms outpouchings (**haustra**) between the teniae.

Feces

The feces contain inorganic material, undigested plant fibers, bacteria, and water. Surprisingly, a large fraction of the feces is of nondietary origin. Of the feces, 75% is water and 25% is solids. Of the total solids, bacteria forms 30%; inorganic material, such as calcium and phosphate, 15%; fat and fat derivatives, 5%; and a variable amount of cellulose and indigestible fiber, mucus, and mucosal cells that have sloughed off from the wall of the gut.

Bacteria and Colon

Although the jejunum contains little or no bacteria, the colon contains large numbers of bacteria. The bacteria in the colon are beneficial because many of them manufacture such vitamins as vitamin K and B complex. Chemicals formed by intestinal bacteria are largely responsible for the odor of the feces. Some bacteria residing in the intestine are harmful and may invade the body when the immunity is particularly low.

Dietary Fiber

Plant materials that reach the large intestine relatively unchanged are known as **dietary fibers.** Fibers are important to increase the bulk of the feces that is required to stretch the walls of the colon and initiate defecation. It has been shown that an intake of large amounts of vegetable fiber decreases the incidence of colon cancer, diabetes mellitus, and some types of heart diseases.

Movement in the Colon and Defecation

The movement in the colon is similar to the small intestine in that peristalsis and a segmentation type of contraction are present. In addition, there is a third type of contraction, **mass action** contraction, in which there is simultaneous contraction of the smooth muscle over a large area. This movement pushes material from one portion of the colon to another and into the rectum. When the rectum is distended, it initiates the **defecation reflex.** When the pressure increases a little, there is a desire to defecate. Beyond a pressure of 55 mm Hg, both the internal and external sphincters relax and the contents of the rectum are expelled. This is the reason for the involuntary expulsion seen in infants and individuals with spinal cord injury.

In humans, sympathetic stimulation causes contraction of the internal anal sphincter and parasympathetic stimulation causes relaxation. The external anal sphincter, which is comprised of skeletal muscle, is supplied by the pudendal nerve. Defecation is primarily a spinal reflex; however, it can be voluntarily initiated by relaxing the external sphincter and contracting the abdominal muscles to increase abdominal pressure.

Distension of the stomach by food also initiates the **gastrocolic reflex.** This reflex is responsible for the defecation soon after meals, often seen in children. In adults, habit and culture play an important role in determining when defecation occurs.

Digestion and Absorption of Food in the Gut

A typical meal contains carbohydrates, fat, protein, water, electrolytes, and vitamins. The gut handles each component differently. Although water, electrolytes, and vitamins do not require special processing, others must be broken down into smaller molecules before they can be absorbed. Also, special transport mechanisms are used for absorption of different types of food. Carbohydrates are fragmented to simple sugars, proteins to amino acids, and fats (lipids) to fatty acids. Special enzymes secreted in specific parts of the gut break down the bondage between the complex molecules and reduce them to their simplest forms. Some enzymes are so specific that they only break up linkages between certain molecules of the components. For example, some break a link only between two glucose molecules and not between glucose and certain other simple sugars.

Many of the enzymes are located in such glands as the salivary gland, glands in the stomach wall, and pancreas and are secreted into the lumen of the gut. Other important enzymes are located in the mucosa of the small intestine.

A summary of the chemical events in digestion is given in Table 11.4.

CARBOHYDRATE DIGESTION AND ABSORPTION

The carbohydrates in the diet are broken down by the enzymes in the mouth, pancreas, and intestinal epithelium.

In the mouth, **amylase,** the enzyme of the saliva, breaks down starches into smaller fragments of two sugars (disaccharides) or three sugars (trisaccharides). The enzyme works best at an alkaline pH (that of the mouth); as long as the pH is adequate, it continues to work even after the food reaches the stomach. It takes about 1 to 2 hours for stomach acid to inactive the salivary enzymes. Amylase secreted by the pancreas begins to work in the duodenum.

The enzymes located in the intestinal epithelium break the disaccharides and trisaccharides into monosaccharides (simple sugars). The enzyme **maltase** breaks the disaccharide maltose into two glucose molecules; **sucrase** breaks sucrose (the sugar we use in coffee) into glucose and fructose; **lactase** breaks down lactose (present in milk) into glucose and galactose.

The monosaccharides are absorbed by facilitated diffusion or active transport into the intestinal epithelium and secreted into the interstitial fluid where they enter the capillaries to reach the liver via the portal system. In the liver, they are further processed and liberated into the blood according to need.

LIPID DIGESTION AND ABSORPTION

Most fat that is consumed is in the form of triglycerides. Triglycerides are three molecules of fatty acids

Lactose Intolerance

Lactose intolerance is a condition in which the enzyme lactase is deficient and proper digestion of milk and dairy products does not take place. As a result, individuals with this condition have digestive problems. For example, the undigested lactose serves as a good energy source for the bacteria living in the colon. This results in gas formation, cramps, and diarrhea in these individuals.

attached to a molecule of glycerol. For absorption to take place, the lipid must be broken into monoglycerides and fatty acids. The digestion of fat begins in the mouth and continues in the small intestine by the action of the enzyme **lipase.** Because they are not water-soluble, the consumed lipids tend to form droplets in the gut. However, because lipases are water-soluble, they are able to only reach the outside of the droplets, with fat molecules deep inside the droplets being unreachable.

The bile salts present in the bile secreted by the liver are important in fat digestion. They break up the large lipid droplets into small droplets, enabling lipase to digest the fat. This process of forming small droplets is known as **emulsification.** In the small intestine, the bile salts emulsify fat and the lipases secreted by the pancreas digest it. The fatty acids and monoglycerides interact with the bile salts to form complexes called **micelles.** The lipids diffuse across the intestinal cell membrane when the micelle comes in contact with the intestinal epithelium. The intestinal cells convert the monoglycerides and fatty acids into triglycerides in the cytoplasm and, after coating them with protein, secrete them into the interstitial tissue. These particles (**chylomicrons**) are absorbed into lymphatic vessels. The lymphatic vessels, seen as blind-ended tubes at the center of the villi, easily absorb the chylomicrons via gaps between the cells lining the vessels. Ultimately, the chylomicrons travel via the lymphatics to the thoracic duct to slowly enter the circulation.

In the absence of bile or pancreatic lipase, fat digestion and absorption are significantly reduced and fat appears in the feces. Other than fat deficiency, the body is deprived of the fat-soluble vitamins A, D, E, and K because they also cannot be absorbed.

PROTEIN DIGESTION AND ABSORPTION

Protein has a complex structure and protein digestion is more time-consuming. The large protein complexes are initially broken down into smaller particles by the teeth. The hydrochloric acid in the stomach helps break down plant cell walls and connective tissue in animal products. The acid in the stomach maintains the pH at the correct level for the enzyme

Table 11.4

Digestion: Enzymes, Regions Secreting the Enzymes, and Actions

Region	Enzymes		
	Protein digestion	*Fat digestion*	*Carbohydrate digestion*
Mouth	–	Lipase	Amylase
Esophagus	–	–	–
Stomach	Pepsin	–	–
Small intestine	Chymotrypsin, trypsin, carboxypeptidase elastase	Bile salts (liver) and pancreatic lipase	Pancreatic amylase, maltase, sucrase, lactase

pepsin, secreted by the stomach, to work efficiently on the proteins. Pepsin breaks down the large polypeptides into smaller ones. When the food enters the intestine, the protein-digesting enzymes liberated by the pancreas begin to work in the more alkaline pH. Each enzyme breaks up special bonds in the proteins to ultimately reduce them to free amino acids.

The surface epithelium of the intestine also has enzymes that break up peptide bonds. The individual amino acids are absorbed into the intestinal epithelium by special transport mechanisms using carriers. From the epithelium, the amino acids enter the interstitial fluid where they then enter the blood capillaries to reach the liver for further processing.

WATER ABSORPTION

The cells of the body cannot absorb or secrete water using active transport; movement of water is solely by osmosis. As previously explained, osmosis depends on concentration gradients of solutes across a semipermeable membrane. Therefore, water is absorbed into the intestinal epithelium and then into the interstitial fluid when the solute concentration is higher in the walls of the intestine. It enters the lumen if the contents of the lumen have more solute. Because the intestines are constantly absorbing solutes, the water moves into the capillaries along the osmotic gradient produced.

About 2–2.5 liters (2.1–2.6 qt) of water are taken in, in the form of food or drink. About 6–7 liters (6.3–7.4 qt) of water enter the lumen of the gut by salivary, gastric, pancreatic, intestinal, and bile secretions. It is remarkable that only about 150 mL (5 oz) of this fluid is lost in the feces.

ELECTROLYTE (ION) ABSORPTION

The ion concentration in the blood must be maintained within a narrow range for proper functioning of various metabolic activities. For example, the correct concentration of sodium and potassium is needed for conduction of impulses along nerve fibers and for muscle contraction, to name just two of the many activities of the body. Calcium, another ion, must be in the right concentration for excitation-contraction coupling to occur. Fluctuation in hydrogen ion or bicarbonate ion levels can drastically change the pH and make enzyme activity chaotic. The absorption of various ions is regulated individually and many of the regulatory mechanisms are poorly understood. Electrolytes are absorbed by active transport or by diffusion.

VITAMIN ABSORPTION

All water-soluble vitamins other than B_{12} are easily absorbed across the intestinal epithelium by diffusion. For adequate quantities of Vitamin B_{12} to be absorbed, it must combine with a glycoprotein intrinsic factor secreted by the stomach. In individuals who have had part of the stomach removed or whose gastric mucosa is atrophied, secretion of intrinsic factor is limited and vitamin B_{12} deficiency results.

Fat-soluble vitamins A, D, E, and K are absorbed like lipids and, therefore, require normal secretion of bile and lipase for absorption.

Metabolism

Food products that are absorbed through the GI tract are in the form of monosaccharides (from carbohydrate); fatty acids, glycerol, and monoglycerides (from fat); and amino acids (from protein). Most of these molecules are used for supplying the energy required for normal functioning, such as muscle contraction, active substance transport, protein synthesis, and cell division. Some are used to synthesize complex molecules, such as enzymes and muscle proteins, and cell repair. Others are changed to storage forms for future use. All of these changes are initiated by metabolism.

Metabolism refers to all of the chemical reactions that take place in the body. Certain reactions result in synthesis, or formation and are known as **anabolism.** Other reactions result in product breakdown (**catabolism**). For example, amino acids may be linked to form proteins or fatty acids used to form phospholipids or glucose molecules linked to form glycogen. This is anabolism. Glycogen may be broken to release glucose. This is catabolism. In both anabolism and catabolism, energy is used or released. The molecule that participates in exchange of energy is **adenosine triphosphate** (ATP).

ATP consists of an adenine and ribose molecule and three phosphate groups. During anabolism, one

---

Excess Ketone Bodies

Normally, ketone bodies are rapidly used by tissue for ATP production and blood levels are low. In conditions such as a triglyceride-rich diet; diabetes mellitus (insulin inhibits lipolysis; in diabetes, lack of insulin facilitates lipolysis; cells use lipids for ATP generation because less glucose enters the cells); starvation (lack of glucose results in use of lipids for energy), ketone levels increase in the blood. This condition is known as ketoacidosis. Because the ketone bodies are acidic, the pH of the body is reduced, affecting normal tissue function.

Individuals with ketoacidosis have a characteristically sweet smell of acetone in their breath.

phosphate group is split, and ATP is converted into ADP, phosphate group, and energy.

$$ATP \rightarrow ADP + P \text{ (phosphate group)} + energy$$

Part of this energy is used for the anabolic reaction, and the remaining energy is in the form of heat.

During catabolism, part of the energy is transferred to ADP to form ATP during the breakdown of complex molecules. The remaining energy is released as heat, which may be used to maintain body temperature.

$$Energy + ADP + P \text{ (phosphate group)} \rightarrow ATP$$

In this way, ATP provides a linkage between anabolism and catabolism.

CARBOHYDRATE METABOLISM

The absorbed carbohydrates in the gut are in the form of glucose, galactose, and fructose (monosaccharides). From here, the monosaccharides are transported to the liver by the portal circulation. In the liver, practically all galactose and fructose is converted to glucose. Glucose is then transported in the blood to various tissue. In the tissue, glucose may be used for (A) production of ATP; (B) formation of amino acids; (C) conversion into glycogen **(glycogenesis)** by the liver and muscle cells; or (D) formation of triglycerides, fat **(lipogenesis).**

Glucose is transported across the plasma membrane of cells by facilitated diffusion (see **page 30**). Therefore, special transport proteins must be present in the cell membrane for glucose to be transported into the cytoplasm. The hormone insulin increases the number of transport proteins in the cell membrane, facilitating the entry of glucose into cells. In the absence of insulin, the entry of glucose into cells is diminished. That is why the lack of insulin (diabetes mellitus) results in increased blood glucose levels. (Note that hepatocytes and neurons do not depend on insulin for glucose entry). Once glucose enters the cytoplasm, it is phosphorylated (combined with phosphate group), which prevents glucose from being removed from the cell.

Inside the cell, glucose is oxidized (process in which electrons are removed) to form ATP. This process, known as **cellular respiration,** involves many steps. Initially, glucose is oxidized to form two pyruvic acid molecules **(glycolysis).** During glycolysis, two ATP molecules are formed. Because oxygen is not required for this step, it is known as **anaerobic respiration.** Depending on the availability of oxygen, pyruvic acid may be converted to lactic acid or may enter the Krebs cycle. In skeletal muscle, for example, pyruvic acid is converted into lactic acid when oxygen availability is scarce. The lactic acid diffuses out of the cell and, on reaching the liver via blood, is again converted to pyruvic acid.

$$Glucose \rightarrow 2 \text{ pyruvic acid} \rightarrow 2 \text{ lactic acid}$$
(anaerobic pathway)

Krebs cycle or the **citric acid cycle** is a series of chemical reactions facilitated by different enzymes that occur in the matrix of the mitochondria. During these reactions, ATP is manufactured, with release of carbon dioxide and water.

$$Glucose \rightarrow 2 \text{ pyruvic acid} \rightarrow Krebs \text{ cycle}$$
(aerobic pathway)

The pyruvic acid is converted to acetyl-coenzyme A before it enters the Krebs cycle inside the mitochondrion. Pyruvic acid is then converted to various intermediate products in the presence of specific enzymes. As a result, the potential energy in the glucose molecule is released in steps and eventually used to form ATP. (Please refer to more advanced textbooks for details of the Krebs cycle.) Special membrane proteins in the wall of the mitochondrion—electron carriers—form the electron transport chain that helps with ATP formation. The net result of glucose entering the Krebs cycle is the formation of carbon dioxide (which is transported to the lungs for exhalation), water, and 36 ATP (only Krebs cycle) or 38 ATP (glycolysis + Krebs cycle).

$$C_6H_{12}O_6 \text{ (Glucose)} + 6 O_2 \text{ (Oxygen)} + 36 ADP \text{ or}$$
$$38 ADP + 36 P \text{ or } 38 P \text{ (phosphate group)} \rightarrow 6$$
$$CO_2 \text{ (Carbon dioxide)} + 6 H_2O \text{ (Water)}$$
$$+ 36 ATP \text{ or } 38 ATP$$

Glycolysis, Krebs cycle, and electron transport chain are sufficient to provide the cell with all the required ATP. Because the Krebs cycle and electron transport chain require oxygen, it is difficult for the cell to perform its functions in the absence of oxygen.

Not all glucose is broken down. Some glucose molecules may undergo anabolism. In cells such as hepatocytes and muscle, glucose is converted to the storage form of glycogen (glycogenesis). When glucose is required, glycogen is broken down to glucose **(glycogenolysis)**. When the glucose supply is low, it may be formed by the breakdown of protein and triglycerides in a process known as **gluconeogenesis.** Gluconeogenesis is stimulated by cortisol and glucagon.

LIPID METABOLISM

Because lipids are not water-soluble, they are transported in the blood by combining with protein particles in the blood. The combination of lipids and proteins is called lipoproteins. Lipoproteins are spherical structures that contain molecules of triglycerides. There are different types of lipoproteins—**chylomicron, low-density lipoprotein** (LDL), **high-density lipoprotein** (HDL), and **very-low-density lipoprotein** (VLDL). Chylomicrons are formed in the gut and absorbed through the lymph before entering the veins. On reaching tissue, fatty acid is released from the triglycerides by the action of the enzyme lipase in tissue. VLDL transport triglycerides from the hepatocytes to the adipose tissue for storage. VLDLs are converted to LDL after the triglycerides are removed by adipose tissue.

LDLs transport triglycerides to the tissues for cell membrane repair and synthesis of bile salts and steroid hormones. It carries most of the total cholesterol in blood. If present in large amounts, LDL deposits in the blood vessels walls to form fatty plaques that predispose individuals to coronary artery disease, thrombus formation, and stroke. That is why LDL is known as "**bad" cholesterol.**

HDL transports the excess cholesterol from body cells to the liver for elimination. Because they inhibit the accumulation of cholesterol in the blood, they decrease the risk of plaque formation; hence, HDL is also known as "**good" cholesterol.**

The lipids absorbed through the gut may be broken down (**lipolysis**) and converted to ATP; stored in the adipose tissue and liver (**lipogenesis**); or used to form other products, such as bile salts, lipoproteins, phospholipids in cell membrane, steroid hormones, and myelin sheath. When lipolysis occurs, triglycerides are converted to fatty acids and glycerol before forming intermediary products that form ATP. During fatty acid catabolism, acetoacetic acid, ß-hydroxybutyric acid, and acetone are formed. These three products, known as **ketone bodies,** easily diffuse out of the cells and en-

Testing Blood Cholesterol Levels

Blood cholesterol levels are measured to assess a person's risk of coronary heart disease. The total blood cholesterol levels (TC), HDL levels, and VLDL levels are measured. The LDL level is calculated from these three values. A TC of less than 200 mg/dL, an HDL higher than 40 mg/dL, and an LDL below 130 mg/dL are considered normal. Deviations from normal increase the risk of heart disease.

Blood cholesterol levels may be reduced by aerobic exercise (increases HDL), diet (low-fat diet), and drugs (increases excretion of bile; decreases synthesis of cholesterol by the liver).

ter the bloodstream. Certain cells, such as cardiac muscle cells and kidney cells, use ketone bodies to form ATP.

PROTEIN METABOLISM

The proteins absorbed in the gut are in the form of amino acids. They are carried by the portal vein to the liver and other tissue where they may be converted to ATP, used to form proteins, or converted to glucose (gluconeogenesis) or triglycerides (lipogenesis). During protein catabolism, one reaction involves removal of the NH_2 group of the amino acid (**deamination**) and formation of ammonia. Ammonia is converted to urea in the liver and excreted in the urine. For gluconeogenesis to take place, the different amino acids are converted to various intermediate products that can enter the Krebs cycle.

Amino acids are linked by peptide bonds in specific sequences to form new proteins. This occurs in the ribosomes of cells. The sequence of amino acids to form new proteins is dictated by DNA and RNA. Protein synthesis is stimulated by hormones such as growth hormone, thyroid hormone, insulin, estrogen, testosterone, and insulinlike growth factor.

Basal Metabolic Rate

The **metabolic rate** is the rate the body uses energy for metabolic reactions. A metabolic rate measured under standard conditions (i.e., when the body is resting, fasting, and quiet) is known as the **basal metabolic rate** (BMR).

As mentioned, some energy is used for ATP production and the rest is converted to heat. The metabolic rate of an individual is calculated in **calories.** A calorie is the amount of heat energy required to raise the temperature of 1 g water from 14°C to 15°C. A kilocalorie (kcal) or Calorie (Cal) is 1,000 calories.

The adult BMR is about 1,200–1,800 kcal/day. The total calories required by an individual depends on

Obesity

Most types of obesity are **regulatory obesity.** Here, there is no organic problem, but there is an imbalance between food intake and utilization. Chronic eating may be associated with psychological and social factors such as stress, habit, family or ethnic traditions, and inactivity. Genetics may play some role.

Rarely, obesity may be the **metabolic obesity** type. In this case, the obesity is secondary to abnormalities in cell metabolism. For example, it may be a result of reduced sensitivity of cells to insulin or hyposecretion or hypersecretion of glucocorticoids and insulin.

It is important to treat obesity because it predisposes individuals to conditions such as hypertension, diabetes mellitus, coronary artery disease, varicose veins, hernias, arthritis, gallstones, and some forms of cancer.

Treatment of obesity includes behavior modification, exercise programs, nutritional counseling, psychotherapy, and surgery. In one type of surgery—gastric stapling—the size of the stomach is reduced, making the person feel full after eating even a small amount of food. Liposuction is another procedure in which the adipose tissue is sucked out through a tube inserted into the subcutaneous layer via a small incision through the skin.

his or her activity and physiologic state. For example, teenage boys and active men need about 2,800 kilocalories per day. The requirement in women is increased during pregnancy and lactation.

To meet the caloric needs of an individual, an adequate diet is required. It is recommended that the distribution of calories in the diet should be: carbohydrates (50% to 60%); fats (about 30% or less), with saturated fat less than 10%; and protein (about 12% to 15%). Metabolism of 1 g of protein or carbohydrate produces about 4 Calories, and 1 g of fat produces 9 Calories.

REGULATION OF METABOLIC RATE

The metabolic rate is regulated by various factors, which depend on the condition of the cells (e.g., availability of ATP and nervous and endocrine stimulus). It also depends on the amount of time after a meal. Soon after a meal and until approximately 4 hours later, when the absorption from the gut is complete, glucose is absorbed from the gut (absorptive state) and is readily available to the tissue. After the absorption is complete (postabsorptive state), the blood glucose levels must be maintained from the body reserves. It is important to maintain normal blood glucose levels because the nervous system and red blood cells depend on glucose for energy production.

Soon after a meal, the rising levels of glucose and certain amino acids stimulate the beta cells of the pancreas to produce insulin. Insulin facilitates entry of glucose into cells, lipogenesis, glycogenesis, and protein synthesis. During the postabsorptive state, blood glucose levels begin to fall. Hormones and sympathetic stimulation maintains the level by breakdown of fat and protein, conversion of fat and protein into glucose, and breakdown of glycogen. The primary hormones involved are glucagon (from alpha cells of the pancreas), epinephrine, norepinephrine, and cortisol.

Age-Related Changes in the Gastrointestinal System

The two major changes that occur in the gastrointestinal tract with aging are the reduction in the proliferation rate of epithelial cells and the loss of neurons from the walls.

ORAL CAVITY

Studies have shown that most changes in the oral cavity in elderly individuals are a result of pathology and not normal aging. There may be shrinkage and fibrosis of the root pulp, and the gums may be retracted.

Some loss of bone density may occur in the jaws. The major change that occurs is the loss of teeth, with resultant impairment of chewing. Salivary flow may be reduced as a result of the reduced sensation of smell and taste and the loss of secretory tissue.

ESOPHAGUS

The function of the esophagus is essentially preserved. The motor activity of the esophagus may be uncoordinated, with delayed entry of food into the stomach and a feeling of substernal fullness.

STOMACH

There is atrophy of the stomach mucosa, with diminished capacity to secrete hydrochloric acid. The motility of the stomach may be reduced, with slower emptying.

SMALL INTESTINE

The villi in the mucosa are atrophied to some extent, becoming broader and shorter with resultant decrease in surface area for absorption. The volume of gastric secretion is decreased with age. There is no evidence that absorption of major nutrients is impaired; however, the effect on the function is still not determined fully.

LARGE INTESTINE

The motility of the colon may be decreased, with some reduction in blood flow. The bowel habits are not significantly affected. It is believed that more distention of the colon is required for discomfort to be felt and this may be one reason for the constipation that is common in elderly persons. Atrophy of muscle, loss of neurons, and changes in collagen are other factors that affect colon motility.

PANCREAS

The pancreas undergoes some changes with age. The ducts are dilated and deposits of calcium and other pigments occur. Fat intolerance in the older age group is sometimes attributed to a decrease in lipase production. However, this seems unlikely because the pancreas has a large functional reserve and the capacity to increase its secretion ten times more than that required to digest normal levels of fat in the diet.

LIVER

The liver diminishes in size, with destruction of hepatocytes. Fibrous tissue replaces the dead cells. The various enzymes and protein synthesis are diminished. The capacity to metabolize drugs also reduces with age.

Aromatherapy and GI Conditions

Digestive stimulants, such as ginger, rosemary, cinnamon leaf, peppermint, citronella, cardamom, and black pepper, have been used to treat constipation.[3] The oils may be added to a warm compress placed over the abdomen to help relieve abdominal pain.

Cinnamon and nutmeg oil have been used to treat diarrhea. They may be added to the bath water, massage oil, or to warm compresses to provide relief.

Lavender has been found to be particularly useful in treating GI disorders such as colic and indigestion.

It is important to note that these essential oils are used externally and should not be taken internally. The supervision and recommendation of a qualified health professional is required for such interventions.

The Gastrointestinal System and Bodywork

Acupuncture and acupressure techniques have been shown to reduce nausea and vomiting resulting from opioid drugs, general anesthesia, cytotoxic drugs, and pregnancy.

Aromatherapy oils are being used for various conditions associated with the GI tract,[3] including constipation, dyspepsia (indigestion), diarrhea, nausea and vomiting, and irritable bowel syndrome.

Massage is beneficial in helping with bowel movements,[4-7] and people with constipation may find mas-

Reflex Areas for GI Tract

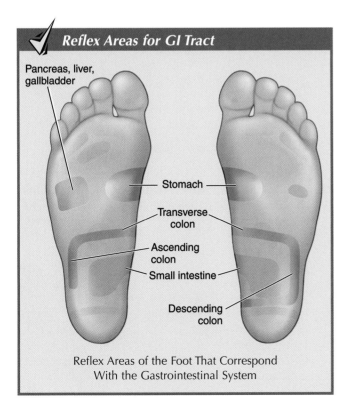

Reflex Areas of the Foot That Correspond With the Gastrointestinal System

Pain Patterns Relating to the Organs of the Gastrointestinal System

Pain originating in different parts of the GI system often has typical characteristics. Some of these characteristics are listed below. These characteristics may be used only as a general guideline because disorders in these regions may present in many other ways. Substernal pain may be a result of esophageal reflux or other disorders associated with the esophagus. Stretching of the liver capsule may present as a dull, aching pain in the upper right quadrant of the abdomen. In the abdomen, inflammation, distention, or stretching of the intestine often presents as a cramping or diffuse pain. Colicky, severe pain may be produced by smooth muscle spasm that may occur with inflammation or obstruction.

Usually, pain arising from the viscera is accompanied by autonomic responses such as pallor, sweating, nausea, and vomiting. Visceral pain is not well localized. If inflammation from the viscera spreads to the parietal peritoneum, the pain becomes well localized. Visceral pain may be accompanied by reflex spasm of the overlying abdominal muscles.

Often, pain from the viscera is referred to another site (referred pain), making diagnosis difficult. Common sites of referred pain are shown in the figure.

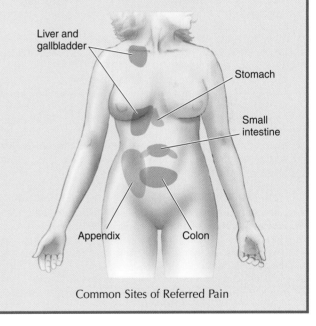

Common Sites of Referred Pain

sage useful. Massage primarily affects the viscera through somatovisceral reflexes. In elderly patients, massage promotes regular bowel movements, reduces the incidence of incontinence, and decreases the use of enemas.[8] Massage may also help relieve intestinal colic, biliary colic, and flatulence. By affecting the parasympathetic system, massage can promote secretion and digestion of food; hence, massage can be useful in programs to retrain bowel function. Abdominal massage is sometimes performed using a tennis ball or other rounded, heavy objects.[9]

Massage is of benefit in other disorders related to the gastrointestinal system, such as anorexia and bulimia.[10,11] Reduced anxiety, improved mood, and decreased stress hormones are some benefits seen in gastrointestinal disorders.

In general, the therapist should avoid massaging the abdomen if the client complains of abdominal pain or diarrhea or if tenderness is detected. The therapist should refer the client to a physician if she or he complains of blood in the stools or vomit, difficulty swallowing, or other unusual symptoms related to the gastrointestinal system. Diarrhea of acute onset is usually a result of infection, and the therapist should avoid treating these clients to prevent spread of infection.

All therapists should ensure that she or he knows enough about the specific conditions (and medications being taken) that clients have been diagnosed with to avoid perpetuating the problem.

REFERENCES

1. Ganong WF. Review of Medical Physiology. 20th Ed. Berkeley, California: McGraw-Hill/Appleton & Lange Medical Publications, 2001.
2. Zang F. An introduction to keeping fit-massage (1). J Trad Chin Med 1993;13(2):120–123.
3. Lawless J. The Complete Illustrated Guide to Aromatherapy. Shaftesbury: Element Books, 1997.
4. Mein EA, Richards DG, McMillin DL, McPartland JM. Physiological regulation through manual therapy. Phys Med/Rehabil: A State of the Art Review 2000;14(1):27–42.
5. Emly M. Abdominal massage. Nurs Times 1993;89(3):34–36.
6. Klauser AG, Flaschentrager J, Gehrke A, et al. Abdominal wall massage: effect on colonic function in healthy volunteers and in patients with chronic constipation. Z Gastroenterol 1992;30:247–251.
7. Ernst E. Abdominal massage therapy for chronic constipation: A systematic review of controlled clinical trials. Forsch Komplementarmed 1999;6:149–151.
8. Resende TL, Brocklehurst JC, O'Neill PA. A pilot study on the effect of exercise and abdominal massage on bowel habit in continuing care patients. Clin Rehabil 1993;7:204–209.
9. Richards A. Hands-on help. Nurs Times 1998;94(32):69–75.
10. Hart S, Field T, Hernandez-Reif M, Nearing G, Shaw S, Schanberg S, Kuhn C. Anorexia symptoms are reduced by massage therapy. Eating Dis 2001;9:289–299.
11. Field T, Shanberg S, Kuhn C, Fierro K, Henteleff T, Mueller C, Yando R, Burman I. Bulimic adolescents benefit from massage therapy. Adolescence 1997;131:555–563.

SUGGESTED READINGS

Holey LAL. The effects of classical massage and connective tissue manipulation on bowel function. Brit J Ther Rehabil 1995;2(11):627–631.
Larsen JH. Infants' colic and belly massage. Practitioner 1990;22(234):396–397.
Premkumar K. Pathology A to Z. 2nd Ed. Calgary: VanPub Books, 1999.
Salvo SG. Massage Therapy. Principles & Practice. Philadelphia: W.B. Saunders, 1999.
Yangoa L. Clinical observations on the treatment of gastrointestinal disorders by massotherapy. J Trad Chin Med 1995;15(4):297–300.

 Review Questions

Multiple Choice
Choose the best answer to the following questions:

1. The layers of the wall of the GI tract outwards from the lumen are the
   A. mucosa, serosa, submucosa, and muscularis externa.
   B. mucosa, submucosa, serosa, and muscularis externa.
   C. serosa, submucosa, muscularis externa, and mucosa.
   D. mucosa, submucosa, muscularis externa, and serosa.

2. Which of the following is an important constituent of hemoglobin?
   A. Copper
   B. Calcium
   C. Iron
   D. Vitamin D

3. Absence of which of the following results in pernicious anemia?
   A. Vitamin B_{12}
   B. Vitamin D
   C. Iron
   D. Calcium

4. All of the following are functions of the liver EXCEPT
   A. bile manufacture.
   B. pathogen removal.
   C. circulating hormone removal.
   D. insulin secretion.

5. The conversion of glucose to glycogen is known as
   A. glycolysis.
   B. glycogenesis.
   C. gluconeogenesis.
   D. glycogenolysis.

6. The organic nutrients needed in minute amounts to maintain normal growth and metabolism are
   A. vitamins.
   B. minerals.
   C. glucose.
   D. proteins

7. The break down of glucose into two pyruvic acid molecules is known as
   A. gluconeogenesis.
   B. glycolysis.
   C. lipogenesis.
   D. deamination.

8. The metabolic rate can be increased by all of the following EXCEPT
   A. thyroid hormones.
   B. epinephrine.
   C. sympathetic stimulation.
   D. parasympathetic stimulation.

9. The largest internal organ is the
   A. pancreas.
   B. spleen.
   C. liver.
   D. gallbladder.

10. The type of innervation associated with the large intestine is/are
    A. sympathetic nerves.
    B. parasympathetic nerves.
    C. both A and B.
    D. none of the above.

11. The cecum is associated with the
    A. esophagus.
    B. stomach.
    C. small intestine.
    D. large intestine.

12. The three pairs of salivary glands that secrete into the oral cavity are the
    A. lingual, labial, and frenulum.
    B. parotid, sublingual, and submandibular.
    C. pharyngeal, palatoglossal, and palatopharyngeal.
    D. vagal, hypoglossal, and facial.

13. A substance absorbed into the lacteals of the lymphatic system within the small intestine walls is
    A. fat.
    B. glucose.
    C. amino acid.
    D. vitamin B_{12}.

14. Mr. Brown has been diagnosed with cirrhosis (chronic liver inflammation) of the liver. If examined and tested, which of the following results may be obtained?
    A. Presence of ascites
    B. A longer blood clotting time
    C. Jaundice
    D. All of the above

Fill in

Complete the following:

1. The _____ peritoneum covers the organs and the _____ peritoneum lines the inside of the abdominal cavity.

2. The wave of muscular contractions that travels the length of the digestive tract is known as _____.

3. The activities of the digestive system are controlled by _____, _____, and _____.

4. The feeding center and the satiety center are located in the _____.

5. Of the various nutrients, _____ are constituents of muscles, enzymes, and antibodies. _____ are the main source of energy, and _____ are needed for formation of steroid hormones.

6. The process of swallowing is known as _____.

7. The elimination of waste products from the GI tract is known as _____.

8. The end product of carbohydrate digestion is _____.

9. The end product of protein digestion is _____.

10. The end product of fat digestion is _____ and _____.

11. The formation of glucose from noncarbohydrate sources is known as _____.

12. The three parts of the small intestine are _____, _____, and _____.

13. Approximately _____% of fat, _____% of protein, and _____% of carbohydrates are normally required in the daily diet.

True–False

(Answer the following questions T, for true; or F, for false):

1. Saliva contains enzymes that begin the digestion of carbohydrates and fats.

2. The function of the large intestine is to absorb water and electrolytes from the chyme.

3. The digestion of starch occurs mainly in the stomach.

4. Vitamin A, D, E, and K are water-soluble vitamins.

5. Intrinsic factor is required for the absorption of vitamin C.

6. The preferred energy source for the brain is polysaccharides.

7. The epiglottis prevents food from entering the nasal cavity during swallowing.

Matching
Match the following. Write a, b, c, d, e, f, g, h, i, and j next to descriptions 1–10.

1. _____ Stores feces
2. _____ Has the lowest pH
3. _____ Secretes insulin
4. _____ Stores and concentrates bile
5. _____ Muscular tube that conducts food to the stomach
6. _____ Manufactures bile
7. _____ Semisolid waste is formed here
8. _____ A common passageway for air and food
9. _____ Contains lymphoid tissue, has no particular function in humans
10. _____ Duct from the pancreas opens here

a. pharynx
b. esophagus
c. stomach
d. duodenum
e. pancreas
f. liver
g. gallbladder
h. appendix
i. colon
j. rectum

Short Answer Questions
1. How is the movement of the digestive tract regulated?
2. How is food intake regulated?
3. What are the functions of the liver?
4. What is the location of the liver? Using your body or your colleague's, trace the location of the liver.
5. How is fat digested?
6. What are the recommended general dietary guidelines?
7. What are the changes that occur with aging in the (a) stomach, (b) liver, and (c) colon?

Case Studies
1. Forty-year-old Ms. Pindel, had been complaining of intermittent abdominal pain for the past two months. The therapist had urged her to see her family physician, and Ms. Pindel had complied and scheduled an appointment for the following month. Her mother and her grandmother had previously had gallstones, and Ms. Pindel was worried that she may be having the same problem. The therapist thought that may be true because Ms. Pindel was beginning to look slightly jaundiced.
   A. What is the function of the gallbladder?
   B. What is the relationship between the gallbladder and jaundice?
   C. What is jaundice?
   D. How is bilirubin produced?
   E. Is jaundice an infection?

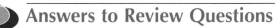

Answers to Review Questions

Multiple Choice
1. D
2. C
3. A
4. D
5. B
6. A
7. B
8. D
9. C
10. C
11. D
12. B
13. A
14. D

Fill-In
1. visceral, parietal
2. peristalsis
3. nerves, hormones, and local mechanisms
4. hypothalamus
5. proteins, carbohydrates, fats
6. deglutition
7. defecation
8. monosaccharides
9. amino acids
10. fatty acid, glycerol
11. gluconeogenesis
12. duodenum, jejunum, and ileum
13. 30%, 15%, and 50% to 55%

True–False
1. True
2. True
3. False
4. False (they are fat-soluble)
5. False (it is secreted by the stomach and is required for the absorption of vitamin B_{12})
6. False
7. False. The epiglottis closes the larynx. It is the soft palate that prevents food from entering the nasal cavity.

Matching
1. j
2. c
3. e
4. g
5. b
6. f
7. i

8. a
9. h
10. d

Short-Answer Questions

1. There are pacesetter cells located in the proximal part of the gut that generate impulses spontaneously. These impulses travel down the gut via the smooth muscle and the network of autonomic nerves in the wall, causing waves of muscle contraction. Nerves, hormones, and local mechanisms also play a part; for example, the sympathetic nerves slow down motility and the parasympathetic speed motility. Hormones, such as gastrin and thyroid, also affect the motility.
2. Food intake is regulated by certain areas located in the hypothalamus. The hypothalamus has two areas—the feeding center and satiety center. Other areas, such as the temporal lobe of the brain, also play a part in determining what is eaten. Food in the gut, amount of fat in the body, culture, and environment are some other factors.
3. The functions of the liver include protein, carbohydrate, and fat metabolism; removal of waste products; removal of pathogen; destruction of circulating hormones; storage of vitamins; and synthesis of bile.
4. Look at Surface Marking on the Liver on **page 590** for details.
5. Fat digestion begins when the mouth comes in contact with the enzyme lipase secreted by the salivary gland. After this, digestion continues in the intestines where it is mixed with bile salts (manufactured by the liver and stored in the gallbladder). The bile salts emulsify the fat and allow the enzyme pancreatic lipase to facilitate breakdown. The final products of fat digestion are then absorbed through the mucosa into the lacteals.
6. The general dietary guidelines are: Decrease total fat intake to less than 30% of calories, saturated fat to less than 10% of total calories, and cholesterol to less than 300 mg per day. Decrease protein intake to approximately 15% of calories. Carbohydrate intake should be about 50% to 55% of calories or more, with more of complex carbohydrates and fiber. Reduce sodium intake to less than 3 g per day. If consuming alcoholic beverages, limit the caloric intake from this source to 15% of total calories (to no more than 50 mL of ethanol per day). Total calories should be sufficient to achieve and maintain body weight within 20% of ideal. Consume sugar in moderation. Eat a wide variety of food.
7. (a) There is atrophy of the mucosa of the stomach, with diminished capacity to secrete hydrochloric acid. The motility of the stomach may be reduced with slower emptying.
   (b) The liver diminishes in size, with destruction of hepatocytes. Fibrous tissue replaces the dead cells. The various enzymes and protein synthesis are diminished. The capacity to metabolize drugs also reduces with age.
   (c) The motility of the colon may be decreased, with some reduction in blood flow. Bowel habits are not significantly affected. It is believed that more colon distention is required for discomfort to be felt; this may be one reason for constipation that is common in elderly individuals. Atrophy of muscle, loss of neurons, and changes in collagen are other factors that affect colon motility.

Case Studies

A. The function of the gallbladder is to concentrate and store bile.
B. The bile contains bile salts, as well as bile pigments. It is excess bile pigment that results in jaundice. Ms. Pindel may have gallstones that are blocking the flow of bile into the duodenum. This may result in damming up of bile and spillage into the circulation.
C. Jaundice is a condition in which the level of bilirubin in the blood is more than normal.
D. Bilirubin is a waste product that is formed when hemoglobin is broken down. The bilirubin is transported to the liver where it is conjugated and secreted into bile and eventually excreted in the feces and urine. Any condition that results in an excessive breakdown of red blood cells or liver dysfunction or blockage of bile in the bile duct would result in jaundice.
E. Jaundice is not an infection; it is a symptom. It is one of the symptoms of viral hepatitis, which is an infection.

Coloring Exercise

Color and Label the Diagrams
The Digestive System

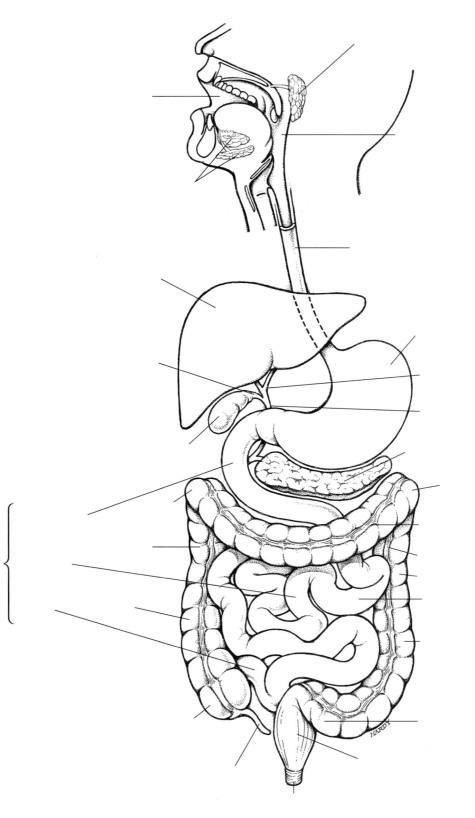

Color and Label the Various Layers in the Wall of the GI Tract

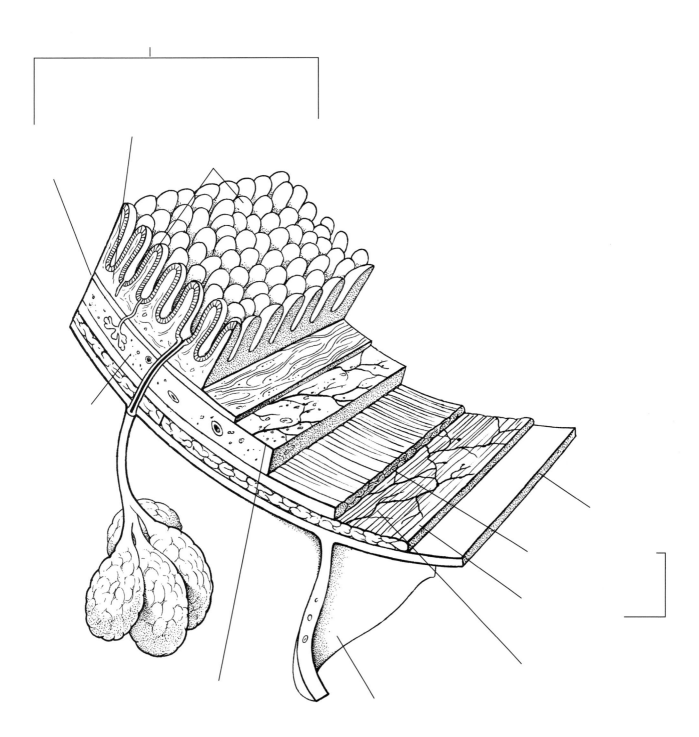

CHAPTER 12

Urinary System

Objectives **On completion of this chapter, the reader should be able to:**

- List the functions of the urinary system.
- Identify the anatomical components of the urinary system.
- Explain how each anatomical component contributes to urinary system functioning.
- Describe the anatomical location of the kidneys.
- Describe the external and internal features of the kidneys.
- Trace the pathway of blood through the kidneys.
- Describe the structure of the nephron.
- Identify the three transport mechanisms involved in kidney function.
- Describe the components of the filtration membrane.
- Explain the role of the juxtaglomerular apparatus in kidney function.
- Explain how urine is formed in the kidney.
- List the composition of urine.
- Describe, in brief, the role of hormones in concentrating and diluting the urine.
- Describe, in brief, the role of kidney in acid-base balance.
- Describe the process of micturition and its control.
- Describe the effects of aging on the anatomical components of the urinary system.
- Describe the effects of massage on the urinary system.

The urinary system, also known as the genitourinary or renal system, works efficiently and silently in the background, ridding the body of waste products via urine. When it fails to function adequately, the urinary system's presence is felt dramatically. On failure, the body has difficulty maintaining homeostasis, with the regulation of pH, blood pressure, blood volume, ion levels, to name a few, being affected. Most often, problems with this system initially present as edema, and it is important to differentiate the edema caused by the urinary system from other causes.

This chapter addresses the components of the urinary system and explains how it performs its various functions.

Functions of the Urinary System

The urinary system consists of organs involved in the *elimination of waste products* produced by the cells of the body. The respiratory system eliminates carbon dioxide—one waste product. All other organic waste products found in the extracellular fluid, such as bilirubin from hemoglobin breakdown, uric acid from nucleic acid in cells, creatinine from creatine phosphate in muscle, urea and ammonia from amino acid metabolism, are taken care of by the urinary system. This system helps *conserve nutrients* by retaining them in the body and excreting only the unwanted products.

In addition to these important functions, the urinary system *regulates blood osmolality, blood volume,* and *blood pressure* by altering the volume of water lost in the urine. It *regulates the levels of sodium, potassium, chloride, calcium,* and *other ions* by altering the quantity excreted in the urine. By monitoring the hydrogen levels in the blood, this system helps *maintain the pH* of the body at an optimal level for enzyme function.

The kidneys—the major components of this system—have *endocrine functions.* They secrete a hormone (renin) that has an effect on blood pressure.

The kidneys also release erythropoietin, a hormone that regulates the production of red blood cells. The kidneys are needed for the *formation of vitamin D,* an important vitamin required for regulating calcium levels in the blood and proper bone formation.

COMPONENTS OF THE URINARY SYSTEM

The urinary system consists of two **kidneys** that produce urine, two **ureters** that convey the urine to the **urinary bladder,** where it is stored, and the **urethra,** which transports the urine out of the body (see Figures 12.1and 12.2)

THE KIDNEYS

The paired kidneys (Figures 12.1, 12.2, and 12.3) are bean-shaped, with the indentation (the **hilum**) facing medially. The renal artery, renal vein, lymphatics, and

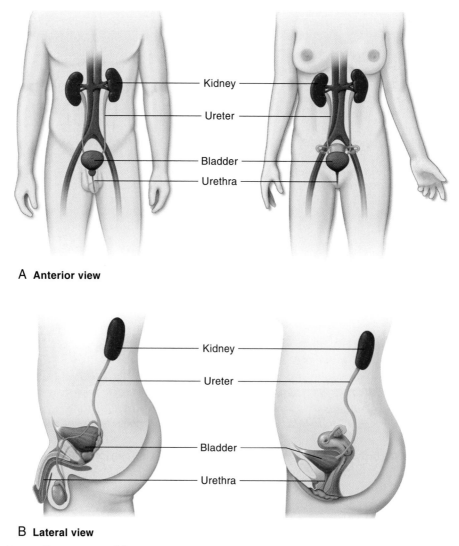

A **Anterior view**

B **Lateral view**

FIGURE **12.1.** Components of the Urinary System in Men and Women. **A,** Anterior View. **B,** Lateral View.

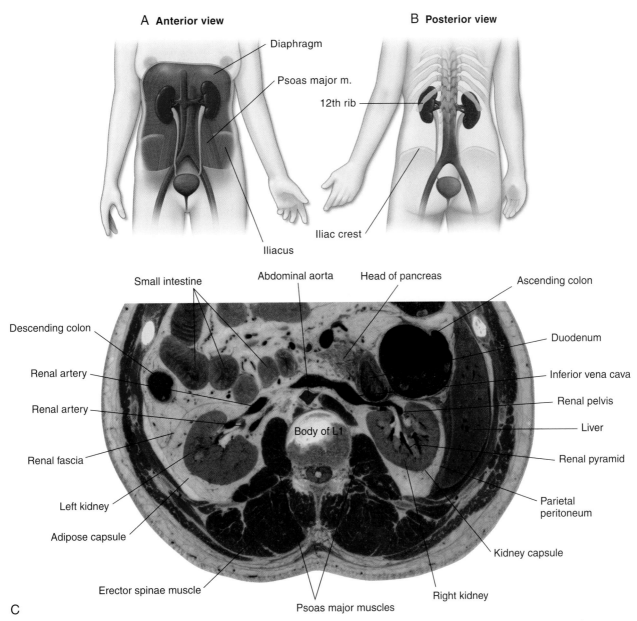

A Anterior view

Diaphragm

Psoas major m.

Iliacus

B Posterior view

12th rib

Iliac crest

C

Small intestine

Descending colon

Renal artery

Renal artery

Renal fascia

Left kidney

Adipose capsule

Erector spinae muscle

Abdominal aorta

Head of pancreas

Body of L1

Psoas major muscles

Ascending colon

Duodenum

Inferior vena cava

Renal pelvis

Liver

Renal pyramid

Parietal peritoneum

Kidney capsule

Right kidney

FIGURE **12.2.**   The Position of the Urinary System Components. **A,** Anterior View of the Kidneys After Removal of the Abdominal Organs. **B,** Posterior View of the Trunk. **C,** Transverse Section of the Abdomen at the Level of First Lumbar Vertebra, Superior View

renal nerves enter and leave at the hilum. An adult kidney is about 11.25 cm (4.43 in) long, 5–7.5 cm (2–3 in) wide, and about 2.5 cm (1 in) thick. The kidneys are located on either side of the vertebral column between the T12 and L3 vertebrae. The right kidney is slightly lower than the left because of the presence of the liver. These organs are *retroperitoneal* (i.e., they are located behind the peritoneum). The anterior aspect of the *right* kidney is related to the liver, the hepatic flexure of the colon, and the duodenum. The *left* kidney is covered by the stomach, pancreas, spleen, jejunum, and splenic flexure of the colon. The superior aspect of both the kidneys is covered by the

adrenal glands. Posteriorly, the kidneys are related to the muscles of the back; the tendon of the transverses abdominis muscle, the quadratus lumborum and the psoas, the diaphragm, the eleventh and twelfth ribs on the left side and the twelfth rib on the right.

The kidneys are held in place, supported, and protected by the surrounding fat and connective tissue. From deep to superficial, the kidney is covered by the **renal capsule, adipose capsule** and **renal fascia.** The renal capsule is a fibrous layer of dense collagen fibers. It forms a smooth and firm covering to the organ. Medially, the renal capsule folds inward at the hilus and lines an internal cavity, the **renal sinus.** The

VISUALIZING THE URINARY TRACT

The urinary tract can be visualized by injecting a radiopaque compound into the circulatory system and then taking x-rays. The compound is filtered by the kidney and transported down the urinary tract. Because it does not allow the x-rays to pass through, the tract is outlined. The tract can be also be visualized by administering the compound through a tube introduced through the urethra.

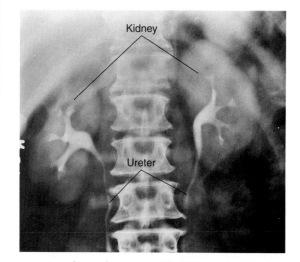

A Radiographic View of the Urinary System.

renal blood vessels and the ureter pass through the hilus and branch in the renal sinus (see Figure 12.3). The kidney and its vessels are embedded in a mass of adipose tissue (**adipose capsule,** or **perirenal fat**).

Surface Marking of the Kidneys, Ureter, and Urinary Bladder

The superior pole of the kidney reaches the level of T12. The inferior pole lies just above the transumbilical plane (the plane at the level of the umbilicus) (i.e., at the level of the upper part of L3). The inferior pole is, therefore, a fingersbreadth superior to the iliac crest. The oblique twelfth rib and the transverse processes of L1 and L2 are located posterior to the kidney. The hilus of the kidney is located in the transpyloric plane (a transverse plane at the level of the disk between L1 and L2). The kidneys are not usually palpable.

The location of the ureter can be visualized by running a line inferiorly from the hilus to the urinary bladder. It is anterior to the tips of the transverse processes of the vertebrae, 3–4 cm (1.2–1.6 in) from midline.

A full urinary bladder can be palpated as a rounded mass superior to the pubis. An empty bladder is located in the pelvic cavity and cannot be palpated through the anterior abdominal wall.

Both the kidneys and the fatty tissue are surrounded by a thick outer layer of fascia, the **renal fascia,** which anchors the kidneys to surrounding structures such as the peritoneum anteriorly and the fascia covering the back muscles posteriorly. Because the kidneys are not directly fixed to the abdominal wall, they move with the diaphragm during respiration.

If a section is made through the kidney, it is found to have two distinctive parts—the outer **cortex** and an inner **medulla.** Medially, the medulla forms 6–18 conical structures known as **renal pyramids.** The part of the cortex that dips between the pyramids is the **renal column.** The apex of the pyramids—the **renal papilla,** located medially—projects into the renal sinus. Urine that is formed is drained by the ducts in the papilla into cup-shaped structures known as **renal calyces** (singular, calyx). Four or five smaller calyces—the **minor calyces**—empty into two to three larger, **major calyces.** The major calyces join and form a large chamber, the **renal pelvis.** The funnel-shaped pelvis, which occupies most of the renal sinus, is continuous with the ureter.

The Nephron

Each kidney is made up of about 1.25 million tubular, microscopic structures known as the **nephrons** (see Figure 12.4). The nephrons are the functional units of the kidney. These nephrons, if laid end to end, would extend about 145 kilometers.

Study of the nephron structure is required to understand the process of urine formation. Each nephron can be considered to be a long tube with one end closed. Imagine the closed end of the tube to be

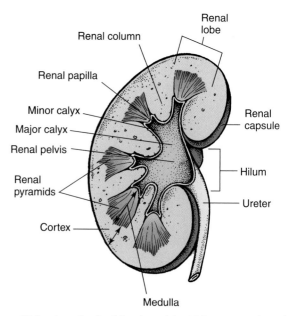

FIGURE **12.3.**   Longitudinal Section of the Kidney, Near the Hilum

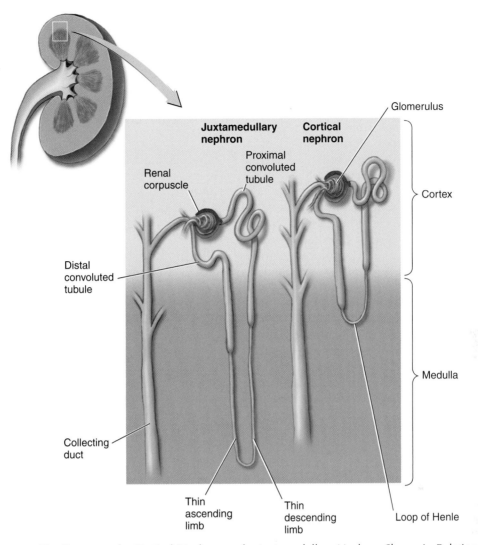

FIGURE **12.4.** The Structure of a Cortical Nephron and a Juxtamedullary Nephron Shown in Relation to the Cortex and Medulla

dilated and indented to form a cup. The long tube is the **renal tubule,** and the cup-shaped end is the **glomerular capsule,** or **Bowman's capsule.** Now imagine a network of capillaries nestled in the cup with both ends of the capillaries continuous with a blood vessel—one bringing blood to the cup and the other taking blood from the capillaries. This network of blood vessels is the **glomerulus** (plural, glomeruli). The blood vessel that brings blood *to* the capillaries is the **afferent arteriole,** and the blood vessel taking the blood *away* is the **efferent arteriole** (not a venule, as one would think). The blood in the afferent arterioles is from the renal artery, which brings blood into the kidney from the abdominal aorta. Together, the glomerular capsule and the glomerulus are known as the **renal corpuscle,** or **malpighian body.**

The glomerular capsule is a double-walled sac. The outer (parietal) wall is continuous with the inner (vis-

ceral) wall where the blood vessels enter. The cavity between the two layers is continuous with the lumen of the tubule. The outer and inner walls are made up of a single layer of epithelium. The visceral layer of the capsule is in close contact with the capillary endothelium and consists of modified epithelial cells (**podocytes**), with footlike processes known as **pedicels.** The pedicels wrap around the capillary endothelial cells and the slits between the pedicels (**filtration slits**) covered by a membrane (**slit membrane**), permitting the passage of small molecules (see Figure 12.5).

The capillary endothelium is leaky, and the endothelial cells contain large pores or **fenestrations.** These two layers (the visceral layer of the glomerular capsule and the capillary endothelium), together with the basement membrane and the gelatinous, glycoprotein matrix between them, filter those specific substances from the blood that enter the lumen of the tubule. This filter, known as the **filtration membrane** or the **endothelial-capsular membrane** (see Figure 12.5), allows water and solutes from the plasma to pass through. However, it does not allow large structures such as proteins.

The blood pressure in the glomerular capillaries forces fluid and solutes from the blood to be filtered through the filtration membrane into the renal tubule. The filtrate, the **glomerular filtrate,** is similar in composition to plasma except for the lack of protein. The composition of the glomerular filtrate changes as it flows through the renal tubule.

The renal tubule is arranged in the cortex and medulla of the kidney in a specific way (Figure 12.4). Most renal corpuscles are located in the renal cortex. Soon after it forms the glomerular capsule, the tubule becomes coiled—the **proximal convoluted tubule.** Then it straightens out and descends into the medulla as the **descending limb** of the **loop of Henle,** forms a loop (loop of Henle) and goes toward the cortex as the **ascending limb.** In the cortex, the ascending limb coils again and forms the **distal convoluted tubule.** The distal convoluted tubule comes in close contact with its own glomerulus before it joins a larger duct, the **collecting duct.** The collecting duct collects urine from many different nephrons. This duct descends into the medulla and opens at the apex of the papilla, emptying the urine into the calyces.

The urine collected from all the nephrons travels, via the pelvis, into the ureter and then into the urinary bladder, where it is temporarily stored until it is

Glomerulonephritis

This is an inflammation of the glomeruli. The most common cause is the immune reaction that occurs 10 to 14 days after a streptococcal infection. The antigen-antibody complexes that result become trapped in the glomeruli and trigger an inflammatory reaction.

emptied in a convenient location and time. This urine is different from the filtrate that is originally present in the renal corpuscle.

Juxtaglomerular Apparatus

The distal convoluted tubule, as mentioned, is in close proximity to its own glomerulus before it straightens and connects with the collecting duct. In this region, the wall of the afferent arteriole, the cells lining the tubule and other cells in the vicinity are modified to form the **juxtaglomerular apparatus** (see Figure12.6). The juxtaglomerular apparatus is an endocrine structure that secretes **erythropoietin** and **renin.** Erythropoietin is a hormone that regulates the production of red blood cells by the bone marrow. The hormone renin is involved with the regulation of blood pressure (see **page 491**). The rate of secretion of these hormones is related to the composition of blood in the afferent arteriole and the tubular fluid in the distal convoluted tubule. In this way, if the oxygen content of blood is low, cell production is stimulated by erythropoietin. Similarly, if the blood pressure drops in the renal vessels, it is brought to normal by the actions of renin.

Juxtamedullary Nephrons

Although 85% of the nephrons are located in the cortex, 15% of the nephrons are located in the junction of the cortex and the medulla. These nephrons, the **juxtamedullary nephrons,** have long loops of Henle that descend deep into the medulla (Figure 12.4). These nephrons, together with the surrounding blood vessels, play an important role in concentrating urine and conserving water.

Blood Supply to the Kidneys

The right and left renal arteries, branches of the abdominal aorta, supply the kidneys. They bring about 20% to 25% of the total cardiac output (the volume of blood pumped every minute by the ventricle of the heart) i.e., about 1,200 mL (73.2 in³) of blood every minute to the kidneys. After entering at the hilus, each artery divides and redivides in a unique manner until it forms numerous **afferent arterioles**

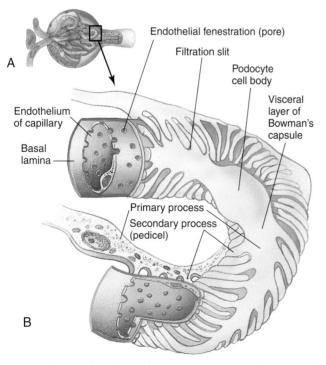

A

Endothelial fenestration (pore)
Filtration slit
Podocyte cell body
Visceral layer of Bowman's capsule
Endothelium of capillary
Basal lamina
Primary process
Secondary process (pedicel)

B

FIGURE 12.5.   **A,** Renal capsule; **B,** the Microscopic Structure of the Filtration Membrane.

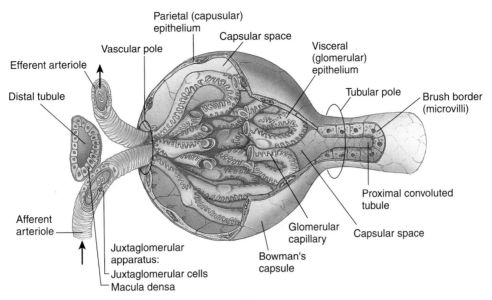

Parietal (capusular) epithelium
Capsular space
Vascular pole
Visceral (glomerular) epithelium
Efferent arteriole
Tubular pole
Distal tubule
Brush border (microvilli)
Proximal convoluted tubule
Afferent arteriole
Capsular space
Juxtaglomerular apparatus:
Glomerular capillary
Juxtaglomerular cells
Bowman's capsule
Macula densa

FIGURE 12.6. Juxtaglomerular Apparatus

(see Figure 12.7). Each afferent arteriole reaches the renal corpuscle to form the network of **glomerular capillaries.** The blood from the capillaries leaves the corpuscle via the **efferent arteriole.** The efferent arterioles descend downward and form **capillaries** again around the loop of Henle. This enables fluid and other substances to be reabsorbed and/or secreted from the renal tubules into the blood and vice versa. These capillaries join and rejoin to form **venules** and **veins** that ultimately empty into the **renal vein.** The renal vein drains into the **inferior vena cava.**

The capillaries around the renal tubules of the juxtamedullary nephrons are different from those of the cortical nephrons in that they form long loops parallel to the loops of Henle. These capillaries are known as the **vasa recta.** This unique arrangement is required for the kidneys to concentrate urine.

Lymphatic Supply to the Kidneys

The kidney has an abundant supply of lymphatic vessels, which drain into the thoracic duct and, ultimately, into the subclavian vein.

Nerve Supply to the Kidneys

The renal nerves of the sympathetic nervous system are the major nerves that supply the kidneys. These nerves regulate the blood flow and pressure in the glomerulus by controlling the diameter of the afferent and efferent arterioles. They also stimulate the release of renin from the juxtaglomerular apparatus when the blood pressure drops in the body. In addi-

tion, they increase the reabsorption of water and sodium in the renal tubules. The latter is especially important when the blood volume drops, as in dehydration or profuse bleeding.

Hormones Affecting Kidney Function

Two hormones play a major part in altering urine concentration. The **antidiuretic hormone** (ADH), also known as **vasopressin,** from the posterior pituitary has an effect on the collecting tubules, increasing the reabsorption of water back into the capillaries. The secretion of ADH is increased when the volume of blood decreases. By reducing the volume of water lost in the urine, the body tries to bring about homeostasis. Antidiuretic hormone, in addition, stimulates the thirst center in the brain to increase water intake and constricts blood vessels to increase blood pressure.

Aldosterone, another hormone secreted by the adrenal cortex, plays an important role in kidney function. This hormone regulates the sodium content in the blood by altering the amount of sodium reabsorbed by the kidney tubules. In conjunction with ADH, by increasing sodium absorption, it draws water back into the renal capillaries by osmosis.

Urine Formation

The filtrate originally formed in the renal corpuscle undergoes many changes as it travels down the renal tubule. These changes are made in different segments

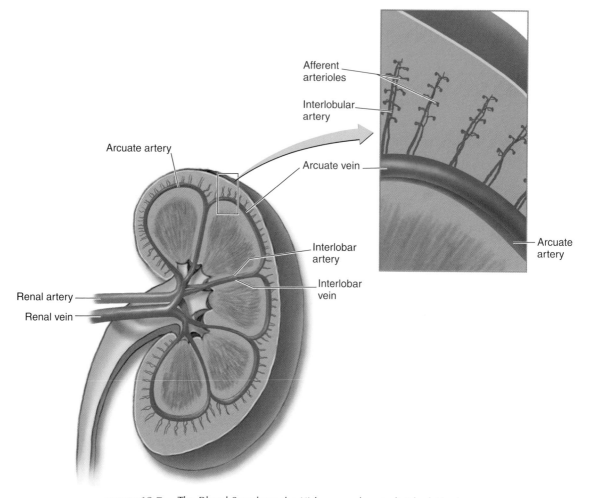

FIGURE 12.7. The Blood Supply to the Kidneys and an Individual Nephron

of the renal tubule, according to the internal environment (i.e., in accordance to the blood volume, blood pressure, plasma concentration, and level of such electrolytes as sodium, potassium, and calcium) The structure of the cells lining the different segments of the tubule is modified according to the functions they perform (see Figure 12.8).

In the renal corpuscle, substances from the blood are allowed to pass passively through the filtration membrane, based on their size. Therefore, solutes, such as glucose, amino acids, and fatty acids, are also filtered. To increase efficiency and avoid waste, useful substances such as these must be reabsorbed. In addition, the large volume of water filtered from the plasma cannot be wasted. To give an idea of the water volume involved, the rate at which the glomeruli filter the plasma—the **glomerular filtration rate** (GFR)—is 125 mL/minute (7.6 in³). This is about 180 liters (10,980 in³ or 47.6 gal) per day. Fortunately, 99% of this fluid is reabsorbed in the renal tubule and only about 1.5 liters (91.5 in³) of urine is excreted a day (see Table 12.1).

GFR can be altered by increasing or decreasing the caliber of the arterioles that enter and leave the glomerulus (e.g., constriction of the afferent arteriole decreases GFR; constriction of the efferent arteriole or dilatation of the afferent arteriole increases GFR) (see Figure 12.9).

The cells of the renal tubule have the ability to *reabsorb* from the lumen as well as *secrete* into the tubule. They reabsorb all useful substances and secrete the waste products that may have escaped filtration. The primary function of different segments of the nephrons is given in Table 12.2.

The rate of water and electrolyte absorption is modified by the action of hormones such as antidiuretic hormone (ADH) and aldosterone. The autonomic nerves are also involved.

In summary, three physical processes—*filtration, secretion,* and *absorption*—are involved in urine formation. The process of concentrating urine and conserving water depends on the differences in the permeability of the cells lining the tubules from segment to segment.

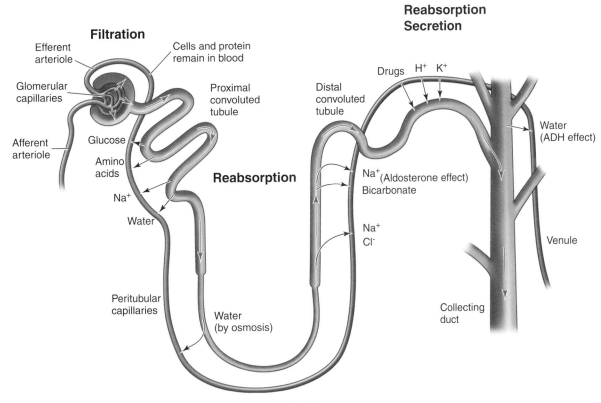

Filtration

Efferent arteriole

Cells and protein remain in blood

Glomerular capillaries

Proximal convoluted tubule

Afferent arteriole

Glucose

Amino acids

Na$^+$

Reabsorption

Water

Peritubular capillaries

Water (by osmosis)

Reabsorption Secretion

Drugs H$^+$ K$^+$

Distal convoluted tubule

Na$^+$(Aldosterone effect)

Bicarbonate

Na$^+$
Cl$^-$

Water (ADH effect)

Venule

Collecting duct

FIGURE **12.8.** Urine Formation

REGULATION OF BODY FLUIDS— THE PROCESS OF CONCENTRATING AND DILUTING URINE

At the glomeruli, filtration occurs; the filtrate, which is similar to plasma other than the lack of plasma protein, travels down the renal tubule. In the proximal convoluted tubule, most ions and organic substances are actively or passively reabsorbed. Some reabsorbed solutes include sodium, potassium, calcium, chloride, phosphate, and bicarbonate. Small proteins and peptides are reabsorbed by pinocytosis. A few substances, such as hydrogen ions, urea, ammonia, and creatinine, may be secreted. Water is reabsorbed by osmosis.

This drastically reduces the volume of the filtrate. As the fluid descends further into the descending limb, more water is reabsorbed and the tubular fluid becomes concentrated. Water and other reabsorbed substances are transported across the lining cells to

Kidney Stones

Kidney stones, nephrolithiasis, or **calculi** may be formed anywhere in the urinary tract by the deposition of calcium salts, magnesium salts, or crystals of uric acid. They may be small or large. Sometimes, large stones with an appearance of a stag's horn (**stag horn calculus**) may form in the renal pelvis. Stones tend to form when there are excessive insoluble salts in the filtrate. These stones may or may not produce symptoms; they may block the tract and produce excruciating pain. Such pain, referred to as **renal colic,** produces spasmodic pain in the flanks that radiate to the groin. Stones may predispose individuals to urinary tract infection because they result in stasis of urine and irritation of tissue.

Small stones may eventually pass. Larger stones may be removed by surgery or noninvasive techniques, such as shockwave lithotripsy or laser lithotripsy, that shatter the stones into smaller fragments. Stone formation can be prevented by treating the underlying condition, altering urine pH, and increasing fluid intake.

Table 12.1

Urinary and Plasma Concentrations of Certain Physiologically Important Substances

Substance	Concentration In Plasma	In Urine
Glucose (mg/dL)	100	0
Sodium (mEq/L)	150	90
Urea (mg/dL)	15	900
Creatinine (mg/dL)	1	150

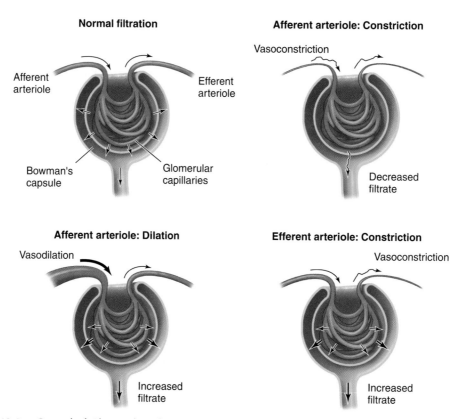

Normal filtration

Afferent arteriole

Efferent arteriole

Bowman's capsule

Glomerular capillaries

Afferent arteriole: Constriction

Vasoconstriction

Decreased filtrate

Afferent arteriole: Dilation

Vasodilation

Increased filtrate

Efferent arteriole: Constriction

Vasoconstriction

Increased filtrate

FIGURE 12.9.   Control of Glomerular Filtration Rate. Normal Filtration; Afferent Arteriole Constriction; Afferent Arteriole Dilatation; Efferent Arteriole Constriction.

the surrounding fluid, where they are absorbed into the blood capillaries that surround the tubules.

The cells in the ascending limb of the loop of Henle are not permeable to water or solutes. The sodium and chloride absorbed here must be actively transported. This process dilutes the tubular fluid (i.e., by removing the solutes alone from the tubular fluid). At the same time, the movement of ions into the interstitial fluid results in concentrating the interstitial fluid surrounding the tubule. As a result, the concentration of interstitial fluid surrounding the loop of Henle progressively increases from the cortex to the deeper parts of the medulla (see Figure 12.10).

Table 12.2

Primary Function of Different Nephron Segments and the Surrounding Capillaries

Region	Primary Function
Renal corpuscle	Filtration of water and inorganic and organic solutes from the plasma; blood cells and plasma proteins remain in the blood; about 180 liters/day (47.6 gal) of filtrate is formed
Proximal convoluted tubule	Reabsorption of ions, organic molecules, vitamins, water, secretion of drugs, toxins and acids. About 60% to 70% of water and 99% to 100% of organic substances are reabsorbed
Loop of Henle	
Descending limb	Reabsorption of about 25% of water from the tubular fluid
Ascending limb	Reabsorption of ions; assists in creation of a concentration gradient in the medulla (needed for concentrating urine)
Distal convoluted tubule	Reabsorption of sodium ions and calcium ions; secretion of acids, ammonia, drugs, and toxins
Collecting duct	Reabsorption of water, sodium ions, secretion or reabsorption of hydrogen ions and bicarbonate ions
Capillaries around the tubules	Return of water and solutes to the general circulation

DIALYSIS OR ARTIFICIAL KIDNEY

When the kidneys cannot function adequately, an artificial kidney may need to be used to remove waste products from the extracellular fluid.

Dialysis involves use of a machine that contains a semipermeable membrane that separates the dialysis fluid and the blood of the individual. Toxic substances that are of a higher concentration in the blood diffuse across the membrane into the dialysis fluid and nutrients and other required ions, which are of a higher concentration in the fluid, diffuse into the blood.

Dialysis can be done in two ways: (1.) shunting blood from an artery through the machine and back into a vein (**hemodialysis**), or (2.) using the peritoneal membrane as a dialysis membrane (**peritoneal dialysis**). Here, the dialysis fluid is infused into the abdominal cavity for a time sufficient to allow substances to diffuse from the blood flowing in the abdominal vessels into the dialysis fluid. The fluid is then removed.

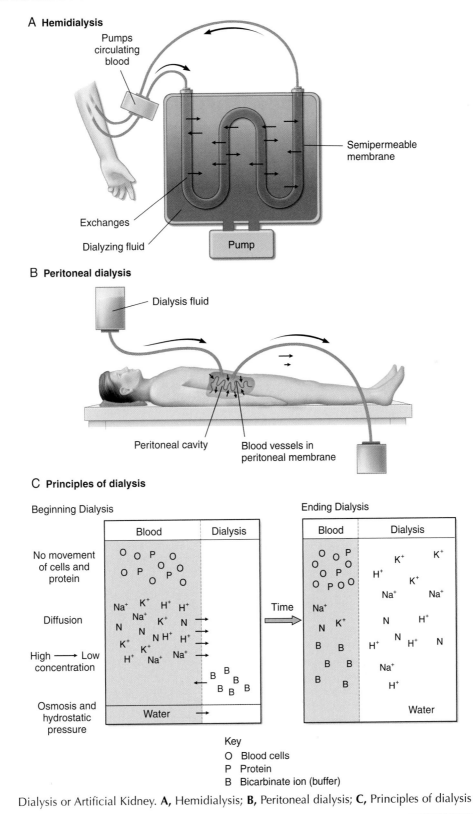

Dialysis or Artificial Kidney. **A,** Hemidialysis; **B,** Peritoneal dialysis; **C,** Principles of dialysis

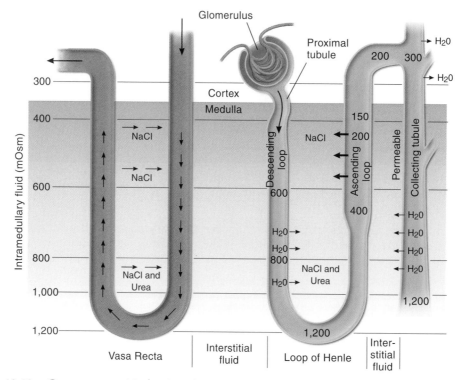

FIGURE **12.10.**   Countercurrent Mechanisms for Concentrating Urine. Antidiuretic hormone (ADH) alters the permeability of the collecting duct to water. When ADH level is increased, more concentrated urine is formed.

The volume of water absorbed from the filtrate as it travels through the rest of the renal tubule—distal convoluted tubule and collecting duct—is determined by the ADH level in the blood. ADH increases the permeability of this segment of the tubule. If a person is dehydrated, more ADH is secreted and the permeability of this segment to water increases and more water moves back into the blood. Water absorption is also increased by the action of aldosterone, which increases sodium reabsorption from the filtrate, and

water moves by osmosis along with the sodium. The fluid from all the nephrons (conveyed by the collecting ducts) that finally reaches the pelvis of the kidney is much less in volume, with a high concentration of waste products. Now referred to as **urine,** from the pelvis, the urine flows into the ureter.

The permeability properties of the ascending and descending limbs (descending permeable to water; ascending, impermeable), the countercurrent (direction of flow opposite in ascending and descending limbs) flow of fluid in the tubule, the countercurrent flow of blood in the vasa recta, the permeability properties of the collecting duct (permeability to water increased by the presence of ADH), and the active and passive transport of solutes across the tubular cells contribute to the ability of the kidneys to concentrate urine. (The process of concentrating urine is complex and beyond the scope of this book. For more details, please refer to more advanced physiology textbooks).

REGULATION OF PH

The kidney is important in acid-base balance. It can regulate the body pH by conserving or eliminating the bases (e.g., bicarbonate) or acids (e.g., hydrogen ions). The kidney has the capacity to secrete hydrogen ions into the tubular fluid. Large quantities of hy-

---

DIURETICS

The term **diuresis** refers to excretion of large volume of urine. **Diuretics** are drugs that increase the volume of urine excreted. They work in different ways. For example, some diuretics are filtered by the glomerulus and draw fluid into the tubules by osmosis (osmotic diuresis). Others may block the ability of the kidney to concentrate urine. Others may inhibit transport of sodium and chloride or block aldosterone. Diuretics are usually given to individuals who have high blood pressure and increased blood volume and to those individuals in cardiac failure.

Caffeine and alcohol also have diuretic effects. Caffeine produces its effects by directly inhibiting the absorption of sodium along the tubules. Alcohol works indirectly by inhibiting ADH secretion by the posterior pituitary.

drogen ions can be eliminated because of the presence of buffers in the urine that combine with the hydrogen ions. (Buffers are substances that combine with hydrogen ions to form weaker acids).

The three major urinary buffers are bicarbonate (HCO_3^-), phosphate (HPO_4^{2-}) and ammonia (NH_3). Bicarbonate present in the filtrate combines with hydrogen ions to form carbonic acid (a weak acid). This acid dissociates into water and carbon dioxide. The carbon dioxide diffuses into the cells and is used to form more bicarbonate ions.

$$H^+ + HCO_3^- \rightarrow H_2CO_3 \rightarrow H_2O + CO_2$$

Hydrogen ion + Bicarbonate ion $\rightarrow$
Carbonic Acid $\rightarrow$ Water + Carbon dioxide

Similarly, filtered phosphate combines with the secreted hydrogen ions to form $H_2PO_4^-$ (dihydrogen phosphate ion) and is excreted. The tubular cells manufacture ammonia from the amino acid glutamine. The ammonia combines with hydrogen ions to form NH_4^+ (ammonium ion) and is also excreted.

When the blood pH is alkaline, fewer hydrogen ions are secreted and more bases excreted.

THE COMPOSITION OF URINE

Urine is composed of 93% to 97% water. Urine pH ranges from 4.5–8.0. Normally, about 1,200 mL (73.2 in³) of urine is excreted each day. Urine is a sterile fluid. It only becomes contaminated with bacteria when it passes through the external genitalia. Some organic substances present include urea, creatinine, ammonia, uric acid, urobilin, and bilirubin.

Urea is derived from the metabolism of amino acids by the liver and kidneys. Its content in the urine would, therefore, increase when protein breakdown is greater than protein buildup. Creatinine is derived from the breakdown of creatine phosphate in skeletal muscle. Its excretion is proportional to the skeletal muscle mass. Ammonia is derived largely from protein breakdown. Uric acid is derived from breakdown of nucleic acid, present in large amounts in the nucleus of cells.

Urobilin and bilirubin are breakdown products of hemoglobin and give urine its yellow color. Increased amounts are excreted when there is liver disease or when there is excessive breakdown of red blood cells. The color of urine may be altered by medications and diet (e.g., beets can cause reddish colored urine).

Urine normally does not contain glucose, or it only contains minute quantities. In conditions in which the blood glucose levels are persistently high, the kidney is unable to reabsorb all the glucose that is filtered. In this case, some glucose is lost in the urine. Glucose is absorbed from the tubules by carriers. When the level of glucose in the filtrate is higher than these carriers can absorb, glucose appears in the urine (**glucosuria**). The upper limit of the rate at which glucose can be transported is known as **transport maximum** (Tm). Tm is measured in milligrams /minute.

The most common cause of glucosuria is diabetes mellitus, in which the blood glucose levels are above normal because of the lack of insulin. Rarely, glucosuria may be found in people whose renal tubules have a low Tm as a result of genetic mutations. One test used to detect and monitor diabetes mellitus is to test the urine for glucose.

Little, if any, protein is lost in the urine. In kidney disease or inflammation or infection of the urinary tract, protein may be detected in the urine.

The excretion of sodium, chloride, potassium, and other ions vary with diet, pH of urine, and effect of hormones.

Normally, no red blood cells can be detected in the urine, and their presence may indicate problems in the urinary tract—anywhere from the kidney to the urethra. Few white blood cells are seen in urine. The presence of an abnormal number of white blood cells indicates urinary tract infection.

The urine can be analyzed to reveal the state of the body. If body metabolism is altered, or if there is kidney dysfunction, substances that are not normally present in the urine may be found or the concentration of normal constituents of urine may be increased to abnormal levels. The status of the kidney can also be analyzed by measuring urea and creatinine levels in blood.

Transportation and Elimination of Urine

THE URETER

Ureters are muscular tubes, about 30 cm (11.8 in) long, that extend from the kidney to the posterior aspect of the urinary bladder. The lumen is lined by transitional epithelium. The walls contain smooth muscle, arranged in spiral, longitudinal, and circular bundles. The ureters convey urine from the kidneys to the bladder. The ureters extend medially and inferiorly from the pelvis of the kidney and pass over the psoas muscles. They lie behind the peritoneum and are attached to the posterior abdominal wall by connective tissue. They then enter the bladder obliquely and open into the bladder by means of slitlike openings—**ureteral openings.** When the bladder contracts, these openings are closed and backflow of urine (reflux) is prevented.

Beginning at the pelvis, the smooth muscle in the wall of the ureters undergoes rhythmic, wavelike contractions every few seconds, which helps force the urine toward the bladder.

THE URINARY BLADDER

The function of the bladder is to temporarily store urine. It is a hollow muscular organ, which is held in place by connective tissue that attaches it to the walls of the pelvic cavity. Superiorly, it is covered by peritoneum; posteriorly, the bladder is related to the rectum in males and the uterus and upper part of the vagina in females (Figure 12.1). When the bladder is empty, the uterus rests on its superior surface. The

---

✚ Common Clinical Terms

Anuria—passage of a low volume of urine (0–50 mL/day)
Cystitis—infection of the bladder
Dysuria—painful or difficult micturition
Frequency—recurrent passage of urine
Hematuria—blood in the urine
Hemoglobinuria—hemoglobin in the urine
Nephrolithiasis—kidney stones
Nocturia—passage of urine at night
Oliguria—production of a low volume of urine (50–500ml/day)
Polyuria—production of excessive amounts of urine
Proteinuria—presence of protein in the urine
Pyelonephritis—infection of the kidney
Pyuria—presence of pus in the urine
Urgency—strong desire to void
Urinary retention—no micturition, with collection of urine in the bladder; renal function is usually normal

---

✚ Urinary Tract Infection (UTI)

Urinary tract infections are common. Infection of the bladder (**cystitis**) and urethra (**urethritis**) are considered lower urinary tract infections, and infection of the kidney (**pyelonephritis**) is considered an upper urinary tract infection. The infection is usually a result of the ascent of organisms from the perineal region. Incontinence, retention of urine, obstruction to urine flow, catheterization, and reduced immunity are a few conditions that predispose to UTI.

Back pain, dysuria, frequency, urgency, hematuria, and cloudy urine are some common symptoms of UTI.

---

bladder is held in position by ligaments that run from its base to the pubis anteriorly and to the rectum and sacrum posteriorly. A fibrous band runs from its superior surface to the anterior abdominal wall and umbilicus. The peritoneum, which covers part of the bladder, also provides some support.

When not distended by urine, the inner lining of the bladder is thrown into folds, except in a triangular region in its posterior part (the **trigone**). The three points of the triangle are made up of the two superior orifices of the ureter and the urethral opening inferiorly. The bladder's inner lining is transitional epithelium, which allows for easy distension and contraction of the bladder. The wall of the bladder is largely smooth muscle—the **detrusor muscle**—arranged in three layers; the inner and outer longitudinal and middle circular. The urethra opens out of the bladder at its most inferior point, the **neck.** The region of the bladder surrounding the urethral opening consists of circular smooth muscle, the **internal urethral sphincter,** or **sphincter vesicae.** The detrusor muscle and the sphincter are controlled by autonomic nerves. The sympathetic nerves relax the detrusor and close the sphincter, and the parasympathetic nerves contract the detrusor and relax the sphincter (the opposite of the sympathetic nerves).

THE URETHRA

The urethra extends from the neck of the bladder to the **external urethral opening,** or **external urethral meatus.** The male urethra is about 18–20 cm (7.1–7.9 in) long as compared with the female urethra, which is only about 3–5 cm (1.2–2 in) long. The shortness of the urethra and its close proximity to the anus, vagina, and exterior and constant irritation to the tissue as a result of tampons and sexual activity, etc., make a woman more prone to urinary tract infections.

The male urethra extends from the neck of the bladder through the center of the prostate gland (**prostatic urethra**) and penetrates through the muscular floor of the pelvis (**membranous urethra**). Finally, it passes through the penis (**penile, or spongiosa urethra**) and opens to the exterior. The urethra in men is a common passage for urine and semen.

In both men and women, a band of circular skeletal muscle surrounds the urethra as it passes through the pelvic floor. This is the **external urethral sphincter,** which is under voluntary control and is relaxed voluntarily when urine is expelled.

Urination or Micturition

As the bladder fills with urine, the walls are stretched and the stretch receptors here are stimulated. Impulses are conducted by sensory nerves (pelvic nerves) to the sacral segment (S2 and S3), the **micturition center** (Figure 12.11).

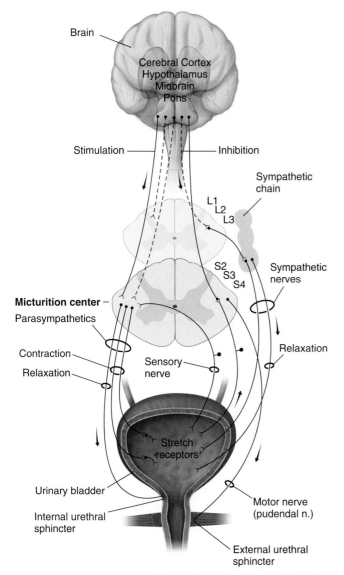

FIGURE **12.11.** Innervation of the Urinary Bladder and the Micturition Reflex

Incontinence and Retention

Incontinence is a condition in which the individual is unable to voluntarily control urination. Loss of muscle tone and problems with innervation are some causes. Stress incontinence is one type that occurs when increased intraabdominal pressure forces urine through the sphincter. It is common in women whose pelvic muscles are weakened by pregnancy or age.

In urinary retention, the production of urine is normal, but urine is retained in the bladder. It is serious because the back pressure can damage the kidney. Common causes of retention are urethral obstruction (e.g., prostatic hyperplasia) or impaired innervation of the bladder. A urinary catheter (a tube inserted into the urethra that drains urine from the bladder) may be used to relieve retention.

The nerves synapse here with parasympathetic nerves, whose action is to contract the detrusor and relax the internal sphincter. The micturition center also communicates with the motor nerves that innervate the skeletal muscles of the external urethral sphincter. The sensory nerves communicate with other nerves that carry impulses to the thalamus, the brainstem, and other areas of the cerebral cortex. The latter is responsible for the conscious awareness of a filled bladder. Communication from higher centers to the micturition center facilitates or inhibits the micturition reflex. Usually, the urge to urinate begins when the bladder is filled with about 200 mL (12.2 in³) of urine (Figure 12.11.)

Both the internal (involuntary control) and external urethral sphincters (voluntary control) must relax for the bladder to be emptied. Infants lack voluntary control, and the bladder is emptied reflexively when the bladder becomes distended. Therefore, micturition is a spinal reflex that can be facilitated or inhibited by higher brain centers. The ability to keep the external urethral sphincter contracted and delay urination is a learned process.

After urination, the female urethra empties by gravity; in males, it empties by contraction of the bulbocavernosus muscle.

Age-Related Changes in the Genitourinary System

KIDNEYS

As one ages, the reserve capacity of the kidney is decreased. This makes the individual more vulnerable to dysfunction if demands on the kidney increase, as in trauma or disease. The number of nephrons decreases, and the length of the tubules decreases. Reduction of blood flow also occurs. As a result, kidney function decreases, with slower rate of filtration in the glomeruli and less production of renin, vitamin D, and erythropoietin. Response to ADH is diminished. All of these changes result in diminished function.

The regulation of blood volume is less efficient, with the ability to concentrate and dilute the urine also diminished. Reduced vitamin D production affects the absorption of calcium from the intestine (a function of the hormone). Reduced production of erythropoietin may contribute to anemia. The tubular changes result in difficulty in maintaining acid-base balance.

One important effect of changes in kidney function is the reduced capacity to excrete drugs. If care is not taken to reduce drug dosages, drugs may accumulate in the body and produce further complications of overdose. Also, when fluids are administered parenterally or diuretics are given to elderly persons, they need to be monitored carefully because such interventions may severely challenge the water and solute balance of the body.

URETERS

There may be reflux of urine into the ureters from the bladder as a result of improper functioning of the junction between the ureter and bladder.

Urinary System and Pain

Pain originating in the abdominal organs is often referred to areas on the surface of the body, not necessarily over the anatomical location of the organ. Often, pain originating in the kidney is felt in the lumbar region or radiating to the right or left upper quadrant of the abdomen.

Bladder infections (cystitis) may present as pain just above the pubis or in the upper inner aspect of the thigh.

The pain produced by cystitis and urethritis (inflammation of the urethra) may be abated by swabbing the urethral opening with a cotton pad soaked in a dilute solution (10–12 drops in 100 mL water, or 6.1 in³ water) of tea tree oil after urination.[4] Note that essential oils are very concentrated and must be diluted before application.

Addition of 8–10 drops of bactericidal oils (e.g., bergamot, lavender, chamomile, tea tree, sandalwood, juniper, frankincense, parsley seed, celery seed, thyme, and yarrow) to bath water can be used as a general disinfectant or as a preventive measure in such conditions.

Oil made of 3–10 drops each of tea tree, sandalwood, bergamot (or lavender) in 25 mL (1.5 in³) of a carrier oil (such as sweet almond or grape seed) may be used to massage over the lower abdomen and back to provide relief from pain originating from the urinary tract.

Reflexology and the Urinary System

Urine output may be altered by applying pressure with the thumb for a few minutes on the kidney, ureter and bladder area of the foot.[5]

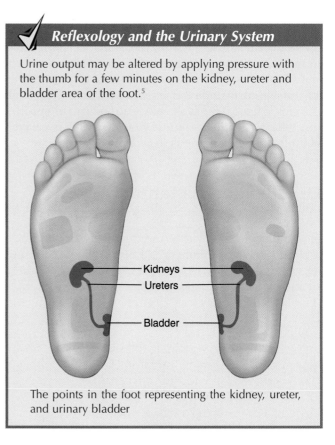

Kidneys
Ureters
Bladder

The points in the foot representing the kidney, ureter, and urinary bladder

URINARY BLADDER AND URETHRA

Smooth muscle and elastic tissue degenerate with time, being replaced with fibrous tissue and a decreased bladder capacity. The muscles become weaker and incomplete emptying of bladder may occur. The decrease in bladder capacity results in increased frequency of urination. In men, prostate hypertrophy is common. Because the urethra passes through the prostate, growth of the prostate may obstruct the urethra, producing difficulty in passing urine. Weakening of the pelvic muscles may result in stress incontinence (i.e., leakage of small quantities of urine when the intra-abdominal pressure is increased).

RELEVANCE TO BODYWORKERS

One common problem faced by elderly individuals is difficulty maintaining bladder control. Individuals with this problem avoid the public or restrict their intake of fluids to avoid embarrassment and it is important for body workers to put them at ease. As a result of incontinence, many elderly individuals may need catheterization or diapers. Rashes and other skin lesions may be present in the lumbar and gluteal regions as a result of irritation of the sensitive skin. Such inflamed areas should be avoided.

Bodyworkers and the Urinary System

One effect of massage is the potential increase of urine production. Massage aids the movement of fluid from the interstitial compartment into the systemic circulation. The resultant increase in blood volume is counteracted by an increase in urine volume. Such effects are more significant in those persons with edema. The increase may be as high as three to four times the normal rate of urine formation. With the increase in urinary volume, an increase in excretion of the products accumulated in the edema fluid can be expected. Massage promotes excretion of nitrogenous wastes and other ions, as evidenced by an increase in urinary levels after treatment.[1,2]

By stimulating large nerve fibers (gate control theory), massage can reduce pain originating from the urinary tract by reducing reflexive muscle spasm and inhibiting pain perception. It has the potential to reduce pain by local reflex mechanisms as well.

It is important for the therapist to elicit a complete history related to the urinary system during the visit. Clients with pain in the low back region associated with fever; those with a history of change in color, frequency, or volume of urine; and those with pain on passing urine should be referred to a physician.[3] History of sudden increase in weight could be a result of fluid reten-tion resulting from kidney malfunction. Because edema can be an early sign of kidney problems, it must be ensured that edema in a client is not caused by kidney disease. Kidney infections often present as tenderness, pain, or swelling in the back, just below the costal margin and adjacent to the vertebrae. Problems with the organs of the urinary system may present as pain that is referred to other areas of the body (see **page 344**).

Polycystic kidney is one condition in which the kidney is enlarged, with or without functional problems. Abdominal massage is contraindicated in this condition.

Floating and movable kidneys are relatively common. Care should be taken when the abdomen is massaged. (It is beyond the scope of this book to give details of the various kidney disorders, and the student is encouraged to refer to pathology textbooks.)

Individuals on dialysis, or those who have had kidney transplants, are usually prescribed antibiotics and drugs that suppress immunity. Care should be taken to prevent these clients from being exposed to any form of infection.

REFERENCES

1. Kurz W, Wittlinger G, Litmanovitch YI, et al. Effect of manual lymph drainage massage on urinary excerption of neurophormones and minerals in chronic lymphedema. Angiology 1978; 29:764–772.
2. Yates J. A Physician's Guide to Therapeutic Massage. 2nd Ed. Vancouver: Massage Therapists' Association of British Columbia, 1999.
3. Premkumar K. Pathology A to Z. A Handbook for Massage Therapists. 2nd Ed. Calgary: VanPub Books, 1999.
4. Lawless J. The Complete Illustrated Guide to Aromatherapy. Shaftesbury, Dorset: Element Books, 1997.
5. Kawashima T. Foot Reflexology. Kyoto: Yamaguchi Seikido, 2001.

SUGGESTED READINGS

Ironson G, Field T, Scafidi F, et al. Massage therapy is associated with enhancement of the immune system's cytotoxic capacity. Int J Neurosci 1996;84:205–217.
Salvo SG. Massage Therapy Principles & Practice. Philadelphia: W.B. Saunders, 1999.

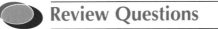 **Review Questions**

Malformations and Displacement of Kidneys

Malformations of the kidneys are common. One kidney may be absent entirely, or congenitally atrophied. At times, the kidneys may be fused only at the lower ends to form a horseshoe-shaped structure, or completely fused to form a disklike kidney.

Occasionally, one or both kidneys may be displaced and fixed in abnormal positions, such as the iliac fossa, over the sacroiliac joint, into the pelvis between the rectum and bladder, or by the side of the uterus.

At times, the kidneys are not fixed in position congenitally and known as **floating kidney.** In some cases, the mobility of the kidney is increased at a later age, especially in those who are emaciated. Such kidneys are known as **movable kidneys.** Floating and movable kidneys may be palpable through the abdomen and may present with gastric, hepatic, and even nervous symptoms.

Abdominal and pelvic massage, together with rest, suitable exercise, and abdominal support, has been found to be beneficial to those with movable kidneys. In such cases, massage should be done with the head and chest at a lower level than the rest of the body. Transient albuminuria may be observed if the kidney is palpated.

Multiple Choice

Choose the best answer to the following questions:

1. A person on a new health regimen drinks 250 mL (15.3 in³) of water, 5 to 8 times a day. His body would respond to this change by
   A. increased production of aldosterone.
   B. increased production of renin.
   C. increased urinary output.
   D. increased production of vasopressin.

2. Which of the following is a normal constituent of urine?
   A. Albumin
   B. Glucose
   C. Blood cells
   D. Urea

3. The function of the urinary bladder is to
   A. store urine.
   B. concentrate urine.
   C. secrete hormones.
   D. reabsorb valuable constituents in the urine.

4. The primary nutrient reabsorption site in the nephron is the
   A. renal corpuscle.
   B. proximal convoluted tubule.
   C. loop of Henle.
   D. distal convoluted tubule.

5. We become consciously aware of increasing pressure in the urinary bladder as a result of sensations relayed to the
   A. sacral region of the spinal cord.
   B. cerebral cortex.
   C. motor neuron.
   D. hypothalamus.

Fill-In

1. The components of the urinary system include the kidneys, _____, _____, and the _____.

2. The _____ (left/right) kidney is located at a lower level because of the presence of the liver.

3. The functional unit of the kidney is the _____.

4. The three processes involved in urine formation are _____, _____, and secretion. Of these, _____ involves selective return of valuable substances from the tubular fluid into blood.

5. The glomerular filtration rate is the _____ _____.

6. _____ percent of cardiac output passes through the kidney each minute. This is approximately _____ mL/minute.

7. Two hormones secreted by the kidney are _____ and _____. The hormone _____ regulates red blood cell production in the bone marrow, and the hormone _____ effects blood pressure.

8. Two other hormones that affect the kidney are _____, secreted by the posterior pituitary, and _____, secreted by the adrenal cortex. _____ helps conserve water, and _____ affects sodium reabsorption.

True–False
(Answer the following questions T, for true; or F, for false):

1. Blood from the glomerular capillaries flow into arterioles, not into venules.

2. A person taking diuretics is likely to excrete larger volume of urine.

3. A ureter is a tube that conveys urine from the urinary bladder to the exterior of the body.

4. Antidiuretic hormone (ADH) decreases the permeability of distal and collecting tubules to water and, thereby, increases urinary volume.

5. The glomerular capsule and the blood vessels it encloses constitute a renal corpuscle.

6. Most water resorption normally takes place in the proximal convoluted tubule.

7. The short, female urethra makes women more prone to urinary tract infection.

8. There is no significant change in the glomerular filtration rate as one ages.

9. Massage has the potential to increase urinary output.

10. The urinary bladder can be palpated above the pubic bone in normal, healthy individuals.

Matching
Match the following with the listed terms (1–12). Not all terms will be used.

a. _____ The outermost layer of connective tissue that anchors the kidney to the abdominal wall.

b. _____ The part of the urinary tract into which urine drains from the collecting ducts.

c. _____ The structure in the kidney that contains cells that secrete erythropoietin and renin.

1. nephrology
2. urology
3. juxtamedullary nephrons
4. juxtaglomerular apparatus.
5. proximal convoluted tubule
6. ascending limb of the loop of Henle
7. collecting duct
8. renal calyx

d. _____ The nephrons that contain long loops of Henle.

e. _____ The part of the nephron that absorbs most of the water.

f. _____ The part of the nephron that is affected by antidiuretic hormone (ADH).

g. _____ The study of kidneys.

9. cortical nephrons
10. glomerulus
11. renal fascia
12. adipose capsule

Short-Answer Questions

1. What is the function of the ureter?

2. What is the function of the urethra (in males and females)?

3. What is meant by micturition reflex? Briefly describe the micturition process.

4. What is the potential effect of massage on the urinary system?

5. How is the fluid in the Bowman's capsule different from that in the renal pelvis?

6. Describe the changes that occur in the kidney and urinary bladder in the elderly.

7. List any three substances in blood not normally found in the urine. Identify conditions that may result in the presence of these substances in urine.

8. Trace the path of a red blood cell from the renal artery to renal vein.

9. Trace the path that you would take to reach the outside of the body if you were a particle in the Bowman's capsule that cannot be absorbed by the tubular cells.

10. Why are urinary tract infections more common in females than males?

11. Describe the structures that separate blood from the fluid in the Bowman's capsule.

Case Studies

1. James is the 19-year-old son of Mrs. Rose, one of your regular clients. Mrs. Rose asked you, the therapist, if you would possibly treat James at their home. After a serious car accident, James almost bled to death and his kidneys failed. He was now on dialysis, waiting to have a kidney transplant. Mrs. Rose felt strongly that massage would help ease James's aches and pain.

On arrival at Mrs. Rose's home, you assess James. His face is puffy; his feet are obviously edematous, twice their original size. Mrs. Rose said that James was being treated with many drugs to help him pass urine. She had been taught to take blood pressure so that she could monitor her son, whose blood pressure had been high following the onset of the kidney problem.

A. Why is James' blood pressure high? What is the role of the kidneys in maintaining blood pressure?

B. Why does James have edema?

C. What is dialysis? Briefly explain the dialysis process.

D. What are diuretics?

E. If James' blood was analyzed, how would it differ from that of a healthy person? Give reasons for your answer.

F. What is the effect of massage on the urinary system? Is James likely to benefit from massage?

2. After a one-hour massage, Mr. Brown feels dizzy soon after getting off the massage table. Fifty-years-old, Mr. Brown is hypertensive and has been on antihypertensive treatment for a long time. Mr. Brown lies back on the table and, after ten minutes, sits up for sometime before getting off. He tells his therapist that this dizziness occurs every time he changes posture quickly and that his physician had mentioned it is one of the adverse effects of the antihypertensive drug he is taking.

A. Why does Mr. Brown feel dizzy?

B. What compensatory mechanisms come into play that restore Mr. Brown's blood pressure when he changes posture?

C. What is the role of kidneys in maintaining blood pressure?

3. Vivian, a 20-year-old model, comes to your clinic for her monthly relaxation massage. On taking a routine medical history, she tells you that she has been urinating frequently and that there is some burning when she passes urine. You are aware that her mother has had recurrent problems with kidney stones.

You advise Vivian to make an appointment with her physician to treat this new urinary tract problem.

A. What are the components of the urinary system?

B. Where are the kidneys located? Identify the location on the surface of the body.

C. Describe the location of pain originating from the different components of the urinary tract.

4. Mr. Logan, a 40-year-old ski instructor, had an accident on a particularly steep ski hill, during training his advanced students. Distracted by a wayward student skiing too close to a precipice, Mr. Logan crashed into a tree. Fortunately, his helmet saved him from severe head injury; however, Mr. Logan suffered a spinal cord injury at the level of the tenth thoracic vertebra.

   Following the accident, Mr. Logan has had problems urinating voluntarily. His physiotherapist trained him to initiate urination by stroking the medial aspect of his thigh.
   A. What is the micturition reflex?
   B. How is micturition regulated?
   C. Why did Mr. Logan lose voluntary control of urination?

5. Tammy had a refreshing treatment at the local spa that included a body wrap session. She was exposed to a high temperature and, although she felt uncomfortable, she did not mind. In fact, despite sweating profusely throughout the session, she thought the session was rejuvenating.

   Later, following the treatment, she noticed that she was passing more concentrated urine, with less volume.
   A. Explain why Tammy is likely to have decreased urinary output.
   B. What mechanisms allow Tammy to alter the concentration of urine when she produces large amounts of sweat?

 ## Answers to Review Questions

Multiple Choice

1. C. The increase in water intake would result in an increase in blood volume and blood pressure. To maintain homeostasis, the blood volume must be brought down. This is accomplished by increasing urinary output. If an increase in aldosterone occurs, sodium and water would be retained, worsening the situation. If renin production is increased, this will result in increased angiotensin II levels, which, in turn, would increase aldosterone production—again, this is undesirable.

   The effect of vasopressin on the kidney is to reabsorb water into the peritubular capillaries. This, too, will worsen matters.

2. D. Urea is a waste product formed by metabolizing protein. Albumin is a protein that is not allowed past the filtration membrane. Glucose, although filtered through the filtration membrane, is completely reabsorbed into the blood. It is only found in the urine if the plasma levels are too high or abnormalities in the kidney tubules prevent reabsorption of glucose, even if the plasma levels are within the normal range. Blood cells are too large to be filtered into the Bowman's capsule; they may be present in urine if the urinary tract is damaged or inflamed.

3. A. The bladder stores urine until it can be expelled voluntarily or involuntarily. No changes occur to the urine in the bladder. The kidney is the only part of the urinary tract that can concentrate urine, secrete hormones, or reabsorb valuable constituents from the tubular fluid.

4. B. Only filtration occurs at the renal corpuscle. Although reabsorption occurs in C. and D., it is maximal in the proximal convoluted tubule.

5. B. Although the micturition center is located in the sacral region, *conscious* awareness occurs only if the sensation is relayed to the cerebral cortex. A motor neuron takes impulses to the effector. The hypothalamus, although situated in the brain, does not play a part in conscious awareness.

Fill-In

1. Ureters, urinary bladder, and the urethra
2. Right kidney
3. Nephron
4. Filtration, absorption, absorption
5. The rate at which fluid is filtered across the filtration membrane from the plasma into the Bowman's capsule. It is normally 125 mL/min.
6. 20% to 25%; 1,200 mL/min (73.2 in^3/min).
7. Erythropoietin, renin. Erythropoietin regulates production of red blood cells, renin has an effect on blood pressure.
8. Antidiuretic hormone (ADH), Aldosterone. ADH is secreted by the posterior pituitary gland and helps conserve water. Aldosterone, secreted by the adrenal cortex, affects reabsorption of sodium.

True–False

1. True
2. True
3. False. The urethra communicates with the exterior.
4. False (decreases urinary output)
5. True
6. True
7. True
8. False. The rate decreases as the number of glomeruli and blood flow decreases with age.
9. True.
10. False. The bladder is located in the pelvis. It can be palpated in the abdomen in newborns.

Matching

a. 11   b. 8   c. 4   d. 3   e. 5   f. 7   g.1

Short-Answer Questions

1. The ureter conveys urine from the kidney to the urinary bladder.
2. The urethra conveys urine from the bladder to the exterior. In males, it also conveys semen.
3. The micturition reflex results in the emptying of the bladder. Like all nerve reflexes, it has a sensory component (stimuli—stretch of bladder, impulses conveyed by the sensory nerve); a center (located in the sacral region); a motor component (the motor nerve that communicates impulses from the center to the effector); and effector(s) (detrusor muscle and the external and internal sphincter). This reflex is facilitated or inhibited by nerves from higher centers located in the brain.
4. The major effects of massage include an increase in urinary volume; an increase in excretion of nitrogenous wastes and ions from the interstitial fluid compartment—particularly in those individuals with edema.
5. The fluid in the Bowman's capsule is an ultrafiltrate of plasma. The ultrafiltrate is modified by secretion and reabsorption as it flows through the tubules. The fluid in the pelvis is what remains after all modifications have taken place in the tubules.
6. The reserve capacity of the kidney is decreased. The number of nephrons decreases. Also, the tubules decrease in length. Reduction of blood flow also occurs. As a result, kidney function decreases, with slower rate of filtration in the glomeruli and less renin, vitamin D, and erythropoietin production. Response to antidiuretic hormone is diminished. The regulation of blood volume is less efficient, with the ability to concentrate and dilute the urine diminished. Reduced vitamin D production affects the absorption of calcium from the intestine (both functions of the hormones). Reduced erythropoietin production may contribute to anemia. The tubular changes result in difficulty maintaining acid-base balance. There is reduced capacity to excrete drugs. The smooth muscle and elastic tissue degenerate with time, replaced with fibrous tissue and decreased capacity of the bladder. The muscles become weaker and incomplete emptying of bladder may occur. The decrease in bladder capacity results in increased frequency of urination.
7. Albumin, glucose, and blood cells are three substances not found in normal urine. Damage to the glomeruli may result in albumin in the blood. Glucose is observed in the urine in those with uncontrolled diabetes mellitus. When the urinary tract is injured or inflamed, blood cells may be detected in the urine.
8. See Figure 12. 7.
9. Bowman's capsule—proximal convoluted tubule—loop of Henle—distal convoluted tubule—collecting duct—renal calyx—renal pelvis—ureter—urinary bladder—urethra.
10. Urinary tract infection is more common in women because of the short urethra, proximity to the anus and vagina, use of tampons, sexual activity, douches, and use of deodorants, etc.
11. Capillary endothelium, basement membrane and matrix, visceral layer of the Bowman's capsule.

Case Studies

1. A, James' blood pressure is high because the kidneys secrete renin, which ultimately results in the formation of angiotensin II, a powerful vasoconstrictor and stimulator of aldosterone. Alteration in the secretion of this hormone results in blood pressure fluctuation.

   B, James has edema because kidney failure affects excretion of fluids and ions.

   C, Dialysis is a procedure used to remove nitrogenous wastes and ions from the plasma and restore it to near normal concentration. In this procedure, plasma is separated from a fluid that contains nutrients and ions in concentrations similar to normal plasma by a semipermeable membrane. Constituents move by diffusion from/to plasma along concentration gradients across the membrane.

   D, Diuretics are chemicals that promote urine formation.

   E, James' blood is likely to contain higher levels of creatinine and urea (normal nitrogenous wastes). The concentration of various ions may be different as their excretion is also affected in kidney failure.

   F, Massage can increase the excretion of nitrogenous wastes and urinary output in healthy individuals. In James' case, the effects would be variable, depending on the functioning of his kidneys. The effect of touch on any person is difficult to quantify. James may, therefore, benefit from a relaxation massage.

2. A, and B. Antihypertensive drugs generally have an effect on the sympathetic nerves, producing vasodilation (and reducing blood pressure). Diuretics may be given, resulting in re-

duced blood volume (and blood pressure). When changes occur in posture, the baroreceptor reflex rapidly produces generalized vasoconstriction and increase in blood flow to the brain when the effect of gravity tends to pool blood in the lower limbs. Other mechanisms include secretion of ADH, aldosterone, and reduced secretion of atrial natriuretic peptide, etc. (see Regulation of Blood Pressure).

In Mr. Brown's case, this does not happen quickly, and he feels dizzy. By sitting up for sometime before getting off the table, Mr. Brown allows sufficient time for his body to compensate for the change in blood pressure.

C, Kidneys increase blood pressure by secreting the hormone renin. Hormones, such as aldosterone and antidiuretic hormone, regulate blood volume and blood pressure by affecting the kidney.

3. A, The components of the urinary system are the kidney, ureter, urinary bladder, and urethra.

B, The kidneys are located retroperitoneally on either side of the vertebral column between vertebrae T12 and L3. The right kidney is slightly lower than the left because of the presence of the liver. On the surface of the body, the superior pole of the kidney is at level T12. The inferior pole lies just above the transumbilical plane, the plane at the level of the umbilicus, (i.e., at the upper part of level L3). The inferior pole is, therefore, a fingers-

breadth superior to the iliac crest. The oblique twelfth rib and the transverse processes of L1 and L2 are located posterior to the kidney. The hilus of the kidney is located in the transpyloric plane (a transverse plane at the level of the disk between L1 and L2).

C, Pain originating in the kidney is felt in the lumbar region (upper back) or radiating to the right or left upper quadrant of the abdomen. Pain from the urinary bladder may present just above the pubis or in the upper inner aspect of the thigh.

4. A, and B. See answer to Short-Answer question 3.

C, Mr. Logan looses voluntary control as the communication is severed from the higher centers to the sacral center. Because the micturition reflex pathway is intact, he can urinate involuntarily.

5. A, Tammy has reduced urinary output because the body is trying to compensate for the water (and blood volume) lost through sweating.

B, To conserve water, Tammy's body secretes antidiuretic hormone (ADH) from the posterior pituitary, which increases water reabsorption in the distal tubule and collecting duct. Aldosterone secretion increases sodium reabsorption. Water is reabsorbed, along with sodium, by osmosis. These are a few mechanisms that help conserve water. Increased thirst is another mechanism that helps increase blood volume by causing the individual to drink more water.

Coloring Exercise

The Position of the Components of the Urinary System. Label and color the diagrams using colors of your choice.

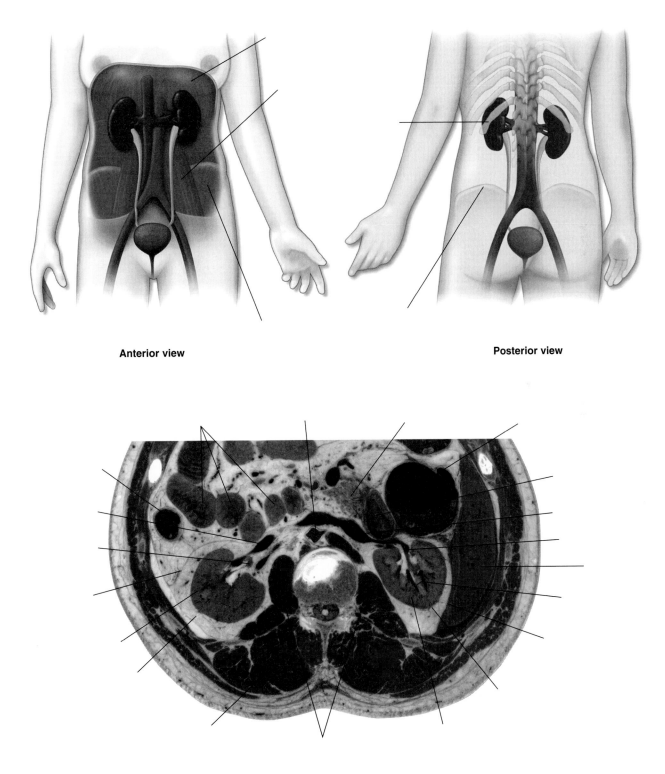

Anterior view

Posterior view

Transverse section

Longitudinal Section Through the Kidney, Near the Hilum. Label and color the various structures, using colors of your choice.

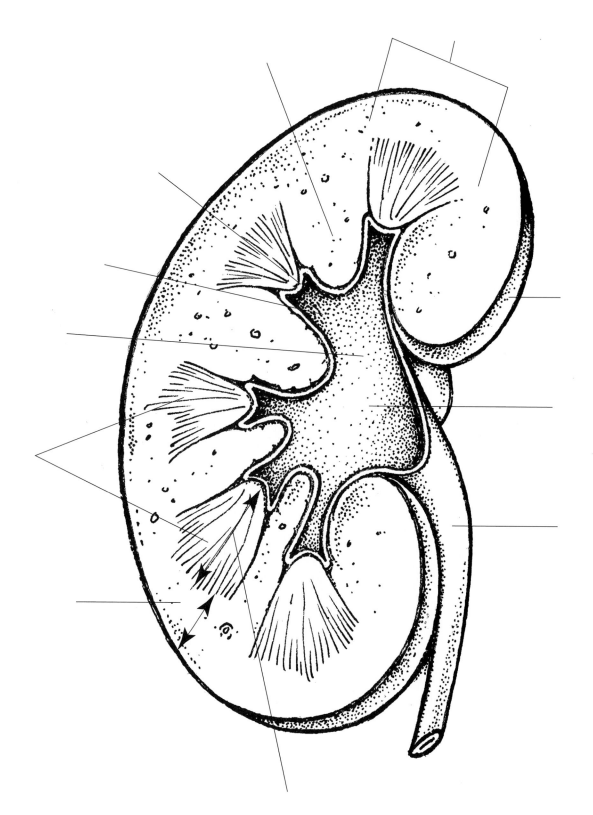

Color the Cortical Nephron and Juxtamedullary Nephron and label the parts.

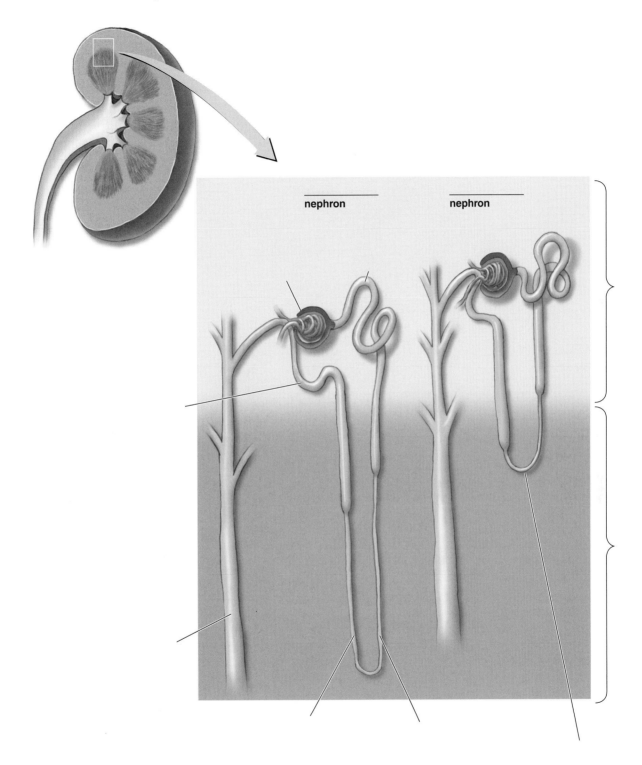

_____ nephron   _____ nephron

Urinary Bladder Innervation and the Micturation Reflex. Label the structures and color them using colors of your choice. Draw arrows to indicate the direction impulses travel in each of the nerves.

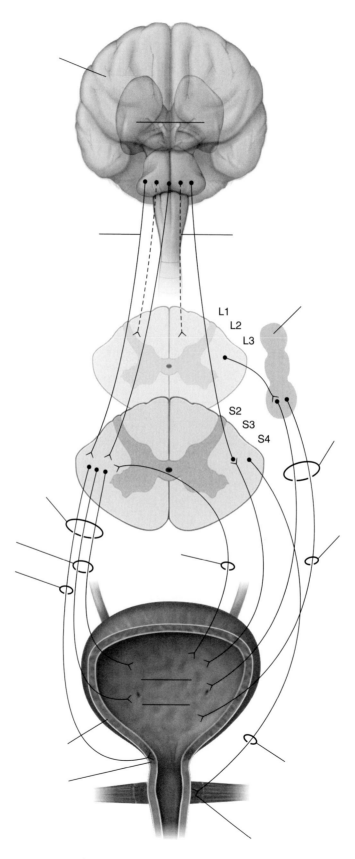

L1
L2
L3

S2
S3
S4

Glossary

A

A band the width of myofibril, occupied by the myosin filaments in a sarcomere of a muscle fiber

abdomen the part of the trunk between the thorax and pelvis

abdominopelvic cavity the space within the abdomen and pelvis

abduction movement in which the articulating bone moves along the frontal/coronal plane, away from the longitudinal axis of the body

abscess collection of pus within a capsule

acetylcholine (ACH) a neurotransmitter

acetylcholinesterase the enzyme that breaks down acetylcholine

Achilles tendon the thick tendon in the heel of the gastrocnemius and soleus muscles; the calcaneus tendon or tendo calcaneus

acid any solute that dissociates in solution and releases hydrogen ions, lowering pH

acidity the state of being acidic; a fluid with more hydrogen ions than water

acinar gland a gland with grapelike-shaped secretory unit(s)

acne a skin condition resulting from blocked sebaceous ducts and inflammation of the sebaceous glands and surrounding area

acquired immune deficiency syndrome (AIDS) an infectious condition caused by the human immunodeficiency virus

acromegaly a condition in which excessive growth of peripheral parts, such as hands and feet, occurs as a result of increased growth hormone levels in adults

actin one myofilament responsible for contraction and relaxation

action the changes produced to the joint by muscle contraction

action potential a rapid change in potential that is propagated along the cell

active immunity immunity in which the body actively manufacture antibodies when in contact with the antigen

active transport transport across the cell membrane in which energy is needed

adaptation the process in which a stimulus applied to a neuron for a prolonged period results in a decline in the frequency of the action potentials generated

Addison disease a condition resulting from decreased adrenal cortex secretion

adduction movement in which the articulating bone moves along the frontal/coronal plane, toward the longitudinal axis of the body

adenoids collection of lymphoid tissue in the nasopharynx; the pharyngeal tonsils

adenosine diphosphate see ADP

adenosine monophosphate a high-energy compound; a product of adenosine with phosphoric acid (AMP)

adenosine triphosphate a high-energy compound; a product of adenosine with triphosphoric acid (ATP)

adequate stimulus the particular form of energy to which the receptor responds

ADH antidiuretic hormone

adhesion the adhering/joining of two surfaces (e.g., the joining of two opposing wound surfaces); the fusion of the parietal and visceral pleura after inflammation

adipocyte a fat cell, with cytoplasm filled with a huge droplet of fat

adolescence the period when final maturation of the reproductive system occurs; puberty

ADP adenosine diphosphate; high energy compound; a product of adenosine with diphosphoric acid

adrenal cortex the outer part of the adrenal gland

adrenal gland one of two endocrine glands located on the superior aspect of the kidneys; suprarenal glands

adrenal medulla the inner part of the adrenal glands

adrenaline hormone secreted by the adrenal medulla; also secreted as a neurotransmitter by certain neurons; also known as epinephrine

adrenocortical steroid   hormone secreted by the adrenal cortex, also known as corticosteroid

adrenocorticotropic hormone (ACTH)   secreted by the anterior pituitary, which regulates hormone secretion by the adrenal cortex

adrenogenital syndrome   a group of disorders resulting from abnormal, excessive secretion of androgens from the adrenal cortex; results in masculinization of women, feminization of men, and precocious puberty in children

afferent arteriole   the arteriole that brings blood to the part (e.g., to glomeruli)

agglutination   the clumping of red blood cells as a result of the antigen-antibody reaction

agglutinin   antibody produced against antigens on the cell membrane of red blood cells; antigen-antibody reactions produce clumping

agglutinogen   antigen on the cell membrane of red blood cells that can provoke antibody formation; antigen-antibody reaction produces clumping

agonist   the main muscle that produces a particular movement; also known as prime mover

agranulocytes   white blood cells that do not have granules in the cytoplasm

albumin   a protein

aldosteronism   a condition with excessive secretion of aldosterone from the adrenal cortex

alkalinity   the state of being alkaline; a fluid with less hydrogen ions than water

allergen   an antigen that induces allergic reaction

alveolar duct   the part of the lung that lies distal to the respiratory bronchiole, extending between the respiratory bronchiole and alveoli

alveolar gland   a gland with saclike secretory unit(s)

alveolar ventilation   the volume of air in the lung that reaches the alveoli

alveoli   small cavities (e.g., alveoli of the lung)

amino acids   organic molecules that link together to form large proteins; organic acid in which one hydrogen atom on a carbon atom has been replaced by NH2

amniotic cavity   the cavity filled with the amniotic fluid surrounding the fetus

amniotic fluid   the fluid in the amniotic sac that surrounds the fetus and protects it from mechanical injury

AMP   a high-energy compound; a product of adenosine with phosphoric acid; adenosine monophosphate

amphiarthrosis   slightly movable joint

ampulla   a saclike dilation of a canal or duct

anabolism   the chemical reaction in which compounds are formed from smaller parts

anaerobic metabolism   metabolism that occurs without the presence of oxygen

anaphylaxis   a condition in which a generalized allergic reaction occurs

anastomosis   direct communication between two blood vessels

anatomic dead space   the volume of air in the conducting passages of the respiratory system, not involved in gas exchange

anatomical position   a standard body position in which the body is erect, with the feet parallel and flat on the floor and the arms at the side, with the palms forward and fingers pointing down

anatomy   study of the external and internal structures of the body and the physical relationship between body parts

anchor   protein in the cell wall that connects the cell membrane to surrounding structures, stabilizing the cell

androgen   hormone secreted by the adrenal cortex that regulates male sex organ activity

anion   negatively charged ion

ankle   the joint region located between the leg and foot

ankylosing spondylitis   a type of arthritis of the spine

anovulatory cycle   ovarian cycle in which ovulation does not occur

antagonist   the main muscle to oppose a particular movement

antebrachium   forearm

anterior   relational term; also known as ventral; a structure lying in front of another

antibody   protein, secreted by B lymphocytes, with the capacity to react with specific antigens

antidiuretic hormone (ADH)   also known as vasopressin; secreted by the posterior lobe of the pituitary gland; stimulates water reabsorption by kidney cells; a powerful vasoconstrictor

antigen   any substance that provokes an immune response

anus   the last part of the digestive tract, from which fecal matter is eliminated from the body

aorta   the largest artery, leading from the left ventricle

aortic bodies   chemoreceptors located near the arch of the aorta

aortic semilunar valve   valve located between the left ventricle and the aorta

apex   upper part or top; in pyramid-shaped structures, the part opposite the base

apex beat   the location on the chest wall where the ventricle hits during every contraction

apical surface   surface of epithelial cells exposed to the external surface, such as the atmosphere or passage they line

apneustic center   area in the medulla of brain that regulates respiration by increasing the duration of inspiration and inhibiting expiration

apocrine sweat gland   sweat gland located in the armpits, around the nipples, bearded region (men), and in the groin area; secretion begins at puberty and produces a cloudy, sticky secretion, with a characteristic odor

aponeurosis   a fibrous sheet of flat, expanded connective tissue that gives attachment to muscular fibers

appendicular skeleton   comprised of bones that form the limbs; includes bones of the shoulder, pelvic girdle, and the upper and lower limbs.

appendix   a wormlike projection from the cecum, containing lymphoid tissue

arachnoid mater   the middle layer of meninges

arrector pili muscle   a strip of smooth muscle in the skin that extends from the upper part of the dermis to connective tissue surrounding the hair; on contraction, makes hair stand on end

artery   blood vessel that carries blood away from the heart

arteriole   smaller artery

arteriovenous anastomosis   direct connections between arterioles and venules

articular cartilage   hyaline cartilage covering the ends of long bones that participates in synovial joint formation

articulation   the process of word formation; requires voluntary movements of lip, cheek, and tongue muscles

arytenoid cartilage   cartilage in the larynx attached to one end of the vocal cord

ascending tract   bundle of neuron axons that carries impulses to the brain

association fibers   axons that interconnect areas of the cerebral cortex in the same hemisphere

association neurons   neurons located between neurons, also known as interneurons

astrocyte   star-shaped neuroglial cell present between the blood capillaries and the brain and spinal cord; monitors substances that enter and leave the brain and prevents sudden changes in the environment around the CNS

ataxia   difficulty coordinating muscle activity during voluntary movement

atom   the smallest particle of matter

atomic number   the number of protons in an atom

atopic disorder   allergy-related condition

ATP   a high-energy compound; a product of adenosine with triphosphoric acid; adenosine triphosphate

atrial natriuretic peptide (ANP)   hormone secreted by the atrial cells of the heart that promotes sodium excretion by the kidneys

atrioventricular valves (AV valves)   valves that separate the atria and the ventricles

atrophy   reduction in muscle size

auditory tube   tube extending from the middle ear to the pharynx; the eustachian tube or pharyngotympanic tube

autoantibody   antibody that attacks antigens of self

automaticity   the capacity of cardiac muscle to contract on its own in the absence of nerve or hormone stimulation

autonomic ganglion   collection of neuron cell bodies belonging to the autonomic nervous system

autonomic nervous system   the part of the nervous system that innervates smooth muscle, cardiac muscle, and glands

autopsy   examination of the organs of a dead body to determine cause of death or for pathologic study

autoregulation   the process in which body activities are regulated by the body itself

axial skeleton   the part of the skeleton made of bone in the central or longitudinal axis; the skull, vertebrae, ribs, sternum ossicles, and the hyoid bone

axillary   relating to the axilla, or armpit region

axon   the neuronal process that takes impulses away from the cell body

B

B (beta) lipotropin   hormone secreted by the anterior pituitary

baroreceptor   stretch receptor in the aortic and carotid bodies; responds to pressure changes

basal surface   surface of epithelial cells exposed to the body

base   solute that removes hydrogen ions from a solution, increasing the pH; the lower part or bottom; in pyramid-shaped structures, the part opposite the apex

basement membrane   thin, fibrous membrane to which the basal surface of the epithelia is attached

basophil   white blood cell with cytoplasm that has blue granules on staining

Bell-Magendie law   law stating that all sensory neurons enter the spinal cord posteriorly and all motor neurons leave the spinal cord anteriorly

belly of muscle   the bulge seen at the center of spindle-shaped muscles

bicuspid valve   valve located between the left atrium and ventricle, also known as mitral valve

bicuspid   eight in number; a tooth with two cusps or points; the premolars

bile ductule   small canal in the liver that carries bile

bilirubin   yellow bile pigment; derived from hemoglobin breakdown

blastocyst   dividing, fertilized mass of cells

blood clot   the sequence that results in the formation of fibrin threads from fibrinogen

blood-brain barrier   mechanism present between the blood capillaries and the brain and spinal cord that monitors substances that enter and leave the brain and prevents sudden environmental changes around the CNS; the astrocytes are responsible

blood-testis barrier   barrier maintained by Sertoli cells in the testis that isolates the seminiferous tubules from the blood

bone   supporting, hard connective tissue, consisting of cells embedded in a matrix of mineralized ground substance and collagen fibers

bone marrow cavity   the bone cavity that contains the soft tissue made up of stroma and cells; the medullary cavity

Bowman's capsule   the cup-shaped end of the renal tubule; the glomerular capsule

brachium   upper arm

brain   the part of the nervous system located in the cranial cavity

brainstem   the part of the CNS that connects the brain to the spinal cord, consisting of the midbrain, pons, and medulla

breathing   moving air in and out of the lungs by increasing and decreasing the size of the thoracic cavity by movement of the chest wall and action of the respiratory muscles; pulmonary ventilation

bronchi   tubes that convey air to and from the lungs to the trachea

bronchiole   subdivision of the bronchi

bronchopulmonary segment   the lung tissue supplied by each tertiary bronchi

buccal cavity   part of the oral cavity between the teeth and gums (posteriorly and medially) and the lips and cheeks (laterally and anteriorly)

buffers   compounds that prevent hydrogen ion concentration from fluctuating too much and too rapidly to alter the pH

bursae fluid-filled cavities found around joints

buttock the region of the bulge formed by the gluteal muscles on each side

C

calcaneus tendon the thick tendon in the heel of the gastrocnemius and soleus muscles; the Achilles tendon or tendo calcaneus

calcification a process in which tissue or noncellular material in the body hardens as a result of deposition of insoluble salts of calcium

calcitonin hormone secreted by the thyroid gland that regulates calcium levels

calcitriol a steroidal hormone; precursor of vitamin D

calf the prominent, muscular part of the lower leg

canaliculi small canals

canine tooth having a thick, cone-shaped crown; two in each jaw; cuspids

capillary the smallest blood vessel in which exchange takes place

capillary hydrostatic pressure pressure exerted by the liquid inside the capillaries that tends to push fluid out

capsule a connective tissue structure that envelops an organ or a joint

carbaminohemoglobin hemoglobin that has combined with carbon dioxide

carbohydrate organic compound that has carbon, hydrogen, and oxygen in the ratio of 1:2:1

cardia part of the stomach close to the esophageal opening

cardiac cycle cyclical or sequential events in the heart that occur between the beginning of one heartbeat and the next

cardiac muscle type of muscle present in the heart

cardiac output volume of blood pumped out of the heart each minute

cardiovascular system organ system responsible for the circulation of blood; includes the heart and the blood vessels

carotid bodies chemoreceptors located at the bifurcation of the carotid arteries

carpal tunnel the tunnel formed between the carpal bones posteriorly and the flexor retinaculum anteriorly; flexor tendons and the median nerve pass through the tunnel

carrier-mediated transport transport across a cell membrane in which integral proteins bind to specific ions or other substances and carry them across the membrane

carriers specific proteins in the cell wall that transport solutes across the cell membrane

cartilage nonvascular, firm, connective tissue found in the ends of long bones and the walls of the thorax and ear, etc.

catabolism chemical reaction in which substances are broken down into smaller parts

catecholamine specific biochemical group; for example, adrenaline, noradrenaline, and dopamine

categoric hemisphere the cerebral hemisphere (left) responsible for language skills, such as reading, writing, speaking, and analytical tasks

cation positively charged ion

cauda equina nerves at the lower end of the spinal cord that look similar to a horse tail

caudal relational term; also known as inferior; structures lying away from the head

cecum the first, dilated part of the large intestine, between the ileocecal valve and the ascending colon

cell physiology study of cell function

cell-mediated immunity immunity in which T lymphocytes are important

cell the smallest living part of the body

cementum bonelike tissue layer that covers the tooth and helps affix the tooth to the jaw

center collection of neuron cell bodies having the same function; located in the CNS

central canal the canal in the middle of the spinal cord filled with cerebrospinal fluid

central nervous system (CNS) system that includes the brain and the spinal cord

centrioles two, short, cylindrical structures made of microtubules located in the cytoplasm of cells that are capable of dividing; at the time of cell division, they help separate DNA material

cephalic relational term; also known as superior or cranial; structures lying toward the head

cerebellum the mass of brain tissue on the inferior and posterior aspect of brain responsible for muscle coordination

cerebral hemispheres large mass of brain tissue on the right and left, separated by the longitudinal fissure

cerebrospinal fluid (CSF) the fluid surrounding the brain and spinal cord

cerumen (ear wax) sticky secretion from the ceruminous glands of the ear that protects the ear from entry of foreign particles

ceruminous glands modified sweat glands found in the external auditory canal that secrete cerumen

cervical relating to the neck

cervical canal in females, the canal located between the uterus and the vagina

cervix necklike structure (e.g., cervix of the uterus)

channels integral proteins in the cell wall that form small paths across the cell membrane and allow water and specific ions to pass through

cheeks the sides of the face that form the lateral walls of the mouth

chemical bonds the force of attraction in a molecule or compound that keeps atoms together

chemoreceptors receptors that respond to chemical stimuli

chemotaxis the process in which white blood cells are attracted to dead/injured/foreign tissue

chest the anterior aspect of the thorax

chondroblast special cell type that results in cartilage formation

chondrocytes cell found in the cartilage matrix

chondroitin sulfate special polysaccharide found in the cartilage matrix

chordae tendineae connective tissue bands that hold mitral and tricuspid valve cusps in place

chromosome structure that bears the genetic material located in the cell nucleus

chylomicrons large, lipid complexes located in the small intestine

chyme semifluid, partly digested food that passes from the stomach into the duodenum

cilia projections from the cell membrane in certain cells, such as those in the respiratory tract; move mucus and other secretions over the cell surface

ciliated epithelium epithelium with cilia

circumcision removal of part or all of the prepuce

circumduction movement in which the part is moved in a circular direction

cisterna chyli a dilated sac at the lower end of the thoracic duct

climacteric the climax of the sexual act; also known as orgasm

clitoris cylindrical, erectile structure located midline of the female external genitalia

clot retraction the process of clot shrinkage

collagen fiber the major protein fiber in connective tissue; made up of strands of polypeptide chains, tightly wound together similar to rope

collaterals branches from the axon

colon the part of the large intestine that extends from the cecum to the rectum

colostrum the first milk secreted soon after childbirth

columnar epithelium epithelium cells that have the appearance of columns (long and slender); located in regions where absorption or secretion occurs

commissural fibers axons that interconnect the two cerebral hemispheres

compact bone the dense, outer layer of bone; also known as cortical bone

compartment syndrome syndrome in which increased pressure in a confined anatomic space affects tissue function and circulation in the space

compound substance formed by the bonding of two or more elements, with different physical characteristics than those of the individual elements

compound gland a gland with larger excretory ducts that branch repeatedly into smaller ducts

concentric contraction a muscle contraction in which the muscle shortens

conception the implantation of the blastocyte in the endometrium

conchae shell-like structures (e.g., bony projections in the nose [superior, middle, and inferior conchae])

conducting system specialized cardiac muscle tissue (autorhythmic cells) in the heart that is responsible for rhythmic contractions

connective tissue tissue that supports and provides framework to the body; made of ground substance, protein fibers, and cells

constriction narrowing

contraction period the duration of muscle contraction in response to a nerve impulse

contracture abnormal muscle shortening as a result of fibrosis or tonic spasm

cornification the transformation process from live cells to dead cells in the superficial layer of skin; keratinization

coronal plane plane running from left to right, dividing the body into front and back portions; frontal plane

coronary circulation circulation of blood that supplies the walls of the heart

coronary sinus vein that drains the walls of the heart

corpus callosum the large bundle of nerves that connects the right and the left cerebral hemispheres

corpus cavernosa two cylindrical columns, consisting of a maze of vascular channels, found in the penis; important in erection

corpus luteum yellow structure formed in the ovary soon after ovulation that secretes hormones

corpus spongiosum cylindrical column of a maze of vascular channels found around the penile urethra; important in erection

corticosteroid hormone secreted by the adrenal cortex, also known as adrenocortical steroid

corticotropin-releasing hormone (CRH) secreted by the hypothalamus that controls corticotropin secretion by the anterior pituitary gland

cortisone hormone (glucocorticoid) secreted by the adrenal cortex

costal surface surface of the lung relating to the ribs

covalent bond bond in which the electrons of atoms are shared

cranial relational term; also known as superior or cephalic; structures lying toward the head

cranial cavity space inside the skull containing the brain, its coverings, and cerebrospinal fluid

cranial nerve nerve attached to the brain/brainstem

cremaster muscle layer of skeletal muscle in the scrotum, deep to the dermis

cretinism hypothyroidism in infants and children

cricoid cartilage signet-shaped cartilage in the lower part of the larynx

crown the part of the tooth covered with enamel

crural relating to the lower leg

cubital relating to the elbow

cubital fossa depression in front of the elbow

cuboidal epithelium cells of this epithelium appear cubelike in section; in areas of absorption or secretion

Cushing's disease condition similar to Cushing's syndrome, resulting from excess ACTH secretion from the anterior pituitary gland

Cushing's syndrome condition resulting from excess glucocorticoid secretion from the adrenal cortex

cuspid tooth with a thick, cone-shaped crown; two in each jaw; also known as canine

cutaneo visceral reflexes reflexes that involve both autonomic nerves and the rich, sensory plexuses in skin

cutaneous membrane combination of epithelia and connective tissue that covers and protects other structures (e.g., outer surface of the body)

cutaneous plexus network of arteries at the junction of the subcutaneous layer with the dermis

cyanosis dark-blue or purplish skin and mucous membrane discoloration as a result of deficient blood oxygenation

cystic duct the duct that carries bile to and from the gallbladder

cytology study of the cell

cytoplasm material enclosed by the cell membrane

cytoskeleton a protein framework located inside the cell, giving the cell flexibility and strength

cytosol another term for cytoplasm

D

dartos muscle layer of smooth muscle in the scrotum responsible for the wrinkled appearance of the skin

dead space the volume of air not involved in gas exchange

decomposition reaction reaction in which compounds are broken down into smaller parts

deep relational term; structures lying away from the surface of the body; internal

defecation reflex nervous reflex resulting in emptying of the rectum

deglutition the swallowing process

deltoid region the lateral aspect of the shoulder over the deltoid muscle

dendrites neuronal processes that bring impulses to the cell body

dentin ivory structure that forms most of the teeth

deoxyribonucleic acid (DNA) acid important for storing and processing information in the cell

depolarization process in which the inside of a cell becomes less negative on stimulation; caused by ion movement changes

depression moving the bone in the inferior direction (e.g., movement in which your jaw opens)

dermal papillae projections of the dermis adjacent to the epidermal ridges

dermatome specific skin area innervated by sensory nerves entering a particular spinal cord segment

dermis layer of connective tissue deep to the epidermis of skin in which the glands, hair, and nails are located

descending colon the part of the colon extending between the splenic flexure and the sigmoid colon

descending tracts bundles of axons that carry impulses from the brain to the spinal cord

desmosomes strong connections between adjacent cells that help maintain the cell layers in sheets

detrusor muscle the smooth muscle found in the wall of the urinary bladder

developmental anatomy study of the changes that occur during physical development

diabetes insipidus a condition that results in production of excessive urine of low specific gravity; results from decreased ADH secretion

diapedesis the movement of neutrophils into tissue space by squeezing between the endothelial cells of the capillaries

diaphysis region of bone between the epiphysis

diarthrosis freely movable joint

diastole the period of relaxation of the heart

diastolic pressure the blood pressure measured during diastole

diffusion movement of ions and molecules from higher concentration areas to lower concentration areas

digestive system the system responsible for breaking food down into a form that can be used

digits the fingers of the hands and toes of the feet

distal relational term; structures away from the trunk (chest and abdomen)

DNA deoxyribonucleic acid

dopamine an epinephrine and norepinephrine precursor; also secreted by certain neurons as a neurotransmitter

dorsal relational term; also known as posterior; a structure lying behind another

dorsal root ganglion collection of the cell bodies of the unipolar sensory neurons that lies just outside the spinal cord

dorsiflexion the ankle movement that occurs when a person stands on their heels

dorsum, foot superior surface of the foot

dorsum, hand posterior surface of hand

ductus deferens a pair of tubules located between the epididymis and the ejaculatory duct that carry semen

duodenum the first part of the small intestine, leading from the stomach

dura mater the outer layer of the meninges

dwarfism condition in which a person's height is below normal; one cause is decreased growth hormone levels

E

eccentric contraction muscle contraction in which the muscle lengthens

eccrine gland a type of sweat gland located over the entire body

effector motor nerve

efferent arteriole the arteriole that removes blood from the part (e.g., from glomeruli)

ejaculation process in which semen is expelled from the male urethra to the exterior

ejaculatory duct duct formed by joining ducts from the seminal vesicles and the vas deferens; opens into the prostatic urethra

elastic cartilage cartilage containing more elastic fibers, making the cartilage springier; located in such regions as the external ear

elastic fiber branched and wavy protein fiber found in connective tissue; contains the protein elastin

elbow the region of the upper limb between the upper arm and forearm; around the elbow joint

electrocardiogram (ECG) the recording of electrical changes that occur in the heart

electron a particle that makes up an atom; carries a negative charge

element substance made of only one kind of atoms (i.e., of identical atomic [proton] number)

elevation moving the bone in the superior direction (e.g., movement in which your jaw closes)

emboli dislodged thrombus, foreign body, or fat, etc., with the potential to clog a blood vessel

embryology study of changes that occur during development in the womb

emigration process of white blood cells squeezing through the widened gap between the cells of the capillary wall, attracted by chemicals liberated by injured tissue

emission the process in which the internal reproductive glands discharge secretions into the male urethra

emulsification the process that breaks up large lipid droplets into small ones, enabling lipase to digest the fat

enamel hard substance that covers the external surface of the tooth

endocardium   the inner lining of the heart

endocrine gland   gland that secretes its products directly into the blood

endocrine system   the system that includes ductless glands that secrete directly into the blood

endocytosis   the process of bringing substances into the cell by forming vesicles

endometrium   innermost layer of the uterus

endomysium   connective tissue that surrounds an individual muscle fiber

endoneurium   layer of connective tissue that surrounds individual nerve axons

endoplasmic reticulum   a network of intracellular membranes in the form of tubes and sacs that is connected to the nuclear membrane; contains enzymes and participates in protein and lipid synthesis

endorphin   opioid peptide located in the brain and other regions with similar effects to morphine

endosteum   the layer of cells that line the medullary cavity

endothelium   simple epithelium lining blood vessels and heart

end-systolic volume   the volume of blood remaining in the ventricle at the end of systole

energy level   the location of the electrons of an atom; also known as the energy shell

enzyme   a protein that facilitates chemical reactions, remaining unchanged in the process

eosinophil   a white blood cell with cytoplasm that has pink granules on staining

ependymal cell   a neuroglial cell that lines the cavities in the brain and spinal cord; responsible for producing, circulating, and monitoring the cerebrospinal fluid

epicardium   the part of the pericardium covering the outer surface of the heart; the visceral pericardium

epidermal growth factor   a peptide that promotes epidermis growth; secreted by various tissue such as salivary glands and glands in the duodenum

epidermal ridges   folds of stratum germinativum of the epidermis of skin that extend into the dermis

epidermis   the cellular, avascular, outer layer of skin

epididymis   a coiled tubule located between the seminiferous tubules and the vas deferens

epidural block   the injection of anesthetic into the epidural space

epidural space   the space between the dura and the vertebral canal

epigastric   the superior and medial part of the abdomen located between the costal margins

epiglottis   a leaf-shaped cartilage found on the posterior aspect of the tongue; closes the larynx during swallowing

epimysium   connective tissue that surrounds the whole muscle

epinephrine   a hormone secreted by the adrenal medulla; secreted as a neurotransmitter by certain neurons; also known as adrenaline

epineurium   the outer layer of connective tissue that surrounds the nerve

epiphyseal plate   a thin region, adjacent to the epiphysis, in which osteoblasts constantly turn cartilage into bone

epiphysis   a part of a long bone (ends) developed from a center of ossification that is initially separated from the shaft by cartilage

epithelial tissue   tissue that covers surfaces exposed to the environment, lines internal passages and chambers, and forms glands

epithelium   the cellular, avascular layer covering all body surfaces (e.g., lining of blood vessel; epidermis)

erection   the process in which blood fills erectile tissue, making the tissue hard (erection of the penis)

erythroblastosis fetalis   a condition of the fetus, resulting from Rh incompatibility

erythrocyte   red blood cell; responsible for carrying oxygen in the blood

erythropoiesis   the process of red blood cell formation

erythropoietin   a hormone secreted by the kidney that regulates hemoglobin synthesis and red blood cell production

esophagus   the tube that conveys the food from the pharynx to the stomach

estrogenic phase   the menstrual cycle phase in which ovarian follicles develop; the preovulatory or follicular phase

estrogen   natural or synthetic hormones that produce effects similar to estrogenic hormones; among many other effects, stimulates development of secondary sexual characteristics

eustachian tube   tube connecting the middle ear to the pharynx; the pharyngotympanic tube

eversion   the movement at the ankle when the sole of the foot is turned outward

exchange pump   special carrier protein in the cell membrane that transports one ion in as another is transported out

exchange reaction   a chemical reaction in which the fragments are shuffled around

exchange vessel   a blood vessel in which exchange takes place i.e., capillary

excitation-contraction coupling   the link between the potential change in the sarcolemma and the contraction of the muscle

exocrine gland   gland that releases secretions on the epithelial surface

exocytosis   the process of transporting substances out of the cell by forming vesicles

expiration   the process of expelling air out of the lungs; also known as exhalation

expiratory reserve volume   the volume of air that a person can breath in after a normal expiration

extension   the opposite movement of flexion in which the angle between the articulating bones is increased in the anterior/posterior plane

external   relational term; structures lying closer to the surface of the body; also known as superficial

external auditory canal   a tube in the temporal bone that leads to the middle ear

external genitalia   the external structures associated with the reproductive system

external nare   opening on the inferior aspect of the nose

external os   the end of the cervical canal that opens into the vagina

external respiration   all processes involved in the absorption of oxygen and the removal of carbon dioxide from the air spaces in the lung and pulmonary capillaries

external rotation   a movement in which the part is moved along its axis in the lateral direction

external urethral meatus   the opening in the urethra that conveys the urine to the outside

external urethral sphincter   a band of circular skeletal muscle that surrounds the urethra as it passes through the pelvic floor

exteroceptor   afferent which senses information in the external environment

extracellular fluid   the fluid that surrounds the cells

extrapulmonary bronchi   bronchi that lie outside the lungs

exudate   fluid that collects outside the cells in an injured area

F

facial   relating to the face

facilitated diffusion   transport across cell membrane facilitated by carriers; movement occurs from a region of higher solute concentration to a region of lower concentration; no energy is required

false ribs   ribs that do not directly articulate with the sternum

fascia   a sheet of fibrous tissue found beneath the skin; around muscles and groups of muscles, separating them into several layers

fast fibers   muscle fibers that rapidly respond to a stimulus

fat   organic compound that has carbon, hydrogen, and oxygen in a different ratio than carbohydrates

fauces   the space between the mouth and the pharynx, bounded by the soft palate superiorly and the base of tongue inferiorly

feedback mechanism   a sequence of events continuously reported to a control center, which, in turn, produces an action to maintain homeostasis.

femoral   relating to the femur or thigh

fertilization   the fusion process of sperm and ova

fibers   protein strands located in the ground substance of connective tissue; refers to a nerve cell axon with its glial cell or Schwann cell envelope; describes elongated, threadlike cells, such as muscle cells

fibrinogen   a protein in plasma needed for blood clotting

fibroblast   most abundant cell in connective tissue that secretes a polysaccharide (hyaluronic acid) and protein fibers into the ground substance that gives connective tissue strength, flexibility, elasticity, and a thick consistency

fibrocartilage   cartilage with little ground substance and more collagen fiber, making the cartilage tough and helping it resist compression and absorb shock; located in intervertebral disks

fibrosis   one process of chronic inflammation resolution, by scar tissue formation

filtration   the movement of water across a semipermeable membrane as a result of hydrostatic pressure

fimbriae   fingerlike structures

first heart sound   the sound heard when the atrioventricular valves close

first-class lever   a lever system with the fulcrum located in the center and the effort and resistance located on either side

fissure   a deep furrow or cleft

fistula   a tract that is open at both ends through which abnormal communication is established between two surfaces

flaccidity   a condition in which there is no muscle tone

flagella   projections from the cell that help move the cell in the surrounding fluid (e.g., sperm cell of the testis)

flare   the diffuse red color observed around the stroke line when stroking the skin with a pointed object

flat bones   bones that are broad and thin with a flattened and/or curved surface

flatfoot   a condition in which the longitudinal arch of the vertebral column is broken

flexion   movement in the anterior/posterior plane that reduces the angle between the articulating bones

flexor retinaculum   a strong, fibrous band in front of the wrist that keeps the tendons in place; helps form the carpal tunnel

floating ribs   ribs that are not attached anteriorly

fluid connective tissue   connective tissue that is fluid (e.g., blood, lymph)

fluid crystal   a substance that can be transformed from one state to another (e.g., by heating or cooling, etc.)

follicle-stimulating hormone (FSH)   secreted by the anterior pituitary and stimulates ova development and female sex hormones secretion

follicular phase   the phase of the menstrual cycle in which ovarian follicles develop; the preovulatory phase

fontanel   the region of membrane between two skull bones in infants

foot   the most distal part of the leg

foramen ovale   an oval opening in the fetus between the two atria

fornix   the part of the vagina surrounding the cervix

friction massage   a technique in which repetitive, nongliding strokes are used to produce movement between connective tissue fiber

frontal plane   plane running from left to right, dividing the body into a front and back portion; the coronal plane

functional residual capacity   residual volume and the expiratory reserve volume combined

fundus   part of a sac away from the opening; in the stomach, the part superior to the esophageal opening

G

galactorrhea   persistent, milky, white discharge from the nipples

ganglia   a collection of cell bodies of neurons

gap junction   the region of cells bound to adjacent cell(s) in which small passages are present that allow movement of substances between adjacent cells

gary mater   regions of the CNS dominated by cell bodies and unmyelinated fibers

gastrocolic reflex   reflex causing movement of the contents of the large intestine when food enters the stomach

gene   the line up of bases that give the sequence of arrangement of amino acids needed to form a specific protein; found in the DNA

genetic code   the genetic information carried by the specific DNA molecules of the chromosomes

gigantism a condition in which the person's height is above normal

gingivae the part of the tissue that surrounds the neck of a tooth; the gums

gland a structure lined with cells that produce secretions

globulin a type of protein

glomerular filtrate the fluids and solutes from the blood that are filtered through the filtration membrane of the glomerulus into the renal tubule

glomerular filtration rate the rate at which the fluids and solutes from the blood are filtered through the filtration membrane of the glomerulus into the renal tubule

glomerulus the network of capillaries that lies inside the Bowman's capsule

glottis the narrow opening of the larynx

glucagon a hormone secreted by the pancreas that regulates carbohydrate, fat, and protein metabolism

glucocorticoid a hormone secreted by the adrenal cortex that regulates glucose metabolism

gluteal relating to the buttock region

glycolysis the process in which glucose is broken into pyruvic acid

goblet cell unicellular gland that secretes mucus

goiter a chronic enlargement of the thyroid gland

golgi apparatus flattened membrane disks in the cytoplasm in which chemicals manufactured by the endoplasmic reticulum are processed, sorted, and packaged in secretory vesicles for storage or for dispatch outside the cell

gonadotropin-releasing hormone (GnRH) secreted by the hypothalamus that controls gonadotropin secretion by the anterior pituitary gland

gonads sex organs that form sperm (males) and ova (females)

granulocytes white blood cells that have granules in the cytoplasm

greater vestibular (Bartholin's) gland mucoid secreting gland located near the vagina

ground substance the medium in connective tissue in which cells and protein fibers are suspended

growth factor peptide found in extracellular fluid that regulates cell division

growth hormone a hormone secreted by the anterior pituitary that regulates growth

growth hormone-inhibiting hormone (GIH) secreted by the hypothalamus that decreases the secretion of growth hormone by the anterior pituitary gland

growth hormone-releasing hormone (GRH) secreted by the hypothalamus that increases the secretion of growth hormone by the anterior pituitary gland

gum the tissue that surrounds the neck of teeth; also known as gingivae

gyrus one of the prominent, rounded elevations found on the cerebral hemispheres

H

H zone the width of the sarcomere in which the myosin and actin filaments do not overlap

hair follicle tubelike invaginations of the epidermis from which the hair shaft develops

haustra pouchlike projections of the wall of the large intestines; resemble buckets in a water wheel

haversian canal special canal in bone that carry blood vessels

haversian system a structure in compact bone made of a central canal containing blood capillaries and the concentric osseous lamellae around it; an osteon

head the upper (anterior in animals) extremity of the body, containing the brain and organs of sight, smell, hearing, taste, and equilibrium; describes the larger, rounded end of any body, bone, organ, or anatomic structure

heel the posterior aspect of the foot

heme part of hemoglobin containing iron that carries oxygen

hemiplegia paralysis of one side of the body

hemoglobin protein in red blood cells with the capacity to combine with oxygen

hemolysis the process of red blood cell destruction

hemolytic disease of the newborn a condition that results in the fetus of a mother with Rh incompatibility

hemophilia a bleeding disorder that results from the lack of antihemophilic factor

hepatic flexure the part of the colon that lies at the junction of the ascending and transverse colon

hepatic portal system venous portal system in which the portal vein receives blood, via its tributaries, from most abdominal viscera capillaries and drains it into the hepatic sinusoids.

hepatocyte liver cell

herniated disk protrusion of the intervertebral disk, or its components, into the vertebral foramen; prolapsed disk or slipped disk

hilum the part of an organ where nerves and blood vessels enter and leave

histology study of the microscopic structure of cells, tissues, and organs

homeostasis the condition of constancy in the internal environment

horizontal fissure a fissure found in the right lung, which separates the upper lobe from the middle

horizontal plane plane running across the body, dividing it into a top and bottom portion; the transverse plane

hormone chemical messenger released in the circulation by an endocrine organ or tissue that has an effect on other tissues

human chorionic gonadotropin (hCG) secreted by the placenta

human immunodeficiency virus a virus that causes acquired immune deficiency syndrome

humoral immunity an immunity in which antibodies are produced

hyaline cartilage cartilage, having a frosted-glass appearance, with closely packed collagen fibers, making it tough and flexible; the most common cartilage, it is located in joints covering the ends of the bones

hydrocele a collection of serous fluid in the tunica vaginalis space of the testis

hydrostatic pressure the pressure exerted by liquid

hydrotherapy the therapeutic application of water

hymen a thin, epithelial fold that partially or fully covers the opening of the vagina

hyperextension   a movement in which the articulating bones are extended beyond the anatomic position

hyperpolarization   the process in which the inside of a cell becomes more negative on stimulation; caused by changes in ion movement

hypertonic   having more tension; one solution possessing a higher osmotic pressure than another

hypertrophy   muscle enlargement as a result of an increase in individual muscle fiber size

hypoaldosteronism   a condition in which there is decreased aldosterone secretion from the adrenal cortex

hypochondriac   relating to the hypochondrium; the region below the ribs laterally

hypodermis   the subcutaneous layer; a layer found deep to the dermis, consisting of loose connective and adipose tissue

hypogastric   the region of the abdomen located in the midline, superior to the pubis and inferior to the umbilicus

hypophysis   an endocrine gland attached to the brain, located in the sella turcica of the sphenoid bone; the pituitary gland;

hypothalamus   part of the brain located inferior to the thalamus

hypothenar eminence   the bulge on the medial aspect of the palmar surface of the hand

hypotonic   having less tension; one solution possessing a lower osmotic pressure than another

I

I band   the width of myofibril, occupied by the actin filaments in a sarcomere of a muscle fiber

icterus   a condition in which there is a yellow discoloration to the skin and mucous membranes; jaundice

identifiers   proteins in the cell wall that serve as recognition proteins

ileocecal valve   separates the ileum from the cecum

ileum   the part of the small intestine between the jejunum and the ileocecal valve

iliac   relating to the groin region; also known as inguinal region

iliotibial tract   a fibrous reinforcement of the fascia lata on the lateral surface of the thigh

immunoglobulin   another term for antibody

impermeable   the cell membrane that does not allow any substance to pass through

incisors   four in number; teeth with a chisel-shaped crown

induced active immunity   deliberate exposure to the modified, harmless organism

inert   atoms with full outer energy shells that are, therefore, stable and do not take part in chemical bond formation

inferior   relational term; also known as caudal; a structure lying away from the head

inferior vena cava   the large vein that drains the lower part of the body

infundibulum   a funnel-shaped structure (e.g., infundibulum of the uterine tube)

inguinal   relating to the groin region; the iliac region

inguinal hernia   abnormal protrusion of a part or structure through the tissue in the inguinal region

inhibin   a hormone secreted by the testis that regulates FSH secretion

inhibitory neurotransmitter   neurotransmitter that results in inhibition of the postsynaptic neuron

inorganic compound   chemical structure that does not have carbon and hydrogen atoms as the primary structure

insensible perspiration   passive loss of water from the interstitial tissue by evaporation; about 500 mL of water is lost via the skin per day; not perceived as moisture on the skin

insertion   the point of attachment of the muscle that is more mobile and moves with the bone

inspiration   the process of drawing air into the lungs; also known as inhalation

inspiratory capacity   the volume of air that a person can breathe in after a normal expiration

inspiratory reserve volume   the volume of air that a person can breath in after a normal inspiration

insulin   a hormone secreted by the pancreas that regulates carbohydrate, fat, and protein metabolism

integral protein   protein in the cell wall that goes completely through the wall

integumentary system   the system that includes the skin and all of its the structures

interatrial septum   the tissue that separates the two atria

intercalated disk   specialized structure between cardiac cells that helps convey the force of contraction and impulses from one cell to another

intermediate fiber   muscle fiber that responds faster to a stimulus than slow fibers but slower than fast fibers

internal   relational term; a structure lying away from the surface of the body; also known as deep

internal environment   the interstitial fluid that surrounds the cells

internal nare   the opening located between the nasal cavity and the nasopharynx; the choanae

internal os   the end of the cervical canal that opens into the uterine cavity

internal respiration   the process of oxygen absorption and carbon dioxide removal from tissue cells by the blood in the surrounding capillaries

internal rotation   a movement in which the part is moved along its axis in the lateral direction

internal urethral sphincter   the circular smooth muscle that regulates flow of urine out of the bladder; the sphincter vesicae

interneurons   neurons located between neurons

internode   gap between the myelin in a nerve axon; also known as node of Ranvier

interoceptors   afferents sensing changes inside the body

interosseous membrane   membrane that stretches across two bones (e.g., between ulna and radius; between tibia and fibula)

interphase   the phase of a cell life cycle when cells do not divide but continue to fully function

interstitial colloid osmotic pressure   the pressure exerted by the particles in the interstitial fluid; tends to pull fluid out of the capillaries

interstitial fluid   fluid that surrounds the cells, lies outside the vascular compartment

interval training   training in which high-intensity exercise is alternated with short rest

intervertebral disk   the disk between two vertebral bones

intracellular fluid   body fluid found inside the cells

intrapulmonary bronchi   bronchi that lie inside the lungs

intrauterine devices (IUD)   plastic or metal pieces, formed in different shapes, that are introduced into the uterine cavity to prevent conception

intravascular fluid   body fluid inside blood vessels

intrinsic factor   a chemical (mucoprotein) secreted in the stomach and needed for vitamin B_{12} absorption

inversion   the movement at the ankle when the sole of the foot is turned inward

inward rotation   a movement in which the part is moved along its axis in the medial direction

ion   an atom, or group of atoms, carrying an electric charge by gaining or losing one or more electrons

ion pumps   cell membrane proteins that facilitate transport of substances against concentration gradient, using energy

ionic bond   a bond formed by the attraction between a cation and anion

irregular bone   bone in various shapes and sizes

islets of Langerhans   cluster of cells in the pancreas that secrete hormones

isotonic   having equal tension; refers to solutions possessing the same osmotic pressure

isotopes   atoms of an element that have different numbers of neutrons in the nucleus; they have the same chemical composition

isthmus   a channel from the uterus between the uterine cavity and the cervical canal

J

jaundice   a condition in which there is yellow discoloration to the skin and mucous membrane

jejunum   the part of the small intestine between the duodenum and the ileum

jugular venous pulse   the pulsation observed if the jugular vein pressure is high

juxtaglomerular apparatus   a structure formed by the wall of the afferent arteriole, the cells lining the tubule, and other cells in the vicinity; secretes erythropoietin and renin

juxtamedullary nephron   nephron located in the deeper part of the cortex of the kidney, closer to the medulla

K

keratin   a tough, fibrous protein found in the superficial layer of skin

keratinization   the transformation process of live cells to dead cells in the superficial layer of skin; cornification

keratinized   refers to epithelia that have keratin

keratinocyte   cell in the skin epidermis that produces a tough fibrous protein (keratin); 90% of the epidermis

keratohyalin   a granular protein in the epidermis of skin that organizes keratin into thicker bundles

ketone bodies   a specific biochemical group (acetone, acetoacetic acid, and ß-hydroxybutyrate are chemicals in this group); they are breakdown products of fat

kidneys   paired, kidney bean–shaped organs, located in the lumbar region, whose functions include regulation of water and electrolytes, blood pressure, and urine formation

kinetic energy   energy, existing in a body as a result of its position or state of existence, which is being exerted at the time

knee   the region of the lower limb located between the thigh and calf

Krebs cycle   a cycle of biochemical events that is the main energy source in the body; the tricarboxylic acid cycle

Kupffer cells   phagocytic cells in the liver

kyphosis   an abnormal anterior concave curvature of the spine

L

labia majora   the two folds of skin in the female external genitalia

labia minora   the two folds of mucous membrane that lie medial to the labia majora in the female external genitalia

labile cells   cells with the capacity to regenerate throughout life, quickly multiply, and produce new cells to take the place of injured or dead tissue

lacrimal   relating to tears

lacrimal duct   the duct that carries tears from the medial aspect of the eye to the nasal cavity

lacteals   the lymph vessels found in the gastrointestinal tract

lacunae   small cavities (e.g., found in bone, cartilage)

lamellae   thin sheets or layers (e.g., layers found around the haversian canal of bone)

lamina propria   layer of connective tissue that lies deep to the epithelium of a mucous membrane

Langerhans cells   cells found in the stratum spinosum layer of the epidermis, which are involved in defense mechanisms

large intestine   the long, wide tube that lies between the ileocecal valve and the anus

laryngopharynx   the part of the pharynx superior to the larynx

larynx   the part of the respiratory tract between the pharynx and the trachea; used for voice production

latent period   the time it takes for a response to occur after the application of a stimulus

lateral   relational term; a structure lying further away from an imaginary line passing through the middle of the body in the sagittal plane

lateral flexion   the movement in which the trunk is turned to the side, as in bending sideways

lateral rotation   a movement in which the part is moved along its axis in the lateral direction

leg   the region located between the knee and the ankle

lesser vestibular gland   mucous-secreting gland located in the vestibule of the female external genitalia

Leydig cells   specialized cells located between the somniferous tubules of the testis that secrete the male sex hormone

ligament   a sheet of fibrous connective tissue that connects two or more bones

ligand-gated channel   protein channel in the cell membrane that is operated by hormones and other chemicals

ligand   specific extracellular molecule that stimulates cell receptors

lines of cleavage   the pattern of collagen and elastic fiber bundles established in the dermis that follow the lines of tension in the skin

lingual tonsils   the tonsils located under the tongue

lipid   organic compound that has carbon, hydrogen, and oxygen in a different ratio than carbohydrates

lobar bronchi   bronchi that enter/leave a lobe of the lung

lobe   subdivision of an organ or part; may be divided by fissures, connective tissue septa, or other form of demarcation

lobule   subdivision of a lobe

long bone   bone with the length greater than the width

lordosis   an abnormal anterior convex curvature of the spine

lower extremity   the lower limb

lower respiratory tract   the part of the respiratory tract below the pharynx that includes the larynx (voice box), trachea (windpipe), bronchi, bronchioles, and the alveoli of the lungs

lumbar   relating to the region of the back and sides that lie between the ribs and pelvis

lumen   the space in the interior of a tubular structure (e.g., artery, intestine)

luteal cell   corpus luteum cell that secretes progesterone and estrogen

luteal phase   the menstrual phase in which there is corpus luteum development; same as the progestational or secretory phase

luteinizing hormone (LH)   secreted by the anterior pituitary; stimulates ovulation and progesterone secretion

lymph   the fluid in the lymph vessels

lymph node   round, oval, or bean-shaped bodies lying along the lymph vessel path; contain lymphocytes

lymphadenitis   inflammation of the lymph nodes

lymphangitis   inflammation of the lymph vessels

lymphatic system   the system, including the lymphatic vessels, lymph, and lymphoid tissue, responsible for defense against infection and disease

lymphatics   pertaining to lymph

lymphocyte   white blood cell that participates in defense

lymphoid tissue   tissue that belongs to the lymphatic system; composed of lymphocytes and connective tissue

lysosome   vesicle found in the cytoplasm that is filled with digestive enzymes

M

macrophage   white blood cell that has the property of phagocytosis

macroscopic anatomy   study of those structures that can be visualized without aid

major histocompatibility complex (MHC)   a group of antigens that determine tissue type and transplant compatibility

mammary   relating to the breasts

mammary gland   breast gland that secretes milk; related to the apocrine sweat glands

manus   hand

margination   the accumulation of white blood cells along the blood vessels walls immediately after injury; also known as pavementing

mass action   simultaneous contraction of the smooth muscle of large intestine over a large area, pushing material from one portion of the colon to another and into the rectum.

mass number   the sum of protons and neutrons in an atom

mast cell   small, connective tissue cell usually found near blood vessels that contains the chemicals histamine and heparin in their cytoplasm

mastication   the chewing process

matrix   the fibers and the ground substance of connective tissue

meatus   external opening of a canal

mechanically-regulated channels   protein channels in the cell membrane that are operated mechanically (e.g., touch)

medial   relational term; a structure lying closer to an imaginary line passing through the middle of the body in the sagittal plane

medial rotation   a movement in which the part is moved along its axis in the medial direction

mediastinal surface   the surface of the lung relating to the mediastinum

mediastinum   the middle part of the thoracic cavity

medullary cavity   the bone marrow cavity; the cavity within bones containing soft tissue made up of stroma and cells

megakaryocyte   large cell in the bone marrow from which platelets are derived

meiosis   the division process in the testis and ovary during the formation of sperm and ova; daughter cells end up with half the number of chromosomes found in somatic cells

melanin   pigment formed by melanocytes that is responsible for the color of skin

melanocytes   pigment cells located in the epidermis that are responsible for skin color

melanocyte-stimulating hormone (MSH)   secreted by the intermediate lobe of the pituitary gland that has an effect on melanocytes (pigment-forming cells) in skin

melanosome   small vesicle containing melanin pigment; found in melanocytes

melatonin   a hormone secreted by the pineal gland

membrane protein   protein in the cell wall that goes completely through the wall or is integrated into the wall, with part of the protein molecules projecting into or out of the cell

membranous urethra   part of the male urethra that passes through the connective tissue in the perineum

memory cell   a lymphocyte that tracks the various microorganisms encountered by the body

menarche   the period when the first menstrual period occurs

meninges   the thick, connective tissue covering the brain and spinal cord

meniscus   a crescent-shaped cartilage found inside certain synovial joints (e.g., knee)

menstrual cycle cyclical changes occurring in females and regarded as periodic preparation for fertilization and pregnancy

menstruation cyclical shedding of the endometrium, along with a bloody fluid, during the menstrual cycle

Merkel cells specialized cells located in the epidermis of skin that are in close contact with touch receptors and stimulate these sensory nerve endings

merocrine gland a sweat gland located over the entire body

mesenchymal cell the mother cell that differentiates into fibroblasts and other cells when there is injury

mesentery the part of the peritoneum that suspends the small intestine in the abdominal cavity

mesothelium epithelium that lines body cavities

metabolism the sum of the chemical and physical changes that take place in tissue

metabolite molecule synthesized or broken down inside the body by chemical reactions

metaphysis the section of bone between the epiphysis and diaphysis

micelles complex formed in the small intestine by the interaction of fatty acids and monoglycerides with bile

microglia neuroglial cells that engulf dead cells and cellular remnants in the CNS

microphage white blood cell attracted to injury and inflammation sites that participates in defense (e.g., neutrophils and eosinophils)

microscopic anatomy study of those structures that cannot be visualized with the naked eye

microvilli small, fingerlike projections from the surface of the cell membrane that increase the surface area; located in cells involved in absorbing substances from the extracellular fluid

milk ejection reflex results in contraction of smooth muscles around the mammary ducts and expulsion of milk; also known as milk let-down reflex

mineralocorticoids hormones secreted by the adrenal cortex that regulate the levels of such minerals as sodium and potassium

mitochondria double-membrane structures in the cytoplasm; contain enzymes required for breaking down nutrients to liberate energy for cellular function

mitosis the division process in somatic cells; involves the separation of the duplicated chromosome into two identical nuclei

mitral valve the bicuspid valve; located between the left atrium and ventricle

mixed gland gland that secretes both serous and mucous secretions

mixed nerve spinal nerve that contains both motor and sensory nerves

molar a tooth having a somewhat quadrangular crown, with four or five cusps on the grinding surface; in the adult, there are six molars in each jaw

molecular formula indicates the elements involved by using their chemical symbol

molecule the product of covalent bonding between elements

monocyte white blood cell with a large, bean-shaped nucleus

monoplegia paralysis of one limb

mons pubis prominence over the pubic symphysis in females

motor end plate portion of the sarcolemma directly under the synaptic knob at the myoneural junction

motor nerve nerve that brings impulses from the spinal cord and brain

motor unit the motor neuron and the muscle fibers it supplies

mucosa the inner lining of various tubular structures (e.g., digestive tract) that secretes mucus

mucous gland gland that secretes the slippery, lubricating glycoprotein (mucus)

mucous membrane combination of epithelia that secrete mucus and connective tissue that cover and protect other structures (e.g., lining of digestive, respiratory, urinary, and reproductive tracts)

mucus the slippery, lubricating glycoprotein secreted by mucous glands

multicellular gland gland made up of many cells that is in the form of simple or more complex tubes that secrete

muscle fatigue condition in which the muscle finds it difficult to contract even when stimulated by the nerve

muscle fiber a single muscle cell

muscle spindle stretch receptor located parallel to muscle fiber that informs other neurons in the brain and spinal cord of muscle length and the rate at which the muscle is stretching

muscle tone the resting tension in a muscle

muscular system system that deals with the structure and function of muscle

muscularis externa a layer of smooth muscle found external to the submucosa

myelin lipo proteinaceous material, made up of regularly alternating membranes of lipid and protein, of the myelin sheath

myelinated nerve nerve whose axons have myelin sheaths around them

myoblast embryonic muscle cell

myocardium the middle part of the heart wall, made up of cardiac muscle

myofascial stretching technique in which nongliding traction is applied to muscle and the associated fascia

myofibril muscle protein located in the cytoplasm of a muscle fiber; made up of a collection of myofilaments

myofilament specialized protein, located in muscle fiber, that is responsible for contraction and relaxation

myometrium the muscular layer of the uterus

myoneural junction junction between the muscle and the motor nerve ending; the neuromuscular junction

myosin one type of myofilament that is responsible for contraction and relaxation

myxedema hypothyroidism; a condition in which there is edema in the subcutaneous tissue

N

nasal relating to the nose

nasal cavity cavity that lies on either side of the nasal septum

nasal septum   structure of bone and cartilage that divides the nose into right and left nasal cavities

nasopharynx   the part of the pharynx that lies posterior to the nasal cavity

natural killer cells   large type of granulocyte

naturally acquired immunity   an immunity in which the body is naturally exposed to antigens (as opposed to artificial exposure)

neck   part of the body which attaches the head to the trunk; also refers to constricted parts of anatomic structures that resemble the neck

neoplasm   uncontrolled cell growth; also known as tumor

nephron   the functional unit of the kidney; the long convoluted tubules of the kidney

nerve plexuses   a network of nerves

nerve   a cordlike structure made up of bundles of nerve fibers

nervous system   system consisting of structures that respond to stimuli both inside and outside the body and structures that integrate the sensed stimuli and produce an appropriate response

neural hormone   hormone secreted by nerve endings into the circulation

neurilemmal cell   neuroglial cell responsible for myelinating nerves in the PNS; also known as Schwann cells

neuroeffector junction   the communication between a neuron and another cell (other than a neuron)

neuroendocrine regulatory function   the regulation of the endocrine system by the nervous system (e.g., the control of the hypothalamus over the pituitary gland)

neuroglandular junction   the communication between a neuron and a gland

neuroglia   non-neuronal cells found in the central and peripheral nervous system

neuromuscular junction   the junction between the muscle and the motor nerve ending; the myoneural junction

neuromuscular junction   the communication between a neuron and muscle fiber

neutron   a particle that makes up an atom; carries no charge

neutrophil   white blood cell with cytoplasm that has tiny granules; the cell appears neutral in color on staining

nodes of Ranvier   the gaps between the myelin in a nerve axon; also known as internodes

nonkeratinized   refers to epithelia that do not have keratin

nonmyelinated nerves   nerves whose axons do not have myelin sheaths around them

noradrenaline   a hormone secreted by the adrenal medulla; also secreted as a neurotransmitter by certain neurons; also known as norepinephrine

norepinephrine   a hormone secreted by the adrenal medulla; also secreted as a neurotransmitter by certain neurons; also known as noradrenaline

nose   the part of the respiratory tract through which air enters the body

nostril   the opening on the inferior aspect of the nose; external nare

nuclear membrane   a membrane that surrounds the nucleus of a cell; also known as nuclear envelope

nucleic acids   large organic molecules with carbon, hydrogen, oxygen, nitrogen, and phosphorus; important for storing and processing information in every cell

nucleus   a rounded or oval mass of protoplasm within the cytoplasm of a cell; the center of the atom; in the nervous system, denotes a group of nerve cell bodies in the brain or spinal cord

nutrient   the essential element and molecule obtained from the diet that are required for normal body function

O

oblique fissure   a fissure in the lungs that runs downward and forward, separating the left lung into an upper and lower lobe and separating the upper and middle lobes from the lower lobe in the right lung

olfactory receptor   receptor in the superior part of the nose responsible for sense of smell

oligodendrocyte   neuroglial cell that forms myelin sheaths in the CNS

oocyte   immature ova

opposition   a special movement that allows the thumb to touch or oppose each of the other fingers

oral cavity   the region located between the mouth and the pharynx; includes the space between the lips and teeth; teeth and gums and the cavity (and its contents) that lie between the cheeks

oral contraceptive   a hormonal preparation, taken orally, that prevents conception

orbit   the cavity that contains the eyeball

organelles   specialized parts of a cell (e.g., mitochondria, Golgi apparatus, nucleus, and centrioles)

organic compound   chemical structure that always has carbon and hydrogen as part of the basic structure

organ   a collection of tissue having the same function

orgasm   the climax of the sexual act

origin   the most stationary point of attachment of the muscle, usually the proximal point

oropharynx   the part of the pharynx posterior to the mouth

orthostatic hypotension   a sudden reduction in blood pressure when changing posture

osmoreceptor   receptor that responds to changes in osmotic pressure in the blood; found in the hypothalamus

osmosis   the net diffusion of water from a region of lower concentration of solute to a region of higher concentration of solute across a semipermeable membrane

osmotic pressure   an indication of the force of water movement into one solution from another solution separated by a semipermeable membrane; the result of the difference in solute concentration between the two solutions

ossification   the process of formation bone

ossification center   the site of earliest bone formation

osteoblast   special cell that forms bone

osteoclast   a cell found in bone that reabsorbs bone

osteocyte   a bone cell located in the lacunae that helps maintain bone

osteomalacia   a disease in adults as a result of vitamin D deficiency, characterized by softening and bending of bone

osteon also known as haversian system; a structure in compact bone made of a central canal containing blood capillaries and the surrounding concentric osseous lamellae

osteoporosis condition in which there is a reduction in the density of bone

outward rotation a movement in which the part is moved along its axis in the lateral direction

ova the reproductive cell produced by the ovaries

ovarian cycle the cyclical changes occurring in the ovary regarded as periodic preparation for fertilization and pregnancy

ovaries pair of organs in the female pelvic region that produce ova and secrete female sex hormones

ovulation the release of ova from the ovarian follicle

oxyhemoglobin hemoglobin that has combined with oxygen

oxytocin a hormone secreted by the posterior lobe of the pituitary gland; stimulates the contraction of smooth muscles of the pregnant uterus and around mammary glands ducts

P

pacemaker any rhythmic center responsible for a pace of activity

palate the bony, muscular part that separates the mouth from the nasal cavity

palatoglossal arch a fold of tissue that passes from the soft palate to the side of the tongue

palatopharyngeal arch a fold of tissue that passes from the soft palate to the lateral wall of the pharynx

palm the anterior aspect of the hand

pancreas a gland in the abdomen that has exocrine and endocrine function

pancreatic islets collection of cells in the pancreas that secrete hormones

pancreatic polypeptide a hormone secreted by the pancreas

papillae any small, nipplelike projections

papillary layer superficial layer of the dermis that has loose connective tissue; the pars papillaris

papillary muscle muscle that projects on the inside of the ventricles that are connected to the mitral and tricuspid valves via the chordae tendineae

papillary plexus the network of arteries at the junction of the dermis and epidermis that follow the contours of the papilla

paranasal sinus air-filled cavities, lined with mucous membrane and located adjacent to the nose that communicate with the nasal cavity

paraplegia paralysis of one half of the body (the lower limbs and trunk)

parasympathetic division the part of the autonomic nervous system that exits from the craniosacral region

parathormone a hormone secreted by the parathyroid gland that regulates calcium levels

parathyroid gland one of four small endocrine glands embedded in the thyroid gland; secretes parathormone

paraurethral gland known as Skene's glands; located near the urethral opening of the female external genitalia

paresis a condition of partial or incomplete paralysis

parietal pericardium the part of the pericardium that is outside the visceral pericardium

parietal peritoneum the part of the peritoneum that lines the abdominal cavity

parietal pleura the layer of the pleural membrane that lines the inside of the thorax

parotid gland a salivary gland that lies anterior to the ears

pars papillaris superficial dermis layer that has loose connective tissue; the papillary layer

pars reticularis the deeper layer of the dermis that contains dense, irregular connective tissue; the reticular layer

parturition the process of labor and delivery of a baby

passive immunity an immunity in which the body is not actively manufacturing antibodies

passive transport a transport across the cell membrane in which no energy is used

patellar relating to the patella or knee cap

pathophysiology study of how disease affects specific functions

pavementing the accumulation process of white blood cells along the blood vessels walls immediately after injury; also known as margination

pelvic relating to the pelvis

pelvic girdle the right and left hip bones, joined at the pubic symphysis

penile urethra the part of the male urethra that passes through the penis

percussion strokes manipulative techniques that alternatively deform and release tissue at varying rhythms and pressure

pericardial cavity space between the two layers (visceral and parietal) of the pericardium

pericardium outer lining of the heart

perichondrium dense, irregular connective tissue membrane around cartilage

perimetrium outer coat of the uterus

perimysium connective tissue that surrounds muscle fascicle

perineum area between the thighs laterally, coccyx and pubis anteroposteriorly

perineurium layer of connective tissue in a nerve that separates axons into bundles

period of gestation the developmental age of a fetus, usually based on the presumed first day of the last normal menstrual period.

periodontal ligament a ligament that is present in relation to a tooth

periosteum the hard, outer shell of bone with blood and nerve supply

peripheral nervous system (PNS) part of the nervous system outside the brain and spinal cord

peripheral protein protein in the cell wall that is integrated into the wall with part of the protein molecule projecting into or out of the cell

peristalsis the special movement of tubular structures, such as the intestine, that results in alternate contraction and relaxation of the smooth muscles, propelling the contents distally

peritoneal fluid fluid secreted by the peritoneum

peritoneum   the sac, made up of mesothelium and thin layer of connective tissue, that lines the abdominal cavity and covers most of the abdominal viscera

permanent cells   cells that cannot divide and the injured and dead cells are replaced by fibrous tissue/scar formation

permeability of capillaries   the property of the capillary wall that determines the movement of substances in and out

peroxisome   vesicle found in the cytoplasm that helps detoxify substances, such as alcohol and hydrogen peroxide, that are produced by the cell

petrissage   a massage technique in which the tissue is repetitively compressed, dragged, lifted, and released against underlying structures

phagocytosis   cell eating; vesicle contents are brought into the cell by endocytosis and digested by enzymes present in the cell

phagosome   a cavity formed by the two extensions of the cytoplasm of a phagocyte that fuse, engulfing the "foreign" tissue into the cytoplasm

pharyngeal tonsils   also known as adenoids; collection of lymphoid tissue in the nasopharynx

pharyngotympanic tube   a tube connecting the middle ear to the pharynx; the eustachian tube

pharynx   the upper widened part of the digestive tract and respiratory system, between the esophagus below and the mouth and nasal cavities above and in front

pheochromocytoma   benign tumor in the adrenal medulla that results in excessive catecholamine secretion

pheromone   a secreted hormone that is perceived by a second individual of the same species

phonation   sound production in the larynx

phospholipid bilayer   the structure of the cell membrane; made up of two layers of phospholipids

physiologic dead space   the volume of air in alveoli not perfused by blood and is not, therefore, involved in gas exchange

physiology   study of the functions of the various body parts

pia mater   the inner layer of the meninges

pineal gland   endocrine gland located in the roof of the third ventricle of the brain; secretes the hormone melatonin

pituitary gland   an endocrine gland attached to the brain, located in the sella turcica of the sphenoid bone, the hypophysis

placenta   organ developed during pregnancy in which metabolic exchange occurs between the fetus and the mother

plantar fasciitis   inflammation of a thick connective tissue on the plantar surface of the foot

plantar flexion   the movement at the ankle when you stand on your toes

plantar surface   the part of the foot that faces the ground; the sole

plasma   the fluid in blood without formed elements

plasma cell   a lymphocyte that manufactures the antibodies

plasma colloid osmotic pressure   osmotic pressure exerted by the particles in plasma; tends to pull fluid into the capillaries

platelet aggregation   the clumping of platelets

platelet plug   clump of platelets that close a break in the blood vessel endothelium

platelet   smallest cell present in the blood; helps stop bleeding at the time of injury

pleural cavity   the space between the two (visceral and parietal) layers of the pleura

pleural fluid   fluid secreted by the pleura

pneumotaxic center   area in the medulla of brain that reduces the duration of inspiration and facilitates the onset of expiration

polypeptide   compound formed by the linkage of a large number of amino acids

popliteal fossa   the depression in the posterior aspect of the knee joint

posterior   relational term; also known as dorsal; a structure lying behind another

postganglionic fiber   autonomic neurons that lead away from a ganglion

postsynaptic neuron   the neuron that is stimulated/ inhibited at the synapse

postural hypotension   sudden reduction in blood pressure when changing posture

potential energy   the energy, existing in a body as a result of its position or state of existence, that is not being exerted at the time

preganglionic fiber   autonomic neurons that lead to a ganglion

premolar   eight in number; a tooth with two cusps or points; bicuspids

preovulatory phase   the menstrual cycle phase in which ovarian follicles develop; the follicular phase

prepuce   the thin, delicate fold of skin that overlies the tip of the penis

presynaptic neuron   the neuron conveying impulses to the synapse

prime mover   the main muscle that produces a particular movement; an agonist

primordial follicle   fluid-filled cavity that forms around the oocyte in the ovary at the beginning of the menstrual cycle

progestational phase   menstrual phase in which there is corpus luteum development; luteal or secretory phase

progesterone   a sex hormone secreted by the corpus luteum and placenta

projection fiber   axon that runs between the cerebral cortex and other structures such as the cerebellum, brain stem, and spinal cord

prolactin   hormone secreted by the anterior pituitary gland that regulates milk production

prolactin-inhibiting hormone (PIH)   secreted by the hypothalamus that decreases prolactin secretion by the anterior pituitary gland

prolactin-releasing hormone (PRH)   secreted by the hypothalamus that increases prolactin secretion by the anterior pituitary gland

proliferative phase   the menstrual phase in which there is development of the ovarian follicles; the preovulatory or follicular phase

pronation   a movement in which the elbow is moved to have the palm of the hand facing the back

proprioceptor   afferent that monitors position and movement of skeletal muscles and joints

prostate gland   located around the proximal part of the male urethra; its secretions are responsible for the milky coloration of semen

prostatic urethra   the part of the male urethra that passes through the prostate

protein   organic compounds that have carbon, hydrogen, oxygen, and nitrogen

proteoglycan   a chemical (mucopolysaccharide) found in the ground substance of connective tissue

proton   a particle that makes up an atom; carries a positive charge

protraction   moving the bone anteriorly in the horizontal plane (e.g., movement in which the jaw juts out)

proximal   relational term; structures closer to the trunk (chest and abdomen)

pseudostratified columnar epithelium   columnar epithelium that, although appears to be in layers, is not in layers

puberty   period when final maturation of the reproductive system occurs; adolescence

pubic   relating to the pubis

pulmonary circulation   blood flow from the right ventricle to the lungs and back to the left ventricle, also known as lesser circulation

pulmonary semilunar valve   valve between the right ventricle and the pulmonary trunk

pulmonary trunk   the large artery that carries blood from the right ventricle to the lungs

pulmonary vein   vein that drains blood from the lungs to the left atrium

pulmonary ventilation   air movement in and out of the lungs by increasing and decreasing the size of the thoracic cavity by movement of the chest wall and action of the respiratory muscles; breathing

pulp cavity   the cavity inside a tooth

pulse   pressure wave felt on palpating the superficial arteries; as it travels, the wave expands the artery walls

pus   yellowish-white fluid that may accumulate in an inflamed area; made up of dead tissue, white blood cells, and their remains and other proteins

pyloric canal   canal in the muscular part of the stomach, adjacent to opening into the duodenum

pyloric sphincter   circular muscle that regulates the passage of contents from the stomach into the duodenum

pylorus   muscular part of the stomach, adjacent to its opening into the duodenum

Q

quadrant   one fourth of a circle; in anatomy, regions are often arbitrarily divided into quadrants (e.g., abdominal region)

quadriplegia   paralysis of all four limbs

R

radioisotope   an isotope that emits radioactive waves

reactive hyperemia   fiery red coloration seen soon after an occlusion to blood flow to the tissue is removed

receptor   special molecule(s) located on the cell membrane that recognize and bind to a ligand. The specialized part of a sensory neuron that responds to an external or internal stimuli is also known as a receptor.

rectum   part of the digestive tract located between the sigmoid colon and the anal canal

red blood cell   cell responsible for carrying oxygen in the blood; erythrocytes

red reaction   red coloration of the skin immediately after stroking the skin with a pointed object

reflex   involuntary reaction in response to a stimulus that is conveyed to the CNS

refractory period   the short time after the first impulse arrives; the muscle is unable to respond to a second stimulus

regional anatomy   study of the superficial and internal features of a specific area

relaxation period   the time taken by muscle fiber to relax after a contraction

relaxin   a hormone secreted by the ovaries and placenta in pregnant women; relaxes the pubic symphysis and other pelvic joints and softens and dilates the uterine cervix

renal corpuscle   the structure that includes the glomerulus and the Bowman's capsule; the malpighian body

renal fascia   thick connective tissue that surrounds the kidney

renal pyramid   pyramid-shaped structure in the renal medulla

renal sinus   the cavity in the kidney containing the calyces, pelvis of kidney, and blood vessels, etc.

renin   enzyme secreted by the kidney that converts angiotensinogen to angiotensin I

repolarization   the process following depolarization, in which the inside of a cell becomes more negative, to reach the resting membrane potential; caused by changes in ion movement

repressor gene   gene that opposes cell division

reproductive system   system responsible for the propagation of species

residual volume   the volume of air that remains in the lungs after forced expiration

resistance vessel   blood vessel that provides greatest resistance to the flow of blood

respiration   the movement of air in and out of the lungs and the exchange of gases

respiratory bronchiole   subdivision of bronchi in which exchange of gases takes place

respiratory center   area of the brainstem involved with regulating respiration

respiratory minute volume   the amount of air breathed in or out per minute

respiratory rate   the frequency of breathing per minute

respiratory system   system that includes all parts from the nose to the lung alveoli; responsible for gas exchange

resting membrane potential   potential inside a resting cell in relation to the outside; transmembrane potential

reticular activating system (RAS)   network of cells in the brain responsible for the conscious, alert state of the body

reticular fibers   a fiber located in loose connective tissue; the fibers are thin, forming branching networks

reticular layer   deeper layer of the dermis containing dense, irregular connective tissue; pars reticularis

retinaculum a retaining connective tissue band

retraction moving the bone posteriorly in the horizontal plane (e.g., movement in which the jaw is pulled in)

Rh factor an special antigen (Rhesus antigen) found on the surface of red blood cells of individuals who are Rh-positive

Rh-negative when an individual's red blood cell membrane does not have Rh antigen

Rh-positive when an individual's red blood cell membrane has the Rh antigen

rhythm method a natural contraceptive method in which intercourse is avoided during the fertile period

ribonucleic acid (RNA) important for storing and processing information in the cell

ribosome tiny organelle in the cytoplasm that manufacture proteins

rickets a disease in children caused by vitamin D deficiency and characterized by softening and bending of bone

RNA ribonucleic acid

root the beginning portion of any part (e.g., root of a tooth)

root canal canal that lies within the root portion of the tooth

rotation a movement in which the part is moved along its axis

S

sacral relating to the sacrum

sagittal plane plane that runs from front to back, cutting the body into a right and a left part

salt compound formed by an interaction between an acid and base

saltatory conduction the rapid propagation of impulse from one node of Ranvier to another

sarcolemma the muscle cell membrane

sarcomere the width between two Z lines in a myofibril; the functional unit of the muscle

sarcoplasm the cytoplasm of a muscle fiber

sarcoplasmic reticulum (SR) endoplasmic reticulum found in the muscle fiber

satellite cell neuroglial cell that surrounds collections of neuronal cell bodies (ganglion) lying outside the CNS; denotes myoblasts seen as individual cells between the muscle fibers

Schwann cells neuroglial cells responsible for myelinating nerves in the PNS; neurilemma cells

scoliosis an abnormal lateral curvature of the spine

scrotum a pouch that lies posterior to the penis and anterior to the anus in which the testis are located

seasonal affective disorder (SAD) condition characterized by depression/mood changes that occur and go away at the same time, year after year; excessive melatonin levels have been implicated

sebum oily secretion (a mixture of lipids, proteins, and electrolytes) secreted by sebaceous glands in the skin; provides lubrication and protects the keratin of the hair, conditions skin, and prevents excess evaporation of water

second heart sound the sound heard when the semilunar valves close

second-class lever a lever system in which the resistance is in the center and the effort and fulcrum are on either side

secretory phase menstrual phase in which there is corpus luteum development; the progestational or luteal phase

segmentation dividing into smaller sections; a special type of movement in the gut

selectively permeable the cell membrane that is impermeable to one substance but freely allows another to pass through

seminal vesicle one of two glands located on the posterior surface of the bladder; the two glands contribute about 60% of the fluid in the semen

seminiferous tubule the tubules of the testis in which sperm are manufactured

sensible perspiration losing water from the interstitial tissue by evaporation; perceived as moisture (sweat) on the skin

sensitization the process of making a person allergic by exposure to an antigen

sensors relating to sensation

sensory nerve nerve that takes impulses to the spinal cord and brain

septal cell special cell in the lungs that secrete surfactant; type II cells or surfactant cells

serosa the outer layer of the viscera that lies in the abdominal or thoracic cavity

serous gland gland that secretes a watery secretion containing enzymes

serous membrane combination of epithelia that secrete serous (watery) fluid and connective tissue that cover and protect other structures (e.g., lining of peritoneal, pleural, and pericardial cavities)

Sertoli cells specialized cells located in the outer layer of the seminiferous tubules that provide nutrition to sperm and secrete hormones; sustentacular cells

serum the fluid portion of blood without blood cells and fibrin clot

sesamoid bones small bones shaped like sesame seeds that develop in tendons exposed to considerable stress

sex cells ova and sperm

sex chromosome chromosome responsible for determining the sex of the individual

sex hormone hormone that regulates sex organ activity

shin the anterior aspect of the tibia

short bone bone with almost equal length, breadth, and height

shoulder the deltoid region; the region over the shoulder joint where the clavicle, scapula, and humerus meet

shunt the diversion of fluid from one part to another

sigmoid colon the part of the colon that extends between the descending colon and the rectum

simple epithelium thin and fragile epithelia that have only one layer of cells over the basement membrane; found only in areas which are relatively protected, such as the heart, blood vessel, and body cavity lining

sinus a tract leading from a cavity to the surface of body; a channel for blood or lymph passage, without the coats of an ordinary vessel (e.g., blood passages in a cavity in bone in the cerebral meninges); (e.g., paranasal sinus)

sinusoid blood vessel that resembles a sinus

skeletal muscle   muscle connected to the bony framework of the body

skeletal system   system that includes the bones, bone marrow, and joints of the body

Skene's glands   located near the urethral opening of the female external genitalia; paraurethral glands

skin rolling   massage technique in which tissue superficial to the deep fascia is grasped and, using gliding strokes, lifted and rolled over in a wavelike motion

skull   the bones of the head, collectively

sliding filament theory   muscle contraction process in which the actin and myosin filaments slide over each other

slow fiber   muscle fiber that slowly responds to a stimulus

small intestine   the long tube located between the stomach and the ileocecal valve

smooth muscle   muscle found in the viscera

sodium-potassium (Na-K) pump   membrane-bound transporter that transports potassium ions into the cytoplasm from the extracellular fluid, simultaneously transporting sodium ions from the cytoplasm to the extracellular fluid using energy; also known as sodium-potassium ATPase or sodium-potassium exchange pumps

sole   the plantar surface; the part of the foot that faces the ground

somatic afferent   neuron that takes impulses to the central nervous system from the skeletal muscle

somatic cells   includes all cells of the body except ova and sperm

somatic motor neuron   efferent that carries impulses to the skeletal muscle

somatic nervous system   the part of the nervous system that innervates skeletal muscle

somatomedin   growth factor produced by the liver and other tissues that interacts with growth hormone

somatostatin   hormone secreted by the pancreas that regulates secretions by the islets of Langerhans

spastic   increased muscle tone

specific compression   massage technique in which pressure is applied to a specific muscle, tendon, or connective tissue in a direction perpendicular to the tissue in question

sperm   the reproductive cell produced by the testis

spermatic cord   the vas deferens along with the blood vessels, lymphatic vessels, nerves, muscles, and connective tissue fascia that surrounds it, located in the inguinal region

spermatogenesis   the formation of sperm

spherocytosis   condition in which the red cells are spherical rather than biconcave

sphincter vesicae   circular smooth muscle that regulates urine flow out of the bladder; the internal urethral sphincter

sphygmomanometer   a device that measures blood pressure

spina bifida   condition in which one or more vertebral arches fail to fuse

spinal cavity   the vertebral cavity; the space within the vertebrae occupied by the spinal cord and its coverings and the cerebrospinal fluid

spinal cord   the part of the nervous system located in the spinal cavity

spinal nerve   nerve attached to the spinal cord

spleen   a large, vascular lymphatic organ located in the left hypochondrium

splenic flexure   part of the colon located at the junction of the transverse and descending colons

spongy bone   bone that is less dense, with bone spicules surrounded by spaces filled with red marrow; trabecular bone

squamous epithelium   epithelium that consists of flat, thin, and somewhat irregularly shaped cells

stable cells   cells that have a low rate of division, but the capacity to regenerate if injured

staircase phenomenon   the steplike increase in muscle tension seen in successive contractions of a muscle; also known as the treppe phenomenon

sterilization   the process in which an individual is made incapable of fertilization or reproduction

sternal   relating to the sternum

stimulatory neurotransmitter   neurotransmitter that results in stimulation of the postsynaptic neuron

stomach   large organ in the upper part of the abdomen that digests and stores food

stratified epithelium   epithelium with many layers that forms an effective protection from mechanical and chemical stress

stratum basale   deepest layer of the epidermis; single-celled layer consisting of cuboidal or columnar epithelium attached to the basement membrane, which separates the epidermis from the dermis; stratum germinativum

stratum corneum   the most superficial epidermal layer, consists mostly of dead cells and keratin

stratum germinativum   deepest epidermal layer; single-celled layer consisting of cuboidal or columnar epithelium attached to the basement membrane, which separates the epidermis from this dermis; stratum basale

stratum granulosum   located immediately above the stratum spinosum of the epidermis; consists of 3–5 layers; when viewed under the microscope, cells in this layer have a granular appearance

stratum lucidum   located immediately above the stratum granulosum of the epidermis; this layer is translucent and consists of flat cells filled with densely packed keratin; more prominent in the palms of the hands and soles of the feet.

stratum spinosum   consists of 8–10 layers of cells located immediately above the stratum germinativum of the epidermis of skin

striated muscle   muscle that has a striated appearance

stripping   a massage technique in which slow, gliding strokes are applied from one attachment of muscle to the other

stroke volume   the volume of blood pumped out of the heart with each contraction

subarachnoid space   space between the arachnoid and pia mater

subcutaneous layer   the hypodermis; a layer found deep to the dermis, consisting of loose connective tissue and adipose tissue

subdural space space between the dura and the arachnoid mater

sublingual gland a salivary gland that lies inferior to the tongue

submandibular gland a salivary gland that lies on the medial aspect of the lower jaw

submucosa layer of connective tissue deep to the mucous membrane

sudoriferous gland sweat gland; coiled, tubular glands surrounded by a network of capillaries in the skin

sulcus one of the grooves or furrows on the surface of the brain

superficial relational term; structures lying closer to the surface of the body; external

superior relational term; also known as cranial or cephalic; a structure lying toward the head

superior vena cava large vein that drains the head, neck, and upper limb regions

supination a movement in which the elbow is moved to have the palm of the hand facing front

supporting connective tissue tissue that provides a strong, solid framework (e.g., cartilage, bone)

suprarenal gland another term for adrenal gland

surface anatomy study of general forms and superficial markings on the surface of the body

surface tension the weak attraction between molecules (e.g., the attraction between water molecules that makes them form a drop)

surfactant oily secretion from septal cells in the lungs that reduces surface tension

surfactant cell special cell in the lungs that secrete surfactant; the septal cell or type II cell

sustentacular cell specialized cell located in the outer layer of the seminiferous tubules that provides nutrition to sperm and secretes hormones; also known as Sertoli cells

sutural bone small, irregularly shaped bone found where two or more other bones meet in the skull; also known as wormian bone

suture a fibrous joint (e.g., coronal suture [skull]); term for stitch or material used for surgery

sympathetic division the part of the autonomic nervous system that exits from the thoracolumbar region

sympathetic tone continuous discharge of impulses in the sympathetic nerves

synaptic cleft space between the nerve and postsynaptic structure, e.g., nerve and muscle; nerve and nerve

synaptic knob the expanded end of the motor nerve at the myoneural junction

synaptic vesicle vesicle present in the axon of neurons; contains neurotransmitters

synarthrosis an immovable joint

synergist muscle that assists a prime mover in performing the movement

synovial fluid fluid found in the joint cavity of synovial joints

synovial joint joint that contains synovial fluid

synovial membrane membrane lining the synovial joint

synovial sheath connective tissue sheath filled with synovial fluid found around certain tendons; tendon sheaths

synthesis a reaction in which compounds are formed from fragments

systemic anatomy study of structures that have the same function(s)

systemic circulation the greater circulation; blood flow from the left ventricle to the body and back to the right ventricle

system a collection of organs that have the same function

systole the period of contraction of the heart

systolic pressure the blood pressure measured during systole

T

T tubule special tubule that runs transversely inside a muscle fiber; the transverse tubules

taste buds chemoreceptors and specialized cells in the tongue that respond to taste

tendo calcaneus thick tendon in the heel of the gastrocnemius and soleus muscles; the calcaneus tendon or Achilles tendon

tendon a cord of connective tissue that connects the contractile part of the muscle with bone

tendon organ receptor located in tendons that respond to muscle tension

tendon sheath connective tissue sheath filled with synovial fluid found around certain tendons; synovial sheath

teniae coli the three muscle bands in the longitudinal axis of the large intestine

terminal bronchiole the last subdivision of bronchi that conducts air

terminal hair heavy, deeply pigmented hair found in the head and eyebrows

testis pair of organs located in the scrotum in males that manufacture sperm and male sex hormones

tetanization the process in which the contraction phase of subsequent contractions fuse and a muscle exhibits sustained contraction on being rapidly stimulated

thenar eminence bulge on the lateral aspect of the palmar surface of the hand

thick filament myosin filament

thigh the region of the lower limb between the hip and the knee

thin filament actin filament

third-class lever a lever system in which the effort is in the center, and the fulcrum and resistance are located on either side

thixotropy the property by which connective tissue becomes more fluid and pliable when exposed to heat, friction, and/or movement and becomes more solid when exposed to cold and/or is unused

thoracic relating to the thorax

thoracic cavity the space within the thorax between the diaphragm inferiorly and neck superiorly

thoracic duct a major vessel that conveys lymph to the left subclavian vein

thorax the upper part of the trunk between the neck and abdomen

thrombocyte platelet

thrombosis   the process of clot formation within a blood vessel

thymosin   hormone secreted by the thymus gland that stimulates lymphocyte synthesis

thymus   gland involved in immune response; located posterior to the sternum in the superior mediastinum

thyroglobulin   a colloid in the thyroid gland that stores thyroid hormones

thyroid cartilage   a shieldlike cartilage that is part of the larynx; posterior and superior to the thyroid gland

thyroid gland   butterfly-shaped endocrine gland located anterior to the trachea, inferior to the cricoid cartilage

thyroid stimulating hormone (TSH, thyrotropin)   secreted by the anterior pituitary that regulates the secretion of hormones by the thyroid

thyrotropin releasing hormone (TRH)   secreted by the hypothalamus that controls the secretion of thyroid-stimulating hormone (TSH) by the anterior pituitary gland

thyroxine   hormone secreted by the thyroid gland

tidal volume   the volume of air that enters and leaves the lung per minute

tight junction   the region of cells bound to each other by cell membrane fusion

tissue   collection of cells having the same function

tongue   fleshy, muscular mass in the floor of the mouth that is covered with mucous membrane and contains taste buds; helps in mastication, swallowing, and speech

tonsillitis   inflammation of the tonsils

tonsils   collection of lymphoid tissue located in the pharyngeal region

total lung capacity   the total volume of air that the lung can hold

trabecular bone   bone that is less dense, with bone spicules surrounded by spaces filled with red marrow; also known as spongy bone

trachea   tube extending from the larynx to the thorax where it divides into the two bronchi

tract   bundle of neuron axons having the same function and destination

transcription   the process by which the genetic code for a specific protein, present in the DNA, is used as a template to copy the sequence of amino acids for that protein; the copy is in the form of RNA

transitional epithelium   epithelium in which the cells seem to change shape; located lining the urinary bladder

translation   with the help of ribosomes and using the RNA template, the process in which amino acids are lined and bonded in the right sequence to form the specific protein in question in the cell cytoplasm

transmembrane potential   the potential inside a resting cell in relation to the outside; resting membrane potential

transverse colon   the part of the colon that extends transversely across the upper part of the abdomen between the hepatic and splenic flexures

transverse plane   plane that runs across the body, dividing it into a top and bottom portion; also known as the horizontal plane

transverse tubule   special tubule that runs transversely inside a muscle fiber; also known as T tubules

treppe phenomenon   the steplike increase in muscle tension seen in successive contractions of a muscle; also known as staircase phenomenon

tributaries   the branches of veins

tricarboxylic acid cycle   a cycle of biochemical events that is the main source of energy in the body; also known as Krebs cycle

tricuspid valve   valve between the right atrium and ventricle

triiodothyronine   hormone secreted by the thyroid gland

trimester   three-month period

triple response   includes the red reaction, wheal, and flare observed when stroking the skin with a pointed object

tropomyosin   a special protein that lies in relation to actin filaments in muscle

troponin   a special protein that lies in relation to actin filaments in muscle; has an affinity for calcium

true ribs   ribs with cartilage directly attached to the sternum

trunk   the body without the head and extremities; the primary part of a nerve or vessel before it divides

tubal ligation   a surgical process that interrupts the continuity of the uterine tubes

tubular gland   gland whose excretory unit(s) are tube-shaped

tumor   uncontrolled cell growth; also known as neoplasm

tunica vaginalis   serous membrane lining the cavity that separates the testis from the inner surface of the scrotum

type II cell   special cell in the lungs that secretes surfactant; the septal cells or surfactant cells

U

ulcer   a lesion formed when an organ's or tissue's surface covering is lost as a result of cell death and is replaced with inflammatory tissue

umbilical   relating to the umbilicus

umbilical cord   the connecting structure between the embryo/fetus and the placenta

umbilicus   the depressed point in the middle of the abdomen that marks the point in which the umbilical cord entered the fetus

unicellular gland   one cell in the epithelia that is secretory

universal donor   an individual with blood type O who can donate blood to all other ABO blood types

universal recipient   an individual with blood type AB who can receive blood transfusions from any other ABO blood type

upper extremity   the upper limb

upper respiratory tract   the part of the respiratory tract that includes the nose, nasal cavity, paranasal sinus, and the pharynx (throat)

ureter   tube that conducts urine from the kidneys to the urinary bladder

urethra   tube that conducts urine from the urinary bladder to the outside

urinary bladder   a pelvic organ that stores urine

urinary system   the system that helps eliminate excess water, salts, and waste products

uterine tube (fallopian tube or oviducts)   one of two tubes that convey the ova from the ovary to the uterus

uterus   pear-shaped muscular organ located in the female pelvic region; where the fetus develops in a pregnant mother

uvula   fleshy mass that projects inferiorly from the posterior aspect of the palate

V

vagal tone   the continuous discharge of impulses in the vagal nerves

vagina   canal located between the uterus and the vulva in females

vas deferens   pair of tubules located between the epididymis and the ejaculatory duct that carry semen; the ductus deferens

vasa recta   special capillary that forms from the efferent arterioles of juxtamedullarynephrons

vascular tone   the tension in the muscle of blood vessels (even at rest)

vasectomy   a surgical procedure that breaks the continuity of the vas deferens

vasomotor center   the area in the brain that regulates circulation

vasopressin   a hormone secreted by the posterior lobe of the pituitary gland that stimulates water reabsorption by the kidney cells; a powerful vasoconstrictor; also known as antidiuretic hormone (ADH)

vein   vessel that takes blood to the heart

vellus hair   fine, fuzzy hair found on the body surface

venous return   the volume of blood returning to the heart

ventral   relational term; anterior; a structure lying in front of another

ventricle   cavity (e.g., in brain, heart)

venule   smaller vein

vertebral   relating to the vertebra(e)

vertebral cavity   the spinal cavity; the space within the vertebrae occupied by the spinal cord and its coverings and the cerebrospinal fluid

vesicular transport   transport in which vesicles or small membrane-lined sacs move substances into or out of the cell

vestibule   small cavity or space found at the entrance of a canal

villi   fingerlike projections from the surface of the mucous membrane

visceral afferent   neuron that takes impulses to the central nervous system from the viscera

visceral motor neuron   efferent that carries impulses to the viscera

visceral pericardium   the part of the pericardium covering the outer surface of the heart; the epicardium

visceral peritoneum   part of the peritoneum that covers the viscera

visceral pleura   layer of the pleural membrane that surrounds the lungs

vital capacity   the volume of air breathed out forcefully after forceful inspiration

vocal cords   the folds of mucous membrane overlying the ligaments that extend between the thyroid and arytenoid cartilage; used for the production of voice

voltage-gated channel   protein channel in the cell membrane operated by changes in voltage

vulva   external female genitalia; includes the mons pubis, labia majora, labia minora, the clitoris, the vestibule of the vagina and its glands, and the urethral and vaginal openings

W

wave summation   increased tension observed in successive muscle contractions

wheal   skin swelling observed after stroking the skin with a pointed object

whiplash   an injury in which there is abnormal movement of the head in any direction

white blood cell   blood cell involved in defense

white mater   regions of the CNS dominated by myelinated axons

work   the movement or change in the physical structure of matter

wormian bone   small, irregularly shaped bones located where two or more other bones meet in the skull; sutural bones

X

X chromosome   two of the female and one of male sex chromosomes

Y

Y chromosome   one of the male sex chromosomes

Z

Z line   zigzag line that passes through the I band of striated muscle myofibrils and anchors the actin filaments at either end of the sarcomere

Index

Page numbers in *italics* denote figures; those followed by a t denote tables